Practical Guide to Equine Colic

Website

This book is accompanied by a companion website:

www.wiley.com/go/southwood

The website includes:

- Quizzes for each chapter
- Additional clinical scenarios
- Video demonstrations of surgical procedures

Practical Guide to Equine Colic

Edited by

Louise L. Southwood

With Illustrations by Joanne Fehr

WILEY-BLACKWELL

A John Wiley & Sons, Inc., Publication

Editorial Offices
2121 State Avenue, Ames, Iowa 50014-8300, USA
The Atrium, Southern Gate, Chichester, West Sussex, PO19 8SQ, UK
9600 Garsington Road, Oxford, OX4 2DQ, UK

For details of our global editorial offices, for customer services and for information about how to apply for permission to reuse the copyright material in this book please see our website at www.wiley.com/wiley-blackwell.

Library of Congress Cataloging-in-Publication Data

Practical guide to equine colic / edited by Louise L. Southwood ; with illustrations by Joanne Fehr.
      p.   cm.
  Includes bibliographical references and index.
  ISBN 978-0-8138-1832-0 (hardcover : alk. paper)
1. Colic in horses.   I. Southwood, Louise L.
   SF959.C6P73 2012
   636.1'089755–dc23

                                    2012010995

A catalogue record for this book is available from the British Library.

Cover design by Modern Alchemy LLC

Set in 9.5/11.5pt Palatino, by SPi Publisher Services, Pondicherry, India
Printed and bound in Malaysia by Vivar Printing Sdn Bhd

1   2013

Dedicated to Eric, Aiden, Kody, and Kylie Parente
Scott, Samantha, and Benjamin Fehr

Contents

Contributors ix
Preface xi
Overview of Practical Guide to Equine Colic xii

1 Patient Signalment and History 1
  Louise L. Southwood

2 Physical Examination 12
  Louise L. Southwood

3 Abdominal Palpation per Rectum 22
  Louise L. Southwood and Joanne Fehr

4 Nasogastric Intubation 38
  Joanne Fehr

5 Management of Mild Colic 45
  Sarah Dukti

6 Analgesia 51
  Luiz C. Santos and Louise L. Southwood

7 Enteral Fluid Therapy 62
  Jennifer A. Brown and Samantha K. Hart

8 Referral of the Horse with Colic 71
  Louise L. Southwood and Joanne Fehr

9 Clinical Laboratory Data 78
  Raquel M. Walton

10 Abdominocentesis and Peritoneal
   Fluid Analysis 87
   Raquel M. Walton and Louise L. Southwood

11 Intravenous Catheterization and
   Fluid Therapy 99
   Louise L. Southwood

12 Abdominal Sonographic
   Evaluation 116
   JoAnn Slack

13 Abdominal Radiographic
   Examination 149
   Sarah M. Puchalski

14 Trocharization 160
   Joanne Fehr

15 Medical versus Surgical Treatment
   of the Horse with Colic 164
   Louise L. Southwood

16 Colic Surgery 173
   Kira L. Epstein and Joanne Fehr

17 Specific Causes of Colic   204
    Eileen S. Hackett

18 Postoperative Patient Care   230
    Samantha K. Hart

19 Postoperative Complications   244
    Diana M. Hassel

20 Biosecurity   262
    Helen W. Aceto

21 Special Considerations   278
    Louise L. Southwood

22 Long-term Recovery and Prevention   292
    Louise L. Southwood

23 Nutrition   301
    Brett S. Tennent-Brown, Kira L. Epstein,
    and Sarah L. Ralston

24 Gastrointestinal Parasitology
    and Anthelmintics   316
    Louise L. Southwood

Appendix A Clinical Scenarios   325
Appendix B Drug Dosages used in the
            Equine Colic Patient   330
Appendix C Normal Ranges for Hematology
            and Plasma Chemistry and
            Conversion Table for Units   339
Index   343

Quizzes for each chapter, additional clinical scenarios, and video demonstrations of surgical procedures are available online at www.wiley.com/go/southwood.

Contributors

Helen W. Aceto, PhD, VMD
Assistant Professor of Veterinary Epidemiology
Director of Biosecurity
Department of Clinical Studies
New Bolton Center
University of Pennsylvania School of Veterinary Medicine
Kennett Square, Pennsylvania, USA

Jennifer A. Brown, DVM, DACVS
Surgeon
Veterinary Relief, Surgical, and Consulting Services
Tampa, Florida, USA

Sarah Dukti, DVM, DACVS, DACVECC
Surgeon and Emergency/Critical Care Clinician
Piedmont Equine Practice
The Plains, Virginia, USA

Kira L. Epstein, DVM, DACVS, DACVECC
Associate Professor
Department of Large Animal Medicine
College of Veterinary Medicine
University of Georgia
Athens, Georgia, USA

Joanne Fehr, DVM, MS, DACVS
Equine Emergency Clinician
Pilchuck Animal Hospital
Snohomish, Washington, USA

Eileen S. Hackett, DVM, PhD, DACVS, DACVECC
Assistant Professor, Equine Surgery and Critical Care
Department of Clinical Sciences
Colorado State University
Fort Collins, Colorado, USA

Samantha K. Hart, BVMS, MS, DACVS, DACVECC
Lecturer, Large Animal Emergency and Critical Care
Department of Clinical Studies, New Bolton Center
University of Pennsylvania School of Veterinary Medicine
Kennett Square, Pennsylvania, USA

Diana M. Hassel, DVM, PhD, DACVS, DACVECC
Associate Professor, Equine Surgery and Critical Care
Department of Clinical Sciences
Colorado State University
Fort Collins, Colorado, USA

Sarah M. Puchalski, DVM, DACVR
Assistant Professor
Department of Surgical and Radiological Sciences
School of Veterinary Medicine
University of California, Davis
Davis, California, USA

Sarah L. Ralston, VMD, PhD, DACVN
Associate Professor
Department of Animal Science
School of Environmental and Biological
Sciences
Rutgers, The State University of New Jersey
New Brunswick, New Jersey, USA

Luiz C. Santos, DVM, MS, DACVA
Research Associate, Large Animal Anesthesia
Department of Clinical Studies
New Bolton Center
University of Pennsylvania School of Veterinary
Medicine
Kennett Square, Pennsylvania, USA

JoAnn Slack, DVM, MS, DACVIM
Assistant Professor, Large Animal Cardiology and
Ultrasound
Department of Clinical Studies
New Bolton Center
University of Pennsylvania School of Veterinary
Medicine
Kennett Square, Pennsylvania, USA

Louise L. Southwood, BVSc, PhD, DACVS,
DACVECC
Associate Professor, Large Animal Emergency and
Critical Care
Department of Clinical Studies
New Bolton Center
University of Pennsylvania School of Veterinary
Medicine
Kennett Square, Pennsylvania, USA

Brett S. Tennent-Brown, BVSc, MS, DACVIM,
DACVECC
Senior Lecturer in Equine Medicine
Equine Center
University of Melbourne Veterinary Hospital
Werribee, Victoria, Australia

Raquel M. Walton, VMD, PhD, DACVP
Assistant Professor, Clinical Pathology
Director Clinical Laboratory, MJR-VHUP
Department of Pathobiology
University of Pennsylvania School of Veterinary
Medicine
Philadelphia, Pennsylvania, USA

Preface

Practical Guide to Equine Colic follows the management of a colic patient from obtaining the history and performing a physical examination through to long-term recovery and an attempt at describing prevention. There are several books available with details of the gastrointestinal anatomy and physiology and the objective of this book was not to duplicate these publications but to present the practical aspect of this information. Our focus as equine veterinarians should be to provide the best possible care for our patients and service to our clients by having up to date knowledge to enable us to best diagnose, treat, and prevent disease. We also have the responsibility to educate the next generation of veterinarians, teach each other by sharing our experience, and to continue to investigate disease processes in order to improve management and prevention. Fiscal responsibility has become increasingly important in recent years. We now more than ever need to weigh the benefit against the expense of a particular diagnostic test or treatment and keep costs in a range where clients can afford to treat their animal while being able to maintain a successful practice. We hope that the book and website will be a useful resource for education of veterinary students, interns, and residents, and provide continuing education for experienced equine practitioners. We encourage equine specialists to use the book and website for teaching and identification of knowledge gaps that should stimulate research ideas to improve equine colic patient management. I personally learned a considerable amount researching the literature to prepare the chapters and reviewing the chapters written by the other authors. While not specifically written for horse owners, the information provided particularly on specific diseases and colic surgery may be of interest to the inquisitive and educated lay-person.

A team-approach was essential for successful completion of this project. When asked by Wiley-Blackwell to write a small 200-page book about equine colic, it seemed like a reasonable endeavor. Thinking I knew something about colic but probably not enough to cover 200 pages (even with large print and a lot of pictures), I sought out several colleagues with expertise in specific areas. I am extremely grateful for the contributing efforts of the chapter authors and the book would not have been feasible without these exceptional veterinarians. Dr. Joanne Fehr, a fellow surgical resident and friend, provided illustrations which give considerable educational value to the material. In all honesty, the chapters would still be in draft form buried somewhere on my desk if it wasn't for Ms. Susan Engelken at Wiley-Blackwell being relentless with ensuring deadlines were met (give or take several months) and my family for giving me the time to meet those deadlines. And we would like to thank the IT support staff at Penn Vet's New Bolton Center, particularly Mr. Tyler Harold, Ms. Linda Lewis, and Mr. Ryan Delaney, for their assistance with video production. Our hope is that this book, which of course is well beyond 200 pages, improves the care of colic patients and the service provided to horse owners through education of equine veterinarians.

Overview of Practical Guide to Equine Colic

The book follows through the basic management of a horse with colic from initial examination (history and physical examination in dark gray) through to long-term recovery and prevention measures including nutritional and parasite management (light olive green). Diagnostic tests are in purple and procedures are in green. The points when these diagnostic tests and procedures are typically performed throughout the course of management are indicated. The key areas of colic patient management (management of mild colic, sedation and analgesia, enteral and intravenous fluid therapy, surgery, and postoperative care including nutrition and postoperative complications) are in orange. It is important to keep in mind that most horses with colic have what is generally considered to be gas colic and will respond to a single dose of flunixin meglumine (or other analgesic) with or without enteral fluids or mineral oil. However, early recognition of the need for referral or surgical intervention is important. Decision-making points (i.e., referral and surgery) are in light gray. Typical lesions seen in horses with colic and special considerations for equine patients with colic of a specific signalment (i.e., specific causes of colic and special considerations) are shown in pink. Because of the importance of infection as a postoperative complication, there is a section on biosecurity. Clinical scenarios illustrating points throughout the text are in Appendix A; dose rates for drugs used in the management of colic patients are in Appendix B; and reference ranges for laboratory data as well as conversion tables for conventional and SI units are in Appendix C. And we would like to thank the IT support staff at Penn Vet's New Bolton Center, particularly Mr. Tyler Harold, Ms. Linda Lewis, and Mr. Ryan Delaney, for their assistance with video production.

Quizzes for each chapter, additional clinical scenarios, and video demonstrations of surgical procedures are available online at www.wiley.com/go/southwood.

Overview of Practical Guide to Equine Colic

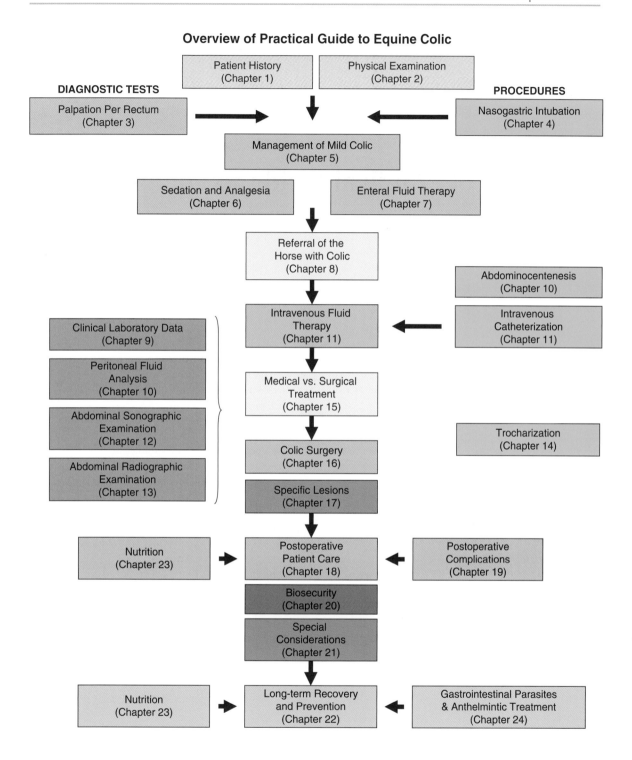

Practical Guide to Equine Colic

1

Patient Signalment and History

Louise L. Southwood

Department of Clinical Studies, New Bolton Center, School of Veterinary Medicine, University of Pennsylvania, Kennett Square, PA, USA

Chapter Outline

Importance of the patient's history	**1**	Exercise regimen, pasture access, and housing	8
Signalment	**4**	Recent transportation	8
Obtaining the patient's history	**4**	Geographical areas in which the horse	
Initial history	5	has been housed	8
Specific signs	5	Gastrointestinal parasite control	8
Duration of colic signs	6	Vaccination	9
Reproductive status of mares	6	Medical history	9
Obtaining a more detailed history	6	Previous colic and colic surgery	9
Appetite, water consumption, defecation,		Other medical problems and current	
and urination	6	medication	9
Management	7	Medical problems of other horses	10
Feeding regimen	7	Crib biting or windsucking	10
Water source	7	**Application of the patient's history**	**10**

Importance of the patient's history

Obtaining a detailed history provides information that can be used to formulate a differential diagnosis list for the horse with colic, direct treatment, and devise a colic prevention plan. Having a standardized history sheet (Figure 1.1) as part of the medical record will streamline the history-taking procedure and ensure details are not omitted. Recording the history as part of the medical record is also important to provide accurate information for referral, for reference in the case of future colic episodes, and as part of a preventative medicine program.

Practical Guide to Equine Colic, First Edition. Edited by Louise L. Southwood.
© 2013 John Wiley & Sons, Inc. Published 2013 by John Wiley & Sons, Inc.

(a)

Colorado
State
University

Veterinary Teaching Hospital
Fort Collins, Colorado 80523

**Equine Colic
History Form**

Client Name: _____

Case #: _____

Signalment: _____

Imprint identification ("blue") card here

Admit date: _____ **time:** _____ **am / pm**

History prior to arrival at CSU-VTH (from rDVM)

1. T:_____ P: _____ R: _____

_____
_____
_____
_____
_____
_____
_____
_____
_____
_____

• **Diagnostics and treatment prior to arrival:**
  - Nasogastric intubation   Y / N   Reflux: Y / N – amount:_____ given via tube: _____
  - Rectal exam   Y / N   Findings: _____
  - Abdominocentesis   Y / N   _____
    _____
    _____
  - Drugs administered: Y / N   Time given, type, route: _____
    _____
    _____
    _____

2. **Time from first signs of colic to arrival at CSU-VTH?**_____

3. **Travel time from point of origin to CSU-VTH?** (time in hours / distance in miles)_____

4. **If mare, currently pregnant / nursing?** (circle all that apply) Days of gestation: _____ Age of foal: _____

5. **Currently eating / drinking normally?** Y / N Describe: _____
   _____

6. **Currently urinating / defecating normally?** Y / N Describe: _____
   _____

Previous History

7. **Previous colic episodes?** Y / N   Describe (include approx. dates): _____
   _____
   _____

Continued on reverse side ⤷

(b)

8. **In the past 30 days has the horse experienced any of the following?**

   ◆ **Diarrhea**   Y / N   Describe: _____

   ◆ **Laminitis** (founder)   Y / N   _____

   ◆ **Temperature** $\geq 102.5°F$ (fever)   Y / N   _____

   ◆ **Received antibiotics / analgesics?**   Y / N   Specify type, schedule, & how given: _____

      (e.g. penicillin, "bute," banamine, etc.)   _____

                           _____

9. **Vaccination:**   *Tetanus / EWE / Influenza / Rhino. / Other:* _____ **Date given:** _____

   (circle all that apply)   Annual schedule:_____

10. **Deworming:**   Product used: _____ **Date given:** _____

                  Annual schedule: _____ Rotate de-wormers? Y / N

11. **Coggins:**   Date of last test: _____

12. **Previous medical problems:** (e.g. respiratory disease, skin problem – **potential for HYPP?**)

   _____

   _____

   _____

13. **Previous surgeries:** (e.g. castration, arthroscopy)   14. **Previous trauma:** (e.g. wounds, lacerations)

   _____   _____

   _____   _____

   _____   _____

   _____   _____

15. **Current diet:** (circle all that apply)

   Grass Hay / Alfalfa / Mix – amount and frequency: _____

   Grain / Pellets / Supplement / Other – type, amount, and frequency: _____

   _____

   ◆ **Is there potential for sand ingestion in the area?**   Y / N   Describe: _____

   ◆ **Diet change in the past 30 days?**   Y / N   Describe: _____

   _____

   ◆ **Water source?** (circle all that apply)   **Well / Municipal / Irrigation / Natural waterway** (stream, lake) **/ Other**

16. **Primary use of the horse?** _____

17. **Current housing?** (circle all that apply) *stall / paddock / pasture / other:* _____

   ◆ **Change in housing in the past 30 days?**   Y / N   Describe: _____

   ◆ **Other horses on property:** number of **adults** _____ **foals** _____

   ◆ **Other horses on property ill?**   Y / N   Describe: _____

18. **Travel history in past 30 days:** _____

19. **Is the horse insured?**   Y / N   Company   Agent   Phone number

                                              (   ) _____

   _____

Student: _____   **Clinician Signature:** _____

colichx.doc: rev. 07/13/1999

Figure 1.1   Example of a detailed patient history sheet. (a) Front and (b) back.
Source: Courtesy of Colorado State University, Fort Collins, Colorado.

Signalment

Knowledge of the patient's signalment, namely, age, breed, and gender, is extremely important during evaluation for colic. While gas colic is by far the most common diagnosis across most age, breed, and gender categories,[28] the signalment is critical for forming a differential diagnoses list. Gas colic can be defined clinically by horses with mild to moderate pain that resolves spontaneously or with a single dose of an analgesic drug and accounts for about 70–80% of colic episodes.[28] Typical differential diagnoses for equine patients of various signalments are shown in Table 1.1.

Signalment is also important because it may direct the history-taking process. For example, (1) if you are presented with a mare showing colic signs, the reproduction status requires investigation; (2) if you have an older horse, underlying diseases should be considered; and (3) in the case of a neonate, questions pertaining to parturition, passive transfer of maternal antibodies, and clinical signs shown by other foals on the farm should be asked. Specific questions are addressed below.

Obtaining the patient's history

Obtaining a thorough and accurate yet succinct patient history is one of the most important and perhaps one of the more difficult aspects of evaluating the colic patient (Table 1.2). It involves

Table 1.1 Differential diagnoses other than gas colic for patients of a specific signalment.

Signalment	Differential diagnoses
Neonate (p. 279)	• Meconium retention (p. 222, 279) • Enterocolitis (p. 215, 279) • Hypoxic-ischemic syndrome (p. 279) • Jejunal intussusceptions (p. 213, 280) • Jejunal volvulus (p. 212, 280) • Atresia coli or jejuni (p. 280)
Geriatric horse (p. 286)	• Strangulating pedunculated lipoma (p. 209) (small intestine or small colon) • Large colon impaction (p. 217)
Pregnant mare (p. 282)	• Uterine torsion (p. 282) • Large colon displacement (p. 220) • Large colon volvulus (p. 220) • Uterine artery hemorrhage (p. 282) • Large colon impaction (p. 217) • Parturition • Discomfort associated with pregnancy
Postpartum mare (p. 284)	• Large colon volvulus (p. 220) • Postpartum hemorrhage including uterine artery hemorrhage (p. 284) • Intestinal ischemia associated with mesenteric rent (p. 284) • Small colon injury (p. 284) • Uterine involution
Stallion (p. 285)	• Inguinal hernia (p. 28, 199)
Miniature horse (p. 287)	• Small colon fecalith (p. 287) • Large colon impaction (p. 217) • Trichobezoar (p. 287)
Yearling	• Ileocecal intussusception (p. 213)
Weanling (p. 280)	• Ascarid impaction (p. 208, 280)

Table 1.2   Pertinent questions to be asked of the owner/caregiver for the equine colic patient.

Initial history
- What specific signs is your horse showing?
- What is the duration of time over which your horse has been showing these signs? Have the signs changed over this time?
- What is the reproductive status of the horse?

Appetite, water consumption, defecation, urination
- Has the horse's appetite and water consumption been within normal limits?
- Has the horse urinated or defecated recently? When was the last time? What was the consistency of feces?

Management
- What is the duration of time the horse has been under the current ownership?
- What is the horse's current feeding regimen? Dental care?
- What is the horse's water source?
- Is the horse stalled or on pasture?
- What is the horse's exercise regimen? What is the intended use of the horse?
- Has there been any change in diet, water source, housing, or exercise regimen?
- Has the horse traveled recently? Where and when?
- What is the horse's vaccination and deworming history?

Medical history
- Has the horse had signs of colic previously? Previous colic surgery?
- Does the horse have any other medical problems?
- Is the horse currently being treated with any medication? Has any medication been administered for this episode of colic?
- Has the horse had a previous surgical procedure?
- Are the other horses on the farm healthy?
- Does the horse have any stable vices such as crib biting or windsucking?

asking a few initial key questions of the owner/caregiver, keeping the owner/caregiver focused on answering the questions thoroughly and concisely during an often stressful situation, and then recognizing areas of the patient's history that require a more in-depth discussion that may take place following the examination.

Meticulous medical records need to be maintained with the historical information. Having a standardized history sheet for horses with colic can assist in obtaining a complete history with each case. Further, owners may be able to complete some parts of the history form while the physical examination is being performed (Figure 1.1).

While history taking is traditionally incorporated into the first part of the patient evaluation, it is important to recognize that the entire history does not need to be obtained prior to examining the patient particularly if the patient is showing severe colic signs. However, there are a few very pertinent historical facts that may alter your initial approach to patient care:

- Specific signs being demonstrated by the patient
- Duration of colic signs
- Reproductive status of mares

Initial history

Specific signs

The owner/caregiver should be able to describe specifically the signs being demonstrated by the horse or foal. The term "colic" is often used to describe any equine patient that is "not quite normal". Recumbency and signs of dull mentation and inappetence are often described as colic. While these signs may be associated with colic, other disease processes should also be considered. Persistent recumbency is more typical of a horse with neurological disease (e.g., equine herpes virus, botulism, or cervical spinal cord injury), severe laminitis, trauma with musculoskeletal injury, debility, or shock from other causes (e.g., blood loss). Dull mentation and inappetence can be associated with any systemic disease process (e.g., colitis, pleuropneumonia, hepatic or renal disease) as well as problems of the head and neck regions.

Signs specific for the horse with colic include pawing at the ground, flank staring, kicking at the abdomen, and rolling. If the horse is not showing any of these signs, the horse is likely to have another problem rather than colic. Colic signs are often described as mild, moderate, or severe:

- Mild colic signs include intermittent flank staring and kicking at the abdomen, inappetence, lying down, and occasional rolling.
- Moderate signs include more persistent rolling but the horse can be distracted and remains standing when walked. The horse may be sweating.
- Severe signs of colic are persistent rolling and thrashing, with difficulty keeping the horse standing when it is walked. The horse is generally covered in sweat and often has multiple abrasions to its head, tuber coxae, and limbs.

Clinical signs shown by the horse should also be interpreted with regard to any analgesic medication (i.e., flunixin meglumine, phenylbutazone, meloxicam, firocoxib) the owner may have administered to the horse that may alter the degree of pain.

The change in clinical signs over time should also be noted, for example, horses with large colon volvulus (p. 220) may have a history of several hours of mild to moderate colic that has recently become markedly more severe; horses with a nephrosplenic ligament entrapment (NSLE) (p. 219) often have periods of moderate pain intermixed with periods of comfort; a horse with an ileocecal intussusception (p. 213) may have a history of chronic intermittent colic with an acute colic episode; and horses with gastric or cecal rupture (p. 206, 215) may have had a history of variable degrees of pain that has progressed to no further signs of pain and shock (sweating, muscle fasciculations, reluctance to move). See Chapter 2 on Physical Examination (p. 12) for further discussion on pain assessment.

Duration of colic signs

While the owner/caregiver can rarely give an accurate time of when the colic signs actually began, they should be able to tell you (1) when the signs were first observed and (2) when the horse or foal was last observed to be normal. Knowledge of at least an approximate duration of signs is important when performing a differential diagnosis list, for example, mild colic for 24 h may indicate a large colon impaction (p. 217) whereas a strangulating lesion (p. 209, 220) may be higher on the differential diagnosis list for horses showing acute severe colic for 1–3 h despite administration of analgesia.

Duration of colic is also vital for determining a diagnostic and treatment plan including the use of diagnostic tests such as abdominal sonographic and radiographic examination in horses with chronic intermittent colic signs, route of fluid therapy (e.g., a horse with a prolonged duration of colic may benefit from intravenous (IV) fluids), and whether or not to refer the horse or manage the horse surgically versus medically (e.g., a long duration of moderate colic that is unresponsive to analgesia is more likely to require surgical management). While other clinical findings, such as heart rate and packed cell volume, are likely more predictive, duration of colic can provide the owner with some information pertaining to prognosis.

Reproductive status of mares

Knowledge of a mare's reproductive status is critical because management of colic in periparturient mares can be particularly challenging from a diagnostic and therapeutic perspective. Specific questions pertaining to the pregnant mare are in Table 1.3. See Chapter 21 on Special Considerations (p. 278).

Obtaining a more detailed history

Appetite, water consumption, defecation, and urination

Whether or not the horse has been eating, drinking, defecating, and urinating can provide an overall impression of general well-being of the patient. This information may not be available if the horse resides at pasture, particularly if the horse is at pasture with other horses.

The owner/caregiver should be asked about the horse's recent feed intake, whether or not the

Table 1.3 Specific history questions pertaining to the broodmare.

- Is the mare pregnant (yes/no)?
  - Days of gestation?
  - Estimated due date?
- Have there been any problems during this pregnancy (yes/no)?
  - If yes, what problems?
- Have there been problems with previous pregnancies (yes/no)?
  - If yes, what problems?
  - Number of previous pregnancies/foals?
- Has the mare recently foaled (yes/no)? When?
- Was parturition normal (yes/no)?
  - If no, what were the problems?
- Did the mare pass her placenta normally (yes/no)?
- Was the foal normal (yes/no)?
  - If no, what were the problems?
- Has the mare had previous colic associated with pregnancy or the periparturient period (yes/no)?
  - If yes, what was the cause?

horse's appetite has been normal and whether or not the horse has been drinking an acceptable volume of water.

Nutritional needs of horses are extremely variable and observation of body condition score (p. 15) is likely the best way to determine the adequacy of nutrition. Whether the horse's appetite has changed and any associated changes in body condition as well as the period of time over which this has occurred are important to note.

Water consumption is variable and dependent on the body weight of the horse, ambient temperature, type of feed (i.e., higher water consumption with hay compared to pasture), activity level, and reproductive status (i.e., pregnancy and in particular lactation increase water requirements). Typically, an adult horse will consume 35–70 L of water a day or about 7–15% of their body weight. Horses require 2–3 L of water per kilogram of dry feed intake. See also Water source.

The last observed defecation amount (e.g., several piles overnight) and consistency (e.g., firm and dry vs. soft or liquid) should be noted. Normal fecal output in an adult horse is 6–8 piles of soft to firm formed feces a day. Whether or not the horse has been observed to urinate or there were several wet areas in the stall should be determined and used to assess hydration status and renal function.

Management

Feeding regimen

Type of feed provided, method of feeding, frequency of feeding, and if there has been any change in feeding regimen should be ascertained and may be related to the colic signs.[2]

Specific hay types have been associated with certain types of colic: Coastal Bermuda grass hay that is fed in the southeastern USA has a strong association with ileal (p. 208)[17] and possibly cecal (p. 214) impactions; enterolithiasis (p. 218) has been associated with feeding alfalfa hay;[7,10,11] and poor quality hay and hay in round bales have been associated with colic.[13,14] Other examples of relationship between feed type and colic include the association between colic and feeding high levels of concentrate (e.g., >2.5kg/day dry matter),[6,14,29] which alters the contents of the colon and may increase tympany and colonic displacements;[18] equine gastric ulcer syndrome and high concentrate diets;[4] and sand colic (p. 217) that has been associated with feeding on the ground in areas with sandy soil (e.g., Arizona, California, Colorado, Delaware, Florida, Michigan, and New Jersey).

Horses typically graze for about 18h each day and management practices of many horses do not necessarily mimic the horses' natural grazing habits. Many studies on colic have found an association between colic and less pasture time.[12,13,29] Alteration in diet and feeding practices (e.g., more time at pasture) may be necessary to manage gastrointestinal problems in some horses.

In several studies, an association between change in feed or feeding regimen and signs of colic has been identified.[3,6,12,13,29] Supporting these findings is the overall higher incidence of colic in the spring and possibly autumn months that tend to be associated with a change in feed particularly for pasture-fed horses.[3,30] Therefore, any change in diet should be made gradually in an attempt to avoid colic signs.

Dental care is also thought to be important in the prevention of colic with an increasing time from last dental care being associated with colonic impactions.[12]

Water source

The water source should be determined, for example, stream, pond, or water bucket. Access to ponds is associated with a decreased risk of colic compared to other water sources.[5] A decrease in water consumption[14] or lack of access to water[24] is also associated with colic. Owners should be aware of the potential consequences of a freezing water source during the winter months. During autumn and winter and early spring, the water source may not necessarily freeze but become cold. Water temperature was found to affect consumption during cold but not hot weather.[16,21] During cold weather, horses with only warm water available drink a greater volume each day than if they have only icy cold water available; however, if they have a choice between warm and icy water simultaneously, they drink almost exclusively from the icy water and drink less volume than if they have only warm water available. While the higher incidence of horses with small (p. 221) and large colon (p. 217) impactions during the winter months[3] may be associated with housing and diet, inadequate water intake during these months may also be a contributing factor. Mineral content of water should also be considered in areas where horses are predisposed to enterolithiasis.[10,11] All horses should have a readily available source of fresh, palatable water available and water intake monitored when possible.

Exercise regimen, pasture access, and housing
An increase in the number of hours in a stall and decrease in exposure pasture and recent change in exercise regimen increased the risk for colic and simple colonic obstruction and distention.[12,13] Horses that are housed for 19–24 h a day are at a particular risk for colic compared to horses at pasture.[5,6,12,13] On the other hand, access to pasture and duration of access have been associated with increased risk of equine grass sickness (p. 209) in certain geographical regions.[20] Large colon (p. 217) and cecal (p. 214) impaction are particularly associated with recent stall confinement. For example, a horse that is normally in the pasture and is stall confined because of an injury is predisposed to cecal impaction. Appetite and fecal output should be monitored closely in these horses.

Recent transportation
Recent transportation has been associated with colic. Horses that had a history of travel in the previous 24 h had an increased risk of simple colonic obstruction and distention compared to horses that had not been transported.[12] Stress, change in diet and water consumption, and possibly restricted movement are likely related to the association between travel and colic. Horses may come into contact with infectious disease during transportation particularly in association with shows or events. There has been also been an association between transportation and salmonellosis: (1) transportation had a major role in reactivating *Salmonella* sp. infection in carrier ponies[22] and (2) horses with a travel time to the hospital >1 h were at an increased risk for shedding salmonella compared to horses with a shorter travel time.[15]

Geographical areas in which the horse has been housed
While there may not be an association between geographical region and occurrence of colic,[30] specific types of colic tend to occur in different regions:

- Equine grass sickness (p. 209) occurs predominantly in the UK, Northern Mainland Europe, and South America.[20]
- Enterolithiasis (p. 218) is particularly common in California.[10,11]
- Ileal impaction (p. 208) is typically associated with horses residing in the southeastern USA.[17]
- Sand colic (p. 217) occurs in horses residing in regions with sandy soils such as Arizona, California, Florida, New Jersey, and Delaware.[2]
- Proximal enteritis (PE) (p. 207) is reported to occur more frequently and with more severity in certain regions. California has a lower incidence of PE compared to other regions and the disease seems to occur with greater severity in the southeastern compared to northeastern USA.[8,9]

It is, therefore, important to know where the horse has previously resided as well as when and for how long the horse was in that region.

Gastrointestinal parasite control
Detailed information is in Chapter 24 on Gastrointestinal Parasitology and Anthelmintics (p. 316). The history of anthelmintic therapy needs to be obtained including the anthelmintic(s) used,

frequency of administration, and results of monitoring of parasite burden.

While historically *Strongylus vulgaris* (large red worm) was associated with colic, with the development of ivermectin-based anthelmintics the role of *S. vulgaris* in colic has diminished.[2] *Anoplocephala perfoliata* (tapeworms) have been associated with many forms of colic including gas colic (p. 45), ileal impaction (p. 208), ileocecal, cecocecal, and cecocolic intussusceptions (p. 213, 214), and cecal impaction (p. 214).[2,19,23] Therefore, treatment with praziquantel tartrate or pyrantel pamoate should be part of the anthelmintic regimen. Cyathostomes (small red worms) have been associated with large colon lesions[2,31] and *Parascaris equorum* (round worms) have been associated with intestinal obstruction, rupture, peritonitis, intussusception, or abscessation in foals.[2,25] Monitoring of resistance of these parasites to routinely used anthelmintics such as ivermectin is recommended.

Horses that were not treated with an ivermectin- or moxidectin-based anthelmintic within the previous 12 months[12] or were not on a regular deworming program[6] were predisposed to colic and horses recently administered an anthelmintic were at a decreased risk of colic.[13] Recent anthelmintic administration, however, within 7–8 days was associated with colic[6] and ascarid impaction.[25]

Vaccination
Vaccination history is also important particularly in cases where it may not be clear that the horse is showing signs of colic. Diseases for which clinical signs can be mistaken for colic and vaccination is available include botulism, rabies, and other neurological diseases. There has only been one study associating vaccination (Potomac horse fever) with colic signs.[20] Research is currently being undertaken to determine the possibility of an equine grass sickness vaccine.[29]

Medical history

Previous colic and colic surgery
Horses that have had previous colic surgery and previous episodes of colic are predisposed to colic.[5,6,12,24,29,30] Horses with a large colon volvulus and displacement necessitating surgical correction were significantly more likely to colic after surgery if they had more than one episode of colic prior to the one necessitating surgery.[26,27]

The specific diagnosis and procedure performed during a previous colic surgery often provides an indication of the cause of colic: for example, colonic displacements (NSLE and right dorsal displacement) and large colon volvulus have a tendency to recur; horses with small intestinal and small colon lesions are predisposed to adhesions; and a previous history of jejunocecostomy may be associated with stenosis at the site of an anastomosis. Often owners/caregivers may be aware of previous colic or colic surgery but with no knowledge of the cause. Owners/caregivers should be encouraged to keep records of the horses under their care so that this information is readily available to the attending veterinarian.

The frequency and severity of previous colic episodes should be recorded. Recurrent intermittent colic warrants a more in-depth diagnostic workup including gastroscopy, radiography (p. 149, e.g., sand or enterolithiasis), sonographic examination (p. 116), and abdominocentesis (p. 87, e.g., neoplasia).

Other medical problems and current medication
Knowledge of current or recent medication including dose rate, route, and frequency of administration that the horse is or was receiving is critical so that

- treatment can be continued should the horse become hospitalized (e.g., administration of antimicrobial drugs for treatment of a wound);
- drug toxicity that may be manifest as signs of colic can be identified (e.g., nonsteroidal anti-inflammatory drug toxicity can manifest as right dorsal colitis and amitraz toxicity can manifest as ileus and impaction); and
- treatment for the signs of colic with potentially toxic drugs (e.g., nonsteroidal anti-inflammatory drugs (NSAIDs) and aminoglycosides) does not result in drug toxicity.

There are certain causes of colic associated with a particular medical history. Acute colitis should be considered in horses with a history of antimicrobial drug administration. Horses with colitis can initially show signs of colic that progress to dull mentation and diarrhea. Colitis should be considered particularly in horses with a fever. Cecal impaction should be considered in horses with a history of recent surgery or stall confinement for an injury. Recent lameness has been associated with colonic impaction.[12]

Whether or not the owner has administered any medication for the current episode of colic, including the route of administration, dose rate, and frequency, should be noted.

Medical problems of other horses
Knowledge of recent medical problems of other horses stabled at the same location may be useful to determine a diagnosis and assist with recommendations for prevention and treatment: for example, in the case where several animals have had problems with colic following treatment with the licicide amitraz; on a farm that has had a problem with strangles, abdominal abscessation should be considered; ileocecal intussusception should be considered on farms with a suspected high incidence of tapeworm infection; and sand colic should be suspected in horses residing in areas particularly if there is a problem with sand colic on the farm.

Crib biting or windsucking
Stable vices, such as crib biting or windsucking, have been recently associated with colonic colic[9] and epiploic foramen entrapment.[1]

Application of the patient's history

Clinical scenarios 1–3, located in Appendix A, are examples of cases where case history is important in determining a tentative diagnosis and case management. Further discussion on the integration of patient history into case management is included in Chapter 8 on Referral of the Horse with Colic (p. 71) and Chapter 15 on Medical versus Surgical Treatment of the Horses with Colic (p. 164). Quizzes for each chapter, additional clinical scenarios, and video demonstrations of surgical procedures are available online at www.wiley.com/go/southwood.

References

1. Archer. D.C., Freeman, D.E., Doyle. A.J., Proudman, C.J. & Edwards, G.B. (2004) Association between cribbing and entrapment of the small intestine in the epiploic foramen in horses: 68 cases (1991–2001). *Journal of the American Veterinary Medical Association*, **15**, 562–564.
2. Archer, D.C. & Proudman, C.J. (2006) Epidemiolical clues to preventing colic. *The Veterinary Journal*, **172**, 29–39.
3. Archer, D.C., Pinchbeck, G.L., Proudman, C.J. & Clough, H.E. (2006) Is equine colic seasonal? Novel application of a model based approach. *BMC Veterinary Research*, **2**, 27.
4. Buchanan, B.R. & Andrews, F.M. (2003) Treatment and prevention of equine gastric ulcer syndrome. *Veterinary Clinics of North America: Equine Practice*, **19**, 575–597.
5. Cohen, N.D., Matejka, P.L., Honnas, C.M. & Hooper, R.N. (1995) Case-control study of the association between various management factors and development of colic in horses. Texas Equine Colic Study Group. *Journal of the American Veterinary Medical Association*, **206**, 667–673.
6. Cohen, N.D., Gibbs, P.G. & Woods, A.M. (1999) Dietary and other management factors associated with colic in horses. *Journal of the American Veterinary Medical Association*, **215**, 53–60.
7. Cohen, N.D., Vontur, C.A. & Rakestraw, P.C. (2000) Risk factors for enterolithiasis among horses in Texas. *Journal of the American Veterinary Medical Association*, **216**, 1787–1794.
8. Edwards, G.B. (2000) Duodenitis-proximal jejunitis (anterior enteritis) as a surgical problem. *Equine Veterinary Education*, **12**, 318–321.
9. Freeman, D.E. (2000) Duodenitis-proximal jejunitis. *Equine Veterinary Education*, **12**, 322–332.
10. Hassel, D.M., Langer, D.L., Snyder. J.R., Drake, C,M., Goodell, M.L. & Wyle, A. (1999) Evaluation of enterolithiasis in equids: 900 cases (1973–1996). *Journal of the American Veterinary Medical Association*, **15**, 233–237.
11. Hassel, D.M., Aldridge, B.M., Drake, C.M. & Snyder, J.R. (2008) Evaluation of dietary and management risk factors for enterolithiasis among horses in California. *Research in Veterinary Science*, **85**, 476–480.
12. Hillyer, M.H., Taylor, F.G., Proudman, C.J., Edwards, G.B., Smith, J.E. & French, N.P. (2002) Case control study to identify risk factors for simple colonic obstruction and distension colic in horses. *Equine Veterinary Journal*, **34**, 455–463.
13. Hudson, J.M., Cohen, N.D., Gibbs, P.G. & Thompson, J.A. (2001) Feeding practices associated with colic

in horses. *Journal of the American Veterinary Medical Association*, **219**, 1419–1425.

14. Kaya, G., Sommerfeld-Stur, I. & Iben, C. (2009) Risk factors of colic in horses in Austria. *Journal of Animal Physiology and Animal Nutrition*, **93**, 339–349.

15. Kim, L.M., Morley, P.S., Traub-Dargatz, J.L., Salman, M.D. & Gentry-Weeks, C. (2001) Factors associated with Salmonella shedding among equine colic patients at a veterinary teaching hospital. *Journal of the American Veterinary Medical Association*, **218**, 740–748.

16. Kristula, M.A. & McDonnell, S.M. (1994) Drinking water temperature affects consumption of water during cold weather in ponies. *Applied Animal Behaviour Science* **41**, 155–160.

17. Little, D. & Blikslager, A.T. (2002) Factors associated with development of ileal impaction in horses with surgical colic: 78 cases (1986–2000). *Equine Veterinary Journal*, **34**, 464–468.

18. Lopes, M.A., White, N.A. 2nd, Crisman, M.V. & Ward, D.L. (2004) Effects of feeding large amounts of grain on colonic contents and feces in horses. *American Journal of Veterinary Research*, **65**, 687–694.

19. Mair, T.S., Sutton, D.G.M. & Love, S. (2000) Caecocaecal and caecocolic intussusceptions associated with larval cyathostomosis in four young horses. *Equine Veterinary Journal*, **32**, 77–80.

20. McCarthy, H.E., Proudman, C.J. & French, N.P. (2001) The epidemiology of equine grass sickness—A literature review (1909–1999). *The Veterinary Record*, **149**, 293–300.

21. McDonnell, S.M. & Kristula, M.A. (1996) No effect of drinking water temperature on consumption of water during hot summer weather in ponies. *Applied Animal Behaviour Science* **49**, 149–163.

22. Owen, R.A., Fullerton, J. & Barnum, D.A. (1983) Effects of transportation, surgery, and antibiotic therapy in ponies infected with Salmonella. *American Journal of Veterinary Research*, **44**, 46–50.

23. Proudman, C.J., French, N.P. & Trees, A.J. (1998) Tapeworm infection is a significant risk factor for spasmodic colic and ileal impaction colic in the horse. *Equine Veterinary Journal*, **30**, 194–199.

24. Reeves, M.J., Salman, M.D. & Smith, G. (1996) Risk factors for equine acute abdominal disease (colic): Results from a multi-centre case-control study. *Preventive Veterinary Medicine*, **26**, 285–301.

25. Southwood, L.L., Ragle, C.A., Snyder, J.R., *et al.* (2002) Surgical treatment of ascarid impactions in foals and horses. In: *Proceedings of the Seventh Equine Colic Research Symposium*, Manchester, U.K., pp. 112–113.

26. Southwood, L.L., Bergslien, K., Jacobi, A., *et al.* (2002) Large colon displacement and volvulus in horses: 495 cases (1987–1999). In: *Proceedings of the Seventh Equine Colic Research Symposium*, Manchester, U.K., pp. 32–33.

27. Southwood, L.L. (2006) Acute abdomen. *Clinical Techniques in Equine Practice*, **5**, 112–126.

28. Tinker, M.K., White, N.A., Lessard, P., *et al.* (1997) Prospective study of equine colic incidence and mortality. *Equine Veterinary Journal*, **29**, 448–453.

29. Tinker, M.K., White, N.A., Lessard, P., *et al.* (1997) Prospective study of equine colic risk factors. *Equine Veterinary Journal*, **29**, 454–458.

30. Traub-Dargatz, J.L., Kopral, C.A., Seitzinger, A.H., Garber, L.P., Forde, K. & White, N.A. (2001) Estimate of the national incidence of and operation-level risk factors for colic among horses in the United States, spring 1998 to spring 1999. *Journal of the American Veterinary Medical Association*, **219**, 67–71.

31. Uhlinger, C. (1990) Effects of three anthelmintic schedules on the incidence of colic in horses. *Equine Veterinary Journal*, **22**, 251–254.

2 Physical Examination

Louise L. Southwood

Department of Clinical Studies, New Bolton Center, School of Veterinary Medicine, University of Pennsylvania, Kennett Square, PA, USA

Chapter Outline

Importance of the physical examination	**12**
Initial patient observation	**14**
Physical examination	**15**
Rapid assessment of the cardiovascular status	15
Heart rate	16
Oral mucous membranes	17
Jugular refill time	18
Extremity temperature	18
Pulse quality	19
Evaluation of the gastrointestinal tract	19
Rectal temperature	19
Respiratory rate and evaluation of the respiratory system	19
Digital pulses	20
Applications of the physical examination	**21**

Importance of the physical examination

Being able to perform a good physical examination is paramount when examining the colic patient. While recent focus has been on more advanced laboratory and imaging diagnostic tools such as blood and peritoneal fluid lactate concentration (p. 81, 92) and abdominal sonographic examination (p. 116), the physical examination along with obtaining a thorough patient history remains the cornerstone of good veterinary medicine.

Information obtained during physical examination of the colic patient is used to confirm that the horse has colic and determine the severity and possible cause, direct analgesic and fluid therapy, make decisions with regard to medical or surgical treatment, and provide the owners with some indication of prognosis.

Meticulous medical records are necessary when examining the horse with colic (Figure 2.1). Often the examination is performed on an emergency basis and at a time of day that is less than convenient. Expecting to recall findings at a later time is unreasonable, at least for most veterinarians. Recording physical examination findings is important so that trends over time can be observed, all abnormal findings can be noted and a problem list formed,

Practical Guide to Equine Colic, First Edition. Edited by Louise L. Southwood.
© 2013 John Wiley & Sons, Inc. Published 2013 by John Wiley & Sons, Inc.

COLIC FLOW SHEET

Duration of colic:_____
Initial degree of pain:_____
Previous history of colic: _____
Mare: # of days pre-/postpartum:_____ # of days since last bred: _____
Previous medication given and time:_____

Severity of pain and mental status:
( )   alert, responsive
( )   depressed, dull
( )   mild - occasionally looks at abdomen, paws, lies down
( )   moderate - frequently looks at abdomen and paws, occasionally lies down and rolls
( )   marked - frequently paws, lies down and rolls
( )   severe - continuous attempts to lie down and roll

Heart rate:_____ Respiratory rate:_____ Capillary refill time_____(sec.) Temperature:_____

Peripheral pulse character: facial: ( ) reduced   ( ) normal   ( ) increased
                              feet: ( ) reduced   ( ) normal   ( ) increased

Mucous membrane color:
( ) normal pink   ( ) pale pink   ( ) bright red, injected
( ) bright pink   ( ) pale, cyanotic   ( ) dark, cyanotic

Borborygmi:

	hyper	normal	hypo	absent
- right side:	( )	( )	( )	( )
- left side:	( )	( )	( )	( )

Nasogastric Tube: NOT DONE ( )
- gas relieved: ( ) none   ( ) slight   ( ) significant
- fluid reflux: ( ) none   ( ) positive   quantity:_____ color:_____

Abdominocentesis:
( ) not done   ( ) difficult   - quantity:_____   opacity:_____
( ) clean   ( ) unsuccessful   - color:_____   cytology:_____

Abdominal distention: ( ) none ( ) slight   ( ) moderate   ( ) severe

Palpation:
- ( ) not done
- male: testicles _____

Rectal findings:

Other diagnostic findings:

Medication administered at admission:

Differential Diagnosis:

Plan:

Figure 2.1   Example of an admission physical examination sheet used for horses with colic.
Source: Courtesy of New Bolton Center, University of Pennsylvania, Kennett Square, Pennsylvania.

and information can be accurately and completely communicated if referral becomes necessary. Should the horse have recurrent bouts of colic, comparison of physical examination findings on each occurrence can be made and trends identified.

Examining the colic patient begins with making several observations during the approach to the horse or foal. The cardiovascular status should be examined first followed by a more thorough examination of pertinent body systems. A checklist of key observations and physical examination findings for the colic patient are provided in Table 2.1.

Initial patient observation

Patient examination begins with a careful 30–60 s observation (Table 2.1). Particular attention should be paid to the horse's body condition (Table 2.2). Poor body condition may be an indication of an underlying disease process (e.g., neoplasia, hepatic or renal disease, right dorsal colitis), inadequate nutrition, or poor dentition.

Mentation or attitude is described as bright, alert, and responsive; quiet and alert; dull or obtunded. Horses with colic are generally bright and alert and will be attentive and even vocalize during the veterinarian's approach. On the other hand, horses with colitis, proximal enteritis (PE), or peritonitis including gastrointestinal rupture tend to have a dull mentation. Abnormal mentation should also be considered with some neurological disease or toxicity. Assessment of mentation should take into consideration any history of the horse being administered a sedative/analgesic drug.

Evidence of inappropriate sweating can be an indication of severe pain or shock. Other disease processes such as equine protozoal myeloencephalitis (EPM) or pituitary pars intermedia dysfunction (Cushing's Disease), can cause inappropriate sweating but should only be considered with other signs that do not fit with colic.

Abdominal distention when mild can be difficult to assess unless the veterinarian is familiar with the horses normal abdominal contour. Moderate to severe abdominal distention is more easily discernible and is generally an indication of a large intestinal obstruction. One exception is a small intestinal mesenteric root volvulus. Asymmetry of abdominal distention can provide some evidence

Table 2.1   Physical examination checklist for the colic patient.

Patient observation	• Mentation or attitude • Signs of pain • Sweating • Evidence of trauma • Abdominal distention • Body Condition

Rapid assessment of the cardiovascular status	• Heart rate
	• Oral mucous membranes
	  ○ Color
	  ○ Moistness
	  ○ CRT
	• Jugular filling
	• Extremity temperature
	• Pulse quality

Other body systems	• Intestinal borborygmi • Rectal temperature • Respiratory rate and effort • Digital pulses • Testes (stallions and colts)

of the type of lesion, for example, horses with a nephrosplenic entrapment may have more distention on the left side of the abdomen and cecal tympany or impaction may result in more apparent distention on the right side. The horse should be standing squarely when symmetry of abdominal distention is assessed.

Abrasions occurring on the head, tuber coxae, and limbs are an indication that the horse at least at some point was showing signs consistent with severe abdominal pain. A strangulating obstruction should be considered in any horse with abrasions associated with colic. Occasionally a horse will be examined for an apparent primary laceration, unbeknown to the owner/caregiver and veterinarian that the horse sustained the injury during an episode of colic. Therefore, when evaluating a horse with trauma of unknown origin, colic should be considered as a potential cause and can be discerned by careful patient observation.

The degree of pain should be assessed. Signs of abdominal pain may be observed initially; however, horses with mild colic are often easily distracted and may not demonstrate signs when being restrained for examination. Once an initial physical examination is completed, it is recommended to allow the horse to be unrestrained in a stall for a brief period so that the signs of colic can

Table 2.2 Body condition score.

1.	Poor	Very prominent withers, dorsal spinous and transverse processes, ribs, shoulder and pelvic bone structure, and tailhead. Thin neck. Emaciated with no fat palpated.
2.	Very thin	Prominent dorsal spinous processes, ribs, pelvic bones, and tailhead. Withers, neck, and shoulder bone structure discernible.
3.	Thin	Prominent dorsal spinous processes but covered by fat to midpoint. Discernible ribs with slight fat covering. Shoulder, withers, and neck are thin and tailhead prominent but individual vertebrae not visible. Tuber coxae visible but tuber sacrale not visible.
4.	Moderately thin	Negative crease along the back and the ribs can barely be seen. Fat around the tailhead. Tuber coxae not seen. Withers, neck, and shoulders not obviously thin.
5.	Moderate	Back level and ribs not seen but can be palpated. Withers rounded and shoulder and neck blend smoothly into the body. Slightly spongy tailhead fat.
6.	Moderately fleshy	Slight crease along the back. Small fat deposits along the sides of the withers, behind the shoulders, and along the sides of the neck. Tailhead fat soft and fat over the ribs palpates spongy.
7.	Fleshy	Maybe crease along the back. Individual ribs palpable but there is fat between the ribs. Soft fat around the tailhead and noticeable fat along the withers, neck and behind the shoulders.
8.	Fat	Obvious crease along the back. Ribs difficult to palpate. Withers and space behind shoulders are filled out with fat. Fat deposits along inner thigh. Very soft tail fat.
9.	Extremely fat	Very obvious crease down back. Ribs not palpable. Bulging fat along neck, shoulder, withers, and tailhead. Fat deposits along inner thigh.

Source: Adapted from Henneke *et al.* (1983).

be carefully observed, prior to administration of analgesia if the horse is not particularly painful. It is often during this observation period that it is determined that the horse truly has colic (more common) or has some other disease process such as a neurological disease. Horses with mild pain will tend to intermittently flank stare, kick at their abdomen, and pace; moderate pain is demonstrated by persistent flank staring, kicking at their abdomen, and rolling but the horse can be distracted; and severe pain is associated with undistractable rolling and thrashing.

Severity of pain along with degree of abdominal distention and frequency of intestinal borborygmi can be used to evaluate the colic gravity.[4,10] Moderate to severe colic observed during the initial examination, persistent colic, and return of colic signs following provision of analgesia is associated with the need for surgery.[6]

It is important to assess the degree of pain in light of any analgesia administered by the owner/caregiver. Although poorly documented, older horses (late teens and older) tend to less readily and less dramatically demonstrate colic signs compared to younger horses (yearlings and 2–3-year-olds) and foals and this should be taken into consideration.

Physical examination

Physical examination should begin with a rapid assessment of the patient's cardiovascular stability. Heart rate and oral mucous membranes can provide much of this information. Once a rapid patient assessment is performed and the horse determined to be cardiovascularly stable or unstable (Table 2.3), the physical examination can be completed. The physical examination for the equine colic patient should focus on intestinal borborygmi, rectal temperature, respiratory rate, and digital pulses.

Rapid assessment of cardiovascular status

The cardiovascular status of the horse can be assessed quickly and thoroughly to determine the severity of disease and the need for emergency resuscitation with intravenous fluids (p. 99). Table 2.3 provides an indication of changes that may be observed as the horse's cardiovascular status deteriorates.

The cardiovascular status of the patient can be rapidly assessed by obtaining a heart rate and examining the oral mucous membrane color, moistness, and capillary refill time (CRT). Jugular vein filling, pulse quality, and extremity temperature can provide more specific information with regard to hydration, vascular volume, and tissue perfusion.

Heart rate

Note: A nasogastric tube should be passed (p. 38) immediately in any horse with a heart rate >60 beats/min because it can be an indication of pending fatal gastric rupture (p. 206).

Heart rate should be evaluated initially either by ausculting the heart on the left side of the cranial thorax immediately behind the point of the elbow or palpating a pulse in the facial or transverse facial artery. The number of beats over 15 or 30 min is counted and the rate calculated in beats/minute. A normal adult horse heart rate is 32–44 beats/min and a neonate is 100–120 beats/min. Older foals and weanlings tend to have a variable heart rate that is slightly higher than that of an adult; however, the heart rate should be within the adult range by 6 months of age.

Tachycardia is generally an indication of pain or shock. In colic patients, tachycardia up to 60 beats/min can be associated with pain alone. Once the heart rate is 70 beats/min or higher, the horse is likely to have some degree of shock. Shock is defined as insufficient oxygen delivery to the cell leading to inadequate cellular ATP production and depletion of ATP supply (see Chapter 11 on Intravenous Catheterization and Fluid Therapy [p. 99]). Failure of the energy (ATP)-dependent Na^+/K^+ pump ultimately results in cell death. Tachycardia is one compensatory mechanism associated with sympathetic stimulation to increase cardiac output and oxygen delivery to the tissues.

Because of its association with pain and shock, heart rate has a strong association with prognosis

Table 2.3   Examples of physical examination findings in horses with various stages of dehydration, hypovolemia, and shock.

Cardiovascular status	Clinical signs
Normal	<ul><li>Bright, alert, and responsive</li><li>Heart rate <48 beats/min</li><li>Mucous membranes pink, moist, CRT <2 s</li><li>Warm extremities</li><li>Good jugular refill</li><li>Good pulse quality</li></ul>
Mild dehydration	<ul><li>Bright or quiet, alert, and responsive</li><li>Heart rate <48 beats/min but if painful up to 60 beats/min</li><li>Mucous membranes pink, tachy, CRT 2–3 s</li><li>Warm extremities</li><li>Good jugular refill</li><li>Good pulse quality</li></ul>
Moderate dehydration and hypovolemia	<ul><li>Quiet but alert and responsive</li><li>Heart rate 62–76 beats/min</li><li>Mucous membranes variable color, tachy to dry, CRT ~3 s</li><li>Cooler extremities</li><li>Slow jugular refill</li><li>Pulse quality variable</li></ul>
Severe dehydration and hypovolemia (shock)	<ul><li>Dull mentation or moribund</li><li>Heart rate 80–120 beats/min</li><li>Dry, injected/toxic (endotoxemia), or pale (hemorrhage) mucous membranes with a CRT >3 s</li><li>Cool extremities</li><li>Poor jugular refill</li><li>Peripheral pulses difficult to palpate</li></ul>

for horses with colic.[1-4,7,8,10] Heart rate along with packed cell volume (PCV) and blood lactate and plasma creatinine concentrations are a good indication of the degree of shock, likelihood of postoperative complications, and prognosis for survival.

Note: When using various physical examination and laboratory findings for patient assessment, observation of trends over time and use of multiple indices is more useful than the use of one index at one point in time.

Alpha-2 agonists (i.e., xylazine and detomidine) cause a reflex bradycardia and heart rate measurements should be interpreted in light of recent medication. The effects of the alpha-2 agonists should have subsided within 1–2 h of administration.

Tachycardia that is inconsistent with other clinical findings (e.g., a horse with a heart rate of 90 beats/min and no other clinical indication of pain or shock) may be associated with an arrhythmia. An electrocardiogram should be obtained if this is observed. Arrhythmias are uncommon in colic patients but may include ventricular tachycardia or atrial fibrillation.

Oral mucous membranes

Oral mucous membranes should be examined after the heart rate is counted. Normal mucous membranes should be pale pink and moist (Figure 2.2). The CRT time should be <2 s.

Injected membranes (Figure 2.3) which are bright pink to red with or without a toxic line are usually associated with endotoxemia (p. 246). Severely injected red to purple mucous membranes are generally associated with gastrointestinal tract

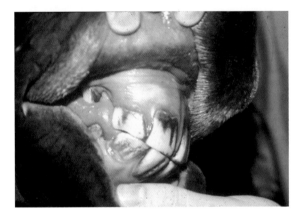

Figure 2.2 Normal oral mucous membranes.
Source: Courtesy of Colorado State University, Fort Collins, Colorado.

(a) (b)

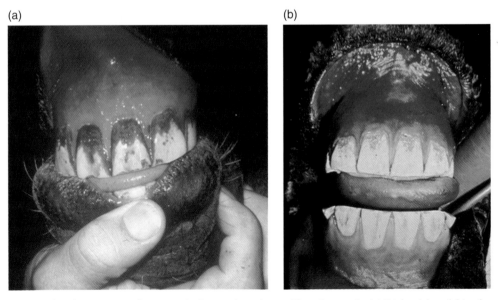

Figure 2.3 Injected oral mucous membranes typically seen in patients with endotoxemia. (a) Bright pink and (b) red.
Source: Courtesy of Colorado State University, Fort Collins, Colorado.

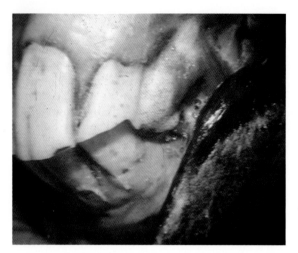

Figure 2.4   Pale oral mucous membranes that may be associated with hemorrhagic shock.
Source: Courtesy of Colorado State University, Fort Collins, Colorado.

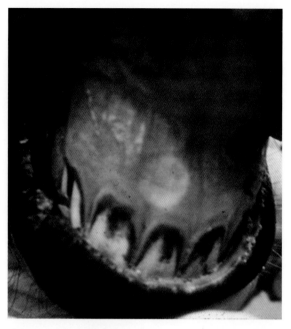

Figure 2.5   Prolonged CRT.
Source: Courtesy of Colorado State University, Fort Collins, Colorado.

rupture, colitis, or an extensive and prolonged strangulating obstruction. Abnormal mucous membranes have been used in models to estimate colic severity score.[11] Tachycardia with pale mucous membranes may be an indication of hemorrhage (e.g., hemoabdomen, Figure 2.4).

Oral mucous membranes should be moist when touched. Tacky mucous membranes are an indication of mild to moderate dehydration (i.e., loss of total body water with loss of water from the interstitial tissue) and may be corrected with either oral or intravenous fluids. Dry mucous membranes are associated with moderate to severe dehydration. Dry mucous membranes may be observed in horses with a prolonged duration of colic that has not been treated appropriately or causes of colic in which a large volume fluid is lost into the gastrointestinal tract. Severe dehydration should be treated with intravenous fluids. See Chapter 7 on Enteral Fluid Therapy (p. 62) and Chapter 11 on Intravenous Catheterization and Fluid Therapy (p. 99).

CRT is measured by applying gentle digital pressure to the mucous membranes, then releasing, and counting the time in seconds for the capillary blanching to disappear. Prolonged CRT (Figure 2.5) is observed in horses with hypovolemia and poor tissue perfusion and is an indica-tion for intravenous fluid therapy. See Chapter 11 on Intravenous Catheterization and Fluid Therapy (p. 99).

Jugular refill time

Jugular refill time is measured by holding off the jugular vein in the lower neck and observing the time taken to fill the vein. Jugular refill time should be <2 s in a well-hydrated horse. Poor jugular refill (>3 s) is generally associated with more serious causes of colic (e.g., large colon volvulus) and indicates hypovolemia and the need for intravenous fluids (p. 99).

Extremity temperature

Extremities (distal limbs, ears, nose) should be warm to the touch. Cool extremities generally represent poor tissue perfusion as a result of peripheral vasoconstriction to maintain circulation of vital organs. Ambient temperature should be taken into consideration when evaluating extremity temperature.

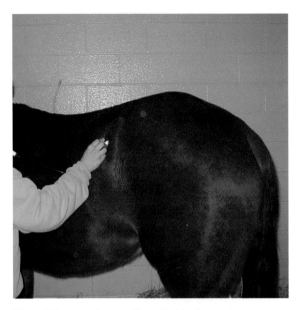

Figure 2.6   Auscultation of intestinal borborygmi.

Pulse quality

The pulse can be palpated in the facial artery and should be easily palpated, regular, and strong. With signs of hypovolemia and poor cardiac output, the pulse quality will deteriorate to become barely palpable. During the hyperdynamic phase of shock bounding pulses may be palpated.

Evaluation of the gastrointestinal tract

The gastrointestinal tract is evaluated initially by ausculting the four abdominal quadrants for borborygmi (Figure 2.6). Normal borborygmi have a constant low-grade rumbling associated with gas and fluid moving through the gastrointestinal tract. Horses that have been inappetent or had feed withheld usually have hypomotile intestinal borborygmi. An absence of intestinal borborygmi is generally associated with the need for abdominal surgery[12] and typically noted in horses with strangulating intestinal obstructions. Hypermotile intestinal borborygmi can occur with mild to moderate colitis. Disparity in intestinal borborygmi between the left and right side of the abdomen may be used to identify the lesion site, for example, intestinal borborygmi may be decreased on the left side in a horse with a nephro-splenic entrapment and the right side in a horse with a cecal impaction. Sand accumulation can be auscultated in some horses on the ventral abdomen caudal to the xiphoid process and is similar to the sound produced if a paper bag were partially filled with sand and slowly rotated.[9]

The gastrointestinal function is also assessed based on historical information and observation. The horse's appetite, fecal output and consistency, and degree of abdominal distention are used with auscultation of borborygmi to complete the initial assessment of gastrointestinal function.

Rectal temperature

Rectal temperature should be performed prior to abdominal palpation per rectum to obtain an accurate measurement. Rectal temperature should be within normal limits for horses (99–101°F [37.2–38.3°C]) and foals (100–102°F [37.8–38.9°C]) with colic. Reasons for a high rectal temperature are hyperthermia (an elevated body temperature due to failed thermoregulation) or fever/pyrexia (elevation of temperature above the normal range due to an increase in the body temperature regulatory set point). Pyrexia is responsive to treatment with anti-inflammatory drugs and is typically more common in horses with colic.

Colitis, enteritis, peritonitis, or a respiratory tract infection should be suspected in horses with pyrexia particularly if the rectal temperature is >102°F (38.9°C). Horses do not typically develop pyrexia associated with stress or pain. Endotoxemia, however, does produce a fever and, therefore, a mild fever may be observed in horses with colic, particularly those with strangulating obstructions.

Respiratory rate and evaluation of the respiratory system

Normal respiratory rate should be 8–12 breaths/ min. Normal respiration in the adult horse is barely visible by observing the nares or thorax/abdomen. Horses with pain, fever, shock, or respiratory tract disease will have a high respiratory rate. The most common reason for a high respiratory rate in a horse with colic is pain. Nostril flare (Figure 2.7) will be observed and is a subtle yet important

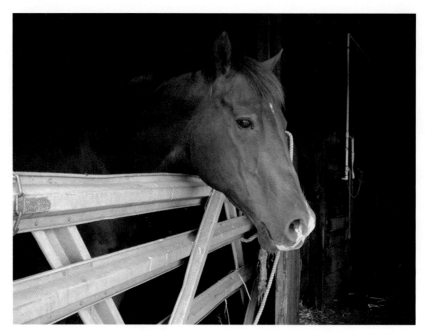

Figure 2.7   Nostril flare can be an important indication of pain in horses with colic.

indication of pain particularly in stoic patients (e.g., geriatric horses). Respiratory rate has been associated with prognosis for short-term survival in a few retrospective studies[1,2,4,10] but is more likely an indication of pain necessitating intensive medical or surgical treatment.

Horses with shock are usually severely tachypneic. Marked abdominal distention can cause inadequate ventilation and tachypnea in an effort to exchange adequate air with a decrease in diaphragm compliance. Trocharization (p. 160) may be indicated in such cases.

Fever can lead to a high respiratory rate. Tachypnea with respiratory rates >40 breaths/min and even >100 breaths/min has been observed in febrile horses administered an alpha-2 adrenergic agonist (i.e., xylazine or detomidine).[6] Tachypnea was observed for at least 1–5 min following drug administration and was also associated with a likely unrelated antipyretic effect.[6] While the response of febrile horses to sedation with xylazine or detomidine can be dramatic, it does not appear to negatively impact the health of the patient.

Occasionally a horse or foal showing signs of colic will have underlying respiratory tract disease (e.g., pneumonia or inflammatory airway disease).

A thorough examination of the respiratory system should be performed in these horses. Complete evaluation of the respiratory system involves examination of the nares for discharge and odor; history of a cough; ability to elicit a cough with tracheal palpation; percussion of the thorax; and thoracic and tracheal auscultation without and then with a rebreathing bag to identify wheezes/crackles and areas with poor air movement. The response to the rebreathing examination should be assessed with most horses not becoming distressed during the examination and having a normal respiratory rate within 1–3 breaths following removal of the rebreathing bag. Distress, coughing, and prolonged recovery should be considered abnormal and warrants further diagnostic tests. Thoracic sonographic and radiographic examination and transtracheal wash to obtain a sample for cytology and bacterial culture and sensitivity testing can be performed if signs are localized to the thorax.

Digital pulses

Laminitis is uncommon in horses with colic and is a relatively rare postoperative complication, the exception being horses with colitis, enteritis, or peritonitis, and those developing a high fever. However, horses with a previous history of laminitis do subjectively appear to be predisposed. Digital pulses should be palpated on the initial examination and the hoof temperature and any signs of lameness noted to establish a baseline to which future assessments can be compared.

Applications of the physical examination

Clinical scenarios 4 and 5, located in Appendix A, illustrate the importance of performing a careful physical examination. Quizzes for each chapter, additional clinical scenarios, and video demonstrations of surgical procedures are available online at www.wiley.com/go/southwood.

References

1. Dukti, S. & White, N.A. (2009) Prognosticating equine colic. *Veterinary Clinics of North America: Equine Practice*, **25**, 217–231.
2. Furr, M.O., Lessard, P. & White, N.A. (1995) Development of a colic severity score for predicting the outcome of equine colic. *Veterinary Surgery*, **24**, 97–101.
3. Garcia-Seco, E., Wilson, D.A., Kramer, J., *et al.* (2005) Prevalence and risk factors associated with outcome of surgical removal of pedunculated lipomas in horses: 102 cases (1987–2002). *Journal of the American Veterinary Medical Association*, **226**, 1529–1537.
4. Grulke, S., Olle, E., Detilleux, J., Gangl, M., Caudron, I. & Serteyn, D. (2001) Determination of a gravity and shock score for prognosis in equine surgical colic. *Journal of Veterinary Medicine A: Physiology, Pathology, Clinical Medicine*, **48**, 465–473.
5. Henneke, D.R., Potter, G.D., Kreider, J.L. & Yeates, B.F. (1983) Relationship between condition score, physical measurements and body fat percentage in mares. *Equine Veterinary Journal*, **15**, 371–372.
6. Kendall, A., Mosley, C. & Bröjer, J. (2010) Tachypnea and antipyresis in febrile horses after sedation with a2-agonists. *Journal of Veterinary Internal Medicine*, **24**, 1008–1011.
7. Mair, T.S. & Smith, L.J. (2005) Survival and complication rates of 300 horses undergoing surgical treatment of colic. Part 1. Short-term survival following a single laparotomy. *Equine Veterinary Journal*, **37**, 296–302.
8. Proudman, C.J., Edwards, G.A., Barnes, J. & French, N.P. (2005) Modelling long-term survival of horses following surgery for large intestinal disease. *Equine Veterinary Journal*, **37**, 366–370.
9. Ragle, C.A., Meagher, D.M., Schrader, J.L. & Honnas, C.M. (1989) Abdominal auscultation in the detection of experimentally induced gastrointestinal sand accumulation. *Journal of Veterinary Internal Medicine*, **3**, 12–14.
10. Southwood, L.L., Gassert, T. & Lindborg, S. (2010) Colic in geriatric compared to mature nongeriatric horses. Part 1: Retrospective review of clinical and laboratory data. *Equine Veterinary Journal*, **42**, 621–627.
11. White, N.A., Elward, A., Moga, K.S., Ward, D.L. & Sampson, D.M. (2005) Use of web-based data collection to evaluate analgesic administration and the decision for surgery in horses with colic. *Equine Veterinary Journal*, **37**, 347–350.

3

Abdominal Palpation per Rectum

Louise L. Southwood[1] and Joanne Fehr[2]

[1]Department of Clinical Studies, New Bolton Center, School of Veterinary Medicine, University of Pennsylvania, Kennett Square, PA, USA
[2]Equine Emergency Department, Pilchuck Animal Hospital, Snohomish, WA, USA

Chapter Outline

Indications	22	Cecum	28
Preparation	23	Large (ascending) colon	28
Restraint	23	Small (descending) colon	33
Rectal sleeve	23	Rectum	33
Lubrication	23	Urogenital tract	34
Relaxation of the rectum	23	Other abdominal structures	35
Sedation	24	Peritoneal cavity	35
Procedure	24	**Complications**	36
Normal anatomy	24	Rectal tear	36
Abnormal findings	26	Emergency first aid	36
Small intestine	27	Management	37

Indications

Abdominal palpation per rectum is used to examine the caudal aspect of the abdominal cavity and pelvic region in horses showing signs of colic. Other indications are for examination of the reproductive and urinary tract as well as abdominal examination for horses with fever of unknown origin, straining to defecate, and nonspecific signs such as weight loss, dull mentation, and inappetence.

Palpation per rectum can be a definitive diagnostic tool for some clinical problems (e.g., ileal, cecal, pelvic flexure [PF], and small colon impactions; uterine torsion in pregnant mares; nephrosplenic ligament entrapment [NSLE]; and broad ligament hematoma in periparturient mares). It can also be used to provide additional information with regard to the likely part of the gastrointestinal tract affected including distended

Practical Guide to Equine Colic, First Edition. Edited by Louise L. Southwood.
© 2013 John Wiley & Sons, Inc. Published 2013 by John Wiley & Sons, Inc.

small intestinal loops which are indicative of a small intestinal lesion; large colon distention which is associated with colonic displacements, volvulus, or intraluminal obstructions; cecal distention or tympany; and abdominal masses. Palpation is also used to examine the rectum in cases of rectal tear, rectal prolapse, and perirectal abscess.

Sonographic examination per rectum can be used to enhance the diagnostic usefulness of palpation per rectum, particularly in horses with abdominal or pelvic masses and periparturient mares with a tentative diagnosis of hemorrhage.

In cases where the patient is small (e.g., weanling, miniature horse) or problems with palpation per rectum are anticipated based on patient demeanor or level of pain, it may be best to avoid palpation per rectum and pursue other diagnostic techniques such as transcutaneous sonographic (p. 116) or radiographic examination (p. 149) or exploratory celiotomy (p. 173). A digital rectal examination with a lubricated gloved hand can be used in foals primarily to determine if there are feces in the rectum.

It is important to recognize limitations associated with this diagnostic technique primarily that only the caudal one-quarter to one-third of the abdominal cavity can be examined and lesions in the cranial abdomen cannot be identified; a definitive diagnosis is usually not obtained but the affected part of the gastrointestinal tract identified; and inherent limitations of blind palpation particularly with an inexperienced examiner should be appreciated.

Preparation

A list of "Things You Will Need" is provided in Table 3.1. Several steps should be taken prior to beginning an abdominal palpation per rectum to facilitate a diagnostic examination and avoid complications including rectal tear (p. 36) and injury to the examining veterinarian.

Restraint

The examination should be performed in a quiet area such as a procedure room or a stall. The horse should be adequately restrained with a halter and lead rope by an experienced and responsible adult.

Table 3.1   "Things You Will Need" for palpation per rectum.

- Quiet area
- Assistant to restrain the horse
- Halter and lead rope
- Rectal sleeve
- Lubrication
- Nose twitch
- ± Stocks
- ± 2% lidocaine (50 mL)
- ± Buscopan®
- ± Sedation

The person restraining the horse should stand on the same side as the examiner. Any movement of the horse while the examiner's arm is in the rectum can result in tearing of the rectum. A nose twitch should be used if the horse responds favorably to this form of restraint. Stocks are recommended, if available, to provide additional restraint of the horse and some degree of protection for the examiner.

Rectal sleeve

There are many choices for rectal sleeves. Selection of a sleeve made from thin, soft plastic without prominent seams is ideal for both palpation as well as avoiding rectal mucosal irritation.

Lubrication

The rectal sleeve should be well lubricated. Sodium carboxymethylcellulose is the most common lubricant used (e.g., 200–500 mL) and should be applied liberally to the arm and reapplied as necessary.

Relaxation of the rectum

Adequate restraint and ample lubrication are the minimal preparation for abdominal palpation per rectum. Often some degree of rectal relaxation is necessary to perform a good quality examination and minimize the risk of rectal injury.

Lidocaine 2% solution (50 mL) can be applied topically per rectum using a syringe and 30 in. (76.2 cm) intravenous (IV) extension set inserted into the rectum using a well-lubricated arm following evacuation of feces from the rectum. Lidocaine is thought to be absorbed into the rectal mucosa and desensitizes the receptors that initiate a contraction response.[10]

N-butylscopolammonium bromide (Buscopan® Injectable Solution) is a short-acting (15–25 min) anticholinergic spasmolytic agent that was shown to be more effective than topical 2% lidocaine at reducing rectal pressure and straining.[11]

Sedation

Sedation is not routinely used; however, it is recommended in young or small patients and horses that have not been palpated previously or are showing resistance to palpation, signs of anxiety, or abdominal pain. An example of a regimen that may be used for sedation is xylazine with or without butorphanol. It is important to recognize that alpha-2 agonists and opiates provide good visceral analgesia which may last for up to 1–2 h and this should be taken into consideration with reevaluating the patient. Examination of the patient prior to sedation for palpation per rectum or other procedures is recommended (see Chapter 2 on Physical Examination [p. 12]).

Procedure

Abdominal palpation per rectum can be performed with either the left or right hand. Many veterinarians prefer to use their nondominant hand in case of injury and so that notes can be taken during the procedure. Developing palpation skills with both hands is ideal. A plastic rectal sleeve is placed over the examiner's hand and arm and then lubricated. The horse's tail is moved to the side. When beginning rectal palpation with the horse not restrained in stocks, it is importation to stand to the side of the horse and as close as possible to the horse's thigh when first inserting the hand into the rectum. It is safe to stand behind the horse if it is restrained in stocks with a back board.

The examiner's hand and then arm are carefully inserted through the anal sphincter (which can be quite tight) and into the caudal rectum.

Attention should be paid to the volume and consistency of feces in the rectum. In a normal horse, there should be several large handfuls of formed fecal balls in the rectum. Feces, however, should not be impacted in the rectum. Time should be taken to completely evacuate the rectum of feces prior to beginning the examination. Topical lidocaine can be applied once the rectum is emptied of feces. Reapplication of lubrication to the examiner's hand and arm several times throughout the procedure is often necessary. The palpation is performed with the fingers together and the hand in a long, narrow formation (fist formation and spreading the fingers apart should be avoided). The examiner's arm is eventually inserted all the way into the horse's rectum to the level of the shoulder. The examiner should allow the arm to move caudally with rectal peristalsis and should never force the arm in a cranial direction against peristalsis. The rectal mucosa is often redundant, and the cranial rectum and distal small colon curve usually to the left and in a ventral direction. Care should be taken to gently navigate the hand through these obstacles and attain a position whereby the abdominal contents can be examined.

Normal anatomy

Abdominal structures that can be palpated per rectum in the normal horse are listed in Table 3.2. Examination of the rectum and pelvic region can be performed initially. The rectum extends from the anus to the level of the pelvic brim where it becomes the small (descending) colon. Lesions in this area are uncommon. The rectal mucosa should be smooth and there should be no masses or defects. The pelvic floor and shaft of the left and right ilium should have left to right symmetry. The bladder is often not identified unless it is distended with urine. The bladder can be distinguished based on its midline location and palpation of the round ligaments on the left and right (Figure 3.1a). The bladder can become extremely large when distended with urine and prohibit further abdominal palpation. If this occurs, the horse should be allowed to urinate (walking the horse to a bedded stall or to a grassy area can be used to encourage urination).

Table 3.2   Abdominal structures that can and cannot be palpated in the normal horse.

Palpable structures	Nonpalpable structures
• Ventral band of the cecum	• Stomach and pylorus
• Great vessels	• Duodenum*
• Caudal pole of left kidney	• Jejunum*
• Caudodorsal aspect of spleen	• Ileum*
• Nephrosplenic space ± ligament	• Right dorsal[1] and ventral colon
• Fecal balls in small colon	• Sternal and diaphragmatic flexure of colon
• Uterus and ovaries (mare)	• Transverse colon
• Inguinal rings (stallion)	• Proximal small colon
• Bladder when distended with urine	• Liver
	• Right kidney
	• Mesenteric root*

*Structures that may be palpated when abnormal.

In the nongravid mare, the uterus and ovaries are palpated in the pelvic region (Figure 3.1b). The uterus is best palpated by putting the hand in the rectum beyond the pelvic brim gently cupping the hand and moving it in a caudal direction. The uterus palpates as a small fold of tissue in the cupped hand. It can be traced to the left and right to identify the left and right ovaries, respectively. The uterus of a gravid mare can be palpated in the pelvic region during the first trimester. During the second trimester and early into the third trimester, the fetus cannot be palpated because of its location cranially and ventrally in the abdomen. The fetus can usually be palpated cranial to the pelvic brim late in gestation. Palpation per rectum of the late-term pregnant mare can be unrewarding because of the large size of the uterus and fetus which may obscure the other abdominal contents.

The inguinal rings can be palpated just over the pelvic brim in stallions but may be difficult to identify in mares and geldings. The spermatic cord (testicular, deferential, and cremaster arteries, cremaster and testicular nerves, ductus deferens, pampiniform plexus, lymphatic vessels, and tunica vaginalis) can be palpated entering the inguinal ring in stallions.

It is important to examine the abdominal cavity systematically. The medial/ventral cecal band can be palpated on the right side of the abdomen (Figure 3.1c). It generally courses from the dorsocaudal aspect on the right side of the abdomen in a cranial and ventral direction toward midline. The cecum is normally empty; however, occasionally soft ingesta and mild tympany may be palpated and generally considered within normal limits. The cecal base is attached to the dorsal body wall and the examiner's hand cannot be moved dorsal to the base of the cecum.

The examiner's hand is then moved toward midline to the dorsal abdominal wall and rotated 180° (palm facing upward) to palpate the aorta and internal and external iliac arteries. These vessels can be identified by their large size and prominent pulse (Figure 3.1c). The root of the mesentery which is on dorsal midline and toward the middle of the abdomen in a cranial to caudal direction is generally not palpable in the normal horse because of its cranial position.

Staying in the dorsal part of the abdomen, the examiner's hand is moved to the left side of the abdomen to palpate the caudal pole of the left kidney (Figure 3.1c). Note that the right kidney is not palpable. The caudodorsal border of the spleen can be palpated immediately adjacent to the left body wall and to the left and slightly ventral to the kidney (Figure 3.1c). The spleen should have a smooth sharp caudodorsal border. The nephrosplenic space is between the left kidney and spleen. The nephrosplenic ligament may be palpable in small horses.

The small colon can be identified usually in the left caudal abdomen based on palpation of fecal balls (Figure 3.1c). The normal small colon has

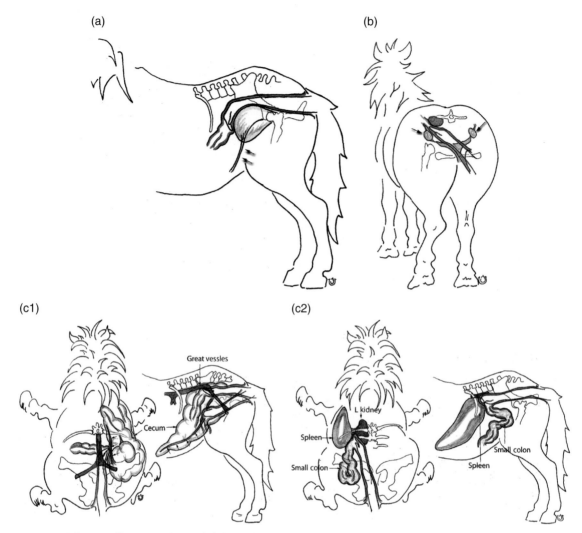

Figure 3.1   Schematic illustration of normal abdominal cavity anatomy as examined by palpation per rectum. (a) Normal urine distended bladder can be palpated on midline and distinguished from other viscera by the round ligaments (arrows). (b) Normal uterus and ovaries (arrows). (c) Palpable structures include medial/ventral cecal band on the right (arrows), great vessels along the dorsal body wall, caudal pole of the left kidney, dorsocaudal border of spleen adjacent to the left body wall, fecal balls in the small colon.

formed fecal balls throughout its length. The broad antimesenteric band and prominent mesenteric band can be palpated.

Normal large colon cannot be definitively identified unless there is ingesta in the region of the PF and it is lying in the caudal abdomen. Failure to identify the PF is not necessarily abnormal. Often several bands (taenia) can be palpated throughout the abdomen and these may be associated with the large or small colon. The small

intestine, including the duodenum, jejunum and ileum, cannot be palpated in the normal horse.

Abnormal findings

Abnormalities that can be found on palpation per rectum with a few differential diagnoses are listed in Table 3.3. Diagnoses that can be made based on palpation per rectum are provided in Table 3.4.

Table 3.3   Abnormal findings on palpation per rectum and some associated differential diagnoses.

Anatomical location	Abnormal finding	Differential diagnoses
Small intestine	A single loop or multiple loops of distended small intestine palpated throughout the abdomen	• Proximal enteritis (p. 207) • Ileus (p. 251) • Epiploic foramen entrapment (p. 211) • Strangulating lipoma (p. 209) • Inguinal hernia (p. 286) • Jejunal volvulus (p. 212) • Jejunal intussusception (p. 213) • Ileocecal intussusception (p. 213) • Ileal impaction (p. 208)
	Thickened loops (uncommon)	• Strangulated small intestine (p. 209) • Lymphoma (p. 233) • Proliferative enteropathy (p. 280) • Distal jejunal or ileal hypertrophy • Infiltrative or inflammatory bowel disease
Cecum	Gas distended or firm viscus on the right side of the abdomen	• Cecal tympany (gas filled) • Cecal impaction (ingesta-filled) (p. 214) • Cecocolic intussusception (firm mass) (p. 214)
Large colon	Gas distention	• Tympany • Impaction (PF or RDC) (p. 217) • Sand impaction (p. 217) • Enterolithiasis (p. 218) • Right dorsal displacement (p. 220) • Nephrosplenic ligament entrapment (p. 219) • Large colon volvulus (p. 220)
Small colon	Gas distention	• Strangulating lipoma (p. 209) • Enterolithiasis (p. 218) • Fecalith (p. 287)

Mass	Single or multiple firm and unindentable mass(es)	• Abscess (usually single)
		  ○ Penetrating foreign body
		  ○ *Streptococcus equi* subspecies *equi*
		• Neoplasia (single or multiple)
		  ○ Lymphoma
		  ○ Adenocarcinoma
		• Hematoma
		  ○ Pelvic injury
		  ○ Broad ligament hematoma

Small intestine

The small intestine is not palpable in the normal horse and finding either gas distended small intestinal loops (Figure 3.2a) or thickened small intestinal is abnormal. The small intestine can be identified based on its small size and smooth surface (i.e., no taenia or haustra) and can be palpated anywhere throughout the abdomen.

Single or multiple loops of gas distended small intestine are indicative of either a functional, strangulating, or nonstrangulating obstruction. Gas distended duodenum can be palpated as it courses right to left around the base of the cecum on the right side of the abdomen (Figure 3.2a). Often a single distended loop of small intestine is identified cranially at the tip of the examiner's fingers and is often missed, which emphasizes the

Table 3.4 Diagnoses that can be made on palpation per rectum.

Anatomical location	Diagnosis
Small intestine	• Ileal impaction (p. 208) • Inguinal hernia (p. 284)
Cecum	• Cecal impaction (p. 214) • Cecal tympany
Large colon	• Pelvic flexure impaction (p. 217) • Right dorsal colon impaction (rarely) (p. 217) • Nephrosplenic ligament entrapment (p. 219)
Small colon	• Small colon impaction (p. 221) • Enterolithiasis (rarely) (p. 218)
Rectum	• Rectal tear (p. 36) • Perirectal abscess (p. 138)

importance of adequate patient preparation and a thorough examination. Gas distended small intestine can be subjectively described as:

- Mild: easily compressible, 2–3 cm diameter, inconsistently distended (motile) loop(s)
- Moderate: somewhat compressible 3–4 cm diameter, consistently distended single or multiple loops
- Marked: multiple >4 cm diameter, consistently distended and taut loops

Mild and inconsistently distended small intestinal may not necessarily be clinically important and the horse should be monitored for signs of worsening pain and palpation per rectum repeated to reassess.

Thickened small intestine is less commonly identified on palpation per rectum and is more likely to be identified on transcutaneous sonographic evaluation (p. 116). The small intestine is distinguished based on its small size and smooth structure.

While in most cases palpation per rectum is limited to identification of distended small intestinal loops, occasionally a definitive diagnosis is made. Ileal impactions can often be palpated early during the course of the disease as a dough-like mass on the right side of the abdomen just medial to the cecum (Figure 3.2b).[8] An inguinal

hernia can be definitively diagnosed in most cases by palpating a distended small intestinal loop entering the inguinal canal (Figure 3.2c).

Cecum

Cecal tympani and cecal impaction (Figure 3.3a and b) can be identified per rectum. Cecal tympany is identified as a mild to severely gas distended cecum on the right side of the abdomen and may be a primary cause of colic but is often associated with an obstruction distal to the cecum (e.g., PF impaction). A cecal impaction is identified as a firm ingesta- and/or liquid-filled structure on the right side of the abdomen. With experience and careful palpation, cecocecal or cecocolic intussusceptions can be tentatively diagnosed when a firm unindentable structure is palpated on the right side of the abdomen and the ventral band in the cecum is not able to be followed along its normal course (Figure 3.3c).

Large (ascending) colon

Large colon distention (Figure 3.4a) is a common finding on palpation per rectum and is also often associated with signs of abdominal distention. The large colon can be identified by its large size as well as the bands (taenia) and sacculations (haustra). Occasionally it can be difficult to distinguish the cecum from the large colon (e.g., cecal impaction versus right dorsal displacement [RDD]). Colonic distention can be described as:

- Mild: colon is barely enlarged, easily compressible and inconsistently distended (motile); generally not associated with signs of abdominal distention.
- Moderate: colon is obviously enlarged, somewhat compressible and consistently distended; may be associated with signs of mild to moderate abdominal distention; the examiner can move their arm around the abdomen.
- Marked: colon is markedly enlarged to the point where it is difficult for the examiner to move their arm around the abdomen; colon is barely compressible and tight; associated with signs of moderate to severe abdominal distention.

A RDD can be tentatively diagnosed by palpating moderately to markedly distended colon

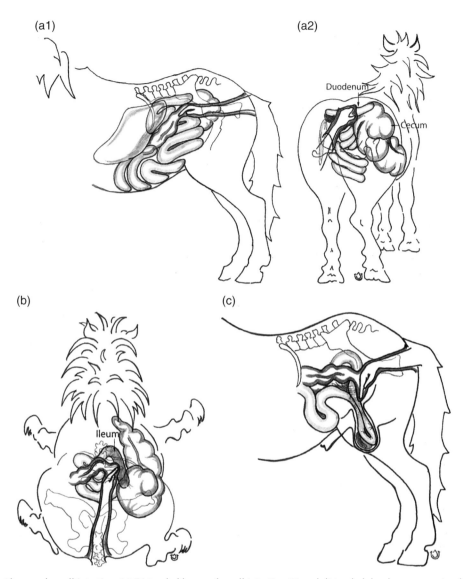

Figure 3.2 Abnormal small intestine. (a) Distended loops of small intestine (1) and distended duodenum coursing from right to left around the base of the cecum (2), (b) ileal impaction, and (c) inguinal hernia.

traversing the abdomen immediately cranial to the pelvic brim. The ventral cecal band cannot be identified with a RDD (Figure 3.4b). Transcutaneous sonographic evaluation can be used to confirm the diagnosis of RDD by identification of colonic vessels coursing along the right side of the abdomen between the 12th and 17th intercostals space at the level of the costochondral junction (see Chapter 12 on Abdominal Sonographic Evaluation [p. 120]).

A NSLE is diagnosed by first identifying the caudal pole of the left kidney. The colon is palpated to the left and slightly ventral to the left kidney between the kidney and caudodorsal border of the spleen. The spleen is usually pulled ventrally and axially off the left body wall in horses with a NSLE (Figure 3.4c) (Clinical scenario 3, located in Appendix A). The entrapped colon can be identified as bands leading to the nephrosplenic space with the entrapped colon palpated over the

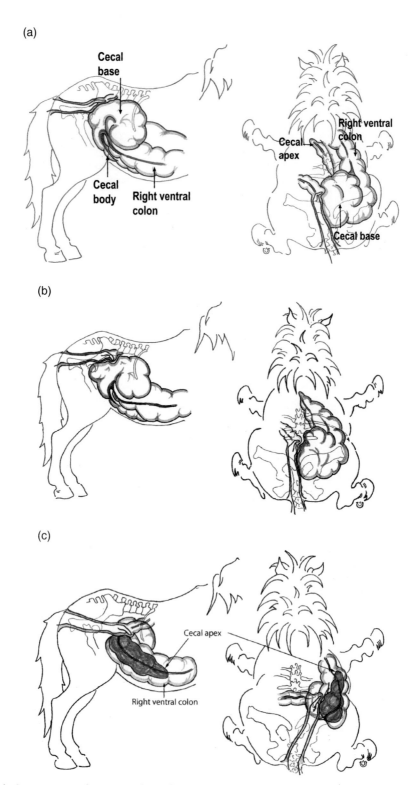

(a)

Cecal
base

Cecal
body

Right ventral
colon

Cecal
apex

Right ventral
colon

Cecal base

(b)

(c)

Cecal apex

Right ventral colon

Figure 3.3   Cecal tympany (a), cecal impaction (b), and cecocecal or cecocolic intussusception (c).

(a)

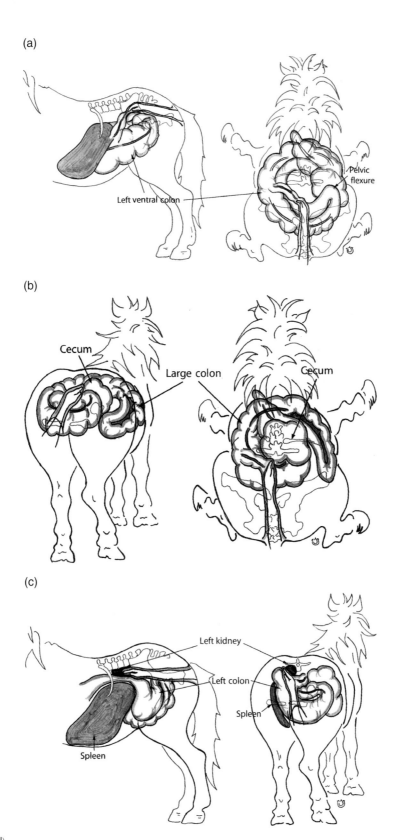

Pelvic flexure

Left ventral colon

(b)

Cecum

Large colon

Cecum

(c)

Left kidney

Left colon

Spleen

Spleen

Figure 3.4 (cont'd)

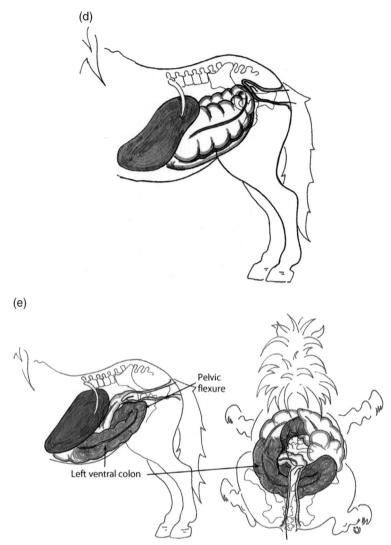

Figure 3.4   Large colon lesions. (a) Large colon gas distention (tympany), (b) RDD, (c) NSLE, (d) LCV, and (e) PF (left ventral colon) impaction.

ligament in the space or as variable gas distended colon in the nephrosplenic region. NSLE is often incorrectly diagnosed on palpation per rectum and the diagnosis cannot be definitively made unless the described relationship between the kidney, colon, and spleen is found. When the findings on palpation per rectum are inconclusive, transcutaneous sonographic evaluation of the nephrosplenic space in the upper left flank region can be used to confirm or refute the diagnosis (p. 121).

It is important to recognize that a large colon volvulus (LCV) is generally not definitively diagnosed on palpation per rectum. In fact, these

horses are often severely painful making palpation per rectum unsafe for the examiner and patient. Marked colonic distention and possibly edema is generally the only abnormality identified per rectum (Figure 3.4d).

PF impactions are readily diagnosed on palpation per rectum as a large, firm, indentable mass in the left caudal abdomen (Figure 3.4e) (Clinical scenario 6, located in Appendix A). The impaction is often 30–40 cm or more in diameter and extends from the pelvic inlet cranially usually as far as can be reached with the examiner's arm. An impaction with ingesta can be distinguished from another type of mass (e.g., tumor or abscess) by its ability to be indented and maintain its indented form.

Right dorsal colon (RDC) impactions are rarely palpated except in small horses or in cases where the impaction is particularly large. The impaction is found on the right side of the abdomen and is located at the most cranial aspect of the palpable region of the abdomen. Sonographic examination may be necessary to distinguish a RDC from a cecal impaction.

Small (descending) colon

Palpation of abnormalities affecting the small colon is uncommon. An absence of normal formed fecal balls in the small colon should be noted and considered abnormal and is indicative of an obstruction of any part of the gastrointestinal tract proximal to the palpable small colon. The small colon is distinguished based on its small size (8–10 cm diameter) and broad and flat antimesenteric band and prominent fibrous mesenteric band.

Impaction is the most common lesion affecting the small colon and can be definitively diagnosed based on palpation per rectum. A small colon impaction is palpated in the caudal abdomen as a long, tubular, indentable, ingesta-filled structure (Figure 3.5).

Occasionally a gas distended loop of small colon can be palpated and is an indication of a mechanical obstruction of the distal small colon. The most common lesion causing this finding is a strangulating pedunculated lipoma which is more likely to occur in older horses. In some cases, the pedicle of the lipoma can be identified encircling the distal small colon/rectum and prohibiting cranial movement of the examiner's hand and arm further into the rectum. Other considerations are an enterolith or fecalith. Rarely are enteroliths or fecaliths identified based on palpation per rectum (Figure 3.6).

Rectum

The most common problem affecting the rectum is rectal tear (Figure 3.7), which can be definitively diagnosed using palpation per rectum. Endoscopic examination may be useful for grading rectal tears. See Complications (p. 36).

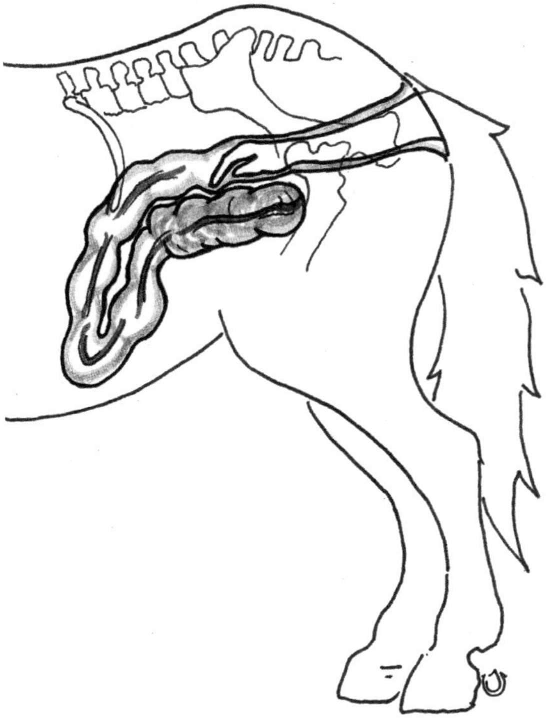

Figure 3.5   Small colon impaction.

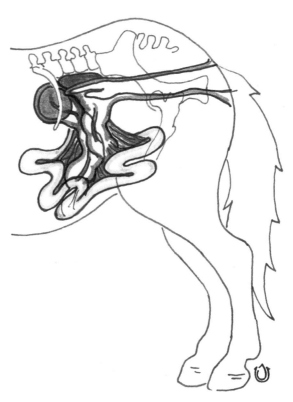

Figure 3.6   Occasionally an enterolith can be palpated in the small colon.

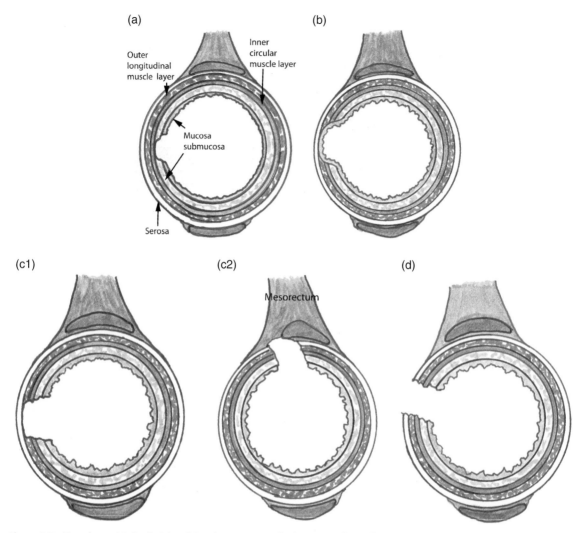

(a)

Outer longitudinal muscle layer

Inner circular muscle layer

Mucosa submucosa

Serosa

(b)

(c1)

(c2)

Mesorectum

(d)

Figure 3.7   Rectal tear. (a) Grade 1 involving the mucosa and submucosa, (b) grade 2 involving the inner circular and outer longitudinal muscle layers only, (c) grade 3A involving all layers with the serosa intact and grade 3B involving all layers with the mesorectum intact, and (d) grade 4 full thickness tear.

Perirectal abscesses that may be associated with lymph nodes can be recognized as a large firm mass in the dorsal caudal rectal wall. The abscess usually has a soft area that can be palpated. Sonography can be used to confirm the diagnosis of abscessation.

Urogenital tract

Lesions affecting the nongravid mare are uncommon. The reproductive tract should always be examined in pregnant mares showing signs of colic. Uterine torsion (Figure 3.8) can be diagnosed by palpating the broad ligaments coursing across the pelvic inlet. Postpartum hemorrhage into the broad ligament is a common cause of colic in postpartum mares[6] and can be identified as a large, firm mass to the left or right of the uterus within the broad ligament (Figure 3.9). Sonographic evaluation per rectum or transcutaneously can be used to confirm the diagnosis. Care should be taken to not dislodge any clot formation when palpating mares with suspected postpartum hemorrhage. Transcutaneous sonographic evaluation flank region can be used to confirm the diagnosis and avoid hematoma disruption.

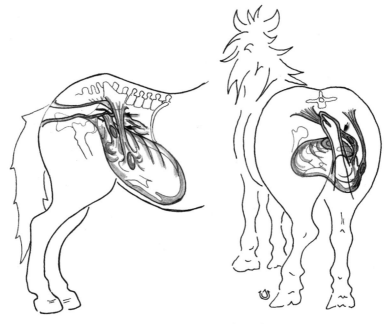

Figure 3.8   Uterine torsion with broad ligaments being pulled across pelvic inlet (arrows).

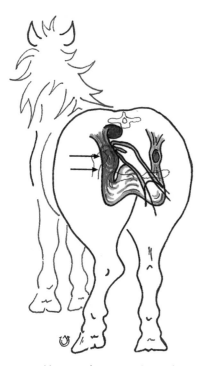

Figure 3.9   Broad ligament hematoma (arrows).

Other abdominal structures

Abnormalities of the kidney and spleen are uncommon. The spleen may be palpable more caudally with gastric distention. Rarely are splenic masses palpated. Thromboembolism of the iliac vessels can be palpated but is a rare occurrence. Urolithiasis is uncommon in horses but uroliths can generally be palpated in the bladder if present. Cystoscopy and renal sonographic examination is also recommended.

Peritoneal cavity

Abscessation of the lymph nodes in the root of the mesentery can often be palpated at the tip of the examiner's fingers. Per rectum sonographic examination can be used to confirm the diagnosis of abscessation. *Streptococcus equi* subspecies *equi* is the most common cause of mesenteric root abscessation (bastard strangles).

Masses within the abdomen are often palpated in horses with neoplasia. The most common neoplastic conditions affecting the equine abdomen are lymphoma, adenocarcinoma, and squamous cell carcinoma.[16]

Pneumoperitoneum is indicative of visceral, usually gastrointestinal, perforation. Pneumoperitoneum is recognized by appreciation of a loss of negative pressure whereby the examiner's hand/arm feel as if it is floating within the abdomen and the rectum sucked down around the arm (Clinical scenario 7, located in Appendix A).

Rarely a large volume of peritoneal fluid (ascites) can be recognized on palpation per rectum. Volumes of fluid in excess of 10 L are necessary for recognition during palpation per rectum. Ascites and hemoabdomen are most often associated with neoplasia.

Transcutaneous sonographic evaluation (p. 116) and abdominocentesis with peritoneal fluid analysis (p. 87) should be performed in horses with apparent intraperitoneal disease.

Complications

Rectal tear

Rectal tear is the most common complication associated with palpation per rectum.[2,13,15] Arabians, American Miniature Horses, mares, and horses >9 years of age were more likely to develop a rectal tear in the most recent study.[5] Rectal tears can be prevented in many cases by using a gentle technique, appropriate restraint, and ample lubrication. The first and most important thing to do if you suspect a rectal tear has occurred is to inform the client[2] of your concern and of the necessity to reexamine the rectum to confirm the presence and determine the severity of the tear. Rectal tears associated with examination of the gastrointestinal tract usually occur dorsally, approximately 30 cm cranial to the rectum, and are variable in size.[5] Prognosis is dependent of the location, size, and grade of the rectal tear, the distance to the referral center, and the extent of abdominal contamination.

Emergency first aid

Examination of the tear is facilitated by sedating the horse (xylazine and butorphanol) and performing a lidocaine enema. A xylazine epidural with or without lidocaine will help prevent the horse from straining (Appendix B, p. 325). The rectum should be completely evacuated of fecal material and the location and grade of the rectal tear assessed (Figure 3.7). Careful assessment of the extent of disruption of the layers of the rectal wall as well as the degree of fecal contamination of the tear with a well-lubricated bare arm is necessary.[15] The tear can also be assessed endoscopically.

Grade 1 rectal tears can generally be managed with broad-spectrum oral antimicrobial drugs (e.g., trimethoprim sulfa) and flunixin meglumine. The feces should be kept soft by feeding either fresh grass, alfalfa hay, or by administering oil with water and electrolytes via a nasogastric tube. The horse should be monitored closely for signs of colic. The prognosis for a horse with a grade 1 tear is excellent.[5] Grade 2 tears are rarely diagnosed and have an excellent prognosis with medical management.[5]

Management of grade 3 and 4 tears is challenging. The prognosis for survival for horses with grade 3 tears is fair (35%) and grade 4 tears poor (2%).[5] Parenteral broad-spectrum antimicrobial drugs (potassium penicillin and gentamicin, or ceftiofur) and oral metronidazole, nonsteroidal anti-inflammatory drugs (flunixin meglumine), and tetanus toxoid should be given.[2,13,15]

A well-lubricated rectal pack may be used that consists of a 3 in. stockinet tied in a knot at one end and of sufficient length to reach from the external anal sphincter to at least several inches cranial to the tear.[1] The stockinet is partially filled with cotton, sprayed with povidone-iodine, and lubricated. The knotted end is placed in the rectum as far cranial as possible to the tear. The lumen of the stockinet is then carefully filled with moistened roll cotton sufficient to prevent passage of feces around the packing. The anus is then clamped with towel clamps or a purse-string suture.[1] The use of a rectal pack is controversial. Rectal packing may not prevent contamination of the tear with fecal material and may make the tear worse if the horse strains against the pack. A rectal pack should only be used if an epidural has been performed and the horse is not straining.

It is recommended to call the referral practice to inform the clinician on duty of the history, physical examination findings, and treatment that has been given, and to get a fee estimate and prognosis for survival prior to referral. It is also recommended to call the malpractice insurance company to get advice on client communication and case management.

Management

Several methods to manage grade 3 and 4 rectal tears have been described and generally consist of medical management (grade 3 tears),[9,12] repair,[10,15] or fecal diversion techniques.[3,7,14,15]

Blind suturing of the tear per rectum using a one-handed technique can be performed with a successful outcome. Blind suturing has the potential to enlarge the lesion and increase contamination and trauma to the region. A technique has been described for repair of rectal tears in postpartum mares by transecting the anal sphincter at the 12 o'clock position, retracting the tear caudally, and stapling across the tear followed by oversewing the staple line.[10] Experimental laparoscopic repair of rectal tears has been described;[4] however, many tears are too caudal for this approach. A laparoscopic-assisted flank approach may be used for more caudal tears (Eric Parente, Personal Communication 2011). Rectal tears may be surgically managed with an exploratory celiotomy and PF enterotomy to evacuate the intestinal contents oral to the tear. Occasionally, the tear can be sutured through a ventral midline incision.

Suturing the tear is often used in combination with a fecal diversion procedure. Fecal diversion techniques include the use of a rectal liner[16] or a temporary loop colostomy.[3,7]

Successful medical management of grade 3 rectal tears has been reported either with[9] or without[12] repeated manual evacuation of the rectum. Unfortunately, medical management can result in progression of the grade 3 to a grade 4 tear with fecal contamination of the peritoneal cavity necessitating euthanasia.

References

1. Baird, A.N., Taylor, T.S. & Watkins, J.P. (1989) Rectal packing as initial management of grade 3 rectal tears. *Equine Veterinary Journal Supplements*, **7**, 121–123.
2. Blikslager, A.T. & Roberts, M.C. (1996) Critical steps in managing equine rectal tears. *Compendium on Continuing Education for the Practicing Veterinarian*, **18**, 1131–1139.
3. Blikslager, A.T., Bristol, D.G., Bowman, K.F. & Engelbert, T.A. (1995) Loop colostomy for treatment of grade-3 rectal tears in horses: Seven cases (1983–1994). *Journal of the American Veterinary Medical Association*, **207**, 1201–1205.
4. Brugmans, F. & Deegen, E. (2001) Laparoscopic surgical technique for repair of rectal and colonic tears in horses: An experimental study. *Veterinary Surgery*, **30**, 409–416.
5. Claes, A., Ball, B.A., Brown, J.A. & Kass, P.H. (2008) Evaluation of risk factors, management, and outcome associated with rectal tears in horses: 99 cases (1985–2006). *Journal of the American Veterinary Medical Association*, **233**, 1605–1609.
6. Dolente, B.A., Sullivan, E.K., Boston, R. & Johnston, J.K. (2005) Mares admitted to a referral hospital forpostpartum emergencies: 163 cases (1992–2002). *Journal of Veterinary Emergency and Critical Care*, **15**, 193–200.
7. Freeman, D.E., Richardson, D.W., Tulleners, E.P., *et al.* (1992) Loop colostomy for management of rectal tears and small-colon injuries in horses: 10 cases (1976–1989). *Journal of the American Veterinary Medical Association*, **200**, 1365–1371.
8. Hanson, R., Schumacher, J., Humburg, J. & Dunkerley, S.C. (1996) Medical treatment of horses with ileal impactions: 10 cases (1990–1994). *Journal of the American Veterinary Medical Association*, **208**, 898–900.
9. Katz, L.M. & Ragle, C.A. (1999) Repeated manual evacuation for treatment of rectal tears in four horses. *Journal of the American Veterinary Medical Association*, **215**, 1473–1477.
10. Kay, A.T., Spirito, M.A., Rodgerson, D.H. & Brown, S.E., 2nd. (2008) Surgical technique to repair grade IV rectal tears in post-parturient mares. *Veterinary Surgery*, **37**, 345–349.
11. Luo, T., Bertone, J.J., Greene, H.M. & Wickler, S.J. (2006) A comparison of N-butylscopolammonium and lidocaine for control of rectal pressure in horses. *Veterinary Therapeutics*, **7**, 243–248.
12. Mair, T.S. (2000) The medical management of eight horses with grade 3 rectal tears. *Equine Veterinary Journal Supplements*, **32**, 104–107.
13. Sayegh, A.I., Adams, S.B., Peter, A.T. & Wilson, D.G. (1996) Equine rectal tears: Causes and management. *Compendium on Continuing Education for the Practicing Veterinarian*, **18**, 1131–1139.
14. Taylor, T.S., Watkins, J.P. & Schumacher, J. (1987) Temporary indwelling rectal liner for use in horses with rectal tears. *Journal of the American Veterinary Medical Association*, **191**, 677–880.
15. Taylor, T.S., Hooper, R.N. & Baird, A.N. (1999) A different perspective of equine rectal tears. *Compendium on Continuing Education for the Practicing Veterinarian*, **21**, 452–454.
16. Taylor, S.D., Pusterla, N., Vaughan, B., Whitcomb, M.B. & Wilson, W.D. (2006) Intestinal neoplasia in horses. *Journal of Veterinary Internal Medicine*, **20**, 1429–1436.

4

Nasogastric Intubation

Joanne Fehr

Equine Emergency Department, Pilchuck Animal Hospital, Snohomish, WA, USA

Chapter Outline

Indications	**38**	Assessing for reflux	42
Preparation	**38**	Information gained by nasogastric intubation	43
Nasogastric tube	39	**Complications**	**43**
Buckets and water	39	Hemorrhage	43
Stomach pump or dose syringe	39	Tracheal intubation	44
Medications	39	Pharyngeal and esophageal trauma	44
Procedure	**39**	Problems with the nasogastric tube	44
Nasogastric intubation	40		

Indications

Nasogastric intubation should be performed in any horse showing signs of colic. A horse showing signs of colic with a heart rate >60 beats/min should have a nasogastric tube (NGT) passed immediately because tachycardia can be an indication of gastric distention and pending fatal gastric rupture. The NGT should be left in place for transportation to a referral hospital if reflux is obtained. Horses can, however, rupture their stomach with a NGT in place. Horses with reflux should be checked often with the frequency dependent on the volume of reflux obtained such that <5 L of reflux is obtained at any one time. Nasogastric intubation is essential in providing diagnostic information as well as providing the ability to perform initial treatments for specific causes of colic.

Preparation

A list of "Things You Will Need" is provided in Table 4.1. Nasogastric intubation should be performed with an experienced horse handler to stabilize the head during intubation and while administering medication. Not surprisingly, horses

Practical Guide to Equine Colic, First Edition. Edited by Louise L. Southwood.
© 2013 John Wiley & Sons, Inc. Published 2013 by John Wiley & Sons, Inc.

Table 4.1   "Things you will need" for nasogastric intubation.

- Assistant to restrain the horse
- Halter and lead rope
- Nasogastric tube
- 2 × 10 L buckets with graduated measurements
  - 1 empty
  - 1 with about 5 L warm water
- Water pump or dose syringe
- ± Sedation
- ± Nose twitch
- Medication

tend to resist intubation by raising their head, backing up and extending their neck, and on occasion rearing and striking. Care should be taken to avoid injury by not standing directly in front of the horse. Ventroflexing the horse's head-neck facilitates passage into the esophagus rather than the trachea. Use of a nose twitch is necessary in many horses to obtain adequate control and sufficient head-neck ventroflexion. If necessary, the use of a short-acting sedative is recommended and a combination of xylazine with butorphanol is effective. While sedation is useful for making the patient more compliant and lowering the head, it can decrease the swallowing reflex and make passage of the NGT into the esophagus more challenging.

Nasogastric tube

NGTs come in multiple lengths and widths and in most cases there are a few choices from the miniature/foal size to the large-bore draft size (Table 4.2). The NGT choice will be based on patient size and personal preference. It is of utmost importance to have a good quality NGT that is moderately stiff with no scratches on the surface; a rough surface can be irritating to the sensitive respiratory mucosa. A NGT with insufficient stiffness may be difficult to get into the esophagus and then through the gastroesophageal sphincter, and a NGT that is too stiff can cause trauma to the nasal passages with resulting hemorrhage.

Permanent marks can be placed on the NGT to indicate (1) the distance to the pharynx/larynx and (2) the point where the tip of the NGT should be within the stomach (Figure 4.1). It is important in most cases, however, to measure these distances

with the NGT against the patient as the head and neck lengths vary between breeds and individual horses.

Buckets and water

Two buckets (10–12 L capacity) with graduated measurements are necessary. One bucket should contain approximately 5 L of fresh warm water. It is important to make note of the volume of water used so that the volume of net reflux can be calculated.

Stomach pump or dose syringe

Use of a stomach pump allows smooth and fast filling of the NGT to form a siphon for evacuation or administration of fluids and medication. The regular stomach pump will provide 7.2 fl oz or 250 mL of fluid with one complete up and down pump. There is a heavy-duty pump available that will pump 700 mL of fluid with one complete up and down pump.

A dose syringe can be used to help remove reflux without the veterinarian needing to place their mouth on the NGT to suck, but must be done with caution to minimize trauma on the gastric mucosa. Veterinarians should recognize the risk of zoonotic infection associated with putting the end of the NGT in their mouth. The dose syringe can also be used to administer treatments of smaller volume such as in the foals and miniature horses. The volume of the common vinyl dose syringes are 400 mL and are graduated so specific volumes can be measured.

Medications

Medications include balanced electrolytes (see Chapter 7 on Enteral Fluid Therapy [p. 62]), mineral oil, and laxatives such as magnesium sulfate and dioctyl sodium sulfosuccinate (DSS).

Procedure

Often it is necessary to sedate the patient prior to NGT placement. This is due to the discomfort of having a NGT inserted into the naris as well as the

Table 4.2   Nasogastric tubes.

Company/tube size	OD	Length	Volume	Material
Jorgensen				
● Large	3/4"	10'	400 mL	Siliconized PVC/blue cuff
● Medium	5/8"	9'	250 mL	Siliconized PVC/blue cuff
● Small	5/16"	9'	60 mL	Siliconized PVC/blue cuff
EZ-swallow	3/4"	10'	400 mL	Vinyl
Jupiter				
● XLarge	5/8"	12'	330 mL	Abrasion resistant/flare with ridge
● Foal/mini	1/4"	5'	20 mL	Abrasion resistant/flare with ridge
Kalayjian				
● Large	3/4"	10'	400 mL	Vinyl
● Medium	5/8"	9'	250 mL	Vinyl
● Mini	3/8"	3.5'	35 mL	Vinyl

OD, outer diameter.

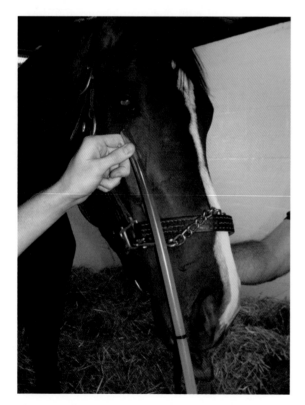

Figure 4.1   Permanent marker can be used to indicate the approximate location along the NGT of when the NGT should be in the pharynx (indicated) and when the NGT should have reached the cardia.

sensitivity of the respiratory mucosa. Most horses are tractable for nasogastric intubation with a combination of an alpha-2 agonist such as xylazine and an opioid such as butorphanol. It is recommended to assess the degree of pain prior to sedation because of the analgesia provided by these drugs and keep in mind that sedation may lessen the swallowing reflex. If the patient is difficult to intubate with sedation, then the added restraint of a nose twitch can help for initial placement. It is important to have an informed and capable handler at the patients head when placing the NGT because too much movement of the patient can cause trauma to the nasal cavity and hemorrhage from the respiratory mucosa or ethmoid turbinates.

Nasogastric intubation[1]

Every practitioner has their preference of side to stand on and naris to intubate. It is recommended, however, to be capable of passing a NGT from either side. When passing a NGT, do not stand directly in front of the horse because it is not uncommon for the horse to strike or rear during the procedure. In order to avoid standing in front of the horse, the NGT should be passed with the right hand when standing on the right side of the horse with the left hand on the nose and used to ventroflex the neck and vice versa (Figure 4.2).

(a) (b)

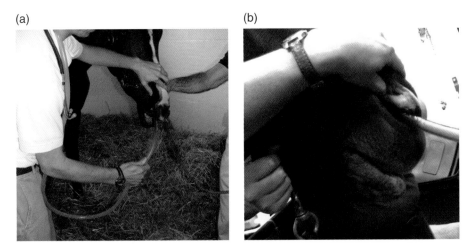

Figure 4.2   (a) The NGT can be passed from the right side of the horse using the right hand with the left hand on the nose and ventroflexing the neck. Avoid standing directly in front of the horse at all times. (b) The thumb is used to guide the NGT into the ventral nasal meatus.

The tip of the NGT should be lubricated with sodium carboxymethylcellulose or mineral oil to minimize friction and trauma when passing the NGT over the respiratory mucosa. As the NGT is introduced into the naris, the tip needs to be directed ventrally into the ventral nasal meatus (Figure 4.2), which can be facilitated by the veterinarian placing their finger inside the external naris and stabilizing the NGT in this location until it has passed into the pharynx. Once the NGT is located in the pharynx, the tip has more space and may flip dorsally. Therefore, it is still important to angle the NGT ventrally and control the horse's head. In this location, the tip of the NGT may either contact the pharyngeal recess (dead end) or touch the larynx either initiating a swallow reflex or a cough (Figure 4.3). Gaining flexion of the head and neck at this point will help position the NGT over the esophageal opening; it is important to wait for the patient to swallow and then slightly rotate the NGT and pass it into the esophagus. Sometimes slight movement back and forth with the tip of the NGT as well as gently blowing into the NGT will initiate a swallow. If the horse is not swallowing the tip of the NGT, changing to the other naris can help on occasion.

Once the patient has swallowed and the NGT has been advanced, determining correct placement is paramount. In some horses, it is easy to observe the tip of the NGT moving back and forth in the cervical

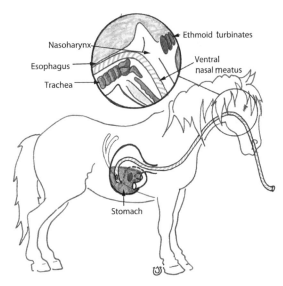

Figure 4.3   Schematic illustration of the nasal passages, pharynx, and stomach demonstrating passage of the NGT.

esophagus on the left ventrolateral aspect of the neck. In other horses it can only be identified by palpation. Gently blowing air into the NGT when the tip is in the esophagus can produce visible esophageal distention. Once the NGT is in the esophagus, there should be negative pressure with suction and there should be slight resistance to passage as the NGT is being passed through a collapsed and nonrigid structure (esophagus). The trachea, on the other hand, is a large diameter rigid structure and there is little resistance to NGT passage. Not all horses will cough when the NGT is placed in the trachea, so it is important to observe and palpate the NGT in the esophagus as well as check for negative pressure and appreciate the slight resistance to passage. To ease movement of the NGT down the esophagus, gently blow in the NGT during passage, especially in a dehydrated patient.

Determining the point at which the NGT has entered the stomach is usually based on identifying an increase in resistance as the NGT passes through the gastroesophageal sphincter. The location can also be determined by assessing the distance the NGT has advanced (close to the second mark on the NGT). Once in the stomach, there should be a release of gas that either smells of fresh or stale acidic feed. Once the tip of the NGT is through the gastric cardia, negative pressure should not be encountered with suction. If there is any question as to the placement of the NGT in the stomach, auscultation over the stomach on the left hemithorax, 14th intercostal space at the level of the shoulder, while blowing in the NGT should elicit the sound of gas bubbling though liquid. When there is marked gastric distention, it can be difficult to pass the NGT through the gastroesophageal sphincter and gastric cardia. Use of lidocaine gel on the tip of the NGT or injection of 10–20 mL of lidocaine through the NGT may facilitate relaxation of the sphincter and passage into the stomach.

Assessing for reflux

To assess for reflux, the NGT will need to be advanced into the fluid in the glandular part of the stomach. The NGT will naturally curve around the side or the top of the nonglandular (squamous) part of the stomach before reaching the fluid (Figure 4.3). Therefore, advancing the NGT 15–20 cm prior to trying to siphon fluid off the stomach is recommended. If the stomach is distended, this may not be necessary initially. However, continued advancement as the fluid is removed should facilitate siphoning. During placement of the NGT, the stomach can become distended with air so removal of this air with the dose syringe will improve the likelihood of placement of the tip of the NGT in the gastric fluid.

To create a siphon, the NGT needs to be primed by filling it with warm water, which usually takes about 1 L (four pumps) with the tip positioned in gastric fluid. Once the NGT is filled with water, the end is lowered and fluid runs out freely. If the flow decreases or stops, the NGT can be gently extracted a few centimeters at a time to try to reposition the tip of the NGT in the fluid and continue flow.

The volume of an average horse's stomach is 8–15 L, but with distention it can hold up to 20 L. The siphoning procedure is continued until it is either determined that the stomach is empty or no more reflux can be obtained (usually indicated by the presence of saliva appearing as a foamy liquid). It is recommended to check 5–10 times for reflux with siphoning. The net reflux (L) is calculated by measuring the total volume of reflux obtained (L) and subtracting the volume of warm water used to create the siphon (L). The decision is then made whether or not to add medications such as electrolytes, water, mineral oil, or laxatives (see Chapter 7 on Enteral Fluid Therapy [p. 62] and Chapter 5 on Management of Mild Colic [p. 45]).

If there was >2 L of net reflux obtained during the exam, distended small intestine palpated per rectum, or the patient was very difficult for NGT placement, consider leaving the NGT in place for further treatment or refluxing. Dry the NGT at the nares and attach white medical tape with long tabs so that the NGT can be secured to the halter. The end of the NGT can be capped with a syringe plunger or a glove finger with the tip cut placed over the end and taped to form a one-way valve. This is done to prevent aspiration of air into the stomach. There is some controversy regarding the degree of trauma associated with leaving the NGT in place versus repeated intubation. If intubation is to be performed every 2–3 h, it is probably less traumatic to leave the NGT in place for a few days only. Complications may arise with a NGT left in place beyond 7 days. There is also somewhat controversial evidence that an indwelling NGT may in fact increase the amount of reflux by delaying gastric emptying.[3,6] If there is a large amount of feed with the reflux consider placing a larger-bore NGT for repeat refluxing.

Removal of the NGT is performed slowly with the patients head under complete control while keeping the NGT directed ventrally in the meatus. The NGT should be empty of liquid and kinked when removed to prevent aspiration of NGT contents into the tracheal.

Information gained by nasogastric intubation

Nasogastric intubation is a diagnostic as well as a therapeutic procedure. Observations that should be noted about the reflux include:

- Volume: if in excess of 2 L, this is suggestive of a gastric outflow problem most often due to ileus, proximal enteritis (PE), or a small intestinal mechanical obstruction. Note that an absence of reflux does not rule out a small intestinal obstruction and horses with large intestinal disease can on occasion have reflux.
- Color: green/brown is considered normal, yellow is consistent with reflux from small intestine, and orange/red may be consistent with hemorrhagic enteritis. Hemorrhage during intubation can result in the horse swallowing blood and the reflux appearing blood tinged or red.
- pH: normal pH is 4–6, and if fluid is from the duodenum and jejunum the pH will increase to 6–8.
- Submit sample of reflux for *Salmonella* spp. culture and toxin screening for *Clostridium difficile*.[2]

Nasogastric intubation can also be used to identify a possible gastric impaction. Gastric impaction should be considered when it is difficult to confirm passage of the NGT into the stomach, when there is discomfort associated with the addition of water into the stomach, and when there is a lot of dense feed and minimal water obtained with siphoning. Horses with severe gastric impaction often will have spontaneous reflux observed from the nares. Sonographic examination (p. 130) can be used to determine the size and content of the stomach.

Horses with proximal enteritis (p. 207) typically have large volumes of reflux (>6 L) and will generally become considerably more comfortable with resolution of colic signs and lowering of the heart rate toward normal following gastric decompression. These clinical findings can support the diagnosis of proximal enteritis in conjunction with peritoneal fluid analysis (p. 90) and sonographic examination (p. 128).

Complications

Hemorrhage

The primary complication encountered during nasogastric intubation is hemorrhage. Hemorrhage can occur either from injury to the respiratory mucosa or from direct trauma to the ethmoid turbinates. Appropriate restraint during placement and removal of the NGT, keeping the tip of the NGT in the ventral nasal meatus, careful NGT selection, and lubrication will reduce the risk of hemorrhage. Particular care should be taken when removing a NGT at the completion of surgery when the horse is under general anesthesia.[7] If hemorrhage is noted at the beginning of intubation, assess restraint and pass the NGT up the contralateral nostril to complete the procedure. Hemorrhage most commonly occurs at the end of the procedure as the NGT is removed and hits the ethmoid turbinates and can be associated with uncontrolled head movement as the tip comes out of the esophagus. Hemorrhage occurring during placement may also not be apparent until extubation.

In most cases, hemorrhage will stop. Cover the nares with dark towels and if the flow does not decrease considerably within 5–10 min consider packing the nasal passage to help the formation of a clot if the patient will allow it. Keep in mind that while blood is not observed coming from the nares when the nasal passages are packed, the horse may be swallowing blood. Elevating the head is contraindicated because of the increased risk of blood aspiration and pneumonia. Sedation is not recommended because lowering the head will increase the blood supply to the nasal passages and prolong hemorrhage. Spraying epinephrine or phenylephrine as far back into the nasal cavity as possible may facilitate vasoconstriction, but it is almost impossible to get the medication back far enough to have any effect without endoscopic guidance. Avoid vasodilatory drugs during hemorrhage. Should future intubation become necessary, the side from which hemorrhage occurred should be avoided at least for several days. The flow should slowly decrease over 15–30 min, but may continue at a slow drip (1 drip per few seconds) for up to an hour. It is recommended to not anesthetize a horse for colic surgery until the hemorrhage has stopped.

Uncontrollable hemorrhage can be treated with procoagulants such as aminocaproic acid which stabilizes the clot; naloxone, an opioid receptor antagonist that blocks shock-associated vasodilation; and Yunnan Baiyao, a Chinese herb observed to control hemorrhage, which may be appropriate. Packing of the entire nasal passage with the horse under general anesthesia may be necessary if hemorrhage is severe and persistent. Blood transfusion is rarely necessary.

Tracheal intubation

Placement of the NGT into the trachea and infusion of fluids into the lungs should not occur if care is taken to ensure correct NGT placement. If there is any question as to the correct placement of the NGT, no fluid should be put through the NGT. A small amount of clean water placed into the lungs will cause coughing and can be withstood; the patient should be placed on anti-inflammatory medication as well as prophylactic antimicrobial drugs to decrease the risk of pneumonia. Even slight contamination of the lungs with mineral oil is fatal.

Pharyngeal and esophageal trauma

Mild pharyngeal trauma occurs with nasogastric intubation and some horses may consequently have a poor appetite. Sucralfate can be given per os to facilitate healing. Clinical signs of more severe esophageal or pharyngeal trauma include salivation, bruxism, coughing, and nasal discharge.[5] Endoscopic evaluation is necessary. Horses may be managed with parenteral nutrition or enteral feeding through a smaller NGT or esophagostomy.[5] Esophageal rupture secondary to traumatic nasogastric intubation is an infrequent complication but can occur in cases where repeat tubing has been performed. Identification of an acute tear would be determined by finding blood on the NGT or noting swelling in the cervical region associate with administration of fluids. Immediate removal of the NGT is advised. Endoscopic examination is used to determine the location and length of the tear and whether it is full or partial thickness. The tear may be repairable depending on the size, location, and duration of time between occurrence and treatment. Most horses, however, are euthanized.[5]

Problems with the nasogastric tube

On a rare occasion, the NGT may break with fragment(s) remaining in the esophagus or stomach. Endoscopic fragment retrieval or gastrotomy may be necessary.[4] The NGT may also form a knot in the pharynx or stomach preventing extubation. Endoscopic-assisted retrieval may be necessary.

References

1. Abutarbush, S.M., Naylor, J.M., Parchoma, G., D'Eon, M., Petrie, L., Carruthers, T. (2006) Evaluation of traditional instruction versus a self-learning computer module in teaching veterinary students how to pass a nasogastric tube in the horse. *Journal of Veterinary Medical Education*, **33**, 447–454.
2. Arroyo, L.G., Stämpfli, H.R. & Weese, J.S. (2006) Potential role of *Clostridium difficile* as a cause of duodenitis-proximal jejunitis in horses. *Journal of Medical Microbiology*, **55**, 605–608.
3. Cruz, A.M., Li, R., Kenney, D.G. & Monteith, G. (2006) Effects of indwelling nasogastric intubation on gastric emptying of a liquid marker in horses. *American Journal of Veterinary Research*, **67**, 1100–1104.
4. DiFranco, B., Schumacher, J. & Morris, D. (1992) Removal of nasogastric tube fragments from three horses. *Journal of the American Veterinary Medical Association*, **201**, 1035–1037.
5. Hardy, J., Stewart, R.H., Beard, W.L. & Yvorchuk-St-Jean, K. (1992) Complications of nasogastric intubation in horses: Nine cases (1987–1989). *Journal of the American Veterinary Medical Association*, **201**, 483–486.
6. Lammers, T.W., Roussel, A.J., Boothe, D.M. & Cohen, N.D. (2005) Effect of an indwelling nasogastric tube on gastric emptying rates of liquids in horses. *American Journal of Veterinary Research*, **66**, 642–645.
7. Trim, C.M., Eaton, S.A. & Parks, A.H. (1997) Severe nasal hemorrhage in an anesthetized horse. *Journal of the American Veterinary Medical Association*, **210**, 1324–1327.

5 Management of Mild Colic

Sarah Dukti

Piedmont Equine Practice, The Plains, VA, USA

Chapter Outline

Practical perspective of colic	45	Laxatives	47
Clinical indications of mild colic	45	Nutrition	48
Management of mild colic	46	**Monitoring**	48
Analgesia	46	**Management changes and prevention**	48
Spasmolytic drugs	47	**When colic is no longer considered mild**	49
Fluid therapy	47		

Practical perspective of colic

Colic is one of the most important clinical problems affecting horses. Annually the frequency of colic is reported to be 4–10% of horses, with great variation between farms, ranging from 0% to 30% of horses per year.[13,16,28,30,31] Notably, the majority of horses with colic, approximately 80%, have gas colic or colic of unknown cause and resolve with no treatment or after only one treatment.[2,22,28] A further 5% of horses have large colon impactions which are usually mild and respond to medical treatment.[22] Fewer than 7% of horses with colic required surgical intervention (see Chapter 15 on Medical versus Surgical Treatment of the Horse with Colic [p. 164] and Chapter 16 on Colic Surgery [p. 173]).[2,22,28] Horses showing mild colic signs have an excellent prognosis for survival.[22,28,32] Recurrence can be a problem for some horses, with 13% of horses in one study having more than one colic episode during the year.[28]

Clinical indications of mild colic

The majority of horses with colic show mild signs that will respond to medical treatment. These signs are usually attributed to gas accumulation or a mild impaction for which there are several predisposing factors.[2,4,5,14,29] Patient history (p. 1) and physical examination findings (p. 12) are used to identify horses with mild colic and include the

Practical Guide to Equine Colic, First Edition. Edited by Louise L. Southwood.
© 2013 John Wiley & Sons, Inc. Published 2013 by John Wiley & Sons, Inc.

short duration of mild signs that are occurring for the first time or recur infrequently (e.g., less than once a year).

Horses with mild colic are cardiovascularly stable, have a normal heart rate or only mild tachycardia, pink mucous membranes that are moist or may be slightly tachy, normal capillary and jugular vein refill time, normal or only slightly increased respiratory rate, and rectal temperature <102°F (38.9°C). Intestinal borborygmi should be present although may be reduced and should improve with initiation of treatment. There should be no net nasogastric reflux (p. 42).

Abdominal palpation per rectum (p. 22) is generally within normal limits; however, mild to moderate cecal or colonic tympany may be identified and should resolve with treatment. Palpation per rectum has been found to be particularly valuable for identification of simple obstructions such as ileal, cecal, or colonic impactions, many of which may be amendable to medical management.

Abdominal sonographic examination (p. 116) is not typically performed on horses with mild colic; however, it is being used with increasing frequency to supplement palpation per rectum. A 2–3.5 MHz transducer should be used in the adult for deeper penetration, or a 5.0–7.5 MHz transducer in foals or for more superficial structures in the adult horse. The small intestine can be evaluated for wall thickness, distention, and motility, and this information may help with early identification of horses with a strangulating lesion.[8] Sonography is also useful in evaluation of large intestinal disease and may be particularly useful in the evaluation of right dorsal colitis.[15]

Diagnostic tests such as clinical laboratory data (p. 78), peritoneal fluid analysis (p. 87), and abdominal radiographic examination (p. 149) are generally not performed on horses showing mild colic for the first time. Horses with severe, persistent, or recurrent signs are generally referred to a hospital for further diagnostic tests and treatment (see Chapter 8 on Referral of the Horse with Colic [p. 71]).

Management of mild colic

Analgesia

See Chapter 6 on Analgesia (p. 51). The use of analgesics in the management of horses with colic is necessary for humane reasons and to reduce the negative impact of pain and sympathetic stimulation on intestinal function and improve motility. Pain management in horses with medical colic is relatively easier to provide than horses that have more severe lesions that may require colic surgery.

Note: Flunixin meglumine (1.1 mg/kg) is typically used as the initial analgesic drug to manage horses with mild colic.

Analgesia is initially provided by the administration of nonsteroidal anti-inflammatory drugs (NSAIDs), such as flunixin meglumine. Phenylbutazone can also be used; however, it appears to be somewhat more toxic to the gastrointestinal tract.[20] NSAIDs work by inhibiting cyclooxygenase (COX), thereby decreasing the production of prostaglandin, prostacyclin, and thromboxane, which in turn interferes with the inflammatory cascade.[21] Flunixin meglumine and phenylbutazone are nonspecific COX inhibitors and, therefore, inhibit both COX-1 (constitutive) and COX-2 (inducible). COX-1 is important for maintenance and repair of the gastrointestinal tract and its inhibition may lead to intestinal injury. More recently, COX-selective or preferential NSAIDs, such as meloxicam and firocoxib, have been developed and the use of these drugs for treatment of mild colic may prove beneficial.[6,17]

Note: Flunixin meglumine at a dose rate of 1.1 mg/kg should not be administered more frequently than every 12 h because of the potential for gastrointestinal and renal toxicity particularly in colic patients.

If NSAIDs are unable to sufficiently control the horse's pain, further analgesia is warranted. It should be noted, however, that if the horse's pain is refractory to analgesic therapy, then medical management may not be an option. Alpha-2 agonist such as xylazine and detomidine are commonly used for sedation and analgesia. Xylazine is most frequently employed as it has a short duration of action (15–120 min) and, therefore, allows for frequent reevaluation.[7]

Opioids are another useful analgesic therapy in horses. Other than butorphanol, opioid use in horses has been limited due to the potential for excitatory behavior or decreased gastrointestinal motility.[26] Butorphanol can be used in combination with alpha-2 agonist to provide neuroleptanalgesia.

The decrease in colonic motility may provide temporary pain relief in horses suffering from gas or impaction colic.

Note: If a horse/foal with colic is unresponsive to flunixin meglumine and sedation with xylazine/butorphanol, referral should be discussed with the owner/caregiver.

Spasmolytic drugs

Spasmolytic drugs may be useful in providing analgesia in horses with mild colic by reducing intestinal spasm for up to 20–30 min.[3,23] Recently, Buscopan® (N-butylscopolammonium bromide) administered at 0.3 mg/kg intravenous (IV) has been approved for use in the USA. Repeat use may be contraindicated as it may prolong ileus. Also, the temporary increase in heart rate for up to 45 min[10] may make monitoring of the patient difficult. Buscopan® is the drug preferred by some practitioners for managing horses with mild colic.

Fluid therapy

Although hypovolemia and dehydration are most rapidly corrected by IV fluid therapy, enteral fluid therapy may be more economical, more easily performed in the field, and more beneficial in certain forms of colic. See Chapter 7 on Enteral Fluid Therapy (p. 62) and Chapter 11 on Intravenous Catheterization and Fluid Therapy (p. 99). One study reported that the use of enteral fluids at 10 L/h for 5 h via a feeding tube produced better hydration of ingesta and feces than the use of IV fluids.[18] In addition, there was a trend toward increased defecation in the horses receiving enteral fluid therapy.[18] It is, therefore, recommended that enteral fluids be administered in horses with mild colic and impactions.

Note: Enteral fluids are typically administered through a nasogastric tube (p. 38) and an initial bolus generally consists of 4–6 L of water for a 400–550 kg horse with or without electrolytes (p. 65).

Laxatives may also be included as part of this initial bolus. Management of impactions with enteral fluids requires repeated administration of 4–6 L of water and electrolytes for a 400–550 kg horse every 2–4 h. Large volumes of fluids (10–12/mL/kg/30–60 min) administered with magnesium sulfate

earlier during the course of treatment resulted in more rapid resolution of large colon impaction (12–36 h) compared to horses administered enteral fluids less frequently or horses receiving only IV fluids (48 h).[11] Continuous enteral fluid administration can also be provided in a hospital setting.

Note: Horses should always be checked for reflux prior to enteral fluid administration because of the risk of fatal gastric rupture.

Enteral fluid administration may not be possible in horses with concurrent ileus and the presence of gastric reflux. High volumes of enteral fluids may not be tolerated in all horses and may cause gastric distention and pain; therefore, frequent reevaluation is warranted and the horse rechecked for nasogastric reflux if painful post administration.

Laxatives

Impactions of both the small and large intestine are frequently diagnosed as the cause of colic. Many horses with impactions have mild colic signs and respond well to medical therapy, which should include the judicious use of laxatives. Laxatives used in horses include mineral oil, magnesium sulfate, dioctyl sodium sulfosuccinate, and psyllium mucilloid. Mineral oil is an intestinal lubricant and can also serve as a marker of intestinal transit. It should be present in the feces of a normal horse 12–24 h after administration.[25]

Enteral magnesium sulfate increased colonic and fecal hydration and when administered with IV fluids caused plasma expansion in horses.[11,18,19] Its mechanism of action is as an osmotic cathartic which promotes water influx into the intestinal lumen.[18,19]

Dioctyl sodium sulfosuccinate (DSS) is an anionic surfactant which facilitates water penetration by decreasing surface tension. There have been reports of toxicity at a dosage of 50 mg/kg.[9] Because of its low margin of safety and questionable efficacy at low dosage, its use is questionable particularly in light of the documented benefits with administration of water and electrolytes.[11]

Psyllium mucilloid has been advocated for use in horses suffering from sand impaction. However, its efficacy is in question and one study found psyllium mucilloid failed to increase evacuation of sand in an experimentally induced model of sand impaction.[12,24]

Nutrition

In general, it is recommended that feed be withheld initially in the management of horses with colic for 4–24h depending on the duration and severity of signs. Withholding feed is generally well tolerated in horses for 24–48h. It is important, however, that if a pregnant mare has feed withheld, IV dextrose is administered, as starvation in the pregnant mare even for a short period of time leads to altered prostaglandin production and fetal loss.[27] Neonates do not tolerate having milk withheld and should be hospitalized and parenteral nutrition provided if the necessity for this becomes apparent.

Once the horse's colic signs have subsided, physical examination parameters have returned to normal, and/or impaction has resolved, it is appropriate to begin reintroduction of feed. The reintroduction of food should be gradual and the type of colic dictates the rate and type of food that the horse is fed. Hand walking and grazing is recommended, if available, to stimulate gastrointestinal motility. Horses with an impaction may also benefit from hand walking and grazing small amounts. Horses with mild colic responding to a single dose of flunixin meglumine can have feed reintroduced after about 4h and be back to full feed by 24h. Feeding may begin prior to defecation, as the gastrocolic reflex may contribute to colonic motility. During the refeeding process, the horse should be monitored closely and if clinical parameters worsen or the horse becomes anorectic or does not produce feces, the horse should be reexamined and the feeding regimen revised. See Chapter 23 on Nutrition (p. 301).

Monitoring

Horses that initially present with signs of mild colic often respond to medical therapy; however, close monitoring is required to identify early indications of clinical deterioration and severity of colic necessitating more aggressive medical or surgical intervention. If the horse is being managed on the farm, it is important to stress to the owner/caregiver that frequently monitoring the horse is essential. While most horses with colic respond to either no treatment or a single treatment, reexamination by the attending veterinarian is not likely to be

necessary but a follow-up telephone conversation should be made to ensure that the horse has completely recovered.

In a hospital setting, hospitals designed with a central island to allow for constant observation are ideal. If this is not available, regular walk bys to check for pain are appropriate. Frequent monitoring of heart rate, respiratory rate, rectal temperature, mucous membrane color, capillary refill time, intestinal borborygmi, and evaluation of fecal production and consistency is necessary until it is apparent that the horse has responded to medical therapy. Feces should be evaluated for presence of sand, gravel, undigested feed material, and consistency. If mineral oil was administered, time until passage can assist the clinician in evaluating intestinal motility and transit. During the management of a horse with mild colic on fluid therapy, it is recommended that the packed cell volume/total plasma protein (PCV/TPP) to be reevaluated every 12h and electrolytes every 24h. If the horse presented with electrolyte abnormalities that are being corrected, monitoring should be more frequent.

If at any point, the horse's condition/physical examination parameters appear to be deteriorating, then reevaluation of the horse should be conducted including passage of a nasogastric tube (p. 38), palpation per rectum (p. 22), and transcutaneous sonographic evaluation (p. 116). See Chapter 8 on Referral of the Horse with Colic (p. 71).

Management changes and prevention

Colic may be encountered on even the best managed farms. Given that risk factors that have identified for colic include crib-biting or wind sucking, changes in routine/exercise program, increasing hours spent in a stall, poor quality hay, lack of appropriate deworming, or lack of a good dentition program, it seems prudent that these may be areas where management may have the most effect. Frequent pasture turn out, feeding good quality hay, feeding off the ground to minimize sand/gravel ingestion, always having freshwater available, minimizing changes in feeding/exercise routine, appropriate deworming program, and routine dental care are recommended to minimize signs of colic.[1,2,14] Older horses with frequent impactions or horses with previous colic surgery may also benefit from a completely pelleted diet or low roughage hay. See Chapter 22 on Long-Term Recovery and Prevention (p. 292).

When colic is no longer considered mild

Management of colic in the field can be difficult. In the majority of horses with gas colic, response will be seen quickly after the administration of an NSAID or a spasmolytic drug. In horses that require further analgesic therapy, it is more likely that the colic may not respond to medical therapy and the horse may benefit from referral to a surgical facility. Furthermore, if abnormalities are identified during evaluation such as an abnormal finding on palpation per rectum (p. 26) or the presence of nasogastric reflux (p. 42), the horse is more likely to require referral. See Chapter 8 on Referral of the Horse with Colic (p. 71).

Enteral and IV fluid therapy may be administered on the farm to manage horses with a large colon impaction (p. 217). However, there is increasing evidence that horses with impactions benefit from frequent or continual administration of enteral fluids which can be challenging without hospitalization. Furthermore, not all horses with an impaction are amendable to medical management; therefore, it may be beneficial for the horse to be at a location with frequent monitoring and where surgery could be performed rapidly if needed prior to clinical deterioration. Clinical scenario 6, located in Appendix A, provides an overview of medical management of an impaction.

Proximal enteritis (p. 207), which is typically treated medically, can be difficult to manage on the farm because of the necessity for close monitoring, frequent refluxing, and high volumes of IV fluids. It can also be difficult to differentiate between proximal enteritis and a strangulating obstruction; therefore, referral for further diagnostic tests and possibly surgery is recommended. Quizzes for each chapter, additional clinical scenarios, and video demonstrations of surgical procedures are available online at www.wiley.com/go/southwood.

References

1. Archer, D.C., Freeman, D.E., Doyle, A.J., Proudman, C.J. & Edwards, G.B. (2004) Association between cribbing and entrapment of the small intestine in the epiploic foramen in horses: 68 cases (1991–2002). *Journal of the American Veterinary Medical Association*, **224**, 562–564.
2. Archer, D.C. & Proudman, C.J. (2006) Epidemiological clues to preventing colic. *Veterinary Journal*, **172**, 29–39.
3. Boatwright, C.E., Fubini, S.L., Grohn, Y.T. & Goossens, L. (1996) A comparison of N-butylscopolammonium bromide and butorphanol tartrate for analgesia using a balloon model of abdominal pain in ponies. *Canadian Journal of Veterinary Research*, **60**, 65–68.
4. Cohen, N.D., Matejka, P.L., Honnas, C.M. & Hooper, R.N. (1995) Case-control study of the association between various management factors and development of colic in horses. Texas Equine Colic Study Group. *Journal of the American Veterinary Medical Association*, **206**, 667–673.
5. Cohen, N.D., Gibbs, P.G. & Woods, A.M. (1999) Dietary and other management factors associated with colic in horses. *Journal of the American Veterinary Medical Association*, **215**, 53–60.
6. Cook, V.L., Meyer, C.T., Campbell, N.B. & Blikslager, A.T. (2009) Effect of firocoxib or flunixin meglumine on recovery of ischemic-injured equine jejunum. *American Journal of Veterinary Research*, **70**, 992–1000.
7. Daunt, D.A. & Steffey, E.P. (2002) Alpha-2 adrenergic agonists as analgesics in horses. *Veterinary Clinics of North America: Equine Practice*, **18**, 39–46.
8. Fisher, A.T. (1997) Advances in diagnostic techniques for horses with colic. *Veterinary Clinics of North America: Equine Practice*, **13**, 203–224.
9. Freeman, D.E., Ferrante, P.L. & Palmer, J.E. (1992) Comparison of the effects of intragastric infusions of equal volumes of water, dioctyl sodium sulfosuccinate, and magnesium sulfate on fecal composition and output in clinically normal horses. *American Journal of Veterinary Research*, **53**, 1347–1353.
10. Geimer, T.R., Ekström, P.M., Ludders, J.W., Erichsen, D.F. & Gleed, R.D. (1995) Haemodynamic effects of hyoscine-N-butylbromide in ponies. *Journal of Veterinary Pharmacology and Therapeutics*, **18**, 13–16.
11. Hallowell, G.D. (2008) Retrospective study assessing efficacy of treatment of large colonic impactions. *Equine Veterinary Journal*, **40**, 411–413.
12. Hammock, P.D., Freeman, D.E. & Baker, G.J. (1998) Failure of psyllium mucilloid to hasten evacuation of sand from the equine large intestine. *Veterinary Surgery*, **27**, 547–554.
13. Hillyer, M.H., Taylor, F.G. & French, N.P. (1997) A cross-sectional study of colic in horses on thoroughbred training premises in the British Isles in 1994. *Equine Veterinary Journal*, **33**, 380–385.
14. Hillyer, M.H., Taylor, F.G., Proudman, C.J., Edwards, G.B., Smith, J.E. & French, N.P. (2002) Case control study to identify risk factors for simple colonic obstruction and distension colic in horses. *Equine Veterinary Journal*, **34**, 455–463.

15. Jones, S.L., Davis, J. & Rowlingson, K. (2003) Ultrasonographic findings in horses with right dorsal colitis: Five cases (2000–2001). *Journal of the American Veterinary Medical Association*, **222**, 1248–1251.

16. Kaneene, J.B., Ross, W.A. & Miller, R. (1997) The Michigan equine monitoring system II. Frequencies and impact of selected health problems. *Preventive Veterinary Medicine*, **29**, 277–292.

17. Little, D., Brown, S.A., Campbell, N.B., Moeser, A.J., Davis, J.L. & Blikslager, A.T. (2007) Effects of the cyclooxygenase inhibitor meloxicam on recovery of ischemia-injured equine jejunum. *American Journal of Veterinary Research*, **68**, 614–624.

18. Lopes, M., Walker, B.L., White, N.A., 2nd & Ward, D.L. (2002) Treatments to promote colonic hydration: Enteral fluid therapy versus intravenous fluid therapy and magnesium sulphate. *Equine Veterinary Journal*, **34**, 505–509.

19. Lopes, M.A., White, N.A., 2nd, Donaldson, L., Crisman, M.V. & Ward, D.L. (2004) Effects of enteral and intravenous fluid therapy, magnesium sulfate, and sodium sulfate on colonic contents and feces in horses. *American Journal of Veterinary Research*, **65**, 695–704.

20. MacAllister, C.G., Morgan, S.J., Borne, A.T. & Pollet, R.A. (1993) Comparison of adverse effects of phenylbutazone, flunixin meglumine, and ketoprofen in horses. *Journal of the American Veterinary Medical Association*, **202**, 71–77.

21. Moses, V.S. & Bertone, A.L. (2002) Nonsteroidal anti-inflammatory drugs. *Veterinary Clinics of North America: Equine Practice*, **18**, 21–37.

22. Proudman, C.J. (1992) A two year, prospective survey of equine colic in general practice. *Equine Veterinary Journal*, **24**, 90–93.

23. Roelvink, M.E., Goossens, L., Kalsbeek, H.C. & Wensing, T. (1991) Analgesic and spasmolytic effects of dipyrone, hyoscine-N-butylbromide and a combination of the two in ponies. *Veterinary Record*, **129**, 378–380.

24. Ruohoniemi, M., Kaikkonen, R., Raekallio, M. & Luukkanen, L. (2001) Abdominal radiography in monitoring the resolution of sand accumulations from the large colon of horses treated medically. *Equine Veterinary Journal*, **33**, 59–64.

25. Schumacher, J., DeGraves, F.J. & Spano, J.S. (1997) Clinical and clinicopathologic effects of large doses of raw linseed oil as compared to mineral oil in healthy horses. *Journal of Veterinary Internal Medicine*, **11**, 296–299.

26. Sellon, D.C., Monroe, V.L., Robers, M.C. & Papich, M.G. (2001) Pharmacokinetics and adverse effects of butorphanol administered by single intravenous injection or continuous infusion in horses. *American Journal of Veterinary Research*, **62**, 183–189.

27. Silver, M. & Fowden, A.L. (1982) Uterine prostaglandin F metabolite production in relation to glucose availability in late pregnancy and a possible influence of diet on time of delivery in the mare. *Journal of Reproduction and Fertility Supplement*, **32**, 511–519.

28. Tinker, M.K., White, N.A., Lessard, P., *et al.* (1997) Prospective study of equine colic incidence and mortality. *Equine Veterinary Journal*, **29**, 448–453.

29. Tinker, M.K., White, N.A., Lessard, P., *et al.* (1997) Prospective study of equine colic risk factors. *Equine Veterinary Journal*, **29**, 454–458.

30. Traub-Dargatz, J.L., Kopral, C.A., Seitzinger, A.G., Garber, L.P., Forde, K. & White, N.A. (2001) Estimate of the national incidence of and operation-level risk factors for colic among horses in the United States, spring 1998 to spring 1999. *Journal of the American Veterinary Medical Association*, **219**, 67–71.

31. Uhlinger, C. (1992) Investigations in to the incidence of field colic. *Equine Veterinary Journal*, **13**, 11–18.

32. White, N.A. (1990) Epidemiology and etiology of colic. In: *The Equine Acute Abdomen* (ed N.A. White), pp. 50–64. Lea and Febiger, Philadelphia, Pennsylvania.

6 Analgesia

Luiz C. Santos and Louise L. Southwood

Department of Clinical Studies, New Bolton Center, School of Veterinary Medicine, University of Pennsylvania, Kennett Square, PA, USA

Chapter Outline

Indications	**51**
Nonsteroidal anti-inflammatory drugs	**52**
Mechanism of action	52
Clinical use	52
Adverse effects and contraindications	53
Alpha-2 adrenergic agonists	**54**
Mechanism of action	54
Clinical use	54
Alpha-2 antagonists	55
Adverse effects and contraindications	55
Opioids	**55**
Mechanism of action	55
Clinical use	56
Opioid antagonists	56
Adverse effects and contraindications	56
Intravenous lidocaine	**57**
Mechanism of action	57
Clinical use	57
Adverse effects and contraindications	58
CNS effects	58
Cardiovascular effects	58
Hyoscine-N-butylbromide	**58**
Mechanism of action	58
Clinical use	58
Adverse effects and contraindications	59

Indications

Analgesic drugs are an important part of the initial treatment of colic pain (p. 45), for treatment of horses with impactions and displacements (p. 217), and postoperative pain management (p. 230). The response of the horse or foal to analgesic drugs is a major determinant of the need for referral and for surgery; therefore, their use is important for patient assessment. While there are really no contraindications to providing analgesia for colic patients, care should be taken when using such drugs in patients that are being monitored closely for response to medical treatment versus the need for surgery. This is particularly important in patients for whom a diagnosis has not yet been

Practical Guide to Equine Colic, First Edition. Edited by Louise L. Southwood.
© 2013 John Wiley & Sons, Inc. Published 2013 by John Wiley & Sons, Inc.

made (see Chapter 8 on Referral of the Horse with Colic [p. 71] and Chapter 15 on Medical versus Surgical Treatment of the Horse with Colic [p. 164]). Anti-inflammatory analgesic drugs such as non-steroidal anti-inflammatory drugs (NSAIDs) are also important in the treatment of ischemia-reperfusion injury (p. 246) and endotoxemia (p. 246). Therefore, they are also used in postoperative treatment and the management of horses/foals with enteritis, colitis, and peritonitis.

Nonsteroidal anti-inflammatory drugs

Mechanism of action

NSAIDs exert their anti-inflammatory and analgesic effects through inhibition of cyclooxygenase (COX). The two isoforms of the COX enzyme are the constitutively expressed COX-1 and inducible COX-2. COX-1 is responsible for normal physiological prostaglandin production in healthy tissue and, while physiologically expressed in healthy tissue at low levels, COX-2 production is upregulated during injury.[26] COX catalyzes the conversion of free essential fatty acids (arachidonic acid) to prostanoids. Prostanoids are important for maintenance of mucosal blood flow and integrity, hind gut fermentation, and volatile fatty acid production as well as restoration of intestinal barrier function following injury.[5] Prostanoids are the prostaglandins (classically considered mediators of inflammation), thromboxanes (mediators of vasoconstriction), and prostacyclins (active in the resolution phase of inflammation). Therefore, the NSAIDs have beneficial anti-inflammatory and analgesic effects; however, nonspecific inhibition of the constitutively expressed COX-1 can have detrimental effects on tissue maintenance and repair (see Adverse effects and contraindications).

The NSAIDs are classified as having nonspecific COX inhibition (e.g., flunixin meglumine [Banamine®, Finadyne®] and phenylbutazone ["bute"]) and COX-1 sparing effects (coxibs, e.g., meloxicam [Metacam®] and firocoxib [Equioxx®]). Meloxicam is reported to have a COX selectivity ratio (50% inhibition (IC[50], microM) COX-1: COX-2) of 3.8 whereas that of firocoxib is 265.[26] While flunixin meglumine is still frequently used in management of colic patients, the COX-1 sparing NSAIDs have been shown to have a less detrimental effect on mucosal repair and will likely be the drugs of choice in the future for use in colic patients.

Clinical use

NSAIDs, particularly flunixin meglumine, are used as the primary analgesic drug for horses with colic. A typical analgesic regimen for the initial management of colic is flunixin meglumine (1.1 mg/kg intravenous [IV]). If there is a lack of response or recurrence of pain then xylazine (0.3–0.4 mg/kg IV) with or without butorphanol (0.01–0.02 mg/kg IV) can be used. Note that flunixin meglumine at maximum dose rate of 1.1 mg/kg cannot be used more frequently than every 12 h. Occasionally a horse will be severely painful and unresponsive to flunixin meglumine or xylazine and treatment with detomidine (0.01–0.02 mg/kg IV) is necessary.

Postoperative colic patients are typically treated with flunixin meglumine (1.1 mg/kg IV every 12 h for 2–3 days then 0.5 mg/kg every 12 h for 1–2 days). Additional analgesia is provided with xylazine or detomidine with or without butorphanol as needed.

Historically, use of flunixin meglumine has been associated with "masking a surgical colic" and "masking signs of endotoxemia" and use of the low dose (0.25 mg/kg) is recommended. Several comments pertain to this notion: (1) veterinarians should become familiar with the analgesic effects of flunixin meglumine and be capable of assessing their patient accordingly; (2) most horses have been treated with at least one dose of flunixin meglumine prior to admission to referral hospitals and this is taken into consideration during patient evaluation and many surgeons would be unlikely to recommend surgery unless an attempt had been made to manage the horse's pain with flunixin meglumine; and (3) treating (as opposed to masking) the signs of endotoxemia is generally considered favorable and an attempt is usually made to surgically correct the lesion prior to the horse becoming severely endotoxemic. However, prudent use of flunixin meglumine, even the low dose, is important when monitoring horses/foals with colic to determine if surgery is indicated (See Chapter 15 on

Medical versus Surgical Treatment of the Horse with Colic [p. 164]).

Meloxicam and firocoxib have been released for equine use relatively recently in Europe and the United States, respectively. Meloxicam is used at a dose rate of 0.6 mg/kg IV every 24 h and firocoxib at a loading dose of 0.27 mg/kg IV and then 0.09 mg/kg IV every 24 h. Firocoxib *cannot* be administered in an aqueous solution including heparinized saline which is often used to flush IV catheters. Administration of firocoxib can be performed by drawing patient blood into the catheter and extension tubing prior to drug administration, using a dimethyl sulfoxide (DMSO)-based solution, or via direct venipuncture.

Other NSAIDs have not gained widespread clinical use for managing equine colic patients.

Adverse effects and contraindications

Complications with the use of NSAIDs primarily pertain to the nonspecific COX inhibition (see Mechanism of action). Prostaglandins are important for maintenance of renal perfusion and renal papillary necrosis leading to renal failure can result from administration of flunixin meglumine or phenylbutazone particularly at high doses or to patients that are dehydrated or showing signs of shock. Therefore, flunixin meglumine and phenylbutazone should be avoided in horses with preexisting renal failure, including prerenal failure which is fairly common in colic patients admitted to referral hospitals. In horses with a persistently high plasma creatinine concentration, urinalysis should be performed to evaluate the presence of renal disease. Use of COX-1 sparing NSAIDs should be considered in these patients if anti-inflammatory analgesic drugs are deemed necessary for optimal patient care.

NSAID use can lead to gastric ulceration (p. 205) and right dorsal colitis (p. 216).[28] NSAIDs are contraindicated in horses with right dorsal colitis, and other analgesic drugs such as a butorphanol (p. 55) and IV lidocaine (p. 57) constant rate infusion (CRI) should be used as alternatives.

Flunixin meglumine has been shown to inhibit recovery of transepithelial barrier function in ischemia-injured jejunum.[11] Restoration of jejunal mucosal barrier function involves three phases:

(1) villus contraction under the control of the enteric nervous system and endogenous prostaglandins; (2) epithelial restitution whereby the epithelial cells produce plasma membrane extensions and migrate into the defect; and (3) closure of the paracellular spaces involving assembly of tight junctions which is also dependent on endogenous prostaglandins.[6] Therefore, prostaglandins are important for restoration of mucosal barrier function. Nonspecific COX inhibition appears to prevent this restoration based on *ex vivo* measurement of transepithelial electrical resistance, mucosal-to-serosal mannitol flux, and mucosal permeability to lipopolysaccharide (endotoxin).[44,45] Neutrophil influx during reperfusion causes further tissue damage and is also detrimental to restoration of mucosal barrier function.[6] Flunixin meglumine and meloxicam administration was associated with an increase in mucosal neutrophil infiltration in a jejunal ischemia model which may further contribute to the effect of these drugs on mucosal repair.[10,22] Interestingly, flunixin meglumine did not appear to affect restoration of colonic mucosal barrier function.[27]

COX-1 sparing NSAIDs (i.e., firocoxib and meloxicam) had fewer toxic effects on the gastrointestinal tract and did not impair recovery of the transepithelial barrier.[11,22] COX-1 sparing NSAIDs such as firocoxib or meloxicam may be used as an alternative to flunixin meglumine for management of postoperative colic patients. Lidocaine IV[9] and misoprostol (prostaglandin E_1 analogue)[44] attenuated the inhibitory effects of flunixin meglumine on restoration of mucosal barrier function in a jejunal ischemia model. Lidocaine IV decreased the jejunal neutrophil infiltration which may explain its apparent beneficial effect.[9,10]

NSAIDs may affect intestinal motility.[26] Nonselective COX inhibitors had an inhibitory effect on colonic[49,50] but in general not ileal[29] contractile activity. Inhibition of tonic ileal contractions was found with flunixin meglumine.[29] There was a decrease in ileal contractile activity with COX-1 sparing NSAIDs (celecoxib).[29] The clinical importance of these findings and application to the equine colic patient is yet to be elucidated.

Perivascular or intramuscular (IM) administration of flunixin meglumine or phenylbutazone creates tissue damage and an anaerobic environment. Clostridial myonecrosis is a serious complication of IM or perivascular injections.[33]

Alpha-2 adrenergic agonists

Mechanism of action

This group of drugs causes depression of the central nervous system (CNS) by occupying alpha-2 adrenergic receptors (α_{2A}, α_{2B}, and α_{2C}) that are found in both central and peripheral nervous systems and are located on both pre- and postsynaptic neurons. Presynaptically, alpha-2 receptors mediate inhibition of the release of substances such as noradrenaline, acetylcholine, serotonin, dopamine, substance P, and possibly other neurotransmitters. In the brain and spinal cord, pre- and postsynaptically located receptors mediate inhibition of neuronal firing, suppression of neuronal excitability, sedation, sleep, antinociception, hypotension, bradycardia, and other responses.[2]

The sedative and anxiolytic effects of alpha-2 agonists are mediated by activation of supraspinal autoreceptors or postsynaptic receptors located in the pons (locus ceraleus), while the analgesic effects are mediated by activation of heteroceptors located in the dorsal horn of the spinal cord.[2] The net effect is a reduction of the sympathetic efflux to the CNS and a reduction of the catecholamines and other substances related to stress.

The physiological effects of alpha-2 agonists are variable according to the receptor subtype occupied, for example, sedation (α_{2A}), somatic and visceral analgesia (α_{2A}, α_{2B}), initial hypertension (α_{2B}) that is followed by hypotension (α_{2A}), and decreased cardiac output (Table 6.1).

Clinical use

Alpha-2 agonists are commonly used with or without butorphanol in colic patients that are unresponsive to treatment with NSAIDs or hyoscine-N-

Table 6.1 α_2: α_1 Selectivity.

Drug	α_2: α_1
Xylazine	160:1
Detomidine	260:1
Dexmedetomidine	1620:1
Romifidine	340:1
Clonidine	220:1

butylbromide (Buscopan®) (see Nonsteroidal anti-inflammatory drugs and Hyoscine-N-butylbromide).

Alpha-2 agonists posses many of the qualities required for an ideal preanesthetic drug, including predictability, anxiolysis, marked sedation, stupor, and indifference to mildly painful procedures. The most widely used alpha-2 agonists in horses are xylazine, detomidine, romifidine, and currently dexmedetomidine has been used. Alpha-2 agonist drugs are also able to decrease minimum alveolar concentration (MAC) of volatile anesthetics. For example, dexmedetomidine (1–1.75 μg/kg/h)[4] and xylazine (1 mg/kg/h)[43] are expected to cause a MAC reduction of nearly 25%.

Alpha-2 agonists can be administered IV, IM, and orally to facilitate anxiolysis, sedation, or induction and maintenance of general anesthesia.[42,43] The IM dose is 2–3 times the IV dose and takes about 15–30 min for the peak effect. Oral or buccal absorption of some alpha-2 agonists, for example, detomidine (60 μg/kg), produces sedation in approximately 45 min. The drug will not be effective if swallowed, due to first-pass hepatic effect. Duration of action may vary according to the drug used; at equipotent doses romifidine > detomidine > xylazine.

Alpha-2 agonists are the agents most widely used to produce standing sedation. Dexmedetomidine, xylazine, and detomidine have being used as a CRI under general anesthesia or during standing surgeries in horses. Detomidine loading dose (7–8μg/kg IV) followed by 0.6μg/kg/min CRI will give heavy sedation and can be combined with opioids and local anesthesia for painful procedures.

Titrating these agents to effect can vary the degree of sedation. The degree and duration of sedation is dose- and drug-dependent. High doses of alpha-2 agonists increase intensity and duration of sedation (not seen with tranquilizers, such as phenothiazines). Sedation persists for many hours following high-dose detomidine (40–60 μg/kg). Ataxia is dose-related, and is more severe with detomidine and xylazine than with romifidine.

Recovery from anesthesia should be a quiet, coordinated, and uneventful process. The administration of reduced doses of alpha-2 agonists immediately before or during the recovery process prolongs recovery by reducing excitement, ataxia, and stress without significant cardiorespiratory consequences.[16]

Alpha-2 agonists may be combined with opioids to induce neuroleptoanalgesia or with phenothiazines to cause a synergistic or additive effect on sedation. Combinations with opioids (e.g., butorphanol) give a more reliable sedation. The horse is also less likely to suddenly react to stimuli. Infusions of alpha-2 agonists can be used in conjunction with other injectable agents, primarily ketamine, to maintain anesthesia. They are also used in conjunction with volatile anesthetics for this purpose.

Epidural administration of alpha-2 agonists are used commonly in horses.[47] These agents can be administered epidurally, alone, with local anesthetics or opioids, to provide analgesia or as an adjunct to general anesthesia. Combination with a local anesthetic or opioids prolong the duration of action.

Alpha-2 antagonists

Alpha-2 antagonists are rarely indicated for reversal of alpha-2 agonist-induced sedation in horses. Exceptions include: cardiorespiratory compromise from overdose of alpha-2 agonists or to shorten the prolonged sedation of high doses given. Drugs such as yohimbine (0.15–0.25 mg/kg, IV) have weak antagonist activity whereas atipamezole (0.15 mg/kg, IV) has potent antagonist activity.

Adverse effects and contraindications

The alpha-2 agonists are known for their cardiovascular effects. Patients with suspected or potential cardiac dysfunction should not be given alpha-2 agonists. Horses should be exercise tolerant at a minimum and should have no signs of cardiopulmonary disease. Because alpha-2 agonists will rapidly increase afterload, horses with dilatative cardiomyopathy and weakened systolic function should not be given an alpha-2 agonist. Similarly, patients with mitral valve disease should not be administered agents that increase afterload. The initial increase in vascular resistance and afterload may reduce cardiac output by 50% or more.

The decrease in blood flow caused by alpha-2 agonists is tolerated quite well in healthy patients, as the largest reductions occur in vascular beds perfusing peripheral tissues, such as the skin and mucous membranes.

Other effects (dose-dependent) that might be seen when alpha-2 agonists are used include respiratory depression (respiratory acidosis), decrease gastrointestinal motility, facial and nasal edema (due to lower head position), and decreased insulin release (associated with stimulation of alpha-2 receptors on pancreatic beta cells). Hyperglycemia is often observed likely as a result of activation of alpha-1 receptors and stimulation of hepatic glucose production. An increase in urine output with decrease in urine specific gravity is seen likely because of interference of alpha-2 agonists with the action of antidiuretic hormone on the renal tubules and collecting duct. Sedated horse may react to noise/stimuli and may kick or bite. Variable degree of ataxia is seen and this depends on the dosage used. There is no evidence that any of the anesthetic drugs commonly used in horses causes fetal damage or loss, although xylazine increases uterine tone and low doses of detomidine are preferable. The importance of alpha-2 agonist induced cardiovascular effects on pregnancy in the horse are unknown. One has to be careful when administering together high doses of phenothiazines and alpha-2 agonists IV, as they might induce recumbency. Recently, transient tachypnea and antipyresis have been observed following sedation of febrile horses with xylazine or detomidine.[20]

Opioids

Mechanism of action

Opioids act by combining reversibly with one or more specific receptor in the brain and spinal cord to induce variable effects including analgesia, sedation, euphoria, dysphoria, and excitation. There are at least three major types of opiate receptors in mammals, designated μ, κ, and σ. Mu receptors are responsible for mediating respiratory depression, supraspinal analgesia, miosis, and sedation. In contrast, κ receptors mediate spinal analgesia, miosis, and sedation, whereas σ receptors mediate dysphoria, hallucinations, and respiratory and vasomotor stimulation.[32]

Clinical use

Opiates are potent analgesic agents that may be underutilized in equine medicine. Opioids are essential for management of various clinical conditions; analgesia is necessary to relieve discomfort associated with injury or surgical procedures, allow for an earlier return to function, facilitate smoother recoveries from general anesthesia, and minimize pain-associated inhibition of gastrointestinal motility. Butorphanol is commonly used in colic patients in combination with xylazine pre- and postoperatively for management of colic signs that are unresponsive to NSAIDs.

In general, opioids cause little sedation in the horse when used alone, but produce excellent results in combination with small doses of sedatives. Indeed, these drugs are often used for sedation in association with alpha-2 agonists for standing restraint. Opioids potentiate the effects of alpha-2 agonists for standing sedation. Dose rates for opioids include morphine (0.15 mg/kg, IV; 0.25 mg/kg, IM), buprenorphine (0.006 mg/kg, IM), butorphanol (0.02–0.05 mg/kg, IV; 0.05–0.1 mg/kg, IM), meperidine (1–2 mg/kg IM—note that an IV administration of meperidine can result in histamine release and hypotension), and methadone (0.1 mg/kg IV, IM). Premedication prior to general anesthesia may be especially helpful in calming a painful horse.

Butorphanol ameliorates signs of superficial and visceral pain in horses when administered as a bolus IV injection but is effective for only 30–90 min.[18,31] Intraoperative administration of butorphanol decreases clinical signs of postoperative pain in horses undergoing orthopedic surgery[17] and a butorphanol CRI (13 μg/kg/h for 24 h after surgery) decreases plasma cortisol concentrations and improves recovery characteristics in horses undergoing abdominal surgery.[41] Postoperative colic patients treated with a butorphanol CRI had delayed in time to first passage of feces compared to saline control horses.[41] Butorphanol CRI has not gained widespread acceptance for managing postoperative colic patients.

Opioids do not consistently reduce the MAC of volatile agent required to prevent purposeful movement in response to a specified stimulus. In horses, MAC may actually be increased.

The epidural route of administration can be used to provide analgesia with morphine (0.1–0.2 mg/kg) while reducing the systemic effects.[47] Recent studies showed that epidural morphine produced pain relief that lasted 20–22 h in horses after orthopedic surgery and decreased discomfort during standing laparoscopic ovariectomy in mares. This may well be the route of choice for this drug, as its solubility characteristics are well suited for epidural administration.

Opioid antagonists

All known opioid agonists and agonist-antagonist are reversible with opioid antagonists; however, they are rarely indicated. The IV administration of naloxone (0.002–0.03 mg/kg) promptly reverses both the central and peripheral effects of opioid agonists, including behavioral and cardiorespiratory effects, locomotor activity, and analgesia. If reversal of an overdose or undesirable effect from a μ-agonist is necessary, but at the same time analgesia is needed, the more logical choice is the administration of an agonist-antagonist drug (e.g., butorphanol).

Adverse effects and contraindications

Unfortunately, the pharmaceutical options for equine clinicians are limited, and opioids (such as morphine) that are available for use can have adverse effects that create additional complications in already compromised animals.[3] Morphine administration delays gastric emptying and decreases peristaltic activity by inhibiting the release of acetylcholine from the myenteric plexus, thereby increasing transit time. Gastrointestinal tract transit time appeared to be modified by morphine in a study of the effects of antidiarrheal drugs.[1] Intestinal myoelectrical activity is substantially suppressed in all segments of the intestinal tract by morphine administration.[37] CNS excitation secondary to morphine administration may play a role in mediating the drug's effect on intestinal function, as has been reported in other species.[24]

A further complication from the use of opioids is the increased risk of postoperative colic, presumably a result of opioid-suppression of normal gut motility. Postoperative colic is more likely to occur with higher doses, and probably with prolonged systemic administration. However, the etiology of postoperative colic is not fully understood; it is likely to be multifactorial, depending also on factors such as preoperative starvation and the administration of other drugs around the time of surgery.

Epidural morphine at a dose of 0.2 mg/kg temporarily reduces gastrointestinal motility but does not cause ileus or colic.[40] One must weigh the negative effects of epidural morphine against the inhibitory effects of pain on gastrointestinal motility through activating a spinal reflex that induces sympathetic hyperactivity.

In ponies and horses, morphine administration (when given alone) elicits increased locomotor activity, signs of apprehension, pawing, headshaking, and restlessness.[8] However, the role of CNS opioid receptors in alteration of gastrointestinal tract function remains unknown. Morphine is a primary μ-receptor agonist that is associated with severe adverse behavioral, cardiovascular, and gastrointestinal tract effects in horses.[34]

Primary κ agonists induce analgesia with little locomotor and sympathetic stimulation. The greater the selectivity for κ receptors, the more favorable the ratio of analgesia to locomotor effects in horses.[19] However κ agonists (e.g., butorphanol) when administered alone to horses can induce headshaking. To avoid this stereotyping behavior an alpha-2 agonist is indicated before administration of butorphanol.

Intravenous lidocaine

Mechanism of action

Lidocaine hydrochloride has variable properties. It reduces the concentration of circulating catecholamines by suppressing the sympathoadrenal responses; suppresses activity of the primary afferent neurons involved in reflex inhibition of gut motility; stimulates smooth muscle directly; and decreases the inflammatory response (alleviating pain).[25]

Lidocaine exerts its analgesic properties by decreasing afferent traffic through small C fibers. The plasma levels necessary for analgesia are much lower than those required to block normal peripheral nerve conduction. Lidocaine has also been shown to decrease reperfusion injury by inhibiting the release of free radicals and decreasing the migration of neutrophils at the site of injury. Experimentally, serosal damage, intestinal distention, endotoxemia, peritonitis, and surgical manipulation have all been associated with enhanced sympathetic stimulation. Lidocaine IV may prevent reflexive inhibition caused by one or several of these factors by blocking transmission through afferent nerves. These factors have been documented to increase the release of nonadrenergic and noncholinergic neurotransmitters with alteration in motility in rats and dogs. Lidocaine may inhibit the release of neurotransmitters rather than alter sympathetic neurotransmission.

Clinical use

Lidocaine IV has been used in horses with colic primarily to treat ileus,[21,25] but is also thought to potentially have favorable analgesic properties. Lidocaine also can have anti-inflammatory action, anti-dysrhythmogenic effect, can provide protection against endotoxemia (e.g., reduction TNF-α production), protection against ischemic and reperfusion injury, reduction in LPS-induced leukocyte-endothelial cell adhesion, and reduction in LPS-induced macromolecular leakage from vasculature.

Lidocaine IV was initially incorporated into the treatment regimen for perioperative colic patients as a visceral analgesic and motility stimulant based on findings in human patients. However, soon after its use continuous infusion of lidocaine was found to actually increase the transit time of feces in normal horses[38] and while it was found to be a good somatic analgesic it did not provide visceral analgesia.[35] More recently, important findings with regards to the beneficial role of IV lidocaine for treating postoperative colic patients include attenuation of ischemia-reperfusion injury in an *in vivo* jejunal model through an anti-inflammatory effect and by ameliorating the inhibitory effects of flunixin meglumine on restoration of the mucosal barrier,[9,10] improvement in smooth muscle contractility and basic cell function following ischemia-reperfusion injury,[15] and a decrease in postoperative ileus in clinical studies of colic patients.[25,46] Lidocaine IV use was associated with decreased postoperative ileus (odds ratio 0.25 [95% confidence interval 0.11–0.56]) and improved short-term survival (odds ration 3.33

[1.02–11.1) in postoperative colic patients.[46] Of the lidocaine-treated horses, 65% stopped refluxing within 30 h whereas 27% of the saline-treated horses stopped within 30 h.[25] Compared with placebo, IV lidocaine treatment resulted in shorter hospitalization time for survivors, equivalent survival to discharge, no clinically significant changes in physical or laboratory variables, and no difference in the rate of incisional infections, jugular thrombosis, laminitis, or diarrhea.[25] Postoperative colic patients treated with IV lidocaine had better jejunal motility based on sonographic examination compared to untreated horses.[7] Therefore, clinical benefit with the use of IV lidocaine has been demonstrated in multiple studies and its beneficial effect is likely though minimizing ischemia-reperfusion injury and inflammation.

Lidocaine IV is typically used postoperatively in horses with strangulating intestinal lesions. The dose rate is 1.3 mg/kg bolus given over 15 min followed by 0.05 mg/kg/min CRI. A fluid pump should be used to administer IV lidocaine to decrease the risk of toxicity (see Adverse effects and contraindications).

When IV lidocaine is intended to be used during general anesthesia, it provides two important properties, analgesia and MAC reduction of volatile anesthetics (by 25–50% depending of the dosage used).[12] Doses recommended are slightly higher than for standing sedation. An initial IV bolus of 2 mg/kg (administered slowly over 10–15 min) can be followed by a continuous IV infusion at a rate of 0.05–0.1 mg/kg/min. It is recommended that lidocaine should be discontinued 30 min before taking the horse to recovery.[48] This is due to the fact that the horse under general anesthesia has a slower metabolism of the drug (decreased hepatic blood flow) and may wake up very disoriented and ataxic if this is not performed.

Adverse effects and contraindications

The likelihood of systemic toxicity with IV lidocaine is related to its plasma concentration. There may also be an increase in incisional infection with its use. We have recently found that there was no association between infection and IV lidocaine use; however, duration of lidocaine use was associated with postoperative infection in colic

patients and in particular incisional infection. Duration of IV lidocaine use was not surprisingly correlated with duration of postoperative reflux and withholding feed which are likely confounding factors.[13]

CNS effects

Low concentrations of IV lidocaine are sedating. Increasing concentrations can result in muscle twitching (fasciculations) and ataxia; the horse may become recumbent temporarily. Seizures (originating in the amygdala) occur at higher doses. Administration of sedatives causes a right shift in dose–response curve. The adverse CNS effects are unlikely to occur under anesthesia. Treatment of seizures using benzodiazepines or thiopental is usually not warranted because seizure activity ceases rapidly once lidocaine administration is stopped.

Cardiovascular effects

Cardiovascular effects occur at higher plasma concentrations than do CNS effects. It results from a delay in impulse transmission by Na^+ channel blockade. This leads to decreased myocardial contractility, vasodilation, and cardiac dysrhythmias. The cardiovascular effects can be seen when animals are under general anesthesia. The treatment of cardiac toxicity can be unrewarding. It is fairly unresponsive to inotropes (e.g., dobutamine) and parasympatholytic drugs (e.g., atropine). Lidocaine infusion should be stopped.

Hyoscine-N-butylbromide

Mechanism of action

Hyoscine-N-butylbromide (Buscopan®) is a derivative of the belladonna alkaloids and causes a spasmolytic effect by blocking the muscarinic acetylcholine receptors of the gastrointestinal tract.[36]

Clinical use

Hyoscine-N-butylbromide is used in horses for alleviation of colic pain through its spasmolytic effects. It is typically used for treatment gas colic and impactions. It is also considered to be beneficial for relaxing the rectum to facilitate palpation.

Hyoscine-N-butylbromide is used in combination dipyrone (metamizole sodium, NSAID of the pyrazolone group) (Buscopan Compositum®) in non-US countries; however, dipyrone has been banned by the United States Federal Drug Administration because of its association with myelotoxicity and development of agranulocytosis. The dose rate of hyoscine-N-butylbromide is 0.3 mg/kg IV.

The effects of hyoscine-N-butylbromide on intestinal motility and visceral analgesia have been variable. In a cecal balloon-dilation colic model, hyoscine-N-butylbromide and hyoscine-N-butylbromide-dipyrone eliminated cecal contractions within 30 s of administration and for approximately 20 min; however, there was no consistent or significant effect on pain relief.[36] In a duodenal and colorectal distention colic model, neither hyoscine-N-butylbromide nor acepromazine or butorphanol had any effect on duodenal distention threshold or duodenal motility. The colorectal distention threshold did increase from 5 to 65 min after hyoscine-N-butylbromide administration; however, overall there were no consistent anti-nociceptive effects observed.[39] On the other hand, administration of hyoscine-N-butylbromide-dipyrone caused a rapid and significant reduction of duodenal, cecal, and left ventral colon contractions evaluated sonographically. Cecal and left ventral colon contractions return to normal after 30 min whereas duodenal contractions did not return to normal until after 120 min. It was concluded that hyoscine-N-butylbromide-dipyrone at its therapeutic dosage has an immediate, potent, short-lived inhibitory effect on cecum and left ventral colon contractions but a minor, longer effect on the duodenal contractions supporting its use for gas and impaction colic.[14] Repeated short-interval administration was not recommended.[14]

Buscopan® decreased rectal pressure and the number of rectal strains compared to intrarectal administration of 50 mL of 2% lidocaine and IV and intrarectal saline indicating that Buscopan® improves the quality and safety of examination per rectum in horses.[23]

Adverse effects and contraindications

Cardiovascular effects of hyoscine-N-butylbromide have been observed clinically and documented experimentally in normal horses.[30,39] Heart rate (sinus tachycardia) and blood pressure are increased immediately following administration of hyoscine-N-butylbromide (0.3 mg/kg IV) or hyoscine-N-butylbromide with xylazine (0.25 mg/kg IV).[30] Peak heart rate (86 ± 2 beats/min) occurred at 5 min following administration and the effect lasted for 50 min. Similarly, an increase in mean arterial blood pressure persisted for 25 min after administration with the peak occurring at 1–2 min (115 ± 7.4 mmHg). Ventricular tachycardia was identified in one horse following hyoscine-N-butylbromide and xylazine administration.[30] Therefore, care should be taken when using hyoscine-N-butylbromide in horses with clinical evidence of cardiovascular compromise and with interpretation of heart rate following administration.

Hyoscine-N-butylbromide can also cause signs of colic with repeated use or high doses. Its use is not recommended in the management of postoperative colic patients.

References

1. Alexander, F. (1978) The effect of some anti-diarrhoeal drugs on intestinal transit and faecal excretion of water and electrolytes in the horse. *Equine Veterinary Journal*, **10**, 229–234.
2. Ansah, O.B. (2004) Use of the alpha-2-adrenoceptor agonists medetomidine and dexmedetomidine in the sedation and analgesia of domestic cats. University of Helsinki, Helsinki, Finland. http://ethesis.helsinki.fi/julkaisut/ela/kliin/vk/ ansah/useofthe.pdf
3. Bennett, R.C. & Steffey, E.P. (2002) Use of opioids for pain and anesthetic management in horses. *Veterinary Clinics of North America: Equine Practice*, **18**, 47–60.
4. Bettschart-Wolfensberger, R., Jäggin-Schmucker, N., Lendl, C., Bettschart, R.W. & Clarke, K.W. (2001) Minimal alveolar concentration of desflurane in combination with an infusion of medetomidine for the anaesthesia of ponies. *Veterinary Record*, **148**, 264–267.
5. Blikslager, A.T., Roberts, M.C. & Argenzio, R.A. (1999) Prostaglandin-induced recovery of barrier function in porcine ileum is triggered by chloride secretion. *American Journal of Physiology*, **276**, G28–G36.

6. Blikslager, A.T., Moeser, A.J., Gookin, J.L., Jones, S.L. & Odle, J. (2007) Restoration of barrier function in injured intestinal mucosa. *Physiological Reviews*, **87**, 545–564.

7. Brianceau, P., Chevalier, H., Karas, A., *et al.* (2002) Intravenous lidocaine and small-intestinal size, abdominal fluid, and outcome after colic surgery in horses. *Journal of Veterinary Internal Medicine*, **16**, 736–741.

8. Combie, J., Dougherty, J., Nugent, E. & Tobin, T. (1979) Pharmacology of narcotic analgesics in the horse. Dose and time response relationships for behavioral-responses to morphine, meperidine, mentazocine, anileridine, methadone, and hydromorphone. *Journal of Equine Medicine and Surgery*, **3**, 377–385.

9. Cook, V.L., Jones Shults, J., McDowell, M., Campbell, N.B., Davis, J.L. & Blikslager, A.T. (2008) Attenuation of ischaemic injury in the equine jejunum by administration of systemic lidocaine. *Equine Veterinary Journal*, **40**, 353–357.

10. Cook, V.L., Jones Shults, J., McDowell, M.R., *et al.* (2009) Anti-inflammatory effects of intravenously administered lidocaine hydrochloride on ischemia-injured jejunum in horses. *American Journal of Veterinary Research*, **70**, 1259–1268.

11. Cook, V.L., Meyer, C.T., Campbell, N.B. & Blikslager, A.T. (2009) Effect of firocoxib or flunixin meglumine on recovery of ischemic-injured equine jejunum. *American Journal of Veterinary Research*, **70**, 992–1000.

12. Dzikiti, T.B., Hellebrekers, L.J. & van Dijk, P. (2003) Effects of intravenous lidocaine on isoflurane concentration, physiological parameters, metabolic parameters and stress-related hormones in horses undergoing surgery. *Journal of Veterinary Medicine A: Physiology, Pathology, Clinical Medicine*, **50**, 190–195.

13. Freeman, K.D., Southwood, L.L., Lane, J., Lindborg, S. & Aceto, H.W. (2012) Post operative infection, pyrexia, and perioperative antimicrobial drug use in surgical colic patients. *Equine Veterinary Journal*, 2011 Dec 11 doi:10.1111/j.2042-3306.2011.00515.x.[Epub ahead of print]

14. Gomaa, N., Uhlig, A. & Schusser, G.F. (2011) Effect of Buscopan compositum on the motility of the duodenum, cecum and left ventral colon in healthy conscious horses. *Berliner und Munchener Tierarztliche Wochenschrift*, **124**, 168–174.

15. Guschlbauer, M., Hoppe, S., Geburek, F., Feige, K. & Huber, K. (2010) In vitro effects of lidocaine on the contractility of equine jejunal smooth muscle challenged by ischaemia-reperfusion injury. *Equine Veterinary Journal*, **42**, 53–58.

16. Hubbell, J.A.E. (1999) Recovery from anaesthesia in horses. *Equine Veterinary Education*, **11**, 160–167.

17. Johnson, C.B., Taylor. P.M., Young, S.S. & Brearley, J.C. (1993) Postoperative analgesia using phenylbutazone, flunixin or carprofen in horses. *Veterinary Record*, **133**, 336–338.

18. Kalpravidh, M., Lumb, W.V., Wright, M. & Heath, R.B. (1984) Analgesic effects of butorphanol in horses: Dose-response studies. *American Journal of Veterinary Research*, **45**, 211–216.

19. Kamerling, S. (1988) Dose related effects of the kappa agonist U-50, 488H on behaviour, nociception and autonomic response in the horse. *Equine Veterinary Journal*, **20**, 114–118.

20. Kendall, A., Mosley, C. & Bröjer, J. (2010) Tachypnea and antipyresis in febrile horses after sedation with alpha-agonists. *Journal of Veterinary Internal Medicine*, **24**, 1008–1011.

21. Koenig, J. & Cote, N. (2006) Equine gastrointestinal motility—Ileus and pharmacological modification. *Canadian Veterinary Journal*, **47**, 551–559.

22. Little, D., Brown, S.A., Campbell, N.B., Moeser, A.J., Davis, J.L. & Blikslager, A.T. (2007) Effects of the cyclooxygenase inhibitor meloxicam on recovery of ischemia-injured equine jejunum. *American Journal of Veterinary Research*, **68**, 614–624.

23. Luo, T., Bertone, J.J., Greene, H.M. & Wickler, S.J. (2006) A comparison of N-butylscopolammonium and lidocaine for control of rectal pressure in horses. *Veterinary Therapeutics*, **7**, 243–248.

24. Mach, T. (2004) The brain-gut axis in irritable bowel syndrome—Clinical aspects. *Medical Science Monitor*, **10**, RA125–RA131.

25. Malone, E., Ensink, J., Turner, T., *et al.* (2006) Intravenous continuous infusion of lidocaine for treatment of equine ileus. *Veterinary Surgery*, **35**, 60–66.

26. Marshall, J.F. & Blikslager, A.T. (2011) The effect of nonsteroidal anti-inflammatory drugs on the equine intestine. *Equine Veterinary Journal*, **43** (Suppl 39), 140–144.

27. Matyjaszek, S.A., Morton, A.J., Freeman, D.E., Grosche, A., Polyak, M.M.R. & Kuck, H. (2009) Effects of flunixin meglumine on recovery of colonic mucosa from ischemia in horses. *American Journal of Veterinary Research*, **70**, 236–246.

28. McConnico, R.S., Morgan, T.W., Williams, C.C., Hubert, J.D. & Moore, R.M. (2008) Pathophysiologic effects of phenylbutazone on the right dorsal colon in horses. *American Journal of Veterinary Research*, **69**, 1496–1505.

29. Menozzi, A., Pozzoli, C., Poli, E., *et al.* (2009) Effects of nonselective and selective cyclooxygenase inhibitors on small intestinal motility in the horse. *Research in Veterinary Science*, **86**, 129–135.

30. Morton, A.J., Varney, C.R., Ekiri, A.B. & Grosche, A. (2011) Cardiovascular effects of N-butylsco-

polammonium bromide and xylazine in horses. *Equine Veterinary Journal*, **43** (Suppl 39), 117–122.

31. Muir, W.W. & Robertson, J.T. (1985) Visceral analgesia: Effects of xylazine, butorphanol, meperidine, and pentazocine in horses. *American Journal of Veterinary Research*, **46**, 2081–2084.

32. Orsini, J.A. (1988) Butorphanol tartrate: Pharmacology and clinical indications. *Compendium of Continuing Education for the Veterinary Practitioner*, **10**, 849–855.

33. Peek, S.F., Semrad, S.D. & Perkins, G.A. (2003) Clostridial myonecrosis in horses (37 cases 1985–2000). *Equine Veterinary Journal*, **35**, 86–92.

34. Roberts, M.C. & Argenzio, A. (1986) Effects of amitraz, several opiate derivatives and anticholinergic agents on intestinal transit in ponies. *Equine Veterinary Journal*, **18**, 256–260.

35. Robertson, S.A., Sanchez, L.C., Merritt, A.M. & Doherty, T.J. (2005) Effect of systemic lidocaine on visceral and somatic nociception in conscious horses. *Equine Veterinary Journal*, **37**, 122–127.

36. Roelvink, M.E.J., Goossens, L., Kalsbeek, H.C. & Wensing. T.H. (1991) Analgesic and spasmolytic effects of dipyrone, hyoscine-N-butylbromide and a combination of the two in ponies. *Veterinary Record*, **129**, 378–380.

37. Roger, T., Bardon, T. & Ruckebusch, Y. (1985) Colonic motor responses in the pony: Relevance of colonic stimulation by opiate antagonists. *American Journal of Veterinary Research*, **46**, 31–35.

38. Rusiecki, K.E., Nieto, J.E., Puchalski, S.M. & Snyder, J.R. (2008) Evaluation of continuous infusion of lidocaine on gastrointestinal tract function in normal horses. *Veterinary Surgery*, **37**, 564–570.

39. Sanchez, L.C., Elfenbein, J.R. & Robertson, S.A. (2008) Effect of acepromazine, butorphanol, or N-butylscopolammonium bromide on visceral and somatic nociception and duodenal motility in conscious horses. *American Journal of Veterinary Research*, **69**, 579–585.

40. Sano, H., Martin-Flores, M., Santos, L.C., Cheetham, J., Araos, J.D. & Gleed, R.D. (2011) Effects of epidural morphine on gastrointestinal transit in unmedicated horses. *Veterinary Anaesthesia and Analgesia*, **38**, 121–126.

41. Sellon, D.C., Roberts, M.C., Blikslager, A.T., Ulibarri, C. & Papich, M.G. (2004) Effects of continuous rate intravenous infusion of butorphanol on physiologic and outcome variables in horses after celiotomy. *Journal of Veterinary Internal Medicine*, **18**, 555–563.

42. Steffey, E.P. & Pascoe, P.J. (2002) Detomidine reduces isoflurane anesthetic requirement (MAC) in horses. *Veterinary Anaesthesia and Analgesia*, **29**, 223–227.

43. Steffey, E.P., Pascoe, P.J., Woliner, M.J., Berryman, E.R. (2000) Effects of xylazine hydrochloride during isoflurane-induced anesthesia in horses. *American Journal of Veterinary Research*, **61**, 1225–1231.

44. Tomlinson, J.E. & Blikslager, A.T. (2005) Effects of cyclooxygenase inhibitors flunixin and deracoxib on permeability of ischaemic-injured equine jejunum. *Equine Veterinary Journal*, **37**, 75–80.

45. Tomlinson, J.E., Wilder, B.O., Young, K.M. & Blikslager, A.T. (2004) Effects of ischemia and the cyclooxygenase inhibitor flunixin on in vitro passage of lipopolysaccharide across equine jejunum. *American Journal of Veterinary Research*, **65**, 1377–1383.

46. Torfs, S., Delesalle, C., Dewulf, J., Devisscher, L. & Deprez, P. (2009) Risk factors for equine postoperative ileus and effectiveness of prophylactic lidocaine. *Journal of Veterinary Internal Medicine*, **23**, 606–611.

47. Valverde, A. & Gunkel, C.I. (2005) Pain management in horses and farm animals. *Journal of Veterinary Emergency and Critical Care*, **15**, 295–307.

48. Valverde, A., Gunkelt, C., Doherty, T.J., Giguère, S. & Pollak, A.S. (2005) Effect of a constant rate infusion of lidocaine on the quality of recovery from sevoflurane or isoflurane general anaesthesia in horses. *Equine Veterinary Journal*, **37**, 559–564.

49. Van Hoogmoed, L.M., Rakestraw, P.C., Snyder, J.R. & Harmon, F. (1999) In vitro effects of nonsteroidal anti-inflammatory agents and prostaglandins I2, E2, and F2 alpha on contractility of taenia of the large colon of horses. *American Journal of Veterinary Research*, **60**, 1004–1009.

50. Van Hoogmoed, L.M., Snyder, J.R. & Harmon, F. (2000) In vitro investigation of the effect of prostaglandins and nonsteroidal anti-inflammatory drugs on contractile activity of the equine smooth muscle of the dorsal colon, ventral colon, and pelvic flexure. *American Journal of Veterinary Research*, **61**, 1259–1266.

7 Enteral Fluid Therapy

Jennifer A. Brown[1] and Samantha K. Hart[2]

[1]Veterinary Relief, Surgical, and Consulting Services, Tampa, FL, USA
[2]Department of Clinical Studies, New Bolton Center, School of Veterinary Medicine, University of Pennsylvania, Kennett Square, PA, USA

Chapter Outline

Indications	62	**Technique**	66
Transit and absorption of fluids and electrolytes	62	Intermittent boluses	66
		Continuous infusion	66
Indications	63	**Complications**	67
Contraindications	64	Colic	67
Preparation	64	Electrolyte disturbances	68
Composition of enteral fluids	64	Diarrhea	68
		Nasogastric tube-associated problems	68

Indications

Although intravenous (IV) fluids remain the primary route of fluid administration in the equine patient with colic, prudent use of enteral fluid therapy can be an important adjunct or alternative treatment. Use of enteral fluids is a low-cost, effective means of treating certain types of colic in the horse. Additionally, the enteral route can be used as a method of rehydration, electrolyte supplementation, and laxative administration. An understanding of the physiology pertaining to enteral fluid therapy is important to relate to indications for its use in the colic patient.

Transit and absorption of fluids and electrolytes

Within minutes of entering the stomach, fluids will rapidly move into and through the small intestine. Gastric emptying of oral rehydration solutions in the adult horse occurs in approximately 15 min.[17] Evaluation of gastrointestinal (GI) transit time has shown that fluids will move from the stomach, through the small intestine, and into the cecum from 30 min to 2 h postadministration.[2,3] When moving from the cecum to the right ventral colon, the transit rate of fluids significantly decreases,

---

Practical Guide to Equine Colic, First Edition. Edited by Louise L. Southwood.
© 2013 John Wiley & Sons, Inc. Published 2013 by John Wiley & Sons, Inc.

with liquid markers taking up to 5h to exit the cecum.[3] From there it can be up to 50h before they exit the large (ascending) colon. This abrupt decrease in transit time is due to the large intestine being the primary site of digestion and water absorption in the horse. Rather than the rapid peristalsis and propulsive motility observed in the small intestine, in the large intestine mixing, propulsion, and retropulsion occur in order to provide adequate time for microbial digestion and absorption of water and electrolytes. It would be expected that enteral fluids administered to a horse with normal motility will move out of the stomach quickly to the sites of the most fluid absorption, the distal small intestine and the large intestine.

The GI tract motility often will be compromised by the cause of colic and potentially by some of the treatments. Functional or mechanical obstructions anywhere along the GI tract will affect transit and can impair the ability to utilize enteral therapies for rehydration. This, however, is generally not a problem for horses with an impaction, for example. Commonly used sedatives and analgesics in the colic patient such as xylazine, detomidine, and butorphanol have been shown to decrease motility in the horse (p. 54, 55).[13,15,18] However, it is unknown how clinically important their effect is on slowing enteral fluid transit. Altered motility does not always preclude the use of enteral fluid therapy, depending on the goal of its use, but it should be taken into consideration.

Intestinal absorption of water is entirely by diffusion.[1] Tied to osmotic changes from sodium transport, water molecules primarily move between the cells through the tight junctions of the intestinal epithelium into the paracellular space, and then across the basolateral membrane into the circulation. Sodium transport is along an electrochemical gradient into the cell, and chloride ions are cotransported with sodium ions. This is an active process relying on the Na^+/K^+ ATPase, ultimately resulting in the movement of ions into the circulation. Bicarbonate ions are secreted and absorbed in varying amounts along the small intestine in exchange for chloride. A considerable amount of bicarbonate is present in the fluids transported into to the large intestine as a buffer for volatile fatty acid absorption.

Each day the large intestine of the horse absorbs a fluid volume equal to its extracellular fluid volume.[3] The cecum and ventral colon are responsible for a majority of the net water absorption of the large intestine, followed by the small and dorsal colons, respectively.[3] In the large intestine, water absorption is driven by sodium transport as well as the absorption of volatile fatty acids present in the ingesta. Sodium absorption is predominantly via a Na^+-H^+ transport mechanism, as well as by diffusion along the electrochemical gradient. Unlike in the small intestine, where sodium is controlled by local electrochemical gradients, in the large colon sodium absorption is also under the influence of aldosterone, especially when the patient is dehydrated. As with changes in motility, some pathology related to colic may also affect the absorption of water and electrolytes from the intestine. For example, inflammation or damage to the GI mucosa may inhibit absorption of fluids and electrolytes when administered orally.

Indications

A benefit of enteral fluid therapy is cost. Treating the colic patient can incur considerable expense for the owner, and often veterinarians are faced with economic issues in making treatment decisions. Basic IV fluid administration (p. 99) requires catheter and supplies, fluid administration sets, fluids suitable for IV administration, and continuous monitoring of fluid rates and the catheter sites to avoid serious complications. Alternate methods of administering fluids that are not only effective but less expensive may be an important and practical consideration for some patients.

The primary indication for use of enteral fluid therapy in horses is in the management of colonic impactions (p. 217). Impactions of the GI tract are a commonly encountered cause of colic in horses. Although most frequently identified in the large colon, impactions are also seen in the stomach (p. 205), ileum (p. 208), and small (descending) colon (p. 221). Impactions are often amenable to medical therapy, and the use of enteral fluids can be a valuable treatment option. A traditional approach to the management of impactions has included the use of both IV fluids and enteral fluids. In these cases, IV fluids are used primarily to maintain systemic hydration of the patient rather than to hydrate the GI contents. However, if the patient appears to be systemically healthy with no apparent fluid deficits, there is no need to administer IV fluids. There does not appear to be a difference in the time to resolution of impactions whether or not IV fluids are administered,[7,14] and the cost is significantly decreased when enteral fluids are used alone.[7] One of the most important factors in resolution of impactions is the large enteral fluid volume necessary, which is often the limiting factor when managing these cases on the farm.

Recently, the use of enteral fluids in the management of large colon displacements (p. 219, 220) has been reported.[14] Although the precise etiology of colonic displacements continues to elude us, it is possible that changes in motility, or an impaction with secondary gas accumulation, contribute to the development of the displacement. Reportedly, 83% of displacements resolved with medical management.[14] Although enteral fluids may not result in resolution of all displacements encountered, use of enteral fluids is a logical first treatment choice. Enteral fluids not only stimulate the gastrocolic reflex and increase GI motility, but also increase the water content of the ingesta and aid in resolution of any impaction that may be present. It is important to recognize that a definitive diagnosis of colonic displacement is difficult without surgery and some of the horses reported to be managed medically may not in fact have had a colonic displacement. Careful monitoring of horses with a suspected displacement is necessary during medical management. See Chapter 15 on Medical versus Surgical Treatment of the Horse with Colic (p. 164).

Enteral fluids using a balanced electrolyte solution may also be an effective adjunct treatment in the management of acute colitis. Although the GI tract is often inflamed, and intestinal absorption may be decreased, the use of low volumes of enteral fluids in conjunction with IV fluids may be useful in maintaining electrolyte balance and preventing villous atrophy.

When the GI tract is relatively normal, there is no nasogastric reflux, and mild hypovolemia and dehydration are evident (e.g., mild colic), enteral fluids can be an effective method of replacing fluid and electrolyte deficits.

Contraindications

Enteral fluid therapy is contraindicated in cases of ileus, when reflux is obtained with nasogatric intubation (p. 38), in severely dehydrated/ hypovolemic animals, or patients with signs of shock (p. 101). When ileus is present, which is usually indicated by nasogastric reflux or lack of motility on abdominal sonographic examination (p. 128), fluids given orally are not likely pass out of the stomach and small intestine. Distending the stomach and small intestine with additional fluids will contribute to colic signs and fail to correct any fluid losses or soften impacted ingesta.

Although the absorption of fluids administered orally in normal horses has been shown to be rapid, horses which are severely hypovolemic or dehydrated will not have adequate absorption of enterally administered fluids. The GI tract is a highly vascular organ and hypovolemia leads to decreases in blood flow, which in turn affects perfusion. Additionally, in patients in shock, blood flow is actively redistributed from the splanchnic circulation to vital organs. This not only affects perfusion of the GI tract, but also has potential effects on motility. In these cases, the use of IV fluids is warranted; however, enteral fluids may be considered once the patient is stable.

Preparation

The equipment needed for enteral fluid administration will depend on whether fluids will be administered by continuous infusion or via intermittent boluses. A list of "Things you will need" is provided in Table 7.1.

Composition of enteral fluids

Plain warm tap water can be used as a source of enteral fluids with caution. Tap water is a hypotonic solution relative to the GI environment, and it contains few if any electrolytes. While it may aid in correcting mild dehydration, it should not be used in horses with severe dehydration or electrolyte imbalances. Electrolytes are normally provided in the feed and tap water may be appropriate when the patient is able to eat. In cases of impaction colic, where feeding is restricted, tap water alone should not be used because it causes hyponatremia and does little to increase the water content of ingesta in the right dorsal colon.[11] Use of plain tap water was less efficient for replacing fluid deficits and restoring body weight after exercise and dehydration compared to a balanced electrolyte solution.[12]

Table 7.1 Things you will need for enteral fluid administration.

Intermittent bolus	● Nose twitch
	● Nasogastric tube
	● 10–15 L bucket with about 5 L plain warm water and empty bucket to check for reflux
	● Dose syringe or pump (reflux check)
	● Electrolytes or laxatives to add to plain warm water once the horse has been checked for reflux
	● Funnel (fluid administration)
Continuous infusion	● Nose twitch
	● Nasogastric tube or feeding tube
	● 10–15 L bucket with about 5 L plain warm water and empty bucket to check for reflux
	● Dose syringe or pump (reflux check)
	● Fluid administration set (may require a Christmas tree connection)
	● Carboy or 5 L fluid bags

Several oral rehydration solutions have been evaluated for use in horses following exercise,[4] but only two have been evaluated either clinically or experimentally for treatment of horses with colic or their affects on softening impactions and fecal matter.[9–11,14] In one study, an isotonic solution made with 6 g of sodium chloride (NaCl) and 3 g of potassium chloride (KCl) per liter of water was used to treat horses with large colon impaction (p. 217) or colonic displacement (p. 219, 220).[14] This solution contained additional potassium to address hypokalemia that can arise with colonic impactions. Experimentally, Lopes and colleagues compared IV fluid therapy, magnesium and sodium sulfate, tap water, and a balanced electrolyte solution on water content of the ingesta, systemic hydration, and electrolyte balance.[11] The balanced electrolyte solution increased the water content of ingesta in the right dorsal colon and fecal matter and did not result in any systemic electrolyte abnormalities compared to tap water and the laxative solutions.[11]

The ideal enteral fluid solution should be formulated so that its constituents closely resemble the electrolyte concentration and tonicity of plasma. Several recipes exist; however, the one based on Lopes' work offers a balanced solution and is easy to prepare (Tables 7.2 and 7.3). Enteral fluid therapy may be tailored to the individual patient by increasing or decreasing a particular electrolyte.

Table 7.2 Recipe for making a balanced electrolyte solution.

	Formulation	g/L water	Teaspoons/L water	mL/L water
NaCl	Table salt	4.9 g	0.75 tsp	3.75 mL
KCl	Lite salt (50:50 NaCl:KCl)	0.74 g	0.074 tsp	0.38 mL
NaHCO3	Baking soda	3.8 g	1 tsp	5 mL

This recipe utilizes Lite salt for the source of KCl in the final solution.
Source: Based on Lopes et al. (2004).

Table 7.3 Recipe for making a balanced electrolyte solution.

	Formulation	g/L water	Teaspoons/L water	mL/L water
NaCl	Table salt	6.0 g	1 tsp	5 mL
KCl	KCL salt (pure)	0.3 g	0.03 tsp	0.15 mL
NaHCO$_3$	Baking soda	3.4 g	1 tsp	5 mL

This recipe utilizes pure KCl salt for the source of the KCl in the final solution.
Source: Based on Lopes et al. (2004).

Based on the etiopathology of the colic (e.g., colonic impaction [p. 217] versus colitis [p. 215]) and suspected or confirmed electrolyte imbalances, the constituents of the solution can be modified.

Laxatives or cathartics can be another component of enteral fluid therapy, particularly in horses with large colon impactions. Cathartics work to either increase the water content within the colon, soften the impacted feces, or facilitate movement of impacted ingesta from the colon. The three main cathartics used in equine patients are magnesium or sodium sulfate, mineral oil, and dioctyl sodium sulfosuccinate (DSS).

Magnesium sulfate (Epsom salts) and sodium sulfate are osmotic cathartics. Both have been shown to increase the water content of the feces; however, sodium sulfate was also shown to increase the water content of ingesta in the right dorsal colon, where magnesium sulfate had no effect.[11] Availability of sodium sulfate and its cost compared to magnesium sulfate makes its use in practice less attractive even though it appears to be a more effective laxative. Magnesium sulfate may be most effective to use in cases of small colon impaction, as it appears to have the most effect on fecal water content.

Mineral oil is thought to act as a lubricating agent for fecal matter, and studies have shown that it also has an effect on the formation of feces. In normal horses administered 10 mL/kg (5 L for a 500 kg horse) twice at a 12 h interval, all horses had unformed feces between 18 and 24 h.[16] Another useful property of mineral oil is its indigestibility. Because it passes through the GI tract unchanged, it can be a reasonable marker of transit. In a normal horse, it should be noted in the feces within 12–24 h after administration; however, when administered to horses with a colonic impaction this transit time may be prolonged. It is possible that mineral oil can pass around an impaction, resulting in mineral oil only being passed from the rectum. When it is observed mixed with fecal matter, this is an indication that some of the ingesta are mixing with the mineral oil and being passed in association with pending resolution of the impaction. Mineral oil is a relatively benign substance, but should only be administered after assuring correct placement of the nasogastric tube into the stomach. Aspiration or accidental administration into the lungs will result in a severe and fatal pneumonia.

DSS is an anionic surfactant commonly used in human medicine as a stool softener (Colace®). It acts by decreasing the surface tension of the ingesta to allow for water to penetrate the fecal mass thereby softening it. In horses there is a limited margin of safety when used, and doses exceeding 65 mg/kg have caused severe complications and death. It is contraindicated to use DSS in any horse with systemic fluid or electrolyte abnormalities as it also acts to stimulate the secretory activities of the small intestine and inhibit absorption of fluids from the distal small intestine. It is recommended that DSS should not be administered concurrently with mineral oil because it may allow for absorption of the mineral oil. However, the importance of systemic absorption of mineral oil is unknown in horses.

Technique

Intermittent boluses

Administration of fluid boluses is typically performed through a standard nasogastric tube (p. 38) in lieu of a continuous rate infusion. Nasogastric tubes can be left in place so that they do not have to be replaced multiple times to administer fluids. The equine stomach has a volume of up to 18 L and boluses of up to 8–10 L every 2 h has shown to be well tolerated.[14] However, the amount of enteral fluids that can be bolused will vary between horses, as some are less tolerant of gastric distention than others. The stomach must be checked for nasogastric reflux prior to administration of each enteral fluid bolus whether the nasogastric tube is left in place or not. Reflux can begin at any time point during treatment. Retrieval of previously administered fluids may be an indication of ileus or intolerance of the enteral fluids. If reflux is obtained, the horse should be checked again in 2–4 h. If at this time <2 L of gastric contents are obtained, enteral boluses can be resumed with careful patient monitoring.

Continuous infusion

Continuous infusions of enteral fluids can also administered using an indwelling nasogastric

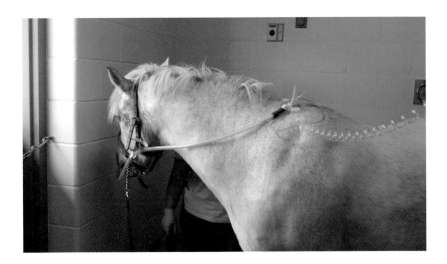

Figure 7.1

tube (Figure 7.1). This can either be via a standard large-bore tube or a small-diameter enteral feeding tube (Veterinary Enteral Feeding Tubes, Mila International, Inc., Florence, Kentucky, USA) as is used with foals. The small-diameter enteral feeding tubes can be difficult to place and maintain and endoscopy may be required to guide placement. The advantage of these feeding tubes, however, is that they are less traumatic to the pharynx, esophagus, and stomach, and the horse may tolerate eating with the tube in place.

Carboys or 5 L fluid bags are used to hold the fluids for continuous administration of an enteral solution. The balanced electrolyte solution can be prepared in a standard 10–20 L bucket and then using a nasogastric tube pumped into the carboy or poured through the top of the fluid bags that have been cut open. The bags are hung as for IV fluid administration to allow for gravity flow of the fluid. Used large-bore coiled IV administration sets are desirable to deliver the fluids to the nasogastric tube so that the fluid rates can be controlled. Other types of solution sets can be used, but it is necessary that the fluid rate is able to be controlled and that there be a large bore in order to deliver sufficient volume. These large-bore sets can be expensive, so to use a new set for enteral administration would be cost prohibitive. A good source for both used fluid bags and IV sets is the area equine referral hospital. Often this equipment is routinely disposed of immediately after IV use and the referral hospital may be amenable for you to recycle it for enteral use.

Once the nasogastric tube is in place and the fluids prepared and in position, the horse should be checked again for reflux before beginning enteral fluid therapy. If >2 L of reflux is obtained, then administration should be postponed. If there is no reflux obtained, starting fluid rates should be slow (1–3 L/h for a 500 kg/horse), to determine if the horse will tolerate enteral fluid therapy. Generally, enteral fluid administration is well tolerated. If after 1–2 h the patient is tolerating the fluids, the rate can be increased up to 5 L/h.

Horses should not be allowed to eat with a large-bore nasogastric tube in place because there is the risk of aspiration pneumonia.

Complications

Enteral fluid therapy can be a highly effective means of managing impactions and mild to moderate dehydration in horses; however, as with any treatment there is the risk of complications.

Colic

Mild colic is the most common complication associated with the use of enteral fluid therapy. In two recent retrospective studies on enteral fluid therapy in horses, 16% and 53% of horses showed signs of mild colic depending on the volume of fluids administered.[7,14] Horses showing signs of mild colic usually responded to discontinuation of the enteral fluids combined with walking and, if required, a single dose of an analgesic drug (p. 51). It has been proposed that mild colic is due to the enteral fluids stimulating the gastrocolic reflex, resulting in contraction of the large colon around the impaction. Some horses may be less tolerant of gastric distention associated with administration of large volumes of fluids irrespective of whether or not an impaction is present.[10] It is also important to keep in mind that horses being treated for an impaction that are receiving large volumes of enteral fluids can show signs of colic associated with the increasing fluid content and expansion of the impaction. It is important to check for nasogastric reflux if a horse that is receiving enteral fluids shows signs of colic. Although most horses tolerate enteral fluids, some can develop nasogastric reflux which is most likely due to compression of the stomach and/or small intestine by the impaction or ileus with delayed gastric emptying. These horses should also be examined via palpation per rectum (p. 22) to assess the consistency of the impaction and feces in the rectum and to determine if gas distention or colonic displacement is present.

Electrolyte disturbances

Horses that are evaluated for colic often have mild electrolyte imbalances, most commonly hypocalcemia and hypomagnesemia. Depending on the composition, administration of enteral fluids also has the potential to result in electrolyte disturbances. The administration of tap water is discouraged, as prolonged administration of this hypotonic solution has the potential to result in severe hyponatremia and hypochloremia. Use of 0.9% NaCl or hypertonic solutions should also be avoided, as these can result in hypernatremia and hyperchloremia. Although these electrolyte disturbances may be tolerated in horses with normal renal function, the potential for complications such as neurologic dysfunction should be

considered. However, even administration of an isotonic, balanced electrolyte solution still has the potential to result in mild electrolyte disturbances, most commonly hypocalcemia, hypokalemia, and hypomagnesemia, which typically resolve once the horse is refed.[10,14] Hypermagnesemia is an uncommon complication following magnesium sulfate administration,[8] which was likely associated with concurrent renal insufficiency, hypocalcemia, or compromise of GI mucosal integrity. It is, therefore, recommended that magnesium sulfate only be administered to horses which are not dehydrated or hypovolemic, that the dose not exceed 1 g/kg, and that it not be given more than twice a day.

Diarrhea

Although undesirable, diarrhea is a well-recognized sequela in horses that are treated with enteral fluids.[6,9] The purpose of enteral fluid therapy is to promote hydration of the ingesta within the GI tract, and it is often difficult to accurately titrate the volume of fluid given so that an impaction, if present, resolves without resulting in loose feces. Importantly, the diarrhea typically resolves within 12–24 h of discontinuing the enteral fluids and is not associated with other clinical signs such as endotoxemia.

Nasogastric tube-associated problems

Although uncommon, complications associated with the passage and maintenance of a nasogastric tube can result in morbidity of horses treated with enteral fluid therapy (see Chapter 4 on Nasogastric Intubation [p. 38]). The most common complication encountered is epistaxis resulting from trauma to the delicate nasal mucosa or ethmoid turbinates, with a variable amount of hemorrhage. Occasionally blood is observed in nasogastric reflux and is usually due to the horse swallowing blood from the nasal passages; however, gastric ulcers, gastroenteritis, and gastric mucosal trauma from the nasogastric tube should also be considered. If this is encountered, gastroscopy and administration of a gastroprotectant may be indicated. Maintenance of an indwelling nasogastric tube will likely reduce the risk of epistaxis; however, it can be associated with other complications. The presence of an indwelling nasogastric tube has the potential to delay gastric emptying,[5] which may mean that decreased volumes of enteral fluids can be administered.

Probably the most serious complication of nasogastric intubation and enteral fluid administration is inadvertent administration into the lungs or aspiration with resultant pneumonia. Careful nasogastric tube placement (p. 39) should avoid such complications. It is also important to ensure that the tip of the nasogastric tube is in the stomach and not the esophagus and not allow the horse to eat with a large-bore tube in place to avoid aspiration.

Other uncommon complications can be encountered associated with the nasogastric tube used for enteral fluid therapy. One such complication is where the tube becomes retroflexed into the oral cavity and is chewed necessitating extraction of the severed tube from the esophagus via an oral approach. Another horse managed with an indwelling nasogastric tube for a large colon impaction, developed severe laryngeal edema, which necessitated placement of an emergency temporary tracheostomy due to the development of respiratory distress. Partial esophageal rupture was discovered in yet another horse that showed signs of dysphagia and coughing soon after the tube was removed.

In order to avoid such complications as colic, nasogastric reflux, electrolyte imbalances, diarrhea, and nasogastric tube problems, enteral fluids should be gradually introduced, the horse should be closely monitored, and adjustments to both the rate and composition of the fluids should be made if required.

References

1. Adair, T.H. (2001) Gastrointestinal physiology. In: *Textbook of Medical Physiology* (eds Arthur C. Guyton & John E. Hall), pp. 754–762. W.B. Saunders Company, Philadelphia, Pennsylvania.
2. Alexander, F. & Benzie, D. (1951) A radiological study of the digestive tract of the foal. *Quarterly Journal of Experimental Physiology and Cognate Medical Sciences*, **36**, 213–217.
3. Argenzio Robert, A., Lowe, J.E., Pickard, D.W. & Sevens, C.E. (1974) Digesta passage and water exchange in the equine large intestine. *American Journal of Physiology*, **226**, 1035–1042.
4. Butudom, P., Schott, H.C., 2nd, Davis, M., Kobe, C.A., Nielsen, B.D. & Eberhart, S.W. (2002) Drinking salt water enhances rehydration in horses dehydrated by frusemide administration and endurance exercise. *Equine Veterinary Journal Supplement*, **34**, 513–518.
5. Cruz, A.M., Li, R., Kenney, D.G. & Monteith, G. (2006) Effects of indwelling nasogastric intubation on gastric emptying of a liquid marker in horses. *American Journal of Veterinary Research*, **67**, 1100–1104.
6. Dabareiner, R.M. & White, N.A., II. (1995) Large colon impactions in horses: 147 cases (1985–1991). *Journal of the American Veterinary Medical Association*, **205**, 679–685.
7. Hallowell, G. (2008) Retrospective study assessing efficacy of treatment of large colonic impactions. *Equine Veterinary Journal*, **40**, 411–413.
8. Henninger, R.W. & Horst, J. (1997) Magnesium toxicosis in two horses. *Journal of Veterinary Medical Association*, **211**, 82–85.
9. Lopes, M.A.F., Moura, G.S. & Filho, J.D. (1999) Treatment of large colon impaction with enteral fluid therapy. In: *Proceedings of the 45th Annual Meeting of the American Association of Equine Practitioners*, Albuquerque, New Mexico, pp. 99–102.
10. Lopes, M.A.F., Walker, B.L., White, N.A., II & Ward, D.L. (2002) Treatments to promote colonic hydration: Enteral fluid therapy versus intravenous fluid therapy and magnesium sulphate. *Equine Veterinary Journal*, **34**, 505–509.
11. Lopes, M.A.F., White, N.A., II, Donaldson, L., Crisman, M.V. & Ward, D.L. (2004) Effects of enteral and intravenous fluid therapy, magnesium sulfate, and sodium sulfate on colonic contents and feces in horses. *American Journal of Veterinary Research*, **65**, 695–703.
12. Marlin, D.J., Scott, C.M., Mills, P.C., Louwes, H. & Vaarten, J. (1998) Rehydration following exercise: Effects of administration of water versus an isotonic oral rehydration solution (ORS). *Veterinary Journal*, **156**, 41–49.
13. Merritt, A.M., Burrow, J.A. & Hartless, C.S. (1998) Effect of xylazine, detomidine, and a combination of xylazine and butorphanol on equine duodenal motility. *American Journal of Veterinary Research*, **59**, 619–623.
14. Monreal, L., Navarro, M., Armengou, L., José-Cunilleras, E., Cesarini, C. & Segura, D. (2010) Enteral fluid therapy in 108 horses with large colon impactions and dorsal displacements. *Veterinary Record*, **166**, 259–263.

15. Rutkowski, J.A., Eades, S.C. & Moore, J.N. (1991) Effects of xylazine butorphanol on cecal arterial blood flow, cecal mechanical activity, and systemic hemodynamics in horses. *American Journal of Veterinary Research*, **52**, 1153–1158.

16. Schumacher, J., DeGraves, F.J. & Spano, J.S. (1997) Clinical and clinicopathologic effects of large doses of raw linseed oil as compared to mineral oil in healthy horses. *Journal of Veterinary Internal Medicine*, **11**, 296–299.

17. Sosa Leon, L.A., Davie, A.J., Hodgson, D.R. & Rose, R.J. (1995) The effects of tonicity, glucose concentration and temperature of an oral rehydration solution on its absorption and elimination. *Equine Veterinary Journal Supplement*, **20**, 140–146.

18. Zullian, C., Menozzi, A., Pozzoli, C., Poli, E. & Bertini, S. (2010) Effects of alpha(2)-adrenergic drugs on small intestinal motility in the horse: An in vitro study. *Veterinary Journal*, **187**, 342–346.

8 Referral of the Horse with Colic

Louise L. Southwood[1] and Joanne Fehr[2]

[1]Department of Clinical Studies, New Bolton Center, School of Veterinary Medicine, University of Pennsylvania, Kennett Square, PA, USA
[2]Equine Emergency Department, Pilchuck Animal Hospital, Snohomish, WA, USA

Chapter Outline

Importance of early referral	**71**	Patient	74
Indications	**72**	Analgesia	74
Signs of abdominal pain	72	Nasogastric intubation	75
Shock	73	Trocharization	75
Tachycardia or increasing heart rate	73	Fluid therapy	75
Nasogastric reflux	73	Transportation	75
Evidence of intestinal obstruction or poor		Client	75
intestinal motility	73	Overview of referral process and what	
Abdominal palpation per rectum	74	happens at the referral hospital	75
Preparation	**74**	Financial considerations	76

Importance of early referral

Colic requires emergency veterinary care and horses/foals that do not respond to initial treatment on the farm should be referred on an emergency basis. Early referral and surgical intervention has probably been the single most important factor contributing to the marked improvement in survival of horses requiring colic surgery. When horses/foals requiring surgery or intensive medical care are treated early, there is improved survival and fewer complications such as shock, ischemia-reperfusion injury, postoperative reflux, adhesion formation, and laminitis. Often very early exploratory surgery of a horse with a small intestinal strangulating obstruction will mean that the lesion can be corrected without resection and anastomosis being necessary and the horse will have an excellent prognosis.

Survival rates for colic surgery in the late 1980s and early 1990s for small intestinal strangulating lesions were as low as 30–50%,[3,7] whereas current survival rates of horses recovering from general anesthesia are reported to be 80–95%.[5,8] Similarly, survival of horses with a large colon volvulus improved from approximately 25% to 60–70% from the late 1980s to the late 1990s[11] and was reported to be as high as 85% at one hospital.[4] While surgical technique and simply recovering the horse from surgery is likely to have played a role in some of these reports,[11] early referral has been shown to be important.[4,14]

Early referral is particularly important for horses with strangulating intestinal lesions. Complete ischemia for a period beyond 3–4 h can lead to irreversible cell damage and tissue injury. Large colon volvulus is a peracute disease that can result in irreversible colonic injury within a few hours and death within several hours. While in most cases of small intestinal strangulating obstruction resection of ischemic tissue is possible, the prolonged distention of the intestine proximal to the strangulating obstruction causes serosal injury and low-flow ischemia with reperfusion injury predisposing the patient to postoperative complications such as ileus and adhesion formation.[1,2]

Early lesion correction also minimizes signs of shock. Shock can be associated with endotoxemia, hypovolemia, and pain. Signs of shock worsen with a prolonged time between lesion occurrence and correction. Clinical and laboratory indices of shock including tachycardia, high packed cell volume (PCV), and hyperlactatemia are associated with prognosis for survival.[6,10–12]

Education of horse owners with regard to the implication of delayed referral is necessary for success. Owners need to understand the importance of having their veterinarian examine the horse with colic. Presentation of information to the owner with regard to the referral process and associated expense will influence their decision making. Information should be presented enthusiastically and positively, yet realistic expectations should be provided.

Indications

While the vast majority of horses with colic can be managed in the field, approximately 10–20%

Table 8.1   Indications for referral.

- Persistent, severe, or recurrent abdominal pain
- Shock
  - Tachycardia (heart rate >70 beats/min)
  - Injected or toxic oral membranes
  - Poor jugular vein refill time
  - Cool extremities
  - Dull mentation
- Tachycardia or increasing heart rate
- Nasogastric reflux, especially large volumes of reflux
- Decreasing or absent intestinal borborygmi
- Severe or increasing abdominal distention
- Absence of fecal production for >24 h and despite treatment
- Palpation per rectum findings (p. 22)
  - Cecal impaction
  - Small colon impaction
  - Colonic displacement (nephrosplenic entrapment or right dorsal displacement)
  - Severe colonic distention
  - Distended small intestinal loops
  - Abdominal mass(es)

will require referral to a hospital or surgical facility.[9,13] Referral does not necessarily mean that surgery is indicated but that

- closer monitoring;
- more thorough diagnostic tests (e.g., hematology and biochemistry [p. 78], abdominocentesis and peritoneal fluid analysis [p. 87], abdominal radiographic [p. 149], or ultrasonographic [p. 116] examination); and
- intensive treatment with intravenous fluids (p. 99) and analgesia (p. 51) is necessary.

There are several factors that go into the decision to refer a horse with colic. Indications for referral are listed in Table 8.1.

Signs of abdominal pain

The main indication for referral on an emergency basis is severe or persistent signs of abdominal pain despite treatment with analgesics. As a guideline, if the horse is treated with a dose of flunixin meglumine, then requires a dose of sedation (xylazine and butorphanol), and is persistently painful through this analgesic regimen, referral is indicated and should be discussed with the owner. Causes of persistent signs of pain despite medical management include strangulating intestinal obstruction, gas distention associated with a mechanical obstruction, or an inflammatory process. See Chapter 17 on Specific Lesions (p. 204).

Often a horse is not particularly painful and is temporarily responsive to analgesics, so other guidelines for referral are necessary. Examples of causes of colic that may have such a response include large colon (p. 217) and cecal impactions (p. 214) and colonic displacements (p. 219, 220). Also of note is the marked individual variability in pain tolerance between horses. Geriatric horses and draft breeds also tend to be less demonstrative of colic pain compared to other horses and this should be considered when evaluating horses in their 20s and older or draft horses.

Chronic recurrent abdominal pain is also an indication for referral, although often these horses do not necessarily need to be referred on an emergency basis. The purpose of referring these horses is predominantly for further diagnostic evaluation including radiographic (p. 149) and sonographic (p. 116) evaluation, abdominocentesis and peritoneal fluid analysis (p. 87), clinical laboratory data (p. 78), gastroscopy (p. 205), and exploratory celiotomy (p. 173) in some instances. Owners should be aware, however, that often the evaluation of the horse with chronic colic is unrewarding. Examples of lesions that may cause such clinical signs include enterolithiasis (p. 218), intermittent nephrosplenic entrapment of the large colon (p. 219), gastric ulceration (p. 205), neoplasia (p. 223), and adhesions (p. 255).

Shock

Shock is defined as inadequate oxygen delivery to the cells leading to insufficient ATP production and ultimately causing cell death. Hypovolemia, endotoxemia, sepsis, and hemorrhage can lead to shock in the horse showing signs of colic.

Signs of shock include tachycardia (heart rate >70 beats/min), injected or toxic oral mucous membranes, prolonged capillary refill time, poor jugular vein refill time, cool extremities, and dull mentation. See Chapter 2 on Physical Examination (p. 12). Referral of horses with shock is generally recommended because of the need of intravenous fluid therapy (p. 99) and the likelihood that they have serious disease.

Tachycardia or increasing heart rate

When treated on the farm, horses should be monitored closely for tachycardia or increasing heart rate. A particularly high heart rate >60 beats/min or a heart rate that is increasing despite medical management is an indication for referral because it suggests worsening of a condition and failure to respond to medical management. The main causes of tachycardia include shock and pain (see Chapter 2 on Physical Examination p. 12). Any horse with a heart rate >60 beats/min is likely to have some signs of either severe pain or shock indicative of a referral.

Nasogastric reflux

Horses with large volumes of nasogastric reflux should be referred because this is often an indication of either proximal enteritis (PE) (p. 207) or a small intestinal obstruction (p. 207) many of which are strangulating obstructions and require surgery. Even if surgery is not necessary (i.e., proximal enteritis or ileus), the horse may benefit from intravenous fluids (p. 99).

Evidence of intestinal obstruction or poor intestinal motility

There are several clinical indications that the horse likely has an intestinal obstruction or is not responding to initial treatment with analgesia and/or oral fluids and mineral oil:

- marked or increasing abdominal distention;
- absent, reduced, or deteriorating intestinal borborygmi; and/or
- absent fecal output despite initial treatment

Of particular note is the association between lack of intestinal borborygmi and the need for colic surgery.[15]

Abdominal palpation per rectum

While not necessarily an overriding clinical feature, findings on palpation per rectum (p. 22) that are indications for referral include:

- cecal impaction because of the risk of cecal perforation;
- small colon impaction because these obstructions are challenging to resolve medically or small colon distention because this is typically associated with a complete obstruction;
- colonic displacement;
- severe colonic distention;
- distended small intestine; and
- abdominal mass(es).

Mild colonic or cecal distention and pelvic flexure/ left ventral colon impaction alone are generally not indications for immediate referral and warrant careful patient monitoring for resolution or deterioration. Findings on palpation per rectum were not necessarily associated with the need for surgery.[15]

Preparation

Referral of the horse with colic on an emergency basis is very often a stressful situation for the horse owner. Encouraging clients to have an emergency plan for their horse(s) and to be prepared will contribute to a favorable outcome. Pertinent information for the clinician at a referral center is outlined in Table 8.2. Table 8.3 has a list of considerations for horse owners.

Referral can also occur on an elective basis. While referral on an elective basis is generally less expensive, it should be reserved for patients with chronic intermittent or recurrent colic.

Veterinarians should be familiar with the referral procedures at a particular hospital. Admission information including client name, address, telephone number(s); horse name, age, breed, gender, and previous admission; and insurance information should be provided.

Table 8.2   Key information to provide to the attending veterinarian at the referral hospital.

History	• Specific signs
	• Duration of colic/previous colic
	• Breeding status of mares
	• Concurrent disease
	• Current medication
Physical examination	• Severity of pain
	• Heart rate
	• Respiratory rate
	• Rectal temperature
	• Oral mucous membrane color, moistness, and capillary refill time
	• Intestinal borborygmi
Drugs administered	• Flunixin meglumine: Time(s)? Dose?
	• Buscopan: Time(s)? Dose?
	• Sedation: Drug used? Time(s)? Dose?
	• Response to analgesia
	• Other drugs
Other	• Who is coming with the horse?
	• Who is the contact person/ decision maker?
	• Is the horse insured?
	• Is surgery an option?
	• Are there financial constraints?
	• What are owner expectations?

Patient

The goal of patient preparation is to have the horse arrive at the referral hospital with as minimal as possible complications or clinical deterioration.

Analgesia

Patient preparation includes providing adequate analgesia (p. 51) for the trailer ride. If the horse is showing mild to moderate pain, xylazine with or without butorphanol is usually adequate; however, in the severely painful horse (e.g., large colon volvulus) detomidine may be necessary. It is important to not use potent long-lasting analgesic drugs such as detomidine in horses that are not particularly painful because this makes patient evaluation upon admission to the referral hospital

Table 8.3   Checklist for horse owners/caregivers for emergency colic preparedness.

- Caregiver should have contact information for horse owner
- Know for which horse/foal referral is an option
- Know for which horse/foal surgery is an option
- Have an idea of the financial outlay that can be made on a particular horse/foal
- Referral hospital information
  - Address
  - Directions
  - Telephone number
- Insurance company information
  - Company name
  - Telephone number
  - Policy information
- Pertinent medical history (see History [p. 1])
- Breeding and foaling dates and information for broodmares

difficult particularly if the horse had a short trailer ride. Analgesic drugs can be given to the owner to administer to the horse during transportation if necessary. Information pertaining to drug used, dose, and time of administration immediately before or during transportation should be provided to the attending veterinarian at the referral hospital.

Nasogastric intubation

If a horse has reflux following nasogastric intubation or distended loops of small intestine on palpation per rectum, then they should be checked for reflux immediately prior to transportation and referred with the nasogastric tube secured in place. While gastric rupture can occur with a nasogastric tube in place, it allows for decompression immediately upon arrival at the referral hospital; and if the end of the tube is left unplugged then fluid under pressure can be expelled. Taping a glove finger over the end of the tube and cutting a hole in the tip can provide a one-way valve whereby gastric contents can be expelled if gastric pressure builds up but aspiration of air into the stomach is prevented. Avoid having the tip of the nasogastric tube near the patient's eye because mechanical damage associated with the nasogastric tube can occur and, more often, chemical injury can result from any expelled gastric contents.

Trocharization

Trocharization (p. 160) is generally not recommended prior to referral. While the procedure is generally safe when the appropriate technique is used, there is still the risk of developing peritonitis or intestinal injury. The only indication for trocharization prior to referral is when the severity of abdominal distention is such that the horse is unable to adequately ventilate and likely to go into respiratory arrest during transportation.

Fluid therapy

Intravenous fluid therapy (p. 99) is generally not necessary prior to referral. The exception to this would be a cardiovascularly unstable horse with a suspected small intestinal strangulating lesion and a long trailer ride. In most cases, the time taken to administer sufficient fluids to stabilize the horse does not warrant the delay in referral. It is not recommended to administer fluids during transportation particularly during winter when the fluid in the bags can freeze.

Transportation

If it is anticipated that the horse may become recumbent during transportation, the dividers should be taken out of the trailer and the horse's head either not tied or tied loosely to facilitate getting the horse off the trailer upon arrival. Horses with large colon volvulus, gastrointestinal rupture, and severe colitis typically become recumbent during transportation. If possible, it can be useful to have the owner/caregiver or transporter give the referral hospital a call when they are 15–30 min from arrival in instances where travel exceeds an hour.

Client

Overview of referral process and what happens at the referral hospital

A list of procedures typically performed at referral hospitals is provided in Table 8.4. The owner should be given an overview of expectations upon arrival at a referral hospital. Procedures and

Table 8.4   Procedures typically performed at referral hospitals.

- History (p. 1)
- Physical examination (p. 12)
- Abdominal palpation per rectum (p. 22)
- Nasogastric intubation (p. 38)
- Intravenous catheterization and fluid therapy (p. 99)
- Clinical laboratory data (venipuncture) (p. 78)
- Abdominocentesis and peritoneal fluid analysis (p. 87)
- Sonographic examination (p. 116)
- Radiographic examination (uncommon in adult horses) (p. 149)
- ± General anesthesia and surgery (p. 173)

Note that the order in which procedures are performed varies and not all procedures are performed at all hospitals or for all cases.

policies vary between hospitals and practitioners should be familiar with such information. Emergency clinicians also have preferences based on clinical experience and practice geographical region regarding procedures and diagnostic tests. Many hospitals have referral packets that can be obtained to have on hand for clients when emergency referral of their horse is necessary.

In most hospitals the client will need to register at the reception desk. The personnel will vary between hospitals and may include interns/residents, emergency clinician or surgeon, nursing or technical staff, and veterinary students.

Typically a history will be taken by a veterinarian, student, or nurse. A physical examination (p. 12) may be performed by multiple veterinarians (and students). Blood may be drawn from the jugular vein for laboratory data (p. 78), a nasogastric tube passed (p. 38), a jugular vein catheter placed, and the horses administered a bolus of intravenous fluids (p. 99). Abdominocentesis (p. 87) may be performed using a needle or teat cannula and it is important to recognize that in some cases peritoneal fluid is not obtained. Abdominal palpation per rectum (p. 22) and in some cases transabdominal sonographic examination (p. 116) is performed. The client may or may not be able to be present during these procedures. The findings will be discussed with the owner and a treatment plan, which will include the decision to manage the horse medically or surgically, with associated expenses and

prognosis outlined. An estimated 40–50% of horses that seek referral for colic require surgery, and it is important to recognize that certain medical diseases (e.g., colitis, enteritis) need intensive management with the associated expense.

Financial considerations

Clients should be aware of the approximate expense associated with emergency (or elective) admission, medical treatment, surgical treatment, as well as required deposits and payment requirements or options. There are considerable regional variations in expenses but some ranges of costs at US hospitals in 2012 are as follows:

- Emergency admission including emergency fee, assessment, intravenous catheterization and fluid bolus, palpation per rectum, laboratory work, and abdominocentesis/peritoneal fluid analysis—$800–1600
- Medical management including emergency admission plus intravenous fluids and analgesia with or without nasogastric intubation for 24–72 h—$1500–3000
- Surgical management including emergency admission plus basic postoperative care—$5 000–$10 000
- A deposit of 50% of the upper or lower end of the estimate is generally required

While it is important that clients have reasonable expectations regarding the expense associated with referral of horses with colic, they should not be deterred because often the components that make up the "standard of care" can be modified. For example, a horse with an impaction that did not respond to initial treatment in the field may not necessarily require laboratory data or intravenous catheterization, and oral fluids are less expensive and likely more beneficial for resolving an impaction than intravenous fluids. These considerations can substantially lower the expense associated with treatment. Client budgetary restrictions should be communicated with the attending emergency clinician at the referral hospital so that every attempt can be made to provide the best possible care for the patient within the client's financial means.

References

1. Dabareiner, R.M., White, N.A. & Donaldson, L.L. (2001) Effects of intraluminal distention and decompression on microvascular permeability and hemodynamics of the equine jejunum. *American Journal of Veterinary Research*, **62**, 225–236.

2. Dabareiner, R.M., Sullins, K.E., White, N.A. & Snyder, J.R. (2001) Serosal injury in the equine jejunum and ascending colon after ischemia-reperfusion or intraluminal distention and decompression. *Veterinary Surgery*, **30**, 114–125.

3. Edwards, G.B. & Proudman, C.J. (1994) An analysis of 75 cases of intestinal obstruction caused by pedunculated lipomas. *Equine Veterinary Journal*, **26**, 18–21.

4. Embertson, R.M., Cook, G., Hance, S.R., Bramlage, L.R., Levine, J. & Smith, S. (1996) Large colon volvulus: Surgical treatment of 204 horses (1986–1995). In: *Proceedings of the 42nd Annual Convention of the American Association of Equine Practitioners*, Denver, Colorado, pp. 254–255.

5. Freeman, D.E. & Schaeffer, D.J. (2005) Short-term survival after surgery for epiploic foramen entrapment compared with other strangulating diseases of the small intestine in horses. *Equine Veterinary Journal*, **37**, 292–295.

6. French, N.P., Smith, J., Edwards, G.B. & Proudman, C.J. (2002) Equine surgical colic: Risk factors for postoperative complications. *Equine Veterinary Journal*, **34**, 444–449.

7. MacDonald, M.H., Pascoe, J.R., Stover, S.M. & Meagher, D.M. (1989) Survival after small intestine resection and anastomosis in horses. *Veterinary Surgery*, **18**, 415–423.

8. Morton, A.J. & Blikslager, A.T. (2002) Surgical and postoperative factors influencing short-term survival of horses following small intestinal resection: 92 cases (1994–2001). *Equine Veterinary Journal*, **34**, 450–454.

9. Proudman, C.J. (1992) A two year, prospective survey of equine colic in general practice. *Equine Veterinary Journal*, **24**, 90–93.

10. Proudman, C.J., Smith, J.E., Edwards, G.B. & French, N.P. (2002) Long-term survival of equine surgical colic cases. Part 2: Modelling postoperative survival. *Equine Veterinary Journal*, **34**, 438–443.

11. Southwood, L.L., Bergslien, K., Jacobi, A., *et al.* (2002) Large colon displacement and volvulus in horses: 495 cases (1987–1999). In: *Proceedings of the 7th International Equine Colic Research Symposium*, Manchester, U.K., pp. 32–33.

12. Southwood, L.L., Gassert, T. & Lindborg, S. (2010) Colic in geriatric compared to mature nongeriatric horses. Part 1: Retrospective review of clinical and laboratory data. *Equine Veterinary Journal*, **42**, 621–627.

13. Tinker, M.K., White, N.A., Lessard, P., *et al.* (1997) Prospective study of equine colic incidence and mortality. *Equine Veterinary Journal*, **29**, 448–453.

14. Van der Linden, M.A., Laffont, C.M. & Sloet van Oldruitenborgh-Oosterbaan, M.M. (2003) Prognosis in equine medical and surgical colic. *Journal of Veterinary Internal Medicine*, **17**, 343–348.

15. White, N.A., Elward, A., Moga, K.S., Ward, D.L. & Sampson, D.M. (2005) Use of web-based data collection to evaluate analgesic administration and the decision for surgery in horses with colic. *Equine Veterinary Journal*, **37**, 347–350.

9 Clinical Laboratory Data

Raquel M. Walton

Department of Pathobiology, School of Veterinary Medicine, University of Pennsylvania, Philadelphia, PA, USA

Chapter Outline

Indications	**78**	Renal parameters	83
Hematology	**79**	Metabolic indicators	83
Erythrogram	79	Glucose	83
Leukogram	79	Triglycerides	83
Clinical chemistry	**80**	**Coagulation**	**83**
Acid-base evaluation	80	Platelets	83
Lactate	81	Secondary hemostasis	84
Electrolytes	82	Coagulation inhibitors	84
Hepatobiliary assessment	82	**Application of clinical pathology findings**	**85**

Indications

Laboratory test results for colic patients typically yield more information pertinent to treatment and prognosis than to diagnosis. Many characteristic clinical laboratory abnormalities are attributable to proximate rather than ultimate causes, for example, sepsis secondary to strangulating intestinal lesions or severe infectious enteritis. The use of blood parameters for prognostication should always take into account the persistence and magnitude of the abnormality as well as clinical context. Table 9.1 offers a summary of common hematologic and biochemical parameters used for prognosticating colic cases.

Hematology and clinical chemistry are usually part of the minimum database for horses presenting to referral hospitals for colic and are generally not performed as part of the initial examination for horses showing mild signs of colic for the first time. A lack of ability to obtain results immediately in field service practice often makes these tests impractical for managing acute colic on the farm. However, some of these tests may be useful for decision-making and management of horses with persistent signs or cardiovascular instability when referral is not an option. Improvements in point-of-care analyzers may make such tests more readily available. Hematology and clinical chemistry are also used to

Practical Guide to Equine Colic, First Edition. Edited by Louise L. Southwood.
© 2013 John Wiley & Sons, Inc. Published 2013 by John Wiley & Sons, Inc.

Table 9.1   Negative prognostic indicators in colic.

Parameter	Change	Bioanalytical significance	Clinical significance
Platelet count	Decreased	Consumption	DIC (thrombosis ± hemorrhage)
MPC	Decreased	Platelet activation	Thrombosis
PT	Increased	Consumption	DIC (thrombosis ± hemorrhage)
aPTT	Increased	Consumption	DIC (thrombosis ± hemorrhage)
AT	Decreased	Consumption ± GI loss	Thrombosis
Fibrinogen	Decreased or normal*	Consumption	DIC (thrombosis ± hemorrhage)
D-dimer	Increased	Marked activation of coagulation system	DIC (thrombosis ± hemorrhage)
PCV	Increased	Dehydration ± catecholamine release	Pain; shock
WBC count	Decreased	Severe acute inflammation	Possible sepsis; endotoxemia
Left-shift	Persistent degenerative	Overwhelming inflammation	Probable sepsis
WBC morphology	Marked toxic change	Severe inflammation	Possible sepsis
pH	Decreased	Hypoperfusion ± ischemia	Thrombosis; shock
Lactate	Increased	Hypoperfusion +/- ischemia	Shock
Ionized Ca, Mg	Marked decrease	GI sequestration; PTH resistance	Possible ileus; severe disease
Creatinine	Persistent azotemia	Renal failure	Thrombosis; ischemia; nephrotoxicity
Glucose	Persistent or marked increase	Insulin resistance	Possible sepsis; severe disease; intestinal strangulation

*Decreases in DIC, but is a positive acute-phase protein; MPC, mean platelet component; PT, prothrombin time; aPTT, activated partial thromboplastin time; AT, antithrombin; DIC, disseminated intravascular coagulation; PTH, parathyroid hormone.

monitor postoperative colic patients routinely (e.g., packed cell volume [PCV], total plasma protein [TPP]) and patients with fever (e.g., fibrinogen concentration and white blood cell (WBC) count), diarrhea (e.g., electrolytes, WBC count), or critical illness (e.g., lactate, creatinine, and glucose concentrations). With the increasing expense associated with diagnostic procedures, clinicians need to be prudent when sel ecting tests so as to not make management of colic patients prohibitively expensive for horse owners. See Appendix C for Reference ranges for Hematology and Plasma Chemistry (p. 339)

Hematology

Erythrogram

The erythrogram is of no diagnostic use in colic, but many groups have shown it has prognostic significance.[17,28,29,37] Increases in PCV are attributable to dehydration and/or splenic contraction; splenic contraction is epinephrine-mediated and may occur with excitement or pain. In a multivariable model that included clinical and laboratory data, the PCV at presentation was the only significant prognostic

indicator for medical colic cases.[17] This model showed that the higher the PCV was at presentation, the higher the probability of a poor outcome. Using this same model for surgical cases, Ihler et al. found increased heart rate, not PCV, to be a significant predictor for poor outcome. However, PCV was eliminated from the model due to its high correlation with heart rate.[17] Similarly, in another study of 649 colic cases no association between PCV and outcome was detected, but heart rate was a significant prognostic indicator.[20] In contrast, other groups reported that risk of postoperative death increased with increasing preoperative PCV in surgical cases involving both small and large intestine.[28,29,37] The use of PCV for determining prognosis is likely to be of most use when considering a specific cause of colic (e.g., large colon volvulus) and when used in conjunction with other clinical findings.

Leukogram

The leukogram provides information regarding the presence and severity of inflammation, thereby impacting treatment strategies. Hematologic indicators of acute inflammation in the horse include

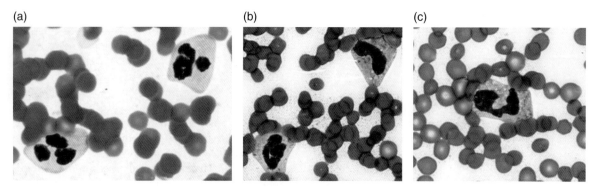

Figure 9.1   (a) Normal neutrophil, (b) a neutrophil and band with mild toxic changes (Dohle bodies, slight foaminess to the band, and increased cytoplasmic basophilia), and (c) toxic neutrophil.

either leukocytosis or leukopenia. Inflammatory leukocytosis is characterized by mature neutrophilia with a left-shift (the presence of immature neutrophils such as bands and metamyelocytes [Figure 9.1]) with or without monocytosis. Leukopenia due to acute inflammation is characterized by neutropenia with or without a left-shift. Typically a leukopenic inflammatory leukogram indicates a more marked inflammatory stimulus.

Severity of inflammation can also be assessed by the presence of toxic changes in neutrophils, especially in conjunction with neutropenia or a degenerative left-shift. "Toxic" neutrophils are characterized by the presence of any or all of the following: cytoplasmic basophilia (often with Dohle bodies), foamy cytoplasm, less condensed chromatin, nuclear hyposegmentation, and larger cell size (Figure 9.1). These changes reflect maturational defects in the bone marrow that are associated with rapid neutropoiesis due to a strong systemic inflammatory stimulus. In general, the more severe the toxic change, the more severe the inflammatory stimulus.

A degenerative left-shift is defined by a normal or decreased WBC count with immature neutrophils (bands, metamyelocytes, myelocytes) exceeding mature neutrophils. Degenerative left-shifts indicate an inflammatory stimulus that is greater than neutrophil production and release. Serial monitoring of the blood is necessary to determine the clinical significance of these changes. A single leukogram characterized by a degenerative left-shift is of little prognostic value, whereas a persistent degenerative left-shift and/or worsening of toxic change are poor prognostic indicators.

The majority of horses with colic have a normal leukogram or a mild neutrophilia and lymphopenia consistent with a stress leukogram. Leukopenia and neutropenia is most often associated with moderate to marked endotoxemia (p. 246) and initiation of the systemic inflammatory response and is most often seen with enterocolitis (p. 215). Interestingly, leukopenia is not typically seen on admission hematology in horses with extensive intestinal ischemia (e.g., small intestinal strangulation or large colon volvulus). Leukopenia, however, can be seen in postoperative colic patients with ischemia-reperfusion injury (p. 246) and endotoxemia (p. 246). Intestinal perforation should be considered in a horse with severe leukopenia (<1500 cells/μL) (Clinical scenario 7, p. 327). An infectious process such as peritonitis, pneumonia, or enterocolitis should be considered in any horse presenting for colic with a left-shift.

Clinical chemistry

Acid-base evaluation

Acid-base imbalances in colic are varied as a result of the varied etiologies with which colic is associated. There are differences in acid-base and electrolyte abnormalities according to type of gastrointestinal disease (e.g., obstruction, ischemia, enteritis, and diarrhea) and even differences in acid-base status within disease groups.[26] Overall, most studies report statistically significant decreases in bicarbonate/TCO_2 and base excess (BE) with normal or decreased blood pH (metabolic acidosis) in colic cases compared to control horses.[24,26] However, metabolic alkalosis may occur more often than acidosis with ischemic intestinal disease, mixed metabolic acid-base disorders can occur with diarrheic colitis, and—especially with obstructive colic—many patients may have a normal acid-base profile.[24,26]

Acid-base status may be evaluated by the traditional method, which assesses bicarbonate, blood pH, BE, and PCO_2, or by a quantitative approach (strong ion difference [SID]). In the quantitative approach, anions (e.g., chloride, proteins) are recognized as acids, and cations (e.g., sodium, potassium, ionized calcium) as bases. Thus, metabolic derangements in these analytes impact acid-base status. In one study, metabolic acid-base abnormalities in over half of diarrheic colic cases with hypoproteinemia/-albuminemia and hyponatremia were not detected using traditional acid-base parameters.[26] Some authors recommend using SID to assess acid-base abnormalities in any patient with electrolyte and/or protein derangements. Because SID is mechanistic, acid-base abnormalities can be broken down into components, thereby facilitating the identification of mixed metabolic acid-base abnormalities.[1,26,41] However, it is also recommended that SID values be interpreted in the context of the traditional blood gas.[32] Since SID formulae vary according to which analytes are included, it should be confirmed that the reference interval is appropriate to the SID formula used. Good reviews of the SID approach to acid-base evaluation are available for veterinary practitioners.[1,41].

Lactate

Increased lactate concentration in the blood reflects anaerobic glycolysis, most often subsequent to tissue hypoxia from hypoperfusion. In addition to tissue hypoxia, other differential etiologies for increased lactate concentration include sepsis (increased metabolic state), endotoxemia (endotoxin interference with pyruvate dehydrogenase), glucose administration, liver disease (decreased lactate clearance), and severe alkalosis.[10] Normal plasma lactate should be <2 mmol/L and normal peritoneal fluid lactate <1 mmol/L with the ratio of peritoneal fluid: plasma lactate being <1. However, plasma lactate concentration should be <1 mmol/L in a well-hydrated patient.[34] Blood lactate concentration is important therapeutically and prognostically in colic cases, but peritoneal fluid lactate concentration is more specific as a marker for intestinal ischemia because blood lactate is affected by systemic hypoperfusion[6] (see Chapter 10 on Abdominocentesis and Peritoneal Fluid Analysis [p. 87]). The odds for surgical intervention, ileus, and nonsurvival increase for each 1 mmol/L increase above the reference limit in blood or peritoneal fluid lactate, but peritoneal fluid lactate is a more sensitive indicator.[6] Blood lactate concentrations >7 mmol/L show strong association with nonsurvival in multiple studies.[6,15,19,37] However, serial assessment of blood lactate is of greater prognostic value than a single determination; persistently high lactate levels or an increasing trend suggest a poorer prognosis than a single high value. When plasma lactate concentration was evaluated in emergency admissions to a referral hospital, nonsurvivors generally had higher blood lactate concentration compared to survivors; however, there was considerable overlap between survivors and nonsurvivors.[34] Both survivors and nonsurvivors also had a rapid decrease in plasma lactate concentration with initial treatment, with the decrease being more rapid in survivors.[34] Plasma lactate appeared to be a better indicator of survival in patients with severe disease (e.g., colitis and large colon volvulus).[34] With the new point-of-care lactate meters, care should be taken to regularly calibrate machines and establish reference ranges and ambient temperature and sample-type should be considered when interpreting results.

The anion gap is traditionally used to detect unmeasured anions (UAs) and increased anion gap correlates well with lactatemia, thus it has been used as a surrogate for lactate measurement.[2] However, for animals with marked electrolyte imbalances and hypo- or hyperproteinemia, the SID approach is more accurate in detecting UAs (e.g., lactate). Hypoproteinemia may cancel out the effect of increased UAs in the anion gap formula, whereas hyperproteinemia may cause an increase in anion gap not attributable to UAs.[2,26] In these patients, direct measurement of lactate concentration or evaluation of UAs with the strong ion approach is advised.

Electrolytes

Electrolyte imbalances observed in colic are varied, usually as a consequence of the diverse causes of colic. However, consistent abnormalities reported in both surgical and medical colic cases include hypocalcemia, hypomagnesemia, and hypokalemia.[5,11,18,24,26,35] The causes of hypocalcemia have been attributed to GI sequestration (reflux), endotoxemia (production of inflammatory cytokines suppresses parathyroid hormone [PTH] and decreases calcium induction set point), or PTH resistance. In humans, concurrent hypomagnesemia can contribute to PTH resistance. The mechanism of hypokalemia and hypomagnesemia is thought to be due to lack of GI absorption and/or decreased intake. However, endotoxemia alone has been shown to be a direct cause of hypokalemia and ionized hypocalcemia and hypomagnesemia.[36] Urinary loss does not appear to contribute to the development of hypocalcemia, hypomagnesemia, or hypokalemia in enterocolitis or endotoxemia because urinary fractional excretions for all three are decreased.[35,36]

Hypokalemia in colic is not correlated with outcome, but several studies show hypocalcemia and hypomagnesemia may have prognostic value.[5,11] Reports are conflicting: while hypocalcemia was significantly correlated with risk of ileus or nonsurvival in one study,[5] another showed that ionized calcium concentration did not correlate with outcome. Garcia-Lopez et al. reported that ionized hypomagnesemia was significantly associated with risk of postoperative ileus and euthanasia at surgery,[11] whereas Johansson et al. found that total serum hypomagnesemia was actually a favorable prognostic indicator for survival although low serum total magnesium at admission was associated with longer hospitalization times.[18]

Hypocalcemia and hypomagnesemia have also been associated with presence of ischemia. The degree of hypocalcemia and hypomagnesemia is significantly lower in strangulating compared with nonstrangulating GI lesions. However, using magnitude of decrease to identify horses with or without strangulating lesions did not have good predictive value.[11] The notion that marked hypocalcemia in colic is more a reflection of disease severity rather than disease type is supported by data showing that the magnitude of ionized calcium decrease correlates with nonsurvival.[5] Note that in horses that are hypoalbuminemic, total calcium is not representative of calcium status.

Hypochloremia is often seen in horses with an intestinal obstruction, particularly a small intestinal functional or strangulating obstruction. The most likely reason for hypochloremia is sequestration of the chloride ion in the gastrointestinal tract (Clinical scenario 5 [p. 327]).

Hepatobiliary assessment

In horses, sorbitol dehydrogenase (SDH) and aspartate transaminase (AST) are commonly measured enzymes associated with hepatocellular injury. SDH is more specific than AST as an indicator of hepatocellular damage due to extrahepatic sources of AST activity (muscle and erythrocytes). Commonly measured parameters associated with cholestasis include gamma glutamyltransferase (GGT) and alkaline phosphatase (ALP), although GGT is much more sensitive than ALP in horses. Because GGT is secreted into milk, reference values for neonatal foals are higher than for adult horses. Common markers of hepatobiliary function include bilirubin and bile acids. Bile acids are more specific indicators of hepatobiliary dysfunction than bilirubin because they are not affected by fasting. In anorexic horses, hyperbilirubinemia is the result of free fatty acids competition for hepatocellular uptake rather than actual cellular dysfunction.[32]

Increases in hepatobiliary indices associated with colic may represent either primary or secondary hepatic dysfunction. In a pilot study of 32 surgical colic cases, increases in SDH, bile acids, and GGT were often noted.[37] GGT activity was not associated with outcome, but increased bile acids concentration at admission was a negative prognostic indicator. Preoperative SDH activity was higher in nonsurvivors than survivors, but the difference was not statistically significant.[37]

In the context of specific disease differentials, GGT may be useful diagnostically. Increases in GGT were shown to occur in nearly half of right dorsal displacements of the large colon (RDD), whereas only 3% of horses with left dorsal displacement of the large colon had increased GGT activity likely because of bile duct compression that may occur in RDD.[12] Similarly, GGT may be helpful in distinguishing proximal enteritis (PE) from small intestinal strangulating obstruction (SISO). While SISO may clinically resemble PE, it does not appear to be associated with hepatic injury, unlike PE.[4] Using a GGT concentration >22 U/L (reference interval 6–22 U/L), the positive predictive value for distinguishing PE from SISO was 84%.[4]

Renal parameters

Azotemia, as reflected by increased creatinine and urea nitrogen concentration, reflects decreased glomerular filtration as a result of decreased renal perfusion (prerenal) and/or damage to nephrons (renal). Urea nitrogen is less sensitive than creatinine as an indicator of glomerular filtration in horses. While azotemia is often prerenal in colic patients, renal ischemia due to hypotension, thromboemboli, and/or nephrotoxic drugs (e.g., flunixin meglumine or gentamicin) can result in primary azotemia. Persistent azotemia has been shown to be a negative prognostic indicator and significantly higher preoperative creatinine concentrations are noted in nonsurvivors compared with survivors.[13,31,37] Rarely postrenal azotemia is observed in colic patients associated with uroabdomen from a ruptured bladder. Ruptured bladder and uroabdomen is more common in neonates.

Metabolic indicators

Glucose

Glucose homeostatic dysfunction is reported in up to half of adult horses with acute abdominal disease.[14,16] Homeostatic abnormalities manifest primarily as hyperglycemia. Hypoglycemia is rarely reported in adult horses with colic. Hyperglycemia is prevalent in critically ill human patients and is attributed to peripheral insulin resistance and increased gluconeogenesis due to the release of epinephrine, cortisol, tumor necrosis factor, and other mediators.[25] Similar mechanisms are likely involved in equine colic patients, but have not been investigated. Measurement of plasma epinephrine and serum cortisol in 35 colic patients revealed that both were significantly higher in nonsurvivors compared with survivors. However, plasma epinephrine was not linearly correlated with serum glucose; the relationship between cortisol and glucose was not investi-

gated.[15] Regardless of the exact pathogenesis, hyperglycemia has negative prognostic significance in colic patients and prognosis worsens with the severity of hyperglycemia.[14,16] Studies addressing the benefits of glycemic control in colic have yet to be performed.

Triglycerides

Measurement of triglycerides can provide an indication of negative energy balance. Hypertriglyceridemia exceeding levels associated with fasting has been reported in colic and enterocolitis cases.[8,9,37,38] Excessive hypertriglyceridemia in these cases may be attributed to increased lipolysis mediated by high concentrations of epinephrine and cortisol, and/or the presence of lipopolysaccharides or inflammatory mediators such as tumor necrosis factor.[9,38] Concurrent azotemia can also interfere with blood triglyceride clearance.[38] Serum triglycerides are often not routinely evaluated in colic; therefore, increases may go undetected since severe hypertriglyceridemia can occur in the absence of serum opacity.[8,9] While studies have shown that parenteral feeding or insulin administration is effective in significantly decreasing serum hypertriglyceridemia, there are currently few data regarding prognostic significance.[9,38] Persistent hypertriglyceridemia, especially if moderate or severe, is an indicator of negative energy balance and as such may adversely affect recovery time or survival.

Coagulation

Platelets

In primary hemostasis, platelets are activated and aggregate to form a plug. Prothrombotic stimuli, especially potent platelet activators such as thrombin and platelet activating factor (PAF), are produced subsequent to endotoxemia and with severe inflammation. Recent studies have shown that platelet activation is associated with inflammatory conditions in humans, dogs, and horses.[23,30,40] Identification of platelet activation may allow early therapeutic intervention for prothrombotic states in colic patients with an inflammatory etiology. Platelet activation can be assessed using automated hematology analyzers that evaluate platelets optically, permitting evaluation of platelet density or granularity (mean platelet component; MPC).[21,23,30] Platelet activation results in a decrease in granularity, which correlates with a decreased MPC. The MPC is readily available on a standard complete blood count (CBC) and has been demonstrated to be a sensitive marker of platelet activation in humans and dogs.[21,23] In horses, MPC is significantly decreased in septic and nonseptic inflammatory disease compared with healthy controls.[30] However, MPC is not a stable parameter in horses and has been reported to significantly decrease after only 2h in EDTA.[27] Thus, clinical use of MPC as an indicator of platelet activation requires immediate evaluation of blood samples and further validation with respect to reference values, but may prove useful in conjunction with other coagulation parameters to identify prothrombotic states.

Systemic activation of the coagulation system associated with severe inflammation and/or endotoxemia may result in thrombocytopenia from platelet activation and consumption. Thrombocytopenia may be present in colic horses with or without disseminated intravascular coagulation (DIC).[7] Postoperative thrombocytopenia is a negative prognostic indicator in large colon volvulus and was reported in 80% of colic horses with DIC.[3,39]

Secondary hemostasis

In colic, hemostatic dysfunction is most often characterized by a hypercoagulable state due to activation of the coagulation system from severe inflammation and/or endotoxemia.[22] Activation may culminate in DIC, which is diagnosed by abnormalities in at least three hemostatic tests in conjunction with hemorrhage or thrombosis at multiple sites.[3,7,22,39] Hemostatic dysfunction in three or more laboratory tests, with or without clinical signs, has a significant negative impact on recovery time and survival.[3,7,39]

Activation of the secondary hemostatic system is primarily initiated by release of tissue factor associated with tissue hypoxia and inflammation and/or endotoxemia, a common occurrence with equine enteritides. Inflammation of a surface area as large as the equine colon may result in enteric loss of anticoagulant proteins antithrombin (AT) and

protein C, and contributes to hemostatic dysfunction in colitis cases. While systemic coagulopathies are frequent in colic cases, actual hemorrhage occurs less frequently and is associated more with severe ischemic/inflammatory disorders. DIC more commonly manifests as thromboembolic disease, which is more difficult to detect clinically.[3,22,33,39]

Readily available laboratory tests of coagulation that should be evaluated to exclude overt or subclinical DIC include tests that evaluate primary and secondary hemostasis as well as the coagulation inhibitory system: platelet concentration, MPC, prothrombin time (PT), activated partial thromboplastin time (aPTT), fibrinogen, AT, fibrin(ogen)-degradation products (FDPs), and D-dimers. Mild to moderate increases in PT and/or aPTT times are among the most commonly reported hemostatic abnormalities associated with DIC in horses.[3,7,33] Prolonged PT times have been significantly associated with nonsurvival in one study of large colon volvulus.[3]

Excessive activation of the coagulation system should produce hypofibrinogenemia, but fibrinogen concentration may be normal or slightly increased in DIC because of fibrinogen's role as a positive acute-phase protein. However, in the face of inflammation, normofibrinogenemia—or a decreasing trend—could be interpreted as an abnormal finding suggestive of a consumptive coagulopathy.

Coagulation inhibitors

FDPs and D-dimers are fibrinolytic products that have an inverse relationship with factor concentration. As factors are consumed to yield fibrin, fibrin is degraded to create FDP and D-dimer fragments. In the horse, increases in FDPs are associated with fibrinolysis, but sensitivity and specificity of FDP assays for diagnosis of equine DIC is low. FDPs were increased in 42% of samples from acute colitis cases without DIC and in nearly 50% of healthy horses.[7,33] Whereas FDP assays test for degradation of either fibrinogen or fibrin by plasmin, D-dimer fragments are specific for fibrin degradation. D-dimer assays tend to have higher sensitivity and specificity than FDP assays for the diagnosis of DIC, but results vary greatly according to the type of antibody used in the assay. In a comparison of four different commercial D-dimer kits, assay sensitivity ranged from 20–50%

and specificity from 57–100%.[33] Neither D-dimer nor FDP concentrations have been shown to have prognostic use in colic, but D-dimers can be useful in the diagnosis of DIC if kits that are properly validated for horses are used.[3,17,33]

AT is a serine protease inhibitor that acts on thrombin, Factor X, and tissue-factor-Factor VII complex to inhibit coagulation. Decreased AT activity is reported to be one of the most common hemostatic abnormalities in colic-associated DIC.[7,33,39] Enterocolitis may result in GI and/or renal loss of AT and decreased AT activity has been correlated with hypoproteinemia in acute colitis cases 48 h after presentation.[7] Thus, decreased AT activity in enterocolitis patients could be attributed to loss rather than consumption. However, in horses with acute colitis, decreased AT activity was more commonly seen in horses with DIC than those without hemostatic dysfunction.[7] In one study that evaluated DIC in severe colic independent of etiology, decreased AT activity was a negative prognostic indicator.[33]

Application of clinical pathology findings

Clinical scenarios 1, 4, 5, and 7 (p. 325–327) provide examples of how clinical pathology findings can be used in evaluating patients presenting with colic.

References

1. Constable, P.D. (2000) Clinical assessment of acid-base status: Comparison of the Henderson-Hasselbalch and strong ion approaches. *Veterinary Clinical Pathology*, **29**, 115–128.
2. Constable, P.D., Hinchcliff, K.W. & Muir, W.W. (1998) Comparison of anion gap and strong ion gap as predictors of unmeasured strong ion concentration in plasma and serum from horses. *American Journal of Veterinary Research*, **59**, 881–887.
3. Dallap, B.L., Dolente, B. & Boston, R. (2003) Coagulation profiles in 27 horses with large colon volvulus. *Journal of Veterinary Emergency and Critical Care*, **13**, 215–225.
4. Davis, J.L., Blikslager, A.T., Catto, K. & Jones, S.L. (2003) A retrospective analysis of hepatic injury in horses with proximal enteritis (1984–2002). *Journal of Veterinary Internal Medicine*, **17**, 896–901.
5. Delesalle, C., Dewulf, J., Lefebvre, R.A., Schuurkes, J.A., Van Vlierbergen, B. & Deprez, P. (2005) Use of plasma ionized calcium levels and Ca²⁺ substitution response patterns as prognostic parameters for ileus and survival in colic horses. *Veterinary Quarterly*, **27**, 157–172.
6. Delesalle, C., Dewulf, J., Lefebvre, R.A., *et al.* (2007) Determination of lactate concentrations in blood plasma and peritoneal fluid in horses with colic by an Accusport analyzer. *Journal of Veterinary Internal Medicine*, **21**, 293–301.
7. Dolente, B.A., Wilkins, P.A. & Boston, R.C. (2002) Clinicopathologic evidence of disseminated intravascular coagulation in horses with acute colitis. *Journal of the American Veterinary Medical Association*, **220**, 1034–1038.
8. Dunkel, B. & McKenzie, H.C. (2003) Severe hypertriglyceridaemia in clinically ill horses: Diagnosis, treatment and outcome. *Equine Veterinary Journal*, **35**, 590–595.
9. Durham, A.E., Phillips, T.J., Walmsley, J.P. & Newton, J.R. (2004) Nutritional and clinicopathological effects of post operative parenteral nutrition following small intestinal resection and anastomosis in the mature horse. *Equine Veterinary Journal*, **36**, 390–396.
10. Feary, D.J. & Hassel, D.M. (2006) Enteritis and colitis in horses. *Veterinary Clinics of North America: Equine Practice*, **22**, 437–479.
11. Garcia-Lopez, J.M., Provost, P.J., Rush, J.E., Zicker, S.C., Burmaster, H. & Freeman, L.M. (2001) Prevalence and prognostic importance of hypomagnesemia and hypocalcemia in horses that have colic surgery. *American Journal of Veterinary Research*, **62**, 7–12.
12. Gardner, R.B., Nydam, D.V., Mohammed, H.O., Ducharme, N.G. & Divers, T.J. (2005) Serum gamma glutamyl transferase activity in horses with right or left dorsal displacements of the large colon. *Journal of Veterinary Internal Medicine*, **19**, 761–764.
13. Groover, E.S., Woolums, A.R., Cole, D.J. & LeRoy, B.E. (2006) Risk factors associated with renal insufficiency in horses with primary gastrointestinal disease: 26 cases (2000–2003). *Journal of the American Veterinary Medical Association*, **228**, 572–577.
14. Hassel, D.M., Hill, A.E. & Rorabeck, R.A. (2009) Association between hyperglycemia and survival in 228 horses with acute gastrointestinal disease. *Journal of Veterinary Internal Medicine*, **23**, 1261–1265.
15. Hinchcliff, K.W., Rush, B.R. & Farris, J.W. (2005) Evaluation of plasma catecholamine and serum cortisol concentrations in horses with colic. *Journal of the American Veterinary Medical Association*, **227**, 276–280.
16. Hollis, A.R., Boston, R.C. & Corley, K.T.T. (2007) Blood glucose in horses with acute abdominal disease. *Journal of Veterinary Internal Medicine*, **21**, 1099–1103.
17. Ihler, C.F., Venter, J.L. & Skjerve, E. (2004) Evaluation of clinical and laboratory variables as prognostic

indicators in hospitalized gastrointestinal colic horses. *Acta Veterinaria Scandinavica*, **45**, 109–118.

18. Johansson, A.M., Gardner, S.Y., Jones, S.L., Fuquay, L.R., Reagan, V.H. & Levine, J.F. (2003) Hypomagnesemia in hospitalized horses. *Journal of Veterinary Internal Medicine*, **17**, 860–867.

19. Johnston, K., Holcombe, S.J. & Hauptman, J.G. (2007) Plasma lactate as a predictor of colonic viability and survival after 360° volvulus of the ascending colon in horses. *Veterinary Surgery*, **36**, 563–567.

20. van der Linden, M.A., Laffont, C.M. & Sloet van Oldruitenborgh-Oosterbaan, M.M. (2003) Prognosis in equine medical and surgical colic. *Journal of Veterinary Internal Medicine*, **17**, 343–348.

21. Macey, M.G., Carty, E., Webb, L., *et al.* (1999) Use of mean platelet component to measure platelet activation in the ADVIA 120 hematology system. *Cytometry*, **38**, 250–255.

22. Monreal, L. & Cesarini, C. (2009) Coagulopathies in horses with colic. *Veterinary Clinics of North America: Equine Practice*, **25**, 247–258.

23. Moritz, A., Walcheck, B.K. & Weiss, D.J. (2005) Evaluation of flow cytometric and automated methods for detection of activated platelets in dogs with inflammatory disease. *American Journal of Veterinary Research*, **66**, 325–329.

24. Nappert, G. & Johnson, P.J. (2001) Determination of the acid-base status in 50 horses admitted with colic between December 1998 and May 1999. *Canadian Veterinary Journal*, **42**, 703–707.

25. Nasraway, S.A. (2006) Hyperglycemia during critical illness. *Journal of Parenteral and Enteral Nutrition*, **30**, 254–258.

26. Navarro, M., Monreal, L., Segura, D., Armengou, L. & Añor, S. (2005) A comparison of traditional and quantitative analysis of acid-base and electrolyte imbalances in horses with gastrointestinal disorders. *Journal of Veterinary Internal Medicine*, **19**, 871–877.

27. Prins, M., van Leeuwen, M.W. & Teske, E. (2009) Stability and reproducibility of ADVIA 120-measured red blood cell and platelet parameters in dogs, cats, and horses, and the use of reticulocyte haemoglobin content (CH(R)) in the diagnosis of iron deficiency. *Tijdschrift voor Diergeneeskunde*, **134**, 272–278.

28. Proudman, C.J., Edwards, G.B., Barnes, J. & French, N.P. (2005) Factors affecting long-term survival of horses recovering from surgery of the small intestine. *Equine Veterinary Journal*, **37**, 360–365.

29. Proudman, C.J., Edwards, G.B., Barnes, J. & French, N.P. (2005) Modelling long-term survival of horses following surgery for large intestinal disease. *Equine Veterinary Journal*, **37**, 366–370.

30. Segura, D., Monreal, L., Armengou, L., Tarancón, I., Brugués, R. & Escolar, G. (2007) Mean platelet component as an indicator of platelet activation in foals and adult horses. *Journal of Veterinary Internal Medicine*, **21**, 1076–1082.

31. Stephen, J.O., Corley, K.T.T., Johnston, J.K. & Pfeiffer D. (2004) Factors associated with mortality and morbidity in small intestinal volvulus in horses. *Veterinary Surgery*, **33**, 340–348.

32. Stockham, S.L. & Scott, M.A. (eds) (2002) Blood gases, blood pH, and strong ion difference. In: *Fundamentals of Veterinary Clinical Pathology*. Blackwell Publishing, Ames, Iowa.

33. Stokol, T., Erb, H.N., De Wilde, L., Tornquist, S.J. & Brooks, M. (2005) Evaluation of latex agglutination kits for detection of fibrin(ogen) degradation products and D-dimer in healthy horses and horses with severe colic. *Veterinary Clinical Pathology*, **34**, 371–382.

34. Tennent-Brown, B.S., Wilkins, P.A., Lindborg, S., Russell, G. & Boston, R.C. (2010) Sequential plasma lactate concentrations as prognostic indicators in adult equine emergencies. *Journal of Veterinary Internal Medicine*, **24**, 198–205.

35. Toribio, R.E., Kohn, C.W., Chew, D.J., Sams, R.A. & Rosol, T.J. (2001) Comparison of serum parathyroid hormone and ionized calcium and magnesium concentrations and fractional urinary clearance of calcium and phosphorus in healthy horses and horses with enterocolitis. *American Journal of Veterinary Research*, **62**, 938–947.

36. Toribio, R.E., Kohn, C.W., Hardy, J. & Rosol, T.J. (2005) Alterations in serum parathyroid hormone and electrolyte concentrations and urinary excretion of electrolytes in horses with induced endotoxemia. *Journal of Veterinary Internal Medicine*, **19**, 223–231.

37. Underwood, C., Southwood, L.L., Walton, R.M. & Johnson, A.L. (2010) Hepatic and metabolic changes in surgical colic patients: A pilot study. *Journal of Veterinary Emergency and Critical Care*, **20**, 578–586.

38. Waitt, L.H. & Cebra, C.K. (2009) Characterization of hypertriglyceridemia and response to treatment with insulin in horses, ponies, and donkeys: 44 cases (1995–2005). *Journal of the American Veterinary Medical Association*, **234**, 915–919.

39. Welch, R.D., Watkins, J.P., Taylor, T.S., Cohen, N.D. & Carter, G.K. (1992) Disseminated intravascular coagulation associated with colic in 23 horses (1984–1989). *Journal of Veterinary Internal Medicine*, **6**, 29–35.

40. Weyrich, A.S., Lindemann, S. & Zimmerman, G.A. (2003) The evolving role of platelets in inflammation. *Journal of Thrombosis and Haemostasis*, **1**, 1897–1905.

41. Whitehair, K.J., Haskins, S.C., Whitehair, J.G. & Pascoe, P.J. (1995) Clinical applications of quantitative acid-base chemistry. *Journal of Veterinary Internal Medicine*, **9**, 1–11.

10 Abdominocentesis and Peritoneal Fluid Analysis

Raquel M. Walton[1] and Louise L. Southwood[2]

[1]Department of Pathobiology, School of Veterinary Medicine, University of Pennsylvania, Philadelphia, PA, USA
[2]Department of Clinical Studies, New Bolton Center, School of Veterinary Medicine, University of Pennsylvania, Kennett Square, PA, USA

Chapter Outline

Indications	**87**	Protein concentration	91
Preparation	**88**	Lactate and glucose concentration and pH	92
Procedure	**88**	D-dimer concentration	92
Needle technique	89	Cells and cell counts	92
Teat cannula technique	89	Erythrocytes	93
Complications	**89**	Nucleated cells	93
Peritoneal fluid analysis	**90**	Interpretation of findings	95
Nonrepresentative sampling	90	Transudates	95
Gross characteristics	90	Exudates	97
Volume	90	Hemorrhagic effusions	97
Color and clarity	90	**Application of peritoneal fluid analysis**	**97**
Biochemical evaluation	91		

Indications

Abdominocentesis refers to the technique of puncture of the abdominal wall and peritoneal cavity with a needle (or teat cannula) and collection of a sample of peritoneal fluid for analysis. Abdominocentesis is performed to obtain peritoneal fluid in cases of colic or enterocolitis as a means of assessing intestinal damage, or horses with a fever of unknown origin to diagnose peritonitis. Neoplastic cells can be seen using cytological evaluation of the peritoneal fluid in approximately 50% of gastrointestinal neoplasia cases and, therefore, peritoneal fluid analysis can also be useful in horses with unexplained weight loss, inappetence, and chronic intermittent colic.

Peritoneal fluid analysis is considered part of the minimum database for colic patients at many

Practical Guide to Equine Colic, First Edition. Edited by Louise L. Southwood.
© 2013 John Wiley & Sons, Inc. Published 2013 by John Wiley & Sons, Inc.

Table 10.1   Things you will need for abdominocentesis.

Needle technique	• Halter and lead rope • ± Stocks • ± Sedation (xylazine/butorphanol) • Clippers • Povidone-iodine or chlorhexidine scrub • Alcohol • Sterile gloves • 3–4 18 gauge 1 1/2 in. needle • EDTA tube (cytology) • Plain tube (bacterial culture and sensitivity testing)
Teat cannula technique	• Halter and lead rope • ± Stocks • ± Sedation (xylazine/butorphanol) • Clippers • Povidone-iodine or chlorhexidine scrub • Alcohol • 3 mL 2% lidocaine in a syringe and 22–25 gauge needle • Sterile gloves • #15 blade • Sterile 4 × 4 gauze sponges • Teat cannula • EDTA tube (cytology) • Plain tube (bacterial culture and sensitivity testing)

referral hospitals. Abdominocentesis and peritoneal fluid analysis is particularly useful when the decision to manage the horse medically versus surgically is not readily apparent (see Chapter 15 on Medical versus Surgical Management of the Horse with Colic [p. 164]) and for monitoring horses that are being managed medically.

Abdominocentesis is generally not performed on the initial examination for colic, particularly with horses showing mild signs (see Chapter 5 on Management of Mild Colic [p. 45]), because it is unlikely to yield results that would alter management and the procedure is not without the potential for complication. The decision to perform abdominocentesis should be made with caution in horses with severe abdominal distention or suspected sand impaction because of the risk for enterocentesis (p. 89). It is also not recommended to perform the procedure on horses with severe uncontrollable pain because of the risk of injury to the veterinarian and in such cases surgery or euthanasia is often indicated.

Indications for abdominocentesis prior to referral include horses with suspected gastrointestinal tract rupture/perforation and horses with clinical signs consistent with a strangulating obstruction where the owners do not chose to pursue referral or surgical treatment. Abdominocentesis and peritoneal fluid analysis in these cases can be used to support the indication for euthanasia.

Preparation

A "List of Things You Will Need" is provided in Table 10.1. Abdominocentesis is performed with the horse restrained in stocks or in a stall with a halter and lead rope. An area of 10 cm × 10 cm to the right of midline at the most dependent aspect of the ventral abdomen is clipped and aseptically prepared using povidone-iodine or chlorhexidine scrub and alcohol. Alternatively, the area on the cranial midline where the pectoral muscles create a V-shape can be used. Sonography (p. 116) can be used to locate abdominal structures that should be avoided (e.g., spleen and colon) and identify an area of peritoneal fluid accumulation; however, it is not particularly sensitive for the latter and abdominocentesis should still be performed when indicated even if peritoneal fluid is not identified sonographically. Abdominocentesis should not be performed to the left of midline because of the potential for splenic injury and subsequent hemoabdomen. Large subcutaneous vessels should be avoided to prevent sample contamination, hematoma formation, and hemorrhage.

Procedure

Abdominocentesis can be performed using an 18 gauge needle or a teat cannula. The use of an 18 gauge needle (see below) is easier and quicker and if an enterocentesis is performed the hole into the intestine is likely to be smaller; however, fluid is obtained more often with a teat cannula because of the more appropriate length and larger bore and proponents suggest that enterocentesis is less likely because of the blunt tip. The needle or teat cannula is manipulated for several minutes in an attempt to obtain a sample from an area of fluid accumulation. The sample is collected into an ethylenediaminetetraacetic acid (EDTA) tube for cytology and a

(a)   (b)

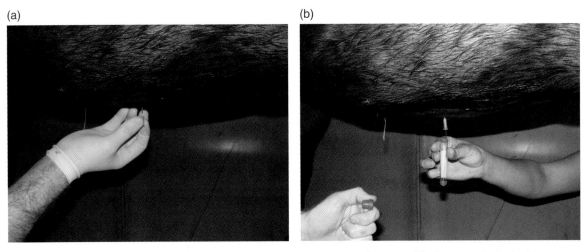

Figure 10.1   Abdominocentesis using the needle technique (a) with collection of peritoneal fluid into an EDTA tube (b).

sterile tube, syringe, or culture vial for bacterial culture and sensitivity testing.

Needle technique

Abdominocentesis using an 18 gauge needle is performed by carefully inserting the needle through the skin, subcutaneous tissue, body wall, and into peritoneal cavity (Figure 10.1). It can be difficult to determine when the tip of the needle is within the peritoneal cavity and in some cases an 18 gauge 1 ½ in. needle may be of insufficient length. Spontaneous movement of the needle is associated with intestinal movement and can be an indication that the needle is correctly positioned. Multiple needles are often needed to obtain a sample.

Teat cannula technique

Abdominocentesis using a teat cannula requires infiltration of the subcutaneous tissue and body wall with 3 mL of 2% lidocaine. A stab incision is made using a #15 blade through the skin and body wall. Gauze sponge is wrapped around the teat cannula to prevent sample contamination. The teat cannula is pushed through the body wall and into the peritoneal cavity; quite a bit of force is usually necessary. Correct positioning of the teat cannula within the peritoneal cavity can be confirmed by filling a 10 mL syringe with air and injecting it

through the teat cannula; if the teat cannula is not in the peritoneal cavity the air will be heard rushing back out of the teat cannula.

Complications

The main complication with abdominocentesis is enterocentesis, which should be suspected when green-brown fluid is obtained in a horse with clinical signs inconsistent with gastrointestinal tract rupture/perforation. In the vast majority of cases, enterocentesis is without clinically apparent consequence. Inadvertent enterocentesis has a reported frequency rate of 2–5%.[4] The incidence of complications directly related to inadvertent enterocentesis was reported to be 0.5% (4/850 abdominocentesis samples).[25] When an enterocentesis occurs, the needle or teat cannula should be removed. Although prophylactic antimicrobial drug administration is recommended, the necessity is unknown. Localized cellulitis and peritonitis are rare consequences of enterocentesis and probably more likely to occur in horses with compromised bowel.

Injury to the spleen can occur and may happen more frequently in horses with a nephrosplenic entrapment whereby the spleen is moved ventrally and across midline. There is usually no consequence except that the results of peritoneal fluid analysis cannot be interpreted.

Omental herniation is a complication of abdominocentesis in foals using the teat cannula technique and occurs with such a frequency that many clinicians will avoid this procedure in neonates. Omental herniation can be corrected by sedating the foal and placing it in dorsal recumbency, aseptically preparing the area, exteriorizing an additional centimeter of the omentum, ligating the exteriorized omentum (if necessary), and placing it back in the abdomen with hemostats or a teat cannula. The skin is apposed using absorbable suture material or a skin staple. Abdominocentesis in foals should be performed with sonographic guidance and using a needle.

Peritoneal fluid analysis

The fluid that bathes the abdominal cavity is an ultrafiltrate of plasma that functions to reduce friction by lubrication. The constituents of peritoneal fluid are affected by the integrity of the mesothelial lining, changes in vascular permeability and lymphatic flow, plasma oncotic pressure, and capillary hydraulic pressure. Thus, changes in the character of the fluid can be attributed to specific disease processes and may yield information in the diagnosis, treatment, and/or prognosis of horses with colic.

Nonrepresentative sampling

When evaluating peritoneal fluid, it is important to determine whether the sample is representative. Two common causes of nonrepresentative peritoneal fluid sampling include blood contamination and enterocentesis. Blood contamination may occur when a peripheral vein or abdominal organ (usually the spleen) is punctured. During abdominocentesis, blood contamination is obvious when the initial sample is clear and becomes bloody or is bloody then clears. As little as 0.05 mL blood in 1 mL of peritoneal fluid (5% contamination) can result in fluid red blood cell (RBC) counts up to 449 000/μL, which is nearly ten times the upper limit of RBC reference values.[4,18] However, white blood cell (WBC) counts and total protein (TP) concentration remain within reference intervals with up to 17% blood contamination.[18] Enterocentesis may manifest grossly as a green to brown discoloration of peritoneal fluid, but

contaminated fluid may also appear grossly normal with contamination only evident upon cytologic evaluation. Peritoneal fluid evaluation alone cannot distinguish between enterocentesis and peracute intestinal leakage or perforation. This distinction is best accomplished in the context of the patient's clinical assessment (p. 171) and sonographic evaluation (p. 133).

Gross characteristics

Volume

In equids, peritoneal fluid volume in health typically ranges from 100 to 300 mL,[1] although it has been estimated that up to 2 L may be present.[4] Although the equine peritoneal cavity normally contains a large volume of fluid, abdominocentesis typically yields <10 mL of fluid and most commonly 3–5 mL.[24] An effusion is defined as an increase in the normal volume of peritoneal fluid, which may or may not have increased protein or cell concentrations. The amount of fluid obtained from abdominocentesis does not necessarily correlate with the presence or absence of effusion. In seriously ill horses with effusion confirmed surgically or postmortem, abdominocentesis may yield only a small volume.[24] Diagnosis of mild to moderate effusions in equids, especially adults, can be difficult due to the constraints on palpation and a large abdominal space that accommodates even moderate effusion volumes. Sonography is often necessary to diagnose effusion (p. 133). In horses, it is convention to classify abnormal peritoneal fluid (i.e., increased protein concentration and/or cell count) as an effusion regardless of whether an increased volume is documented. In contrast, a fluid with a normal cell count and protein concentration is only classified as an effusion if there is a confirmed increase in volume.

Color and clarity

The physical characteristics of peritoneal fluid may provide hints as to its cellularity or biochemical composition. Normal peritoneal fluid is yellow and transparent. Discoloration of the fluid may reflect hemorrhage (orange to red), gastrointestinal tract rupture/perforation (green or brown), bile peritonitis (dark green), or vascular compromise (orange to reddish brown). Abnormal abdominal fluid color has been used in studies to predict the need for surgical treatment. The sensitivity and specificity of subjectively discolored fluid for predicting the need for surgical intervention varies in different reports: 92% and 74%,[19] 78% and 48%,[10] and 51% and 95%, respectively.[27] Weimann et al. used hemoglobin concentration as an objective measurement of discoloration from hemolysis and found that when peritoneal hemoglobin concentration was >0.01 mmol/L (0.02 g/dL), the test was 80% sensitive and 82% specific for selecting surgical treatment.[27] While discolored fluid, especially serosanguinous, supports the need for surgical treatment,[10,19,27] an interpretation of discolored fluid should only be made when the possibility of enterocentesis or blood contamination has been excluded and should be formulated in the context of clinical findings.

The clarity of abdominal fluid in health reflects low cellularity. Increased turbidity is usually reported in terms of cloudy/hazy or opaque, and suggests increased cellularity, presence of plant material, or, rarely, lipid (i.e., chyloabdomen). While turbidity is abnormal, measurement of cell numbers and cytologic evaluation of the fluid are necessary to determine its cause.

Biochemical evaluation

Many peritoneal fluid biochemical parameters have been assessed to determine their use in diagnosis and prognosis. Only tests that are readily available are discussed.

Protein concentration

Because peritoneal fluid is an ultrafiltrate of plasma, protein concentrations are much lower than plasma. Protein can be rapidly and accurately measured by handheld refractometers. Protein measured by refractometer for body cavity fluids is linearly related to protein measured by biochemical methods and results are accurate to at least 0.6 g/dL.[13] Many references cite the reference interval for normal peritoneal fluid protein concentration as <2.5 g/dL,[4] which is the lowest protein reading on many refractometers. To report values below the lower end of the protein scale, the value measured using either refractive index, refraction, or urine specific gravity (SG) scales can be converted to TP with published conversion tables.[12] When abdominal fluid protein was calculated using conversion tables or measured biochemically, normal values were typically ≤2.0 g/dL.[1,14,17] Increases in peritoneal fluid protein concentration above reference values indicate either increased permeability of the capillaries due to inflammatory mediators or increased hydraulic pressure within hepatic sinusoids. An increase in protein concentration due to inflammatory mediators is typically accompanied by an increase in nucleated cell count (NCCs).

Because refractometers measure protein via a total solids (TS)-based technique, the total dissolved solids in the sample affect light refraction.[12] In addition to protein, TS include electrolytes, glucose, urea, and lipids. While the altered refraction of body fluid is mostly due to protein content, increases in lipid, glucose, or urea content interfere with refractometric protein measurements. However, marked increases in urea or glucose (273 and 649 mg/dL, respectively) are needed to increase protein measurement by 0.4–0.5 g/dL.[20] Unlike glucose and urea, lipid does not freely diffuse into peritoneal fluid from plasma; increased concentrations of lipid in peritoneal fluid only occur in cases of chylous effusion (chyloabdomen).

Another potential cause of erroneous refractometer readings is the addition of EDTA from K_3EDTA anticoagulant tubes. At the standard concentration of EDTA (5 μmol/mL), K_3EDTA by itself has minimal effect on the fluid's refraction (≤0.1 g/dL increase). At higher concentrations of EDTA (10 and 20 μmol/mL), EDTA can increase refractometer total protein (TP_{Ref}) by 0.9–1.0 g/dL. Underfilling of EDTA tubes has the effect of increasing the EDTA concentration and will cause spurious increases in the TP_{Ref}. Some commercial tubes with K_3EDTA anticoagulant may also contain additives to prevent crystallization of the EDTA. Tubes that contain the additive may increase TP_{Ref} readings by up to 0.9 g/dL, even when properly filled.[9] It is recommended that TP_{Ref} readings should be performed on either fluid collected in serum tubes or in properly filled K_3EDTA tubes containing no additives. While sodium heparin anticoagulant has no effect on TP_{Ref},[9] heparin has deleterious effects on cellular morphology and is not recommended for samples that will be evaluated cytologically.

The term "total solids" has caused much confusion in the reporting of refractometric protein results. TP and TS are not synonymous. Currently the majority of all refractometers incorporate a conversion factor in their design so that the scales report TP and not TS. Contributing to the confusion is the fact that at least one refractometer is named the "TS meter" (AO Corporation) when it is in fact calibrated to report TP.[12] Today nearly all refractometers report TP and not TS, so comparisons between peritoneal fluid samples are appropriate.

(SG) has also been used to estimate protein concentration in equine peritoneal fluid. However, use of the refractometer SG scale will yield erroneous results because the SG scale is calibrated specifically for urine. Urea, not protein, is the principal constituent of urine, thus SG calibrated for urine gives falsely high results for body fluids.[12] A caveat applies to low protein peritoneal fluid (<1.0 g/dL); in this instance, the urine SG scale more accurately estimates true SG because the fluid's refractive index is more similar to urine.[23]

Lactate and glucose concentration and pH

Lactate is the end product of anaerobic glycolysis and has been used as a marker for ischemia in colic. Normal peritoneal fluid lactate concentrations vary with respect to methodology, but are usually <1.0 mmol/L and the ratio of peritoneal fluid: plasma lactate concentration <1:1.[5,17] Peritoneal lactate, TP, NCC, and glucose concentrations were significantly increased in peritoneal fluid of horses with colic compared to clinically normal horses.[5,17] Peritoneal lactate concentrations were significantly higher in horses with strangulating compared to nonstrangulating lesions,[5,17] with the exception of strangulating small colon obstructions.[17] Increases in fluid lactate, decreases in fluid pH, and abnormal fluid color and/or turbidity were most strongly correlated with ischemic strangulating lesions. Peritoneal fluid lactate concentrations were shown to be more sensitive than blood lactate concentrations in detecting early ischemic lesions.[5,17] The prognosis becomes progressively poorer for horses with strangulating and nonstrangulating lesions as peritoneal fluid lactate concentration increases. One study showed the probability of death of horses with nonstrangulating lesions to be 63% for peritoneal lactate concentrations of 12 mmol/L and 82% for lactate concentrations of 16 mmol/L; the same concentrations of peritoneal fluid lactate had 82% and 92% probabilities of death, respectively, in strangulating lesions.[5] An increase in the peritoneal fluid lactate concentration with serial measurements several hours apart has been associated with the need for surgical treatment.[21]

Peritoneal glucose concentrations have been shown to be useful as a relatively rapid test for distinguishing septic from nonseptic exudates.[26] Positive bacterial culture or cytologic identification of intracellular bacteria in abdominal fluid is a definitive indicator of abdominal sepsis, but false-negatives do occur, especially with antimicrobial therapy. In one study of 36 peritonitis cases, peritoneal fluid glucose concentration and pH were significantly lower in horses with septic versus nonseptic peritonitis.[26] Serum to peritoneal fluid glucose concentration differences >50 mg/dL were most diagnostically useful in confirming sepsis.

D-dimer concentration

Mesothelial cells play an important role in the initiation and resolution of inflammation by secretion of immunomodulatory mediators, which impact coagulant and fibrinolytic factors such as D-dimer.[3,6] D-dimer concentrations in normal peritoneal fluid are reported to be <88 ng/mL,[6,7] whereas in horses with colic, median peritoneal fluid D-dimer concentrations ranged from 2023 to 24301 ng/mL depending upon diagnosis. In horses with colic, median fluid D-dimer concentrations were highest with enteritis, ischemic lesions, and septic peritonitis (8028, 16181, and 24301 ng/mL, respectively) compared with large colon obstructions (2023 ng/mL).[6] Blood contamination <20% does not alter peritoneal fluid D-dimer concentrations.[7] These studies show that peritoneal fluid D-dimer concentration appears to be a useful indicator of fibrinolytic activity and higher concentrations are correlated with greater disease severity.

Cells and cell counts

Cytologic evaluation of peritoneal fluid can yield important information that may even be diagnostic (e.g., large cell lymphoma, carcinoma, uroabdomen, septic inflammation). However, cytology should be interpreted in the context of clinical signs, cell counts, and biochemical evaluation.

Erythrocytes

Erythrocytes are not normally present in peritoneal fluid in health, but blood contamination during abdominocentesis results in RBC counts that range from <5000/μL to <43200/μL in healthy horses.[4,18,23] Visual assessment of discoloration attributable to RBCs was not detected for samples with <40000 RBCs/μL,[15] thus typical amounts of blood contamination associated with abdominocentesis should not change the fluid color. Erythrocyte counts will increase above reference values because of minor blood vessel damage associated with necrosis and/or inflammation. See Hemorrhagic effusions (p. 97).

Nucleated cells

Total NCCs for abdominal fluid are performed with automated blood count analyzers or manually with a hemocytometer. Generally, NCC reference values in normal peritoneal fluid are reported as <10000/μL,[4,23] and often <5000/μL.[1,4,26] Many equine clinicians and clinical pathologists consider values <5000/μL normal, values between 5000 and 10000/μL to be ambiguous, and values >10000/μL as abnormal. Reference values for foals are <1500/μL.[14] The cells normally present within the peritoneal cavity comprise leucocytes and mesothelial lining cells. Nucleated cells in cytologic differentials are categorized as neutrophils, lymphocytes, and large mononuclear cells (monocytes/macrophages and mesothelial cells).

In horses, mature neutrophils comprise the predominant cell in the differential evaluation (typically 50–80% of nucleated cells). Because neutrophils do not return to the vasculature, but age and die in body cavity fluid, pycnotic and hypersegmented neutrophils are normally noted in a proportion of the population. Increased numbers of neutrophils enter the peritoneal cavity in response to chemotactic inflammatory mediators. During inflammation, the ability of neutrophils to respond to stimuli and migrate into tissue increases with maturation.

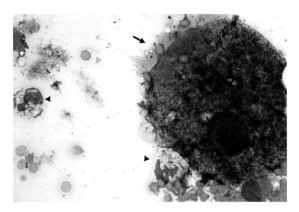

Figure 10.2 Peritoneal fluid from a horse with a septic abdomen. Neutrophils are degenerate and contain many cytoplasmic bacterial rods and cocci (arrowheads). The presence of a large ciliated protozoal organism indicates that there has been intestinal rupture or leakage (arrow).

Consequently, mature neutrophils arrive first and immature forms (i.e., bands, metamyelocytes) are only present in tissue when mature neutrophils have been severely depleted. Thus, the presence of band or earlier forms of neutrophils in peritoneal fluid indicates severe inflammation; a caveat would be if the immature forms originate from blood and there is significant blood contamination of the sample. If blood contamination is not apparent, the presence of immature neutrophils in peritoneal fluid is associated with a poorer prognosis (i.e., need for surgical intervention and increased mortality rates).[11]

Degenerate change in neutrophils is characterized by swollen, pale-staining chromatin and loss of membrane integrity (Figure 10.2). While degenerate change is not pathognomonic for infection, the presence of degenerate neutrophils warrants a more thorough search for organisms. These changes occur *after* the cell has left the blood and indicate release of neutrophil enzymes and/or exposure to bacterial cytotoxins. In contrast, "toxic" neutrophils are characterized by the presence of cytoplasmic basophilia (often with Dohle bodies), foamy cytoplasm, less condensed chromatin, nuclear hyposegmentation, and larger cell size. These changes reflect maturational defects in the bone marrow that are associated with rapid neutropoiesis due to a strong systemic inflammatory stimulus. Toxic change exists in neutrophils *before* they enter the peritoneal cavity. Toxic change is often associated with severe bacterial infections or significant tissue necrosis.

Large mononuclear cells encompass both monocytes/macrophages and mesothelial cells. When monocytes exit the vasculature, they differentiate into macrophages; both forms will be present in body cavities (Figure 10.3). Macrophages will occasionally contain senescent neutrophils. As with neutrophils, increases in monocyte/macrophage concentrations in fluid are attributable to inflammation and usually accompany neutrophil increases; neutrophil proportions typically exceed those of monocyte/macrophages in acute inflammation, whereas mononuclear cells may predominate with chronic effusions and certain disease processes (e.g., fungal infection).

Mesothelial cells are readily identified when they are present in cohesive aggregates (Figure 10.4), and in horses they are rare in both normal fluid and effusions. Although included in the large mononuclear cell group, they comprise only a minor fraction of the large mononuclear cell differential.

The lymphocytes in normal peritoneal fluid are small to medium sized (7–10 μm diameter) and constitute the smallest proportion of the three main cell types in normal peritoneal fluid. Increases in lymphocytes may be associated with chronic inflammatory conditions, parasitism, or

chyloabdomen. In chronic inflammation, the lymphocyte population is often a mixture of small lymphocytes, medium lymphocytes (prolymphocytes), reactive lymphocytes, and plasma cells. Reactive lymphocytes are usually slightly larger than small lymphocytes (9–11 μm diameter) and are characterized as having deeply basophilic cytoplasm and a mature chromatin. Lymphoblasts are large lymphocytes (12–16 μm diameter) whose nuclei have immature chromatin and usually contain a nucleolus or nucleoli. The presence of lymphoblasts is abnormal and is usually associated with large cell lymphoma. However, in the context of reactive lymphocytes and plasma cells, rare lymphoblasts may be part of the inflammatory response.

Other cell types such as eosinophils, basophils, and mast cells do not contribute to the cellular differential in normal abdominal fluid. The largest increases in eosinophil numbers can be associated with parasitic infections (including larval migration), but smaller increases may be seen with inflammation due to any etiology. Eosinophilia in peritoneal fluid (Figure 10.5) may also be seen with focal eosinophilic enteritis[22] and, rarely, lymphoma.[16] Basophils and mast cells can increase concurrently with eosinophils, though both are rare findings, even in inflammation.

Neoplastic cells can occasionally be found in peritoneal fluid. Lymphoma (Figure 10.6) and carcinoma (Figure 10.7) are the most common neoplasms identified in peritoneal effusions.

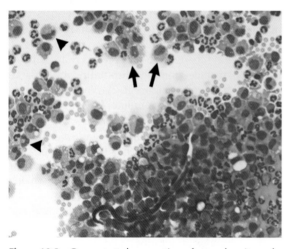

Figure 10.3 Concentrated preparation of normal peritoneal fluid containing both monocytes (arrowheads) and macrophages (arrows). Note the presence of a microfilarial organism in the bottom center. *Setaria* spp. are an incidental finding, especially in horses that have not been routinely dewormed.

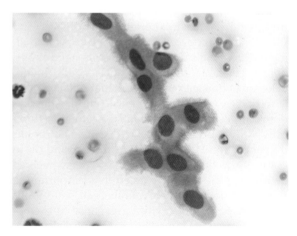

Figure 10.4 Mesothelial cell cluster. Mesothelial cells are round to polygonal, uniform, and cohesive.

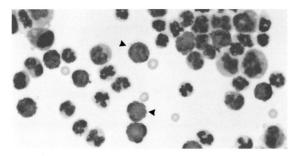

Figure 10.5   Eosinophilic inflammation in peritoneal fluid. Neutrophils comprise the predominant leukocyte, but significant numbers of eosinophils are present (arrowheads).

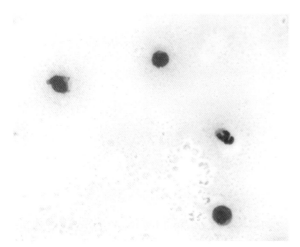

Figure 10.6   Peritoneal fluid from a horse with large cell lymphoma. Three large immature lymphocytes are present; note the size of the three lymphocytes compared to the neutrophil.

Interpretation of findings

The main categories of effusion are formulated to provide insight into the general pathophysiologic mechanism responsible for an increase in the volume of body cavity fluid. Effusions are caused mainly by transudative, exudative, or hemorrhagic processes (Table 10.2). A fourth category, which is uncommon in horses, is lymphorrhagic effusion caused by leakage of lymph from lymphatic vessels (e.g., chyloabdomen).[23]

Transudates

Transudates are caused by increased hydraulic pressure or increased hydraulic and decreased oncotic pressure. These effusions have low protein concentrations and NCCs. In horses, normal peritoneal fluid is distinguished from a transudate only by documenting an increase in fluid volume. The most common causes of transudates are the per-acute/acute phase of any lesion causing decreased venous/lymphatic drainage in the portal system (e.g., volvulus/torsion, neoplasia, granuloma), lymphatic obstruction, acute uroabdomen, and protein-losing nephropathies and enteropathies. Diagnosis of uroabdomen in the horse is facilitated by the characteristic presence of calcium carbonate crystals in equine urine, which are present extracellularly and within neutrophils (Figure 10.8). Suspicion of uroabdomen should be confirmed by measuring fluid creatinine concentration.

(a)   (b)

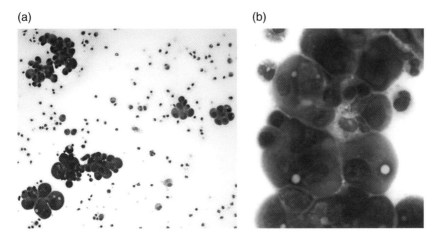

Figure 10.7   (a) Many clusters of large, cohesive cells in abdominal fluid. (b) The marked variability in cell and nuclear sizes, multinucleation, and prominent nucleoli are criteria of malignancy. The cohesive nature implies either an epithelial (carcinoma) or mesothelial (mesothelioma) phenotype.

Table 10.2   Effusion classifications.

Classification	TP$_{Ref}$	NCC	RBC	Mechanism	Disorder
Transudate	<2.0	<5×10³	<4×10⁴	↑Hydraulic and ↓oncotic pressure	• Nephrotic syndrome • Cirrhosis • Acute uroabdomen
High-protein transudate ("modified")	≥2.0	<5×10³	<4×10⁴	↓Hydraulic and ↓oncotic pressure in postsinusoidal or sinusoidal hepatic vessels	• Congestive heart failure • Portal hypertension (postsinusoidal)
Exudate	>2.0	>5×10³	4×10⁴–5×10⁵	↑Vascular permeability due to inflammatory mediators	*Septic:* • Bacterial, fungal, or parasitic infection *Nonseptic:* • Neoplasia • Ischemic necrosis • Pancreatitis • Bile peritonitis • Chronic uroabdomen
Hemorrhage (acute)	≥2.0	≥ or ≤5×10³	≥1×10⁶	Loss of blood from vessels	• Trauma • Neoplasia • Hemostatic defects • Uterine artery rupture

TP$_{Ref}$, total protein by refractometer (g/dL); NCC, nucleated cell count/μL; RBC, red blood cells/μL.

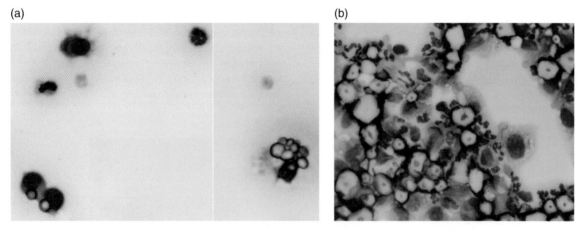

Figure 10.8   (a) Peritoneal fluid from an adult male horse with colic. Note the presence of round to oval calcium carbonate crystals within three macrophages. (b) Concentrated preparation of normal peritoneal fluid. There are many round to polygonal crystals with a characteristic central divet consistent with starch granules from surgical gloves. These are common contaminants that should not be mistaken for calcium carbonate crystals.

Plasma protein permeability of vessels within the hepatic sinuses is higher than that for vessels elsewhere in the peritoneal cavity. Consequently, increases in hydraulic pressure that involve the hepatic sinuses (i.e., sinusoidal or postsinusoidal increases) will produce a higher protein transudate with a normal NCC. Congestive heart failure and any lesion that produces postsinusoidal portal hypertension are the most common causes of high-protein transudates in the peritoneal cavity.

Exudates

Exudates are characterized by increased vascular permeability due to inflammatory mediators and therefore are attributable to inflammation. Inflammation may be caused by infectious or non-infectious processes (Table 10.2). The absence of microorganisms on cytologic examination does not preclude an infectious process. If clinical findings are suspicious of an infectious process, biochemical evaluation of the fluid (for lactate, glucose, and pH) and bacterial culture are warranted.

Hemorrhagic effusions

Uniformly hemorrhagic specimens or consistently hemorrhagic specimens from different abdominocentesis sites suggest true abdominal hemorrhage, which may be confirmed via cytology and/or sonographic evaluation of the abdomen (p. 134). Because platelets (and coagulation factors) are consumed during hemorrhage, hemorrhagic fluid contains no platelets and does not clot, whereas fluid with blood from peripheral or splenic vessels will contain platelets and will clot. A hemorrhagic effusion is defined by the fluid RBC count (Table 10.2); acute hemorrhagic effusions usually have RBC counts >1 000 000/μL and packed cell volumes >3%.[23] Erythrocytes and plasma from hemorrhage will be resorbed by lymphatics so the fluid TP and RBC counts vary with time; in dogs ~65% of RBCs are resorbed within 2 days of hemorrhage.[2]

Cytologic evaluation of abdominal fluid can be helpful in determining whether there is true hemorrhage. In fluids with high RBC counts, the presence of platelets indicates a component of blood contamination since platelets are not present in hemorrhagic effusions. However, the absence of platelets does not preclude peripheral blood contamination if the sample was collected into a non-anticoagulant tube (e.g., red top tube) and subsequently clotted *in vitro*. Cytologic findings that support hemoabdomen include the presence of erythrocytes and/or hemosiderin within macrophages. If there is a delay in sample processing (>3–4 h), RBC phagocytosis can occur *in vitro* in the transport tube. Conversely, erythrophagocytosis can be absent in samples from true hemorrhage if there has been insufficient time for RBC phagocytosis within the peritoneal cavity (i.e., peracute hemorrhage). In general, it takes several hours for erythrophagocytosis to occur; subsequent RBC breakdown into hemosiderin usually takes at least 3 days.[8] Thus, cytologic interpretations of hemorrhagic fluid should be undertaken with knowledge of the type of collection tube used as well as the amount of time before the sample was processed.

Application of peritoneal fluid analysis

Abdominocentesis is a valuable clinical tool whose sensitivity and specificity are highest when all components of fluid evaluation are considered together in conjunction with clinical findings and initial response to treatment (Clinical scenarios 5, 7–9, located in Appendix A). All fluid evaluations should include assessment of gross appearance, TP concentration, cell counts (or estimation of cellularity), and cytology. If this is not possible, the minimum testing for fluid evaluation should include measurement of TP and measurement (or estimation) of cellularity, because effusions are defined by these parameters.

References

1. Brownlow, M.A., Hutchins, D.R. & Johnston, K.G. (1981) Reference values for equine peritoneal fluid. *Equine Veterinary Journal*, **13**, 127–130.
2. Clark, C.H. & Woodley, C.H. (1959) The absorption of red blood cells after parenteral injection at various sites. *American Journal of Veterinary Research*, **20**, 1062–1066.
3. Collatos, C., Barton, M.H., Prasse, K.W. & Moore, J.N. (1995) Intravascular and peritoneal coagulation and fibrinolysis in horses with acute gastrointestinal tract diseases. *Journal of the American Veterinary Medical Association*, **207**, 465–470.
4. DeHeer, H.L., Parry, B.W. & Grindem, C.B. (2002) Peritoneal fluid. In: *Diagnostic Cytology and Hematology of the Horse* (eds R.L. Cowell & R.D. Tyler), 2nd edn., pp. 127–162. Mosby, St. Louis, Missouri.
5. Delesalle, C., Dewulf, J., Lefebvre, R.A., *et al.* (2007) Determination of lactate concentrations in blood plasma and peritoneal fluid in horses with colic by an Accusport analyzer. *Journal of Veterinary Internal Medicine*, **21**, 293–301.

6. Delgado, M.A., Monreal, L., Armengou, L., Ríos, J. & Segura, D. (2009) Peritoneal D-dimer concentration for assessing peritoneal fibrinolytic activity in horses with colic. *Journal of Veterinary Internal Medicine*, **23**, 882–889.

7. Delgado, M.A., Monreal, L., Armengou, L., Segura, D. & Ríos, J. (2009) Effects of blood contamination on peritoneal D-dimer concentration in horses with colic. *Journal of Veterinary Internal Medicine*, **23**, 1232–1238.

8. Epstein, C.E., Elidemir, O., Colasurdo, G.N. & Fan, L.L. (2001) Time course of hemosiderin production by alveolar macrophages in a murine model. *Chest*, **120**, 2013–2020.

9. Estepa, J.C., Lopez, I., Mayer-Valor, R., Rodriguez, M. & Aguilera-Tejero, E. (2006) The influence of anticoagulants on the measurement of total protein concentration in equine peritoneal fluid. *Research in Veterinary Science*, **80**, 5–10.

10. Freden, G.O., Provost, P.J. & Rand, W.M. (1998) Reliability of using results of abdominal fluid analysis to determine treatment and predict lesion type and outcome for horses with colic: 218 cases (1991–1994). *Journal of the American Veterinary Medical Association*, **213**, 1012–1015.

11. Garma-Avina, A. (1998) Cytology of 100 samples of abdominal fluid from 100 horses with abdominal disease. *Equine Veterinary Journal*, **30**, 435–444.

12. George, J.W. (2001) The usefulness and limitations of hand-held refractometers in veterinary laboratory medicine: An historical and technical review. *Veterinary Clinical Pathology*, **30**, 201–210.

13. George, J.W. & O'Neill, S.L. (2001) Comparison of refractometer and biuret methods for total protein measurement in body cavity fluids. *Veterinary Clinical Pathology*, **30**, 16–18.

14. Grindem, C.B., Fairley, N.M., Uhlinger, C.A. & Crane, S.A. (1990) Peritoneal fluid values from healthy foals. *Equine Veterinary Journal*, **22**, 359–361.

15. Hunt, E., Tennant, B.C. & Whitlock, R.H. (1985) Interpretation of peritoneal fluid erythrocyte counts in horses with abdominal disease. In: *Proceedings of the Second Equine Colic Research Symposium*, University of Georgia, Athens, Georgia, pp. 168–174.

16. La Perle, K.M.D., Piercy, R.J. & Blomme, E.A.G. (1998) Multisystemic, eosinophilic, epitheliotropic disease with intestinal lymphosarcoma in a horse. *Veterinary Pathology*, **35**, 144–146.

17. Latson, K.M., Nieto, J.E., Beldomenico, P.M. & Snyder, J.R. (2005) Evaluation of peritoneal fluid lactate as a marker of intestinal ischaemia in equine colic. *Equine Veterinary Journal*, **37**, 342–346.

18. Malark, J.A., Peyton, L.C. & Galvin, M.J. (1992) Effects of blood contamination on equine peritoneal fluid analysis. *Journal of the American Veterinary Medical Association*, **201**, 1545–1548.

19. Matthews, A., Dart, A.J., Reid, S.W., Dowling, B.A. & Hodgson, D.R. (2002) Predictive values, sensitivity and specificity of abdominal fluid variables in determining the need for surgery in horses with an acute abdominal crisis. *Australian Veterinary Journal*, **80**, 132–136.

20. McSherry, B.J. & Al-Baker, J. (1976) Comparison of total serum protein determined by T/S meter and biuret technique. *Bulletin of the American Society of Veterinary Clinical Pathologists*, **3**, 4–12.

21. Peloso, J.G. & Cohen, N.D. (2012) Use of serial measurements of peritoneal fluid lactate concentration to identify strangulating intestinal lesions in referred horses with signs of colic. *Journal of the American Veterinary Medical Association*, **240**, 1208–1217.

22. Southwood, L.L., Kawcak, C.E., Trotter, G.W., Stashak, T.S. & Frisbie, D.D. (2000) Idiopathic focal eosinophilic enteritis associated with small intestinal obstruction in 6 horses. *Veterinary Surgery*, **29**, 415–419.

23. Stockham, S.L. & Scott, M.A. (2008) Cavitary effusions. In: *Fundamentals of Veterinary Clinical* (eds S.L. Stockham & M.A. Scott), 2nd edn., pp. 831–868. Blackwell Publishing, Ames, Iowa.

24. Swansick, R.A. & Wilkinson, J.S. (1976) A clinical evaluation of abdominal paracentesis in the horse. *Australian Veterinary Journal*, **52**, 109–116.

25. Tulleners, E.P. (1983) Complications of abdominocentesis in the horse. *Journal of the American Veterinary Medical Association*, **182**, 232–234.

26. Van Hoogmoed, L., Rodger, L.D., Spier, S.J., Gardner, I.A., Yarbrough, T.B. & Snyder, J.R. (1999) Evaluation of peritoneal fluid pH, glucose concentration, and lactate dehydrogenase activity for detection of septic peritonitis in horses. *Journal of the American Veterinary Medical Association*, **214**, 1032–1036.

27. Weimann, C.D., Thoefner, M.B. & Jensen, A.L. (2002) Spectrophotometric assessment of peritoneal fluid haemoglobin in colic horses: An aid to selecting medical vs. surgical treatment. *Equine Veterinary Journal*, **34**, 523–527.

11 Intravenous Catheterization and Fluid Therapy

Louise L. Southwood

Department of Clinical Studies, New Bolton Center, School of Veterinary Medicine, University of Pennsylvania, Kennett Square, PA, USA

Chapter Outline

Basics of fluid distribution throughout the body	**99**
Oxygen delivery to the cells	**101**
IV catheterization	**103**
Indications	103
Preparation	103
Catheters	103
Skin preparation	103
Procedure	105
Over-the-needle technique	105
Over-the-wire (Seldinger) technique	106
Care of the IV catheter	106
Complications	107
IV fluid therapy	**109**
Isotonic crystalloids	109
Replacement or resuscitation	109
Maintenance	110
Electrolytes	110
Hypertonic saline solution (HSS)	111
Colloids	112
Plasma	112
Hydroxyethyl starch (HES)	113

Basics of fluid distribution throughout the body

The total body water of the adult horse is ~60% of the body weight (300 L for a 500 kg horse). The total body water is divided by the cell membrane into the intracellular (66%, 200 L for a 500 kg horse) and extracellular (33%, 100 L) compartments. The principle intracellular cation is potassium and anion is bicarbonate and the principle extracellular cation is sodium and anion is chloride. The cell membrane is impermeable to electrolytes and molecules which cross the cell membrane through channels or pumps. Water moves across the cell membrane by osmosis from high to low osmolality to maintain isotonicity of ~300 mEq in the intra- and extracellular compartments. In addition to isotonicity, electroneutrality and pH are maintained using the various channels and pumps. Water typically moves across membranes and capillaries in tandem with the sodium ion. The intracellular and extracellular electrolyte difference is important for cellular function especially for nerve and muscle cells. The movement of water across the cell membrane is clinically important in patients with hypo- and hypernatremia (see Electrolytes [p. 110]).

The capillary membrane separates the extracellular fluid into the intra- and extravascular spaces (intravascular 25% [25 L for a 500 kg horse] and extravascular 75% [75 L for a 500 kg horse]). Water and electrolytes move freely across the capillary membrane and are distributed equally across the capillary membrane throughout the extracellular fluid space. Water moves across the capillary membrane according the Starling-Landis equation which describes the balance between intravascular and interstitial oncotic and hydrostatic pressure as well as the capillary permeability:

$$J_v = K_f \left([P_c - P_i] - \sigma[\pi_c - \pi_i] \right)$$

where

$([P_c - P_i] - \sigma[\pi_c - \pi_i])$ is the net driving force

σ is the reflection coefficient of the capillary membrane (i.e., the ability of the capillary to maintain molecules such as albumin within the intravascular space)

P_c and P_i are the capillary and interstitial hydrostatic pressures, respectively

π_c and π_i are the capillary and interstitial oncotic pressures, respectively

K_f is the filtration coefficient which is the proportionality constant; K_f is a product of the capillary surface area and the capillary hydraulic conductance (i.e., the ease with which water can move across the capillary)

J_v is the net fluid movement between compartments

There is normally a net movement of fluid from the intravascular into the extravascular compartment which is absorbed by the lymphatics and returned to the intravascular compartment via the lymphatic ducts.

The importance of Starling's equation is that it can be used to understand fluid distribution in endotoxemia, hypoproteinemia, and with high fluid loads. The reflection coefficient of the capillary membrane (σ) decreases in shock and endotoxemia

when the endothelial cell tight junctions separate and the vessels become leaky with loss of albumin and water from the intravascular space resulting in inadequate colloid oncotic pressure (COP) and hypovolemia. Albumin (~67 kDa) is responsible for ~75% of the intravascular COP through attraction of water to the anionic albumin molecules as well as the Gibbs–Donnan effect whereby positively charged sodium molecules are also attracted to the negatively charged albumin and draw additional water across the capillary membrane. Loss of albumin and other proteins from the gastrointestinal tract and damaged vascular endothelium leads to hypoproteinemia and insufficient COP to maintain water within the vascular space resulting in hypovolemia. When the interstitial water accumulation exceeds the absorption capability of the lymphatics, interstitial edema occurs. Edema formation can impair organ function and oxygen delivery to cells. Maintenance of total plasma protein (TPP) >4 g/dL (40 g/L), albumin >2 g/dL (20 g/L), and COP > 15 mmHg is critical to maintain intravascular water and prevent edema formation. Normal plasma COP is ~20–30 mmHg for adult horses and ~15–25 mmHg for neonatal foals.[23] COP can be calculated using formulas or measured directly using a colloid osmometer. Direct measurement is recommended for hypoproteinemic colic patients and following administration of synthetic colloids.

Landis–Pappenheimer equation for healthy foals:[37,44]

$$COP = 2.1\,TPP + (0.16\,TPP^2) + (0.009\,TPP^3)$$

Equations for healthy adult horses:[4,44]

$$COP = 0.986 + 2.029\,A + 0.175\,A^2$$
$$COP = -0.059 + 0.618\,G + 0.028\,G^2$$
$$COP = 0.028 + 1.542\,TPP + 0.219\,TPP^2$$
$$COP = -1.989 + 1.068\,TPP + 0.176\,TPP^2$$
$$COP = -4.384 + 5.501\,A + 2.475\,G$$

where TPP is total plasma protein (g/dL), A is albumin concentration (g/dL), and G is globulin (g/dL).

Excessively high fluid loads can increase capillary hydrostatic pressure and cause interstitial edema

Table 11.1   Clinical findings associated with dehydration.

%	Mentation	Heart rate (bpm)	Mucous membranes	CRT (s)	PCV/TPP (%/g/dL)	Cr (mg/dL)
<5*	BAR	<44	WNL	<2	WNL	WNL
6	BAR	44–60	Tachy	2	40/7	1.5–2
8	Quiet	60–80	Tachy to dry	3	45/7.5	2–3
10†	Dull	80–100	Dry	4	50/8	3–4
12†	Moribund	>100	Dry	>4	>50/>8	>4

BAR, bright, alert, and responsive; bpm, beats per minute; WNL, within normal limits.
*Clinically undetectable.
†Associated with signs of shock including poor jugular refill, cool extremities, and weak pulse.
Source: Modified from Hardy (2010).

in the pulmonary and systemic tissues. It is critical to maintain COP in equine colic patients (see Colloids [p. 112]) and to avoid excessive intravenous (IV) fluid administration (see Isotonic crystalloids [p. 109]).

Dehydration is defined as loss of total body water primarily from the interstitial fluid compartment and is manifest clinically by tacky to dry oral mucous and prolonged skin tent (not particularly reliable in the horse) (Table 11.1). Isotonic crystalloid fluids are ideal for correcting dehydration (p. 109). Hypovolemia is inadequate fluid volume within the vascular space. Clinical features of hypovolemia include prolonged capillary refill time and poor jugular refill. While isotonic crystalloids are often satisfactory for correcting mild hypovolemia, hypertonic solutions (p. 111) and colloids (p. 112) are better for improving vascular volume in moderate and severe hypovolemia. When dehydration and hypovolemia are prolonged or moderate to severe, oxygen delivery to cells is impaired.

Oxygen delivery to the cells

The goal of fluid therapy is to maintain oxygen delivery to the tissues. Shock is defined as inadequate tissue perfusion and is characterized by poor tissue oxygenation causing inadequate cellular ATP production and ultimately cell dysfunction and death. It results from as an imbalance between tissue oxygen delivery (DO_2) and oxygen consumption (VO_2). In general, VO_2 is not pathologically increased in colic patients and the limiting factor is DO_2. DO_2 is the product of cardiac output (Q) and arterial oxygen content (CaO_2). Cardiac output (Q) is the product of heart rate (HR) and stroke volume (SV) and CaO_2 is primarily based on the hemoglobin concentration ([Hb]) and arterial hemoglobin oxygen saturation (SaO_2). The arterial oxygen tension (PaO_2) comprises a small proportion of CaO_2; however, its importance lies in its relationship to hemoglobin saturation with oxygen based on the oxygen dissociation curve. In summary:

$$Shock = DO_2 < VO_2$$
$$DO_2 = Q \times CaO_2$$
$$Q = HR \times SV$$
$$CaO_2 = ([HB] \times SaO_2 \times 1.34)$$
$$+ (PaO_2 \times 0.0031)$$
$$VO_2 = Q \times [Hb] \times 13.4 \times (SaO_2 - SvO_2)$$

SvO_2 is the venous oxygen saturation. Note that cardiac index (CI) and stroke volume index (SVI) are Q and SV expressed per kilogram of body weight, respectively.

In adult colic patients, pulmonary function is generally normal and SaO_2 adequate. Except in horses or foals with moderate to severe hemorrhage, the hemoglobin concentration should also be within normal limits. Therefore, the CaO_2 is unlikely to contribute to shock in colic patients except in complicated cases. Hypovolemic and distributive shock are classically observed in colic patients. Hypovolemia is caused by inadequate water intake and loss of water into the gastrointestinal tract and intestinal wall (edema formation). Distributive shock creates a "relative hypovolemia" associated with vasodilation and is typically associated with endotoxemia (p. 246). Resuscitation and maintenance of cardiovascular function during the postoperative period is dependent on administration of crystalloid and colloid fluid therapy using a goal-directed approach.

Phases of shock are compensated, early decompensated, and late decompensated leading to death. Compensatory mechanisms involve stimulation of the sympathetic nervous system, activation of the rennin-angiotensin-aldersterone system, and release of antidiuretic hormone (ADH, vasopressin) and adrenocorticotropic hormone. These mechanisms serve to improve blood supply to the vital organs through increasing heart rate and cardiac contractility and causing vasoconstriction and water retention to increase the venous return to the heart and direct blood flow to the vital organs.

Clinical features associated with shock include tachycardia, abnormal mucous membrane color, prolonged capillary refill time, poor jugular refill, cool extremities, hypotension, and oliguria/azotemia reflective of the disease process and compensatory mechanisms.

In states of hypoxia, cellular metabolism switches from efficient aerobic to less efficient anaerobic glucose metabolism to maintain ATP production which is important for ion pumps (e.g., sodium-potassium ATPase function) and cell maintenance. Lactate is produced as the end product of anaerobic glucose metabolism and accumulates in the blood. Blood lactate concentration can be used as an estimate of adequacy of tissue perfusion and shock and should be <1.0 mmol/L in an adequately hydrated horse.[24]

Plasma creatinine concentration can also be used as a measure of tissue perfusion and should be <1.5 mg/dL (15 mg/L) in a well-hydrated adult horse. Urine output can be estimated in adult horses and should be 15–30 mL/kg/day (7.5–15 L for a 500 kg horse, i.e., there should be several wet areas throughout the stall).[24] Urine output in equine neonates can be measured using an indwelling urinary catheter and should be 4–8 mL/kg/h.[24]

SvO_2 and venous oxygen tension (PvO_2) can be used to determine whether tissue oxygen demand is being met and is a measure of tissue oxygen tension rather than pulmonary function. Normal adult jugular PvO_2 is 40–50 mmHg and SvO_2 65–75%.[23] In neonatal foals, mixed venous PvO_2 is ~35–42 mmHg.[24] SvO_2 is low in states of shock when the tissue oxygen supply is not being met.

Intravascular volume is important to maintain SV and Q. Central venous pressure (CVP) is the intraluminal blood pressure within the cranial vena cava and can be used as an approximation of preload and right ventricular filling pressure.[24] Normal CVP is 8–12 cmH₂O and an attempt should be made to maintain CVP>5 cmH₂O. CVP is measured using a water manometer attached using extension tubing to a ~26 in. (~60 cm) IV catheter inserted in the jugular vein with the catheter tip located within the intrathoracic cranial vena cava.[24] All bubbles should be removed from the fluid lines. The water manometer is zeroed at the point of the shoulder. CVP measurement is particularly useful for guiding IV fluid therapy in postoperative colic patients showing signs of shock (e.g., large colon volvulus), with moderate to marked hypoproteinemia (e.g., colitis, large colon volvulus), or with large volumes of nasogastric reflux.

Mean arterial blood pressure (MAP) is used as an estimate of tissue blood flow and can be measured directly or indirectly.[24] While direct blood pressure measurement may seem impractical at first glance, most horses and foals have a facial or a transverse facial arterial catheter placed during general anesthesia which can be sutured and glued into place for recovery and maintained for several days. Direct pressure is measured using noncompliant tubing attached to the arterial catheter, a pressure transducer, and a continuous recorder.[24] Direct blood pressure measurement is more accurate than indirect methods. Normal direct pressure measurements in adult horses are 110–133 mmHg.[24] Blood pressure values in foals vary with age, size, and breed.[24] Indirect blood pressure is typically measured using the oscillometric method with an occlusion cuff placed over the coccygeal artery (tail cuff) in adult horses. The dorsal metatarsal, median, or digital arteries on the limb can be used in neonates. The bladder width should be 20–25% of the tail circumference (40–50% of the limb circumference) and the bladder length 80% of the tail/limb circumference. Inadequate cuff size or too loose or too tight placement results in false readings. The horse should be quiet with its head at a resting level and heart rate recorded should be the same as that obtained with auscultation. Normal MAP measured using the oscillometric method and coccygeal artery is 85–95 mmHg in the adult horse (note the lower value compared with direct measurement because the coccygeal artery is above heart level).[24] MAP should be maintained

>60 mmHg to ensure adequate perfusion of vital organs. It is important to recognize that MAP is maintained until decompensation and is not as sensitive as other measurements for directing fluid therapy. Inotropes and pressors are not typically used in colic patients beyond the intraoperative period primarily because horses with that degree of cardiovascular compromise likely have nonviable intestine, and pressors tend to redirect blood from the gastrointestinal tract to vital organs.

IV catheterization

Catheterization of the left or right jugular vein is generally considered the standard of care for horses and foals admitted to referral hospitals for colic. Catheterization of the lateral thoracic or cephalic vein can also be performed in horses with damage to the jugular vein or inflammation of the perivascular tissue.[5] These techniques are rarely necessary in colic patients.

Indications

Obtaining venous access is an important component of emergency case management. However, IV catheterization is in fact indicated in a small percentage of horses with colic (<20%). Indications for IV catheterization include

- dehydration;
- shock;
- prior to general anesthesia for colic surgery;
- recurrent or persist signs of pain despite analgesia; and/or
- pain or difficult behavior making administration of medication difficult.

IV catheterization of the colic patient is recommended primarily for administration of IV fluids to correct water and electrolyte disturbances. Many horses with mild signs of dehydration (Table 11.1) can be managed with enteral fluids and electrolytes (see Chapter 7 on Enteral Fluid Therapy [p. 62]). Horses that have not been drinking for 24 h or longer are likely to be moderately dehydrated especially if signs of colic are associated with excessive sweating and inadequate water intake. These

horses may benefit from IV fluids. Horses showing signs of shock including tachycardia, injected or toxic membranes, prolonged capillary refill time, cool extremities, poor pulse quality, and poor jugular refill require IV catheterization and resuscitation fluid therapy with crystalloids and possibly colloids.

An IV catheter can also facilitate administration of medications in a horse or foal that is particularly painful or difficult to treat and is recommended for administration of anesthetic drugs for colic surgery.

Preparation

A list of materials necessary for IV catheterization is provided in Table 11.2.

Catheters

There are typically three types of IV catheters used in equine patients:

- Polytetrafluoroethylene (PTFE, Teflon®): for example, Abbocath, Abbott Laboratories, Abbott Park, IL, 14-gauge 5 1/2 in. (Figure 11.1)
- Polyurethane: over-the-needle, for example, Mila International, Florence, KY, 14-gauge 5 1/4 in. (Figure 11.5)
- Polyurethane: over-the-wire, for example, Mila International, Florence, KY, 14-gauge 8 in. (Figure 11.5)

Table 11.2   Materials required for IV catheterization.

- Clippers (optional)
- Povidone-iodine or chlorhexidine scrub and alcohol
- 2 mL 2% lidocaine (optional)
- Sterile gloves (optional)
- #15 blade for small skin stab incision (optional)
- 14- or 16-gauge IV catheter (flushed with heparinized saline)
- Injection cap, T-port, or extension set
- 2-0 nylon on straight needle
- 1 in. white tape to make butterfly on extension tubing for suturing to neck skin (optional)
- Suture scissors
- Cyanoacrylate adhesive (optional)
- Heparin flush in 20 mL syringe with 20-gauge needle
- Fluid administration set and IV fluids

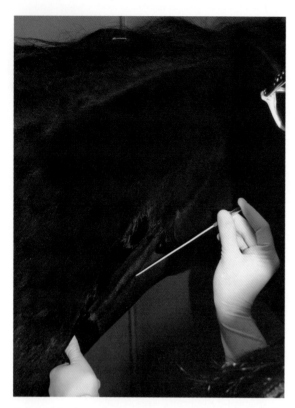

Figure 11.1 An area over jugular vein in the upper third of the neck is clipped and aseptically prepared. The vein is occluded using the left (or right) hand and a 14-gauge 5 1/2 in. (14 cm) catheter inserted through the skin parallel to the vein and at an angle of about 45°. Care should be taken to ensure that the stylet and catheter do not separate at this point during placement.

A 14-gauge catheter is typically used in an adult horse and a 16-gauge catheter in foals. Occasionally a larger bore catheter (e.g., 10- or 12-gauge) is needed to resuscitate adult horses. The catheter type used should be selected based on the anticipated duration of IV catheterization and the critical illness of the patient. For example, a horse with a large colon displacement is cardiovascularly stable, unlikely to have complications with coagulopathy or sepsis, and should require IV fluids for <24 h postoperatively. A PTFE catheter is suitable for this type of patient and is economical and easy to place. On the other hand, a horse with colitis or large colon volvulus is likely to require ongoing fluid therapy and have catheter-associated problems.[7]

An injection cap, T-port, or extension set (7 or 30 in.) can be inserted into the hub of the catheter to seal the end and provide a site for injection. A T-port or 7 in. extension set is recommended in the colic patient. Fluids are usually administered through a wide-bore fluid set with a 10 ft coil (STAT Large Animal IV Set, International WIN, Kennett Square, PA). Fluids are hung from a free-rotating fluid hanger (GYRO Fluid Hanger, International WIN, Kennett Square, PA) that allows four 5 L bags to be hung at one time.[5] The flow of fluids is dependent on the Hagen–Poiseuille equation with volumetric flow rate

$$= \frac{\pi R^4}{8\eta} \frac{|\Delta P|}{L}$$

where
   R is the internal radius of the tube (m)
   ΔP is the pressure difference between the two ends
   η is the dynamic fluid viscosity
   L is the length of the tube in the direction of flow

Therefore, hanging the fluids higher and using a large bore and short catheter will result in faster fluid administration; for example, a flow rate of 12 L/h can be achieved through a 14-gauge catheter by hanging fluids 50 in. (127 cm) above the catheter, using the wide-bore administration set.[5]

Skin preparation

The catheter site, most commonly the left or right jugular vein in the upper one third of the neck, is aseptically prepared. It is generally recommended to clip the site and the area clipped can vary from 2 cm × 2 cm to 10 cm × 10 cm (Figure 11.1). If the IV catheter is to be left in for only a few hours, the site can be prepared without clipping the hair. The skin (and hair) should be cleaned using a chlorhexidine- or povidone-iodine-based scrub and alcohol with care being taken to not drag the sponge used for cleaning from the dirty to the clean area. The sterile preparation should begin once the skin is clean. The site is sprayed with chlorhexidine solution and alcohol or alcohol only when a chlorhexidine- or povidone-iodine-based prep is used, respectively.

(a)   (b)

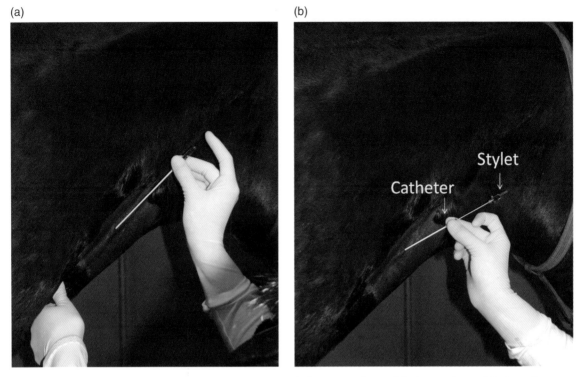

Figure 11.2   (a) Once blood is observed, the catheter and stylet hub are moved toward the horse's skin and (b) the catheter is slid over the stylet and into the vein to the level of the catheter hub. Care is taken to not advance the stylet with the catheter to avoid damage to the vessel.

Procedure

IV catheterization should be performed

- aseptically,
- atraumatically, and
- the catheter secured in place to prevent kinking or dislodgement of the catheter.

Sterile gloves may or may not be worn depending on the experience of the individual placing the IV catheter and the technique used. If gloves are not worn, particular care should be taken to avoid handling the shaft of the catheter or any material entering the vein.

Over-the-needle technique

Using the right hand (for right handed individuals), the thumb and middle finger are placed on the hub while the index finger is placed over the stylet hub to secure it in place (Figure 11.1). The vein is distended with the left hand which will likely result in contamination of this hand. A sterile 4×4 gauze sponge can be used to avoid contamination. The catheter is inserted through the skin parallel and at 45° to the jugular vein (Figure 11.1) and then directed into the distended vein. It is important to avoid tunneling the catheter in the subcutaneous tissue prior to entering the vein because this can cause kinking and problems with fluid administration. The catheter and stylet hub is then moved toward the horse's neck so that the shaft of the catheter and stylet are parallel to the vein. Ensure that the catheter and stylet are seated well within the vessel. The left hand is then used to slide the catheter over the stylet and into the vein (Figure 11.2). It is important to hold the stylet with the other hand and not advance the stylet further into the vein while placing the catheter to avoid

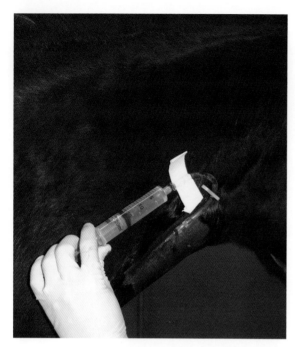

Figure 11.3 The extension set or tubing is placed onto the hub of the catheter and the catheter is flushed with heparinized saline. Care should be taken to avoid air aspiration into vein through the catheter once the stylet is removed and before the extension set is secured by occluding the jugular vein below the level of the catheter tip.

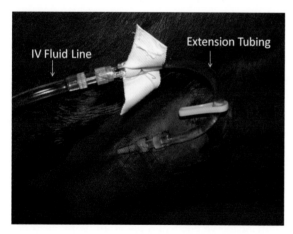

Figure 11.4 The catheter and extension set or tubing are sutured in place using 2-0 synthetic absorbable suture material.

damage to the vein. The catheter is inserted into the vein to the level of the catheter hub. Once inserted, the vein should be held off to avoid air aspiration.

The injection cap, T-port, or extension set is placed (Figure 11.3). The catheter is flushed with heparinized saline and then secured in place using 2-0 nylon (Figure 11.4) with or without cyanoacrylate adhesive. Nylon suture is placed around the indentation in the catheter hub and a butterfly is used to secure the extension set or tubing to the skin on the neck.

Polyurethane catheters are less rigid and can be somewhat more challenging to place using the over-the-needle technique. A small (2 mL) subcutaneous lidocaine bleb can be used so that a stab incision through the skin can be made to prevent damage to the catheter tip. Inserting the catheter and stylet shaft further down the vein before the catheter is slid over the stylet for final placement can prevent kinking of the softer material during placement.

Over-the-wire (Seldinger) technique

These types of catheters are typically used in critically ill patients (Figure 11.5). The 14- (adult) or 16-gauge (foal) needle is inserted into the vein. The wire is placed through the needle into the jugular vein and then the needle removed from the vein by sliding it back out over the needle. A dilator is placed over the wire to enlarge the hole in the skin to facilitate catheter insertion. The catheter is inserted over the wire. It is absolutely critical that the wire is not let go during the procedure to avoid it slipping into the vein and being lost. Once the catheter is inserted into the vein, the wire is removed. The jugular vein should be occluded during wire removal to prevent air aspiration. Extension tubing and a one-way valve are part of the catheter (Figure 11.5). The catheter is flushed with heparinized saline. The catheter is secured into the vein using 2-0 nylon in the places provided with the catheter (Figure 11.5).

Care of the IV catheter

The catheter site should be kept clean and flushed with heparinized saline at least every 6 h. The IV catheter should be removed as soon as it is no longer necessary; maintaining an IV catheter "in case it is needed" can result in complications. PTFE catheters and lines should be changed every 72 h. The polyurethane over-the-needle catheters can be

(a)   (b)

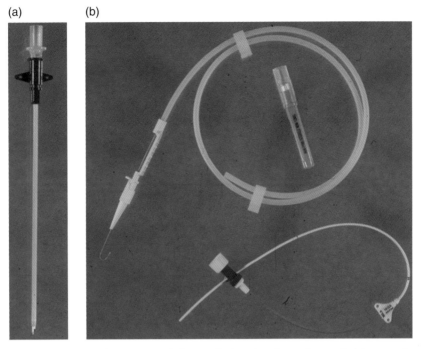

Figure 11.5   Polyurethane catheters (Mila International) that can be introduced over-the-needle (a) or over-the-wire (b).

maintained for up to 7 days and the over-the-wire catheters can be maintained for several weeks with proper care.

The catheter site should be monitored for swelling at the insertion site, venous thrombosis, or perivascular swelling. The IV catheter should be monitored for kinking at the insertion site, dislodgment, and particular care should be taken to ensure that the extension set does not become disconnected from the catheter hub.

Complications

The IV catheter should be monitored for signs of perivascular infection (heat, pain, swelling, redness, drainage at the insertion site), thrombophlebitis (thickening and thrombosis of the catheterized vein with or without heat, pain, and swelling indicative of septic thrombophlebitis), kinking of the catheter, and hemorrhage or aspiration of air associated with the extension set becoming dislodged or being transected. Air aspiration can be fatal. Adult horses usually do not exsanguinate from a catheter

because the blood usually clots in the catheter; however, having the site open can increase the risk of sepsis particularly in foals.

Adult horses with endotoxemia, salmonellosis, hypoproteinemia, and large colon disease are at considerably higher risk for developing thrombophlebitis compared to horses without these problems.[7] Horses with a high rectal temperature when the IV catheter is placed are more likely to develop thrombophlebitis than horses with a normal rectal temperature, and NSAID administration is reported to be protective.[9] A polyurethane long-term catheter should be used in these patients. Should catheter-associated infection or thrombophlebitis develop, the catheter should be removed, the tip submitted for bacterial culture and sensitivity testing, and the area kept cleaned and managed with hot compresses. Topic medications such as dimethylsulfoxide or 1% diclofenac sodium (Surpass®) may reduce the inflammation and alleviate patient discomfort. Rarely is thrombectomy necessary.[38] If IV access is remains necessary, use of the lateral thoracic (or cephalic) vein is recommended.

Table 11.3 Intravenous fluids.

Fluid	Na+ (mEq/L)	Cl− (mEq/L)	K+ (mEq/L)	Ca2+ (mEq/L)	Mg2+ (mEq/L)	mOsm/LpH
Plasma	140	100	4	~3	~1	300 7.38
Resuscitation and maintenance[a]						
Lactated Ringer's solution[c]	130	109	4	3	0	273 6.6
Normasol R[d] Abbott Laboratories	140	98	5	0	3	294 6.6
Plasmalyte A[d] Baxter Healthcare	140	98	5	0	3	294 7.4
0.9% Saline	154	154	0	0	0	308 5.0
Resuscitation						
7.2% Saline	1196	1196	0	0	0	2400 4.0
Maintenance						
Normasol-M and 5% dextrose[d] Abbott Laboratories	40	40	13	0	3	363 5.0
Plasmalyte-56 and 5% dextrose[d] Baxter Healthcare	40	40	~3	0	3	363 5.0
Colloids						
Hetastarch, Hospira	154	154	0	0	0	308
Hextend, Hospira	143	124	3	5	0.9	307

[a] These fluids are not typically considered maintenance fluids because of the high sodium and low potassium concentration; however, they are the fluids typically used for maintenance in adult horses because of their availability in 5 L bags.
[b] Buffer—bicarbonate.
[c] Buffer—lactate.
[d] Buffer—acetate or gluconate.
[e] Calcium containing fluids cannot be administered with blood products because of binding to the anticoagulant.
Source: Modified from Pantaleon (2010) and Cook and Bain (2003).

Repeated kinking of PTFE catheters can cause damage to the catheter and leakage at the insertion site or into the subcutaneous tissue. On rare occasions, a catheter can break off from the hub into the vein and become lodged in the heart or lung. These catheters can be removed if identified before they enter the lung.[1,13,21,22,37]

IV fluid therapy

The goal of IV fluid therapy is to volume replete the intravascular space thereby improving cardiac output, tissue perfusion, and oxygen delivery and ultimately restoring aerobic metabolism. IV fluids are also necessary for maintenance of patients that cannot or will not drink sufficient water and when oral fluid administration is insufficient. The mainstay of IV fluid therapy is polyionic isotonic crystalloid solutions. However, some patients require rapid intravascular expansion with hypertonic solutions and/or synthetic colloids and maintenance of COP with plasma or synthetic colloids.

Isotonic crystalloids

Polyionic isotonic fluids are most commonly used for resuscitation and maintenance of colic patients. Typically used fluids are listed in Table 11.3. The fluids available in 5 L bags for administration to adult horses are replacement or resuscitation fluids because the electrolyte concentration is similar to that of plasma. Maintenance fluids have lower sodium and chloride concentrations and higher potassium concentration. Adult horses with normal renal function are capable of maintaining the plasma sodium concentration within normal limits despite the high sodium concentration of the fluids; however, neonates may not and can accumulate sodium and water.

Fluid therapy can be considered in several phases:

- Replacement or resuscitation
- Maintenance
- Electrolyte replacement
- Colloid replacement

Replacement or resuscitation

Fluids are initially administered to correct dehydration and shock. Large volumes of IV fluids are necessary to correct water losses in adult horses:

500 kg horse that is 5% dehydrated has a fluid deficit of 25 L fluids:

$$500 \times 0.05 = 25\,L$$

In most patients, a 20 mL/kg bolus of a resuscitation or replacement fluid is administered and then careful reassessment performed (adult horses 10–20 L bolus and foals 1 L bolus). Fluid boluses can be given until improved signs of perfusion are observed (lower heart rate, improved jugular vein and capillary refill, moist mucous membranes, warmer extremities, brighter mentation, urination). Instances in which this may not be considered safe include hemorrhage, marked hypoproteinemia, renal failure (rare), heart failure (rare), and hyponatremia or hypernatremia. Hemorrhage is uncommon in the colic patient (except for postpartum mares); however, hemoabdomen may occur as a result of the primary lesion or postoperatively. Plasma lactate concentration and blood pressure can be monitored using direct or indirect pressure to guide resuscitation in these patients. Hypoproteinemia is not uncommon in the postoperative colic patient, particularly horses with large colon volvulus or colitis. Overhydration should be avoided in these patients and the adequacy of fluid therapy can be monitored using CVP and serial measurement of blood lactate concentration. TPP and COP should be monitored in these patients to guide colloid fluid therapy. Hyponatremia is more common in horses with diarrhea than in colic patients. Hypo- and hypernatremia should be corrected slowly if the problem is considered "chronic" (probably >48 h). Neurological complications associated with too rapid sodium correction are likely more of a problem in foals (see Electrolytes [p. 110]).

The limitation with isotonic crystalloids is that large volumes are necessary and the fluids are rapidly redistributed from the intravascular space following administration. Therefore, these fluids are ideal for correcting dehydration but not necessarily hypovolemia. Small volume resuscitation is often beneficial for equine colic patients prior to general anesthesia for more rapid cardiovascular stability. Hypertonic saline solution (HSS) (p. 111) and hydroxyethyl starch (HES) (p. 113) are the main fluids used for small volume resuscitation.

Maintenance

The maintenance fluid rate for an adult horse is 2 mL/kg/h. Therefore, for a 500 kg horse, the maintenance fluid rate would be ~1 L/h. Maintenance fluid rates for pregnant and lactating mares may be 1 $1/2$–3 times this rate, respectively. The fluids that are most commonly used for maintenance in adult horses are replacement fluids. Maintenance fluids have a lower sodium and higher potassium, calcium, and magnesium concentration (Table 11.3). The adult horse kidney is capable of excreting the sodium; however, neonates are often unable to because of concurrent disease, and care should be taken to avoid excessive sodium in neonates. The addition of 20 mEq/L of KCl can provide sufficient potassium for maintenance. Calcium borogluconate (23%) can be added to the fluids at 20 mL/L (100 mL/5 L bag) to supplement calcium in patients with hypocalcemia and lactating or pregnant mares.

Maintenance fluid rates for neonatal foals can be calculated from the Holliday–Segar formula[30]:

1–10 kg body weight	100 mL/kg/day
11–20 kg body weight	1000 mL + 50 mL for each kg >10 kg/day
>20 kg body weight	1500 mL + 25 mL for each kg >20 kg/day

Therefore, for a 50 kg foal, the rate would be:

$$1500\,ml + 25\,ml \times 30\,kg = 2250\,mL/day\ or\ 94\,mL/h$$

(see Electrolytes).

Fluids are usually administered using a fluid pump to ensure that the precise volume is being administered. Equine neonates have a requirement of dextrose at 4–8 mg/kg/min, which can be met with a 5–10% dextrose solution (50–100 mg/mL of dextrose) (see Chapter 23 on Nutrition [p. 301]).

Ongoing losses need to be factored into the maintenance fluid requirements. The most common source of fluid loss in colic patients is nasogastric reflux and diarrhea. Nasogastric reflux can be quantified and the rate of loss calcu-

lated on a L/h basis and added to the standard maintenance rate. Diarrhea can be difficult to quantify with some adult horses losing up to 5 L/h. Typically, 2–3 times the maintenance fluid rate is administered to horses with diarrhea and the adequacy of fluid therapy monitored (see previously).

Electrolytes

In general, severe electrolyte abnormalities are uncommon in colic patients. The key to electrolyte replacement is selecting a reasonable fluid concentration and then monitoring plasma levels closely and adjusting supplementation accordingly.

Horses with diarrhea can develop hyponatremia. In chronic (>48 h), severe hyponatremia, the rate of correction should not exceed 0.5–1 mEq/L/h, with a total increase not to exceed 8–12 mEq/L/d and no more than 18 mEq/L in the first 48 h because of the risk of osmotic demyelination syndrome (central pontine demyelination). It is necessary to correct the hyponatremia to a safe range (usually to no greater than 120 mEq/L) rather than to a normal value. Spontaneous diuresis secondary to ADH suppression with intravascular volume repletion could lead to unintended overcorrection. Neurological signs associated with too rapid correction of hyponatremia are more likely to be observed in neonates than adult horses. Similar guidelines should be followed with chronic severe hypernatremia, which is less commonly observed in patients with gastrointestinal disease.

Sodium requirements of neonates are 1–3 mg/kg/day, which is ~1 L of polyionic isotonic fluids for a 50 kg foal.[30] While adult horses may be able to manage the high sodium load associated with replacement fluids, neonates are often less able to and can retain water. Therefore, it is recommended to use a 5% dextrose solution as a source of free water with polyionic isotonic fluid.

Potassium supplementation is necessary for maintenance, particularly in horses and foals that are not eating. Maintenance fluid for adult horses can also be supplemented at 20 mEq/L of KCl. Electrolytes should be monitored, particularly in horses with complications. It is important to remember that potassium cannot be administered at more than 0.5 mEq/kg/h. Neonatal foals can also receive potassium supplementation at 20–60 mEq/L KCl depending on the fluid rate.[30]

Hypocalcemia is more commonly observed in colic patients. It is important to determine whether or not low total calcium can be attributed to hypo-albuminemia or if it is truly the ionized calcium that is low. Supplementation of calcium in patients with endotoxemia and ischemia-reperfusion injury is controversial. Inflammatory mediators, inter-leukin (IL)-1 and -6, and tumor necrosis factor (TNF)-α released during endotoxemia suppress the response of parathyroid hormone to hypocal-cemia. On the other hand, the importance of calcium in the production of inflammatory cyto-kines (e.g., TNF-α) is being recognized.[14] During ischemia-reperfusion injury, there are large increases in the cytosolic Ca^{2+} concentration which is initially sequestered in the mitochondria; mitochondrial Ca^{2+} handling has emerged as a key regulator in the progression to cell death during ischemia-reperfusion injury.[26] Calcium supplemen-tation (23% calcium borogluconate at 100mL/5L) is recommended in hypocalcemic patients following cardiovascular stabilization particularly if associated with hypotension during general anesthesia or poor motility during the postopera-tive period and can be important in lactating and late-term pregnant mares.

Magnesium can be low in colic patients and is not routinely supplemented in addition to that available in some of the polyionic isotonic fluids (Table 11.3); however, it is likely an overlooked electrolyte that may have a beneficial effect in colic patients. Magnesium sulfate is reported to have anti-inflammatory effects during endotoxemia and may be protective during ischemia-reperfusion injury.[18,20] Further research is necessary to under-stand the role of calcium and magnesium in ischemia-reperfusion injury and endotoxemia in equine colic patients as well as the benefit or detri-ment of supplementing with these electrolytes.

Acidosis/acidemia that does not respond to IV fluid therapy with restoration of tissue perfusion is uncommon in colic patients unless complicated by colitis which is associated with loss of bicarbonate from the gastrointestinal tract. Horses and foals with severe diarrhea can occasionally require bicarbonate supplementation because of moderate to severe losses from the gastrointestinal tract. Care should be taken when correcting bicarbonate and the sodium concentration (i.e., sodium bicarbonate) should also taken into consideration (see above). The bicarbonate deficit is calculated:

Bicarbonated deficit (mEq/L) = 0.4 × body weight (kg) × 24− patients bicarbonate concentration (mEq/L).

Half of the bicarbonate deficit is corrected over several hours and then the remaining deficit corrected gradually. Plasma sodium and bicarbonate concentrations should be monitored frequently.

Hypertonic saline solution (HSS)

HSS (7.2–7.5% sodium chloride, Table 11.3) can be given to horses showing severe signs of shock at a rate of 3–6mL/kg (1 $^1/_2$–3L [usually 2L] for a 500kg horse). HSS transiently increases intravascular volume, improves cardiac contractility and cardiac output, decreases endothelial and tissue edema, causes arteriolar vasodilation reducing systemic vascular resistance, and improves microcirculation, oxygen transport, and blood viscosity; HSS may also have an effect on immunomodulation.[2,18,19,28,29,31] The hemodynamic effects of HSS are short lived (~30min). The increase in intravascular volume is attributed to the high osmolarity attracting fluid from the interstitial and intracellular (endothelium and erythrocyte) space. Therefore, intravascular volume increases at the expense of the interstitial and intracellular compartments. HSS should, therefore, be followed within 1h with 10L of polyionic isotonic fluids per liter of HSS administered. The observed beneficial effect of HSS on intravascular volume may also be associated with ADH release and activation of aquaporin channels in the renal collecting duct responsible for water resorption.[2,35] HSS also report-edly inhibits leukocyte-endothelium interactions minimizing the capillary leakage and improving cardiac preload.[34] Anti-inflammatory effects may also reduce tissue damage and organ failure.[29,31]

HSS provided faster resolution of hypovolemia compared to isotonic saline in endurance horses eliminated from the ride; however, it was associ-ated with more marked but transient electrolyte disturbances.[8] Plasma volume expansion was estimated to be 29 ± 4% following 2L HSS and 5L lactated Ringer's solution (LRS) compared to 12 ± 15% following administration of 2L isotonic saline and 5L LRS with an estimated increase in the extracellular fluid volume of 8–10L beyond the volume of fluid administered.[8]

HSS has been reported to have a concentration-dependent anticoagulant and antiplatelet effect, likely related to the effect of high sodium load and ionic strength altering enzyme function and coagulation mechanisms.[47] Clotting function deteriorates with increasing ionic strength (plasma Na+ and Cl- concentration). The sodium concentration that leads to impairment coagulation and platelet function is unknown and likely to be high (plasma sodium concentration of 250 mEq/L or administration dose rate of 20 mL/kg HSS);[36] an administration dose rate of 5 mL/kg results in a plasma sodium concentration of 155 mEq/L and, therefore, a clinically important impact on coagulation is unlikely. Importantly in an equine endotoxemia model, there were no differences in coagulation measurements between horses treated with isotonic saline and a combination of HSS (7.2% NaCl 5 mL/kg) and HES (6% HES 10 mL/kg). The HSS-HES treated horses had less observed effect on ionized calcium and not surprisingly did have a transient increase in NaCl.[33] Concerns with coagulation arise in colic patients because of the effects of endotoxin on coagulation through cytokine release: (1) stimulating macrophage and endothelial tissue factor expression which activates the extrinsic (tissue factor-factor VII) coagulation pathway; (2) attenuating antithrombin III, protein C, and tissue factor inhibitor; (3) increasing plasma concentrations of plasminogen activator inhibitor impairing fibrinolysis through plasmin; and (4) activating platelets causing thrombosis and consumption of coagulation factor leading to disseminated intravascular coagulopathy in severely affected patients. Based on clinical experience and experimental data, the effect of HSS (7.2% 4 mL/kg) on coagulation is negligible.

Colloids

Colloids used most often in colic patients are plasma and HES (hetastarch or pentastarch) (Table 11.3). Dextrans are rarely used because of their negative effect on coagulation and hypersensitivity reactions. Dextran anticoagulant effect is attributed to platelet coating, inhibition of platelet, neutrophil and erythrocyte agglutination, clotting factor dilution, and decreased von Willebrand's factor and factor VIII activity. Dextrans also interfere with cross-matching of blood products.[23] While benefits with albumin have been observed in some human patients and animal models,[12] their use for providing colloidal support in colic patients has not gained widespread acceptance. Blood transfusions are rarely needed in equine colic patients.

Colloids are used in resuscitation because of their ability to draw water into the vascular space and for maintenance of COP in patients with protein loss into the gastrointestinal tract and interstitial space through leaky endothelium. COP < 15 mmHg during general anesthesia can increase intestinal edema which can be attenuated by colloid administration.[12] Typically a combination of plasma (2–8 L for a 500 kg horse) and HES (10 mL/kg/d or 5 L/day for a 500 kg horse) is used.

Plasma

Equine plasma is typically provided as fresh frozen plasma (frozen within 6 h of collection without prior refrigeration and stored for <1 year) or stored plasma (frozen for >1 year). Fresh plasma is defined as that administered to the patient within 6 h of collection.[23] Fresh and fresh frozen plasma can provide stable (II, VII, IX, and X) and labile (V, VIII, von Willebrand's factor) coagulation factors and stored plasma can only provide stable clotting factors. Platelets are not provided in routinely prepared plasma. Other proteins such as globulin, fibronectin, complement, antithrombin III, and protein C as well as anti-endotoxin antibodies when collected from immunized horses can be provided with plasma. The beneficial effects of hyperimmune plasma in endotoxemia have been inconsistent. Albumin is the primary determinant of COP in plasma. Albumin is also an important carrier protein for drugs, toxins, and hormones. Albumin, because of its small size, is distributed to the extracellular space, limiting its use in restoring intravascular COP. The COP of plasma (20–25 mmHg) is also lower than that of the synthetic colloids, which means it has less effect on drawing large volumes of fluid into the intravascular space and improving intravascular COP. In fact, in the adult horse 5–10 L or more are required to increase plasma total protein by only 0.5–1 g/dL. Plasma is expensive compared to synthetic colloids, particularly with the large volumes required. Plasma is not typically used for resuscitation because it requires slow thawing in warm water. Plasma should be administered through a blood administration set with a filtration device and patients should be monitored for hypersensitivity reaction (urticaria, pyrexia, tachycardia, tachypnea, muscle tremors, colic, anaphylaxis) during administration.[23]

Hydroxyethyl starch (HES)

HES is a synthetic modified branched-chain glucose polymer (amylopectin) and is described based on its average molecular weight and molar substitution ratio (attachment of hydroxyethyl ether groups to carbons 2, 3, and 6 of the glucose moieties).[23,31] The molecular size determines the colloidal activity with smaller molecules having a higher colloidal activity. The degree of substitution affects the metabolism by amylase and circulating half-life with more highly substituted products having a slower metabolism and longer effect. Hetastarch, the product used in the USA, has a weight average molecular weight of 450–480 kDa (number average molecular weight 69 kDa) and a molar substitution rate of seven hydroxyethyl groups per ten molecules of glucose (450/0.7). Whereas pentastarch, which is used in Europe and Australia, has a weight average molecular weight of 250–280 kDa (number average molecular weight of 120 kDa) and a molar substitution of five hydroxyethyl groups per ten molecules of glucose (250/0.5). Pentastarch is a more homogeneous product than hetastarch with regard to molecular size. The COP of hetastarch ranges from 29 to 32 mmHg and that of pentastarch is higher (~40 mmHg) than that of hetastarch because of the smaller and more numerous molecules making it a better plasma expander. The larger molecules of HES compared to albumin (~67 kDa) increase the likelihood of retention within the vascular space particularly with the associated increase in capillary permeability associated with endotoxemia. HES is reported to attenuate reperfusion injury and seal leaky capillaries[25,27,48] and reduce adhesion molecule expression which reduces leukocyte-endothelial interactions and decreases microvascular permeability with reduced tissue injury.[3,25,34,41] Because of the its more ideal molecular size, pentastarch is thought to have more beneficial effects with regard to capillary leak syndromes.[24] The increase in blood volume following hetastarch administration is 110% of the volume infused after 240 min in dogs.[42] Therefore, HES may provide intravascular volume expansion in addition to oncotic support.

HES is eliminated in several phases: (1) molecules <50 kDa are rapidly eliminated through glomerular filtration, (2) larger molecules are hydrolyzed by serum amylase and then excreted by the kidney, and (3) some molecules are taken up by the reticuloendothelial system.[31] Because of its higher molecular weight and molar substitution ratio, hetastarch is more slowly eliminated than pentastarch, with the oncotic effect lasting <24 h.[10,40]

HES is available as a 6% solution in saline (hetastarch, Hespan®) or LRS (hetastarch, Hextend®) or 10% solution in saline (pentastarch, Pentaspan®). HES is typically administered as 10 mL/kg (5 L for a 500 kg horse) no more than once a day. Recently, Abbott Laboratories has launched VetStarch™, a 6% HES in saline with 130/0.4 which reportedly has less impact on coagulation and is more resistant to degradation compared to hetastarch. There is no information on clinical use of this product in horses at this time.

In a small prospective randomized clinical trial comparing HSS and pentastarch for preoperative cardiovascular stabilization of colic patients, pentastarch administration resulted in a higher CI for 150 min and SVI for 60 min following anesthesia induction.[10] Pentastarch decreased packed cell volume and TPP better and for longer than HSS or isotonic saline.[40] Hetastarch administration was shown to have a significant oncotic effect in hypoproteinemic patients for 24 h[16] and normal ponies for 120 h.[15] However, resuscitation with HSS and hetastarch failed to ameliorate the deleterious hemodynamic response in an equine endotoxemia model[32] and administration of 2.5 mL/kg 6% HES to horses during general anesthesia did not attenuate the decline in COP observed with administration of 7.5 mL/kg/h of LRS.[46]

Hetastarch has been shown to alter activated partial thromboplastin time (aPTT), prothrombin time (PT), fibrinogen concentration, and coagulation activities[6] and has potent anticoagulant and antiplatelet effects in vitro.[47] HES causes a dose-dependent decrease in plasma factor VIII and von Willebrand's factor which is thought to be the main mechanism by which it affects coagulation.[15] The impact of HES on coagulation is dependent on the volume infused, molecular weight and elimination kinetics, frequency and number of infusions, concurrent administration of other fluids, and patient status.[33] Doses of HES <20 mL/kg are associated with minimal clinically important effects on coagulation.[15,45] In an equine endotoxemia model, there were no differences in coagulation measurements between horses treated with isotonic saline and a combination of HSS (7.2% NaCl 5 mL/kg) and HES (10 mL/kg). The HSS-HES treated horses had less effect on ionized calcium and did have a transient increase in NaCl.[33] Ponies administered 20 mL/kg HES did have a decrease in platelet count; however, absolute thrombocytopenia was not observed and the mild alterations in hemostasis were attributed to hemodilution.[15] Pentastarch has less profound effects on coagulation than hetastarch.[43] Adverse clinical effects were not observed in clinical cases administered pentastarch.[10,40] HES appears to be safe when administered at 10 mL/kg/day; however, care should be taken with administration of higher doses.

References

1. Ames, T.R., Hunter, D.W. & Caywood, D.D. (1991) Percutaneous transvenous removal of a broken jugular catheter from the right ventricle of a foal. *Equine Veterinary Journal*, **23**, 392–393.
2. Batista, M.B., Bravin, A.C., Lopes, L.M., *et al.* (2009) Pressor response to fluid resuscitation in endotoxic shock: Involvement of vasopressin. *Critical Care Medicine*, **37**, 2968–2972.
3. Boldt, J., Muller, M., Heesen, M. Neumann, K. & Hempelmann, G.G. (1996) Influence of different volume therapies and pentoxifylline infusion on circulating soluble adhesion molecules in critically ill patients. *Critical Care Medicine*, **24**, 385–391.
4. Brown, S.A., Dusza, K. & Boehmer, J. (1994) Comparison of measured and calculated values for colloid osmotic pressure in hospitalized animals. *American Journal of Veterinary Research*, **55**, 910–915.
5. Cook, V.L. & Bain, F.T. (2003) Volume (crystalloid) replacement in the ICU patient. *Clinical Techniques in Equine Practice*, **2**, 122–129.
6. De Jonge, E. & Levi, M. (2001) Effects of different plasma substitutes on blood coagulation: A comparative review. *Critical Care Medicine*, **29**, 1261–1267.
7. Dolente, B.A., Beech, J., Lindborg, S. & Smith, G. (2005) Evaluation of risk factors for development of catheter-associated jugular thrombophlebitis in horses: 50 cases (1993–1998). *Journal of the American Veterinary Medical Association*, **227**, 1134–1141.
8. Fielding, C.L. & Magdesian, K.G. (2011) A comparison of hypertonic (7.2%) and isotonic (0.9%) saline for fluid resuscitation in horses: A randomized, double-blinded, clinical trial. *Journal of Veterinary Internal Medicine*, **25**, 1138–1143.
9. Geraghty, T.E., Love, S., Taylor, D.J., Mellor, D.J. & Hughes, K.K. (2009) Assessment of subclinical venous catheter-related diseases in horses and associated risk factors. *Veterinary Record*, **164**, 227–231.
10. Hallowell, G.D. & Corley, K.T. (2006) Preoperative administration of hydroxyethyl starch or hypertonic saline to horses with colic. *Journal of Veterinary Internal Medicine*, **20**, 980–986.
11. Hardy, J. (2010) Basic procedures in adult equine critical care. In: *Equine Internal Medicine* (eds S.M. Reed, W.M. Bayly & D.C. Sellon), 3rd edn., pp. 249–258. WB Saunders, St. Louis, Missouri.
12. Haynes, G.R., Navickis, R.J. & Wilkes, M.M. (2003) Albumin administration—What is the evidence of clinical benefit? A systematic review of randomized controlled trials. *European Journal of Anaesthesiology*, **20**, 771–793.
13. Hoskinson, J.J., Wooten, P. & Evans, R. (1991) Nonsurgical removal of a catheter embolus from the heart of a foal. *Journal of the American Veterinary Medical Association*, **199**, 233–235.
14. Hotchkiss, R.S. & Karl, I.E. (1996) Calcium: A regulator of the inflammatory response in endotoxemia and sepsis. *New Horizons*, **4**, 58–71.
15. Jones, P.A., Tomasic, M. & Gentry, P.A. (1997) Oncotic, hemodilutional, and hemostatic effects of isotonic saline and hydroxyethyl starch solutions in clinically normal ponies. *American Journal of Veterinary Research*, **58**, 541–548.
16. Jones, P.A., Bain, F.T., Byars, T.D., David, J.B. & Boston, R.C. (2001) Effect of hydroxyethyl starch infusion on colloid oncotic pressure in hypoproteinemic horses. *American Journal of Veterinary Research*, **218**, 1130–1135.
17. Kien, N.D. (1998) Hypertonic saline: Current research and clinical implications. *Seminars in Anesthesia, Perioperative Medicine and Pain*, **17**, 167–173.
18. Kim, J.E., Jeon, J.P., No, H.C., *et al.* (2011) The effects of magnesium pretreatment on reperfusion injury during living donor liver transplantation. *Korean Journal of Anesthesiology*, **60**, 408–415.
19. Kreimeier, U., Thiel, M., Peter, K. & Messmer, K. (1997) Small-volume hyperosmolar resuscitation. *Acta Anaesthesiologica Scandinavica Supplementum*, **111**, 302–306.
20. Lee, C.Y., Woan-Ching Jan, W.C., Pei-Shan Tsai, P.S. & Huang, C.J. (2011) Magnesium sulfate mitigates acute lung injury in endotoxemia rats. *Journal of Trauma*, **70**, 1177–1185.
21. Lees, M.J., Read, R.A., Klein, K.T., Chennel, K.R., Clark, W.T. & Weldon, A. (1989) Surgical retrieval of a broken jugular catheter from the right ventricle of a foal. *Equine Veterinary Journal*, **21**, 384–387.
22. Little, D., Keene, B.W., Bruton, C., Smith, L.J., Powell, S. & Jones, S.L. (2002) Percutaneous retrieval of a jugular catheter fragment from the pulmonary artery of a foal. *Journal of the American Veterinary Medical Association*, **220**, 212–214.
23. Magdesian, K.G. (2003) Colloid replacement in the ICU. *Clinical Techniques in Equine Practice*, **2**, 130–137.

24. Magdesian, K.G. (2004) Monitoring the critically ill equine patient. *Veterinary Clinics of North America: Equine Practice*, **20**, 11–39.

25. Marik, P.E. & Iglesias, J. (2000) Would the colloid detractors please sit down. *Critical Care Medicine*, **28**, 2652–2654.

26. Nicoud, I.B., Knox, C.D., Jones, C.M., *et al.* (2007) 2-APB protects against liver ischemia-reperfusion injury by reducing cellular and mitochondrial calcium uptake. *American Journal of Physiology: Gastrointestinal and Liver Physiology*, **293**, G623–G630.

27. Nielsen, V.G., Tan, S., Brix, A.E., Baird, M.S. & Parks, D.A. (1997) Hextend (hetastarch solution) decreases multiple organ injury and xanthine oxidase release after hepatoenteric ischemia-reperfusion in rabbits. *Critical Care Medicine*, **25**, 1565–1574.

28. Oliveira, R.P., Velasco, I., Soriano, F. & Friedman, G. (2002) Clinical review: Hypertonic saline resuscitation in sepsis. *Critical Care*, **6**, 418–423.

29. Oliveira, R.P., Weingartner, R., Ribas, E.O., Moraes, R.S. & Friedman, G. (2002) Acute haemodynamic effects of a hypertonic saline/dextran solution in stable patients with severe sepsis. *Intensive Care Medicine*, **28**, 1574–1581.

30. Palmer, J.E. (2004) Fluid therapy in the neonate: Not your mother's fluid space. *Veterinary Clinics of North America: Equine Practice*, **20**, 63–75.

31. Pantaleon, L. (2010) Fluid therapy in equine patients: Small-volume fluid resuscitation. *Compendium on Continuing Education for the Practicing Veterinarian*, **32**, E1–E7.

32. Pantaleon, L.G., Furr, M.O., McKenzie, H.C., 2nd & Donaldson, L. (2006) Cardiovascular and pulmonary effects of hetastarch plus hypertonic saline solutions during experimental endotoxemia in anesthetized horses. *Journal of Veterinary Internal Medicine*, **20**, 1422–1428.

33. Pantaleon, L.G., Furr, M.O., McKenzie, H.C. & Donaldson, L. (2007) Effects of small- and large-volume resuscitation on coagulation and electrolytes during experimental endotoxemia in anesthetized horses. *Journal of Veterinary Internal Medicine*, **21**, 1374–1379.

34. Pascual, J.L., Khwaja, K.A., Chaudhury, P. & Christou, N.V. (2003) Hypertonic saline and the microcirculation. *Journal of Trauma*, **54**, S133–S140.

35. Radhakrishnan, R.S., Shah, S.K., Lance, S.H., *et al.* (2009) Hypertonic saline alters hydraulic conductivity and up-regulates mucosal/submucosal aquaporin 4 in resuscitation-induced intestinal edema. *Critical Care Medicine*, **37**, 2946–2952.

36. Reed, R.L., Johnston, T.D., Chen, Y. & Fischer, R.P. (1991) Hypertonic saline alters plasma clotting times and platelet aggregation. *Journal of Trauma*, **31**, 8–14.

37. Runk, D.T., Madigan, J.E., Rahal, C.J., Allison, D.N. & Fredrickson, K. (2000) Measurement of plasma colloid osmotic pressure in normal thoroughbred neonatal foals. *Journal of Veterinary Internal Medicine*, **14**, 475–478.

38. Russell, T.M., Kearney, C. & Pollock, P.J. (2010) Surgical treatment of septic jugular thrombophlebitis in nine horses. *Veterinary Surgery*, **39**, 627–630.

39. Scarratt, W.K., Moll, D.H. & Pleasant, S.R. (1997) Fragmentation of intravenous catheters in three horses. *Journal of Equine Veterinary Science*, **17**, 608–611.

40. Schusser, G.F., Rieckhoff, K., Ungemach, F.R., Huskamp, N.H. & Scheidemann, W. (2007) Effect of hydroxyethyl starch solution in normal horses and horses with colic or acute colitis. *Journal of Veterinary Medicine A: Physiology, Pathology, Clinical Medicine*, **54**, 592–598.

41. Shields, C.J., O'Sullivan, A.W., Wang, J.H., Winter, D.C., Kirwan, W.O. & Redmond, H.P. (2003) Hypertonic saline enhances host response to bacterial challenge by augmenting receptor-independent neutrophil intracellular superoxide formation. *Annals of Surgery*, **238**, 249–257.

42. Silverstein, D.C., Aldrich, J., Haskins, S.C., Drobatz, K. & Cowgill, L. (2005) Assessment of changes in blood volume in response to resuscitative fluid administration in dogs. *Journal of Veterinary Emergency and Critical Care*, **15**, 185–192.

43. Strauss, R.G., Stansfield, C., Henricksen, R.A. & Villhauer, P.J. (1988) Pentastarch may cause fewer effects on coagulation than hetastarch. *Transfusion*, **28**, 257–260.

44. Thomas, L.A. & Brown, S.A. (1992) Relationship between colloid osmotic pressure and plasma protein concentration in cattle, horses, dogs, and cats. *American Journal of Veterinary Research*, **53**, 2241–2244.

45. Trieb, J., Baron, J.F., Grauer, M.T. & Strauss, R.G. (1999) An international view of hydroxyethyl starches. *Intensive Care Medicine*, **25**, 258–268.

46. Wendt-Hornickle, E., Snyder, L.B.C., Tang, R. & Johnson, R.A. (2011) The effects of lactate Ringer's solution (LRS) or LRS and 6% hetastarch on the colloid osmotic pressure, total protein and osmolality in healthy horses under general anesthesia. *Veterinary Anaesthesia and Analgesia*, **38**, 336–343.

47. Wilder, D.M., Reid, T.J. & Bakaltcheva, I.B. (2002) Hypertonic resuscitation and blood coagulation: In vitro comparison of several hypertonic solutions for their action on platelets and plasma coagulation. *Thrombosis Research*, **107**, 255–261.

48. Zikria, B.A., Subbarao, C., Oz, M.C., *et al.* (1989) Macromolecules reduce abnormal microvascular permeability in rat limb ischemia-reperfusion injury. *Critical Care Medicine*, **17**, 1306–1309.

12 Abdominal Sonographic Evaluation

JoAnn Slack

Department of Clinical Studies, New Bolton Center, School of Veterinary Medicine, University of Pennsylvania, Kennett Square, PA, USA

Chapter Outline

Indications	**117**
Preparation	**117**
Patient	117
Transducer selection	117
Procedure	**118**
Fast localized abdominal sonography of horses (FLASH)	118
Complete abdominal examination	118
Transrectal examination	120
Application of abdominal sonography to the colic patient	**120**
Large colon displacements	120
Right dorsal displacement (RDD)	120
Left dorsal displacement with and without Nephrosplenic ligament entrapment (NSLE)	121
Large colon volvulus (LCV)	122
Large intestinal impactions	123
Large colon or cecal impaction	123
Sand impactions	124
Small colon impaction	124
Meconium retention or impaction	125
Right dorsal colitis	125
Intussusceptions	127
Jejunojejunal intussusception	127
Ileocecal intussusception	127
Cecocecal and cecocolic	127
Small intestinal lesions	128
Strangulating vs. nonstrangulating obstruction	128
Idiopathic small intestinal muscular hypertrophy	130
Adhesions	130
Gastric distention and impaction	131
Peritoneal fluid, peritonitis, and gastrointestinal rupture	133
Hemoperitoneum	134
Hernias	136
Diaphragmatic hernia	136
Other hernias	137
Masses	138
Abscesses	138
Hematomas	140
Enterolithiasis	141
Neoplasia	141
Alimentary lymphoma	141
Hemangiosarcoma	142
Gastric neoplasia	142
Gastrointestinal stromal cell tumors (GIST)	143
Ovarian tumors	143
Other	143
Urolithiasis	143
Cholelithiasis	145

Indications

Sonographic evaluation of the abdomen is a complementary diagnostic procedure in the workup of horses with colic. When applied transcutaneously, sonographic examination permits noninvasive evaluation of abdominal organs and gastrointestinal viscera that are otherwise difficult to image or examine directly. The sonographic evaluation can be used to localize the lesion, help determine if medical or surgical treatment is indicated, monitor response to treatment, and aid in formulating a prognosis. Sonographic findings are most valuable when interpreted together with physical examination (p. 12) and clinicopathological findings (p. 78, 87) and not in isolation of this information.

Preparation

Patient

Sonographic evaluations are typically well tolerated and best performed with the horse standing. Evaluation of the recumbent adult horse is challenging as intraluminal gas will rise to the dorsal portions of the abdomen obscuring visibility of much of the abdominal contents. Unless the horse has a very short hair-coat, the best images are obtained by removing the horse's hair with a #40 clipper blade. The skin should then be cleaned and coupling gel applied. Warmed gel is usually better tolerated by foals. In instances where clipping is not possible or practical, the hair can be soaked with water or alcohol. Frequent reapplication of water or alcohol may be needed throughout the examination. Complete examination of the abdomen typically yields the best information and is recommended if the patient is reasonably comfortable. Otherwise, physical examination findings (p. 12), abnormalities on palpation per rectum (p. 22), the presence or absence of reflux (p. 38), and serum biochemical findings (p. 78) may aid in determining the area of the abdomen that should be examined.

Common interventions in the colic patient may affect sonographic findings and interpretation. Fasting has been shown to increase jejunal visibility, decrease jejunal, cecal, and colonic activity, and cause the stomach to be visible ventral to the costochondral junction.[29] Xylazine sedation causes decreased jejunal and cecal activity in fasted horses but has no effect on the stomach in fed or fasted horses. Hyoscine n-butylbromide (Buscopan®) administration results in an immediate reduction in contractility of the duodenum, cecum, and left ventral colon.[18] Cecal and left ventral colon motility return to normal after 30 min, while duodenal motility returns to normal after 120 min. Nasogastric intubation introduces air into the duodenum but has no effects on intestinal activity in fasted horses.[29] Gastroscopy with air insufflation results in dorsal expansion of the stomach immediately following gastroscopy, gas accumulation within the duodenum, and more prominent rugal folding 2–4 h after completion of the procedure.[25] Bowel handling during abdominal exploration of normal ponies causes a mild functional ileus immediately postoperatively and mild bowel wall thickening in the first 5 days postoperatively.[15] The effects of these common interventions should be considered when interpreting the sonographic examination.

Transducer selection

Transducer selection will vary depending on the structure under evaluation and whether the examination is being performed transcutaneously or transrectally. Transrectal evaluation can be performed with a rectal linear transducer or a microconvex transducer. The microconvex transducer has several advantages over the linear rectal transducer, specifically an increased depth of penetration, a wider pie-shaped image, and the ability to be manipulated to obtain images in two planes. Complete transcutaneous evaluation of the adult horse will require a range of transducer frequencies including a low-frequency transducer (2.5–3.5 MHz) for imaging deeper structures. Use of the higher frequency transducers (5.0–13.5 MHz) will provide better resolution of more superficial structures and is critical for evaluation of intestinal wall thickness and layering abnormalities.[41] Neonatal foals are best examined with very high-frequency transducers (8.0–13.5 MHz).

Procedure

Fast localized abdominal sonography of horses (FLASH)

Rapid evaluation of the equine abdomen may be indicated in cases of severe abdominal pain, and a protocol for fast localized abdominal sonography of horses (FLASH) has been developed.[6] The abdomen is evaluated in seven locations including the ventral abdomen, gastric window, splenorenal window, left middle third of the abdomen, duodenal window, right middle third of the abdomen, and thoracic window. The abdomen is evaluated for the presence of free peritoneal fluid, ability to see the left kidney, small intestinal distension, motility and contents, and large intestinal contents. The procedure is completed in less than 15 min. Using this method, the positive and negative predictive values of dilated turgid loops of small intestine for the need for surgery are 89% and 81%, respectively (Clinical scenario 5, located in Appendix A).[6] The utility of FLASH to differentiate specific small intestinal lesions or large intestinal diseases is unknown. The FLASH method has not been evaluated in foals.

Complete abdominal examination

In cases of chronic colic or stabilized acute colic, a complete abdominal examination should be performed. A systematic approach to evaluating the abdomen will optimize the chances of identifying abnormalities, especially when the clinical signs and physical examination do not localize the problem to a specific abdominal structure.

One approach includes starting in the right dorsocaudal paralumbar fossa and scanning the right lateral abdomen in a dorsal to ventral and caudal to cranial fashion until the 6th intercostal space is reached. The exam should extend dorsally enough to evaluate the diaphragm and ventral thorax. The costochondral junction can be used as a ventral landmark or dividing line between the lateral and ventral abdomen. This approach will permit the sonographer to first evaluate the motility, contents, and wall thickness of the base of the cecum, which can typically be seen in the right paralumbar fossa and flank and followed cranially 2–3 intercostal spaces. The lateral cecal mesentery and associated vasculature can be followed in the right flank. Occasionally, the small intestine can also be identified in the right flank region. The right kidney can then be seen in the dorsal aspect of the right 17th through the 15th intercostal spaces. Kidney size, shape, corticomedullary distinction, pelvic contents, and vascular pattern can be evaluated as can ureteral contents and contractility. The normal duodenum is visible caudal to the caudal pole of the right kidney and ventral and medial to the liver over approximately 3 intercostal spaces, most commonly the 14th through the 12th. Duodenal motility, distention, contents, and wall thickness should be evaluated. The right lobe of the liver is typically seen from the 14th through the 7th intercostal spaces, although the degree of gastrointestinal distension will affect visibility and more or less of the right lobe may be seen. The right liver lobe should not extend ventral to the costochondral junction. Increasing age is associated with right liver lobe atrophy and late pregnancy may obscure portions of or the entire right liver lobe. Besides size, the right liver lobe should be evaluated for echogenicity, architecture, biliary distension, and vascular pattern. Echogenicity may be compared to the right kidney or the spleen by freezing an image of the liver, splitting the view screen, and then evaluating the other structures. Frequency and gain should be kept the same when comparing structures. The normal liver is hypoechogenic relative to the spleen and hyperechogenic relative to the cortex of the kidney. The intrahepatic bile ducts and common bile duct are not visible in the normal horse. With biliary obstruction, the intrahepatic bile ducts will appear as channels that run parallel to the hepatic veins and the obstructed common bile duct will become visible in the region of the porta hepatis. The dilated common bile duct can be distinguished from the portal vein by Doppler interrogation. The right dorsal colon is seen ventral and medial to the right liver lobe typically from the 10th to the 14th intercostal spaces depending on the degree of colonic distention. It should be evaluated for wall thickness, contents, and motility. The right ventral colon is often visible along the right ventrolateral abdomen at or slightly above the level of the costochondral junction and can be followed onto the ventral abdomen. It too should be evaluated for motility, contents, and wall thickness (Table 12.1).

The left side of the abdomen can be evaluated in the same dorsal to ventral and caudal to cranial manner, taking care to evaluate the diaphragm and ventral thorax. The spleen occupies the majority of the left abdomen and is typically seen against the diaphragm and/or abdominal wall from the paralumbar fossa region to the 7th or 8th intercostal spaces. On occasion, loops of small intestine and/or peritoneal fluid may be between the body wall and spleen in the paralumbar fossa or caudal intercostal spaces and the greater curvature of the stomach may sometimes be immediately adjacent to the diaphragm in the mid aspect of the left lateral abdomen. The spleen should be evaluated for size, echogenicity, and architecture keeping in mind the large variation in normal splenic size.

The left kidney is quite variable in its dorsal to ventral positioning but can usually be seen in the left paralumbar fossa or flank region and in the 17th and 16th intercostal spaces. Because of its position deep into the spleen, it is often more difficult to evaluate the architecture of the left kidney. On occasion, the caudal intestinal tract will be positioned between the body wall and left kidney, and its view will be obscured by the gas contents of the intestinal tract. For this reason, the inability to see the left kidney should never be used as the sole criteria for nephrosplenic ligament entrapment (NSLE).

Small colon and left dorsal colon are seen in the left lateral flank region. Occasionally these structures can be followed caudally by scanning through the cranial left thigh/hip region. As one scans the more cranial intercostal spaces, the left dorsal colon and loops of small intestine will be seen medial to the spleen. The stomach is typically seen in the mid

portion of the abdomen over 3–4 intercostal spaces. It can be recognized by its thicker wall and location adjacent to the gastrosplenic vein. Small intestine and peritoneal fluid may sometimes be seen between the stomach and spleen. The stomach should be evaluated for contents and wall thickness. The left liver lobe is present from the 9th to the 6th intercostal spaces and should be hypoechoic relative to the adjacent spleen. It can occasionally be followed onto the cranioventral abdomen but should otherwise be evaluated similarly to the right liver lobe. The left liver lobe does not seem to atrophy with age or colonic distension and the inability to see the left liver lobe should raise suspicion for colonic displacement or left liver lobe torsion.

Evaluation of the ventral abdomen should be performed in both longitudinal and transverse planes in multiple cranial to caudal or caudal to cranial sweeps. The ventral abdomen should be evaluated from the sternum to the caudal inguinal regions and laterally to the level of the costochondral junctions. Peritoneal fluid is often pocketed in the cranioventral abdomen between the spleen and apex of the cecum. The spleen typically occupies the majority of the left ventral abdomen and the cranial portion of the spleen may extend to the right of midline or even dorsal to the costochondral junction in the right 8th–6th intercostal spaces. The cecum is present along ventral midline and should be followed from apex to base. The left ventral colon is often deep to the spleen. The small intestine is typically seen in the caudoventral abdomen with occasional loops present between the spleen and cecum in the mid to cranioventral abdomen. The bladder may be seen in the caudoventral abdomen of adult horses and typically contains very echogenic urine.

The method for evaluating juvenile and adult horses can easily be applied to neonatal foals with the exception that neonates are typically scanned in lateral recumbency. The "down side" of the foal should always be examined by placing the transducer under the dependent side of the foal. This is important because abnormal portions of the intestine tend to fall to the dependent portion of the abdomen. Very high-frequency transducers should be used to evaluate intestinal walls, which tend to measure approximately 2.0 mm or slightly less in the normal foal (unpublished, personal

Table 12.1 Normal sonographic measurements in adult horses.

	Adult horses
Duodenal and jejunal wall thickness (mm)	3.0
Ileal wall thickness (mm)	5.0
Colonic wall thickness (mm)	3.0
Gastric wall thickness (mm)	7.5

observation). Special attention should be paid to determine if gas is present within the intestinal wall, suggestive of necrotizing enterocolitis.[33] The large and small colon should be evaluated for the presence of meconium. The umbilical remnants rarely play a role in abdominal pain unless there is herniation or extension of infection into the abdomen.

Other differences in the sonographic appearance of the neonatal foal abdomen include heterechoic fluid within the stomach consistent with milk clots and the ability to see the stomach from the ventral abdominal window. Also in contrast to adults, neonatal foal urine is typically anechoic although echogenic material may be seen in foals as young as a couple of weeks of age. The bladder may extend as far cranially as the external umbilical remnant, especially in sick, recumbent foals. The renal pelvis may be dilated without cortical thinning (pyelectasis) in foals receiving intravenous fluid therapy. Lastly, it is not unusual to be able to see the kidneys from the caudoventral abdominal window.

Transrectal examination

Transrectal examination of the caudal intestinal and urogenital tracts can be performed with the patient restrained as for transrectal palpation. A microconvex or linear rectal transducer can be used. Use of a microconvex transducer increases the depth of penetration and allows evaluation in two perpendicular planes. Because it can be positioned with the footprint facing cranial to the examiner's hand, it allows one to see portions of the abdomen cranial to the examiner's reach. From a transrectal window, the following structures can be evaluated: root of the mesentery, caudal margin of the spleen, caudal pole of left kidney, entire left ureter, caudal portion of right ureter, entrance of ureters into bladder with urine emptying into the bladder, urethra, uterus, ovaries, region of broad ligament, inguinal rings, caudally positioned small and large intestine, small colon, rectal wall, terminal aorta, and iliac arteries. The ileocecal junction is not typically identified in the normal horse but may become evident with intussusception. Because of the risk of rectal perforation with prolonged transrectal manipulation, complete

evaluation of all visible structures is rarely performed. Instead, physical examination findings, rectal examination findings, or clinicopathological data direct the areas that are to be evaluated.

Application of abdominal sonography to the colic patient

Large colon displacements

Displacement of the large colon can be a difficult sonographic diagnosis to make as there are no sonographic characteristics that allow reliable identification of the various portions of the ascending (large) colon. Detection of haustra is an unreliable means of distinguishing the dorsal from the ventral colon in the normal horse.[21] Colonic displacement may be suspected based on an unusual location of the colon relative to other abdominal structures such as spleen, kidney, liver, stomach, small intestine, or diaphragm or based on identification of structures not normally seen such as medially positioned mesocolonic vessels.

Right dorsal displacement (RDD)

Sonographic detection of a distended mesenteric vessel along the right lateral body wall has been seen in two horses with RDD (p. 220) and 180° colonic volvulus confirmed at surgery. In these cases, a distended vessel (2 cm in diameter) was seen in the 12th and 13th intercostal spaces just ventral to the diaphragm or liver and followed caudoventrally toward the right flank (Figure 12.1). In one horse, fluid-filled small intestine and a pocket of peritoneal fluid were present dorsal to the distended colonic vessel in the 13th intercostal space (Figure 12.2). In the same horse, the right liver lobe was obscured by the presence of gas-filled colon along the right body wall; there was an impaction of the ventrally positioned colon (identified as the right dorsal colon at surgery) and mild hypoechoic, edematous thickening of the colonic wall. The duodenum could not be identified in either horse.

Subsequent to this case a large retrospective study revealed that 100% of horses with colonic vessels identified along the right body wall

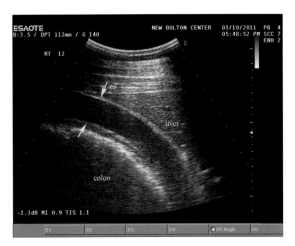

Figure 12.1 Right dorsal displacement with 180° torsion. Image obtained in the right 12th intercostal space; dorsal is to the right. Note the distended mesocolonic vessel (between arrows) ventral and medial to the right liver lobe. The vessel could be followed in a craniodorsal to caudoventral direction from the 12th intercostal space to the right flank.

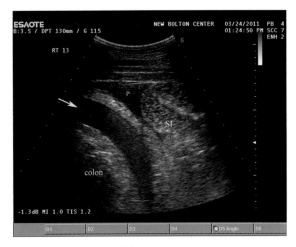

Figure 12.2 Right dorsal displacement with 180° torsion in a late gestation mare. Image was obtained in the dorsal aspect of the right 13th intercostal space, just ventral to the diaphragm. Dorsal is to the right. Note the distended mesocolonic vessel (between arrows), fluid-filled small intestine (SI) dorsal to the colon, and pocket of peritoneal fluid (P).

sonographically had surgical lesions localized to the large colon and that these horses were 32.5 times more likely to have a RDD or 180° large colon volvulus (LCV).[34] Colonic vessels were not seen in this location in horses with NSLE or a small

intestinal lesion.[34] These sonographic findings are consistent with visibility of the mesocolonic veins that are normally positioned along the medial aspect of the large colon. Gas within the colon prevents sonographic visibility of these vessels when the colon is normally positioned. In horses with a RDD with 180° colonic volvulus, the mesocolon and associated vessels become positioned along the right body wall. Venous obstruction results in distension of the mesenteric vein and edema of the colon wall. Because gas-filled colon is immediately adjacent to the right body wall, the liver and duodenum may be medially displaced and obscured from view. The small intestine can become displaced between the colon and diaphragm. Concurrent impaction of the right dorsal colon is not unusual in cases of RDD. It is probable that the sonographic findings for RDD will vary depending on the location of the pelvic flexure and degree of rotation of the colon as these factors will affect the amount of gas distension and venous congestion.

Left dorsal displacement with and without Nephrosplenic ligament entrapment (NSLE)

The sonographic findings of NSLE (p. 219) of the left colon include the presence of gas- or ingesta-filled large colon along the dorsal aspect of the left abdomen preventing visibility of the left kidney and dorsal portions of the spleen.[45] The hyperechoic reflection of the displaced large colon creates a horizontal border along the most dorsal margin of the spleen. This border can typically be followed from the paralumbar fossa to the 10th–12th intercostal spaces at which point the colon is no longer visible due to overlying lung. Peritoneal fluid or small intestine is occasionally observed between the colon and spleen (Figure 12.3). The spleen is ventrally displaced and the gastrosplenic vein and stomach may be identified along the ventral abdomen. The inability to identify the left kidney should not be used as the sole criteria for the diagnosis of NSLE. Follow-up sonographic examination can be used to determine the response to phenylephrine, exercise, or rolling.[45]

Left dorsal displacement without NSLE can also be identified sonographically. The findings are similar to NSLE in that the colon is dorsal to the spleen creating the same horizontal border

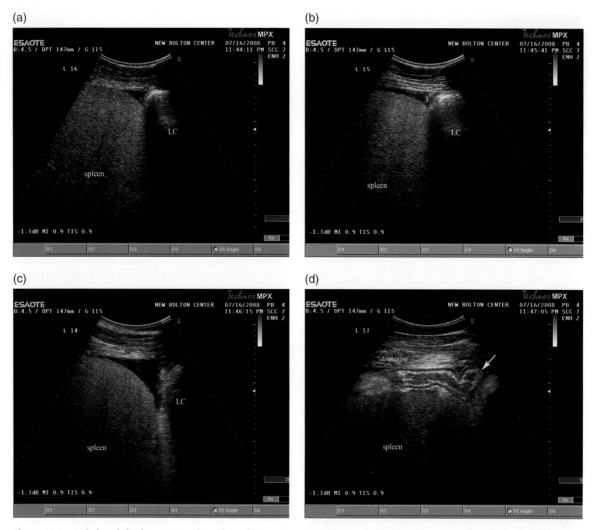

Figure 12.3   Left dorsal displacement with nephrosplenic entrapment. Images are obtained from the left 16th through the 13th intercostal spaces; dorsal is to the right. (a) Gas within the large colon (LC) creates a shadow over the dorsal aspect of the spleen preventing visualization of the left kidney. A small amount of fluid can be seen between the colon and the spleen. This appearance continues in the 15th (b) and 14th (c) intercostal spaces. (d) In the 13th intercostal space, a loop of small intestine (arrow) can be seen between the spleen and the diaphragm.

along the dorsal margin of the spleen. There is ventral displacement of the spleen and the stomach may be seen from the left ventral abdominal window. Without entrapment, the left kidney is still visible.

Large colon volvulus (LCV)

Some horses with LCV (p. 220) may have equivocal examination per rectum findings or uncommonly show insufficient pain to warrant immediate surgical intervention. In these cases, sonographic evaluation may help support a diagnosis of LCV. A colon wall thickness ≥9 mm obtained from a ventral abdominal window has been shown to accurately predict LCV in horses with colic localized to the large colon.[38] The intestinal wall in these cases may appear diffusely hypoechoic or heteroechoic with loss of layering. The colonic mesentery may be thickened and

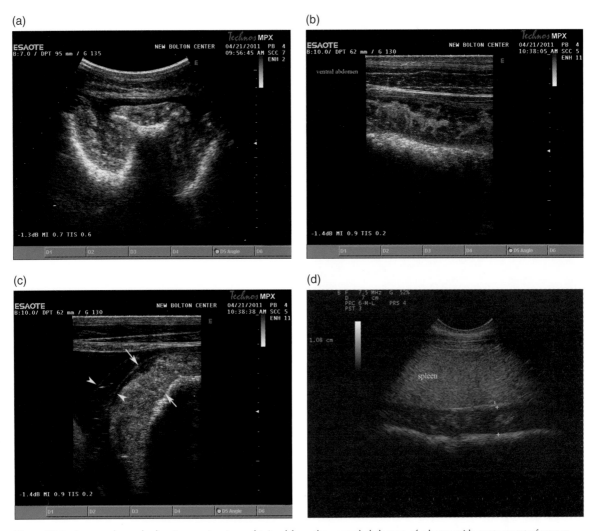

Figure 12.4   Large colon volvulus. Images (a–c) are obtained from the ventral abdomen of a horse with acute onset of severe abdominal pain. (a) Note marked thickening and folding of the wall of the large colon. (b) High-frequency image shows the colon wall to be echoic with loss of normal layering. (c) Hypoechoic edematous mesentery (between arrowheads) can be seen along the echoic colon wall (between arrows). (d) Image obtained from ventral abdomen of horse with colitis. Note similar sonographic appearance to the colon wall with marked thickening (1.08 cm) and loss of layering.

hypoechoic due to edema (Figure 12.4). The primary differential for this sonographic finding is colitis (p. 215), and case history, physical examination, and clinicopathologic findings are critical for differentiation (Clinical scenario 1, located in Appendix A). Cases of RDD with significant vascular obstruction may also have markedly thickened colon visible from the ventral abdominal window.

Large intestinal impactions

Large colon or cecal impaction

Sonography is useful for confirming the diagnosis of cecal impaction (p. 214), differentiating cecal from right dorsal colon impactions (p. 217), and identifying impactions that cannot be palpated per rectum either due to size of patient or cranial location of the impaction. Impactions of the cecum and large colon are typically seen as hyperechoic intraluminal material that cast a strong acoustic shadow (Figure 12.5). The distended colon or cecum takes on a more flattened appearance and the wall thickness is typically normal to thin. Gas, fluid, and ingesta layers can occasionally be seen. Fluid distension of the more proximal portions of large colon or small intestine may be appreciated, particularly if enteral fluids have been administered. The distended small intestine in these cases will have a normal wall thickness and may exhibit normal, increased, or decreased motility.

Sand impactions

Sand impactions (p. 217) are best identified along the ventral aspect of the abdomen.[26] The large colon takes on a flattened appearance and peristaltic activity is markedly reduced or absent. Sand along the mucosal surface appears as hyperechoic pinpoint material and can cast acoustic shadows (Figure 12.6). Quantifying the amount of sand is best performed radiographically (p. 156).[26]

Small colon impaction

Small colon impactions (p. 221) in adult horses are best examined transrectally. Small colon impactions in miniature horses may be seen transcutaneously by imaging the caudoventral abdomen and identifying the small colon dorsal to the bladder. The impaction typically appears as hyperechoic intraluminal contents that cast an acoustic shadow.

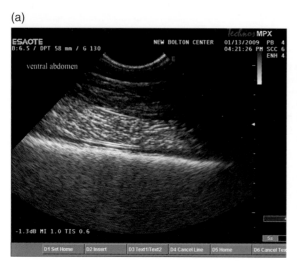

Figure 12.5   Cecal impaction. Image is obtained from right paralumbar fossa; dorsal is to the right. Note the echoic ingesta casting an acoustic shadow. Wall thickness is near normal at 3.6 mm.

(a)

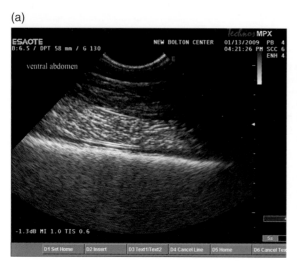

(b)

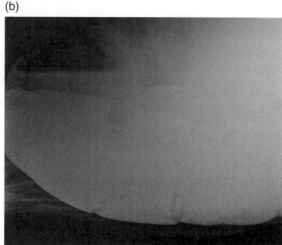

Figure 12.6   Sand impaction. (a) Sonographic image is obtained from the ventral abdomen. Note echoic ingesta and flattening of the wall of the large colon. (b) Radiographic image of the cranioventral abdomen of the same horse in (a). There is significant sand accumulation in large colon.

Meconium retention or impaction

Meconium retention (p. 222) within the large colon of foals can take on a variety of sonographic appearances. The most recognizable appearance is that of hyperechoic pinpoint speckling within hypoechoic material all surrounded by echogenic material. Impaction of the small colon with meconium is best diagnosed by scanning the caudoventral abdomen and identifying the small colon dorsal to the bladder. In these cases, the meconium is usually very echogenic and the small colon indents the bladder wall (Figure 12.7).

Right dorsal colitis

Right dorsal colitis (p. 216) can be diagnosed by identifying a thickened right dorsal colon wall in the right 10th–14th intercostal spaces just ventral and medial to the liver.[24] The right dorsal colon can occasionally be seen cranial to the 10th and/or the 15th intercostal space. The appearance of the colonic wall can be variable depending on the amount of edema versus inflammatory infiltrate that is present. The wall thickness will be greater than 3 mm and can be up to several centimeters thick.[24] Often,

(a)

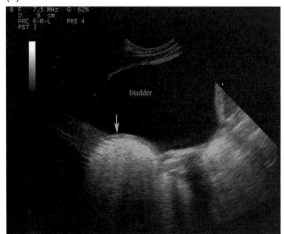

(b)

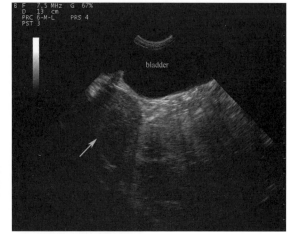

(c)

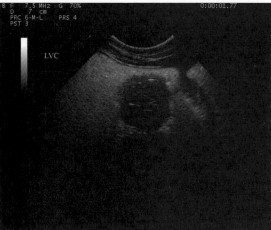

Figure 12.7 Meconium retention and impaction. Images are obtained from ventral abdomens of three foals with mild to moderate abdominal pain. (a) Firm echogenic meconium in small colon is indenting dorsal bladder wall. (b) Hypoechoic meconium within small colon dorsal to bladder. (c) Hypoechoic speckled meconium surrounded by more echogenic material within left ventral colon.

(a)

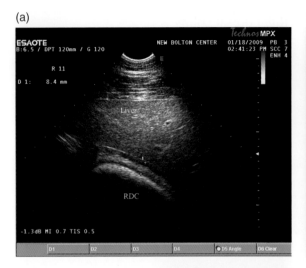

(b)

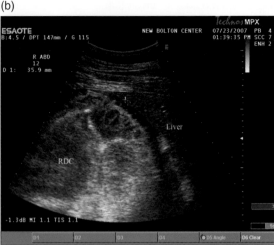

(c)

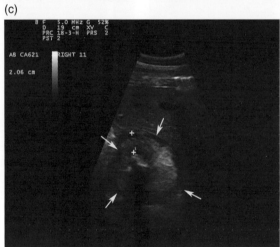

Figure 12.8   Right dorsal colitis. Each image is obtained from a different horse; dorsal is to the right for all images. (a) Image obtained in the right 11th intercostal space. Note the thickening and echoic infiltrate of the right dorsal colon wall. (b) Image obtained from the right 12th intercostal space. Note the marked thickening and heteroechoic appearance of the wall of the right dorsal colon. (c) Image obtained from right 11th intercostal space. Note marked narrowing of the lumen and thickening of the wall of the right dorsal colon. Severe right dorsal colitis with stricture was confirmed at surgery.

there is a central echoic layer consistent with cellular infiltrate within the submucosa of the colon wall (Figure 12.8). At other times, the wall is diffusely echoic with no distinction between wall layers or a mixture of hypoechoic edema and echoic infiltrate may be present. In severe cases, there may be marked narrowing of the lumen of the right dorsal colon (Figure 12.8). Peritoneal fluid may be pocketed between the right dorsal colon and liver and concurrent peritonitis should be considered if the fluid is increased in echogenicity. Significant

hypoproteinemia may result in a large peritoneal effusion, edema of the colonic mesentery, and/or edema of walls of other portions of the intestinal tract. Other differentials such as lymphoma or inflammatory bowel disease should be considered if there is thickening and echogenic infiltrate within the walls of other portions of the large intestine or small intestine. Right dorsal colitis should not be completely ruled out by normal sonographic findings as disease may be localized to the medial portions of the right dorsal colon in some cases.

Intussusceptions

An intussusception has a complex sonographic appearance composed of the intussuscipiens (the receiving loop) and the intussusceptum (the donor loop). The intussusceptum has both an entering limb and a returning limb. The attached mesentery along with mesenteric vessels, lymphatics, and fat are dragged between the two limbs. The thickest portion of the intussusceptum is typically the everted returning limb which, together with the thin intussuscipiens, forms the hypoechoic outer ring on short axis scans. The center of the intussusception contains the central or entering limb which is eccentrically surrounded by echoic mesentery. The appearance of the intussusception is variable depending on the amount of enclosed mesentery, degree of vascular compromise and resulting edema or necrosis of the intestinal wall, the presence of fluid and fibrin between the intussuscipiens and intussusceptum or between the two limbs of the intussusceptum, and whether gas and/or ingesta are visible within the lumen. The appearance also changes along the length of the intussusception with mesentery being absent at the apex of the intussusception and increasing toward the base.

Jejunojejunal intussusception

Jejunojejunal intussusception (p. 213) is a common cause of colic in foals but rare in adult horses.[5,16] Because the abnormal intestine becomes heavy, these are best identified by scanning the most ventral aspect of the abdomen.[5] For laterally recumbent foals this means placing the transducer under the dependent side of the foal. The transverse sonographic image of a small intestinal intussusception has been described as concentric rings that resemble a target or bull's eye–like image (Figure 12.9).[5] The exact appearance can be variable. Proximal to the intussusception, the small intestine is fluid distended and has normal wall thickness. There may be fluid distension of the stomach if not recently decompressed. In foals, small intestinal intussusceptions may be intermittent or self-resolving and repeated sonographic examination may be indicated to determine if there is need for surgical intervention.[5]

Ileocecal intussusception

Ileocecal intussusceptions (p. 213) are best seen via transrectal sonographic evaluation of the right caudal abdomen. Evaluation of a young horse with mild to moderate colic signs and/or palpation of a mass alongside the medial aspect of the cecum are the usual prompts for performing a transrectal sonographic examination. The telescoped ileum is identified as a target-like structure in the short axis plane (Figure 12.10). Transcutaneous evaluation will reveal fluid-distended small intestine proximal to the intussusception. The wall thickness of the proximal small intestine is usually normal unless the intussusception is chronic in which case the proximal ileum and distal jejunum may become hypertrophied.[13] In some cases the cecal contents will be fluidy and the intussusception can be seen via transcutaneous sonographic evaluation of the paralumbar fossa and flank region (Figure 12.10). More commonly gas within the cecum prevents transcutaneous visibility and this approach should not be used to rule out ileocecal intussusception.

Cecocecal and cecocolic

Cecocecal and cecocolic intussusceptions (p. 214) are the most common types of large intestinal intussusceptions.[4,51] Colocolic and small colon intussusceptions are rarely reported.[1,44] Colonic intussusceptions typically occur in young or adult horses and only rarely in foals. Cecocecal intussusceptions can be found via transcutaneous sonographic evaluation of the mid to right ventral abdomen. Cecocolic intussusceptions are found along the right ventrolateral abdomen or flank region. Like intussusceptions involving the small intestine, the appearance can be variable from base to apex and depends on the amount of incorporated mesentery and degree of vascular compromise. Still, the most common description is that of a target-like mass consisting of concentric rings (Figure 12.11).[51] Large intestinal intussusceptions can occasionally be mistaken for neoplastic masses or abscesses particularly if there is significant edema or if the intussusception is necrotic with gas within the intestinal wall. The sonographic appearances of colocolic and small colon intussusceptions have not yet been described but they are likely to have a target-like appearance, and differentiation from other types of intussusceptions would be based on location within the abdomen.

(a)

(b)

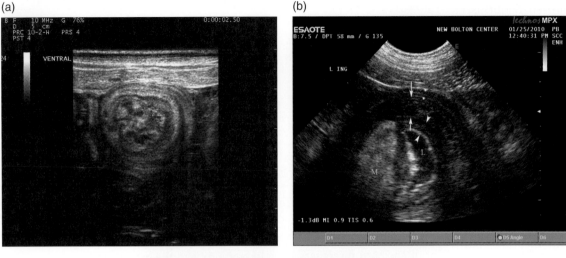

(c)

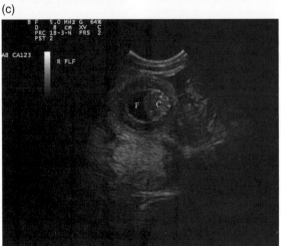

Figure 12.9 Small intestinal intussusception. All images obtained from ventral abdomen. (a) Typical target appearance of the transverse image of a small intestinal intussusception in a foal. (b) Transverse image of a small intestinal intussusception in an adult horse on prokinetics following small intestinal surgery. Note the thin intussuscipiens (between stars), the thickened, edematous returning limb (between arrows) of the intussusceptum, and the edematous entering or central limb (between arrow heads) of the intussusceptum. There is mesentery (M) that has been dragged between the two limbs of the intussusceptum and fluid within the lumen (L) of the returning limb of the intussusceptum. (c) Transverse image of intussusception showing peritoneal fluid (F) between the central (C) limb of the intussusceptum and the hypoechoic returning limb of the intussusceptum. The intussuscipiens is the echogenic outer layer.

Small intestinal lesions

Strangulating vs. nonstrangulating obstruction

One of the most common indications for sonographic evaluation of the horse with colic is to aid in the differentiation between small intestinal lesions that require surgical intervention and those that are likely to respond to medical management. The diagnosis of a strangulating small intestinal lesion (p. 209) is typically based on identification of turgid, amotile loops of small intestine with thickened walls. The loss of motility results in ingesta with a layered appearance. The presence of two populations of small intestine (one collapsed and of normal wall thickness, the other dilated, amotile, and thick-walled) and

(a)

(b)

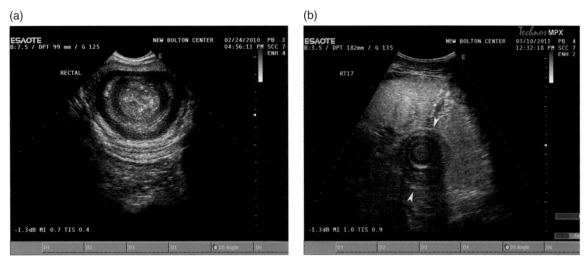

(c)

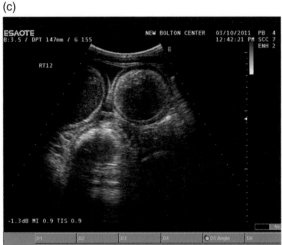

Figure 12.10 Ileocecal intussusception. (a) Image of palpable right caudal abdominal mass. Note the target-like appearance of the intussusception. The image was obtained transrectally using a microconvex curvilinear transducer. (b) Transcutaneous image from the same horse. The cecum contains echoic fluid rather than gas thus permitting visualization of the ileal intussusception (between arrowheads). Image was obtained in the right 17th intercostal space, dorsal is to the right of the image. (c) Image obtained from same horse as in (b). Note thick-walled dilated loops of small intestine proximal to the intussusception. The muscular layers of the walls are hypoechoic consistent with muscular hypertrophy. This appearance should not be confused with a strangulating obstruction but should prompt further evaluation for a nonstrangulating, chronic partial obstruction.

progressive peritoneal fluid accumulation are often considered supportive findings (Figure 12.12). In contrast, small intestinal ileus or simple obstruction typically results in small intestine that is hypomotile and dilated but not necessarily turgid and is of normal wall thickness (Figure 12.13). The problem with these criteria is that there is considerable overlap in sonographic findings between strangulating and nonstrangulating lesions. For example,

cases of proximal enteritis (p. 207) may have marked wall thickening while strangulated small intestine may initially have normal wall thickness before congestion and edema develop. Cases of proximal enteritis may have thickened and distended proximal small intestine as well as collapsed, normal thickness distal small intestine, giving the appearance of two populations of small intestine. For these reasons, the sonographic findings should be interpreted with

(a)

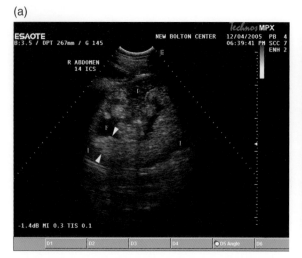

(b)

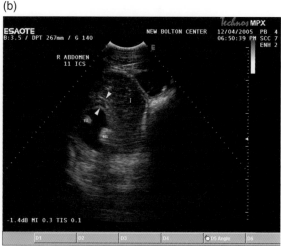

Figure 12.11   Cecocolic intussusception. (a) Image obtained in right 14th intercostal space, dorsal to the costochondral junction, along the ventrolateral abdomen. The thick-walled, folded intussusceptum (arrowheads) can be seen surrounded by ingesta (I) within the lumen of the intussuscipiens. The entering and returning portions of the intussusceptum are not clearly delineated. Fluid within the center of the intussusception (F) is peritoneal fluid. (b) Same horse as in (a). This image is obtained in a more cranial location closer to the base of the intussusception. In this image, mesentery (m) can be seen attached to the serosal surface of the intussusceptum. Peritoneal fluid (F) in the center of the intussusception and the intussusceptum can be seen between the arrowheads. Ingesta (I) is present between the intussuscipiens and the intussusceptum.

caution and in light of the physical examination and clinicopathologic data, especially in areas where proximal enteritis and/or ileal impactions (p. 208) are common.

Idiopathic small intestinal muscular hypertrophy

Ileal muscular hypertrophy is uncommon. Horses with ileal muscular hypertrophy usually present with a chronic history of recurrent, mild colic. The sonographic features of muscular hypertrophy of the small intestine include hypoechoic circumferential thickening of the muscularis layer of the small intestine (Figure 12.14).[10] Thickening may be focal, diffuse, or multifocal and involve ileum, jejunum, and/or duodenum.[7] Motility is usually reduced to absent in severely affected portions of small intestine and increased anechoic or hypoechoic peritoneal fluid is often present.[10] The large intestine is unaffected and lymphadenopathy is not a feature of this disease.[7] Side-to-side jejuno- or ileocecostomy with (complete) or without (incomplete) transaction (or resection) of the affected ileum is reported to be successful.

Adhesions

Adhesions (p. 255) are a common cause of postoperative colic and repeat laparotomy in the horse.[19] Small intestinal adhesions can occur following small intestinal or large intestinal surgery. Common sites of adhesion formation following small intestinal surgery include adhesions of adjacent loops of small intestine distal to the surgery site, adhesions of small intestine to the mesenteric stump, and adhesions of small intestine to the anastomosis site.[19] Adhesions of the spleen to the ventral body wall may occur following surgical correction of left dorsal displacement of the large colon.[30] In horses with a history of incisional infection, adhesions of small intestine or spleen to the peritoneum may occur in the region of the incision. Adhesions are suspected by the lack of normal gliding of the small intestine or spleen against the peritoneum, other intestinal loops, or abdominal organs in association with intestinal peristalsis or respiratory motions. The presence of hypoechoic fibrin tethering the serosa of small intestinal loops to other loops of intestine, abdominal organs, or peritoneum confirms the diagnosis (Figure 12.15). The small intestine may show peristaltic activity or may

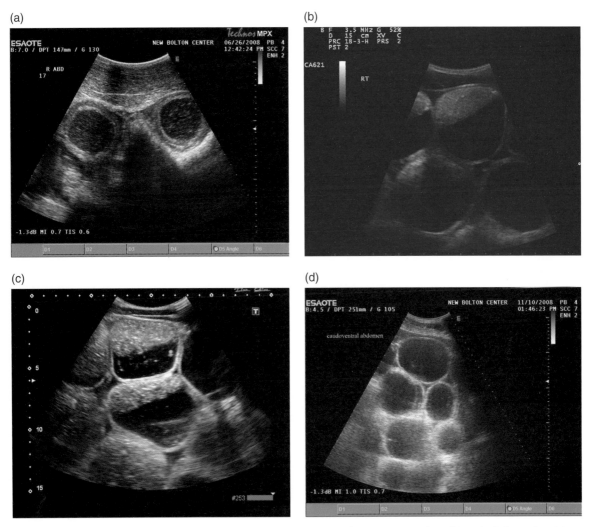

Figure 12.12   Small intestinal obstruction. Images obtained from horses with various types of small intestinal obstruction. (a) Image from horse with strangulating lipoma. Note thick-walled dilated small intestine. Loops were hypomotile and horse had significant gastric reflux. (b) Image obtained from a horse 3 days following correction of small intestinal volvulus. Note sedimentation of ingesta within dilated, stacked loops of small intestine. Small intestinal wall thickness is within normal limits. (c) Image obtained from yearling with small intestinal volvulus. Note sedimented ingesta within stacked but compressible loops of small intestine with normal wall thicknesses. (d) Image obtained from horse with postoperative ileus. Note stacked loops of dilated small intestine with normal wall thickness.

be distended and amotile due to concurrent ileus or mechanical obstruction by the adhesions.

Gastric distension and impaction

The sonographic appearance of the stomach is often altered by various factors including anorexia or hypophagia, the passage of a nasogastric tube and gastric lavage, or previous gastroscopy. Interpretation of the sonographic findings should be made with these factors in mind. In normal adult horses on full feed the stomach has a curved appearance, typically spans 3–4 intercostal spaces, and cannot be seen from the ventral or right side of the abdomen. With gastric distension the stomach loses its curved shape, extends over 5 or more intercostal spaces, and on rare occasions can be seen from the

(a)

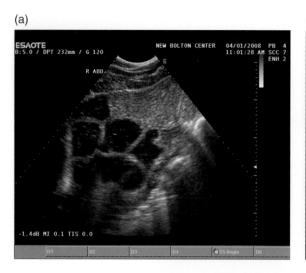

(b)

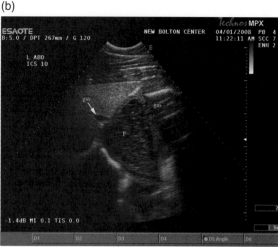

(c)

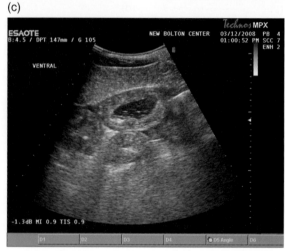

Figure 12.13   Enteritis. (a) Transcutaneous image obtained in the right flank region from a horse with abdominal pain and a large volume of gastric reflux. Note fluid-filled, compressible loops of small intestine with normal wall thickness. These loops were hypomotile to amotile in real-time imaging. This horse's colic resolved with medical management. (b) Same horse as in (a). Note ventral fluid (F) accumulation and dorsal gas within the stomach. Identification of the adjacent gastrosplenic vein (GSV) within the spleen confirms that this structure is the stomach and not fluid-filled colon. Image obtained in left 10th intercostal space, dorsal is to the right of the image. (c) Transcutaneous image of thick-walled echoic loops of small intestine along the ventral abdominal wall of a postpartum mare. Intestinal loops were hypomotile. The mare was presented because of moderate abdominal pain and large volume gastric reflux. Peritonitis was diagnosed by abdominocentesis and fluid analysis. The peritonitis and enteritis resolved with medical therapy.

ventral or right side of the abdomen. In horses with small intestinal lesions and gastric reflux, there may be marked fluid distension or a combination of fluid, gas, and solid ingesta. With feed impactions the gastric contents appear hyperechoic along the mucosal surface and typically cast a dense acoustic shadow (Figure 12.16). The spleen may become ventrally or caudally displaced with gastric impac-

tions.[50] Gastric impaction (p. 205)[35,50] has been associated with inflammatory bowel disease in a small number of horses and sonographic evaluation of the small and large intestine may be indicated in these cases. Gastric ulcers are not typically apparent on sonographic examination but have been identified in at least one horse with severe gastric impaction due to outflow obstruction (Figure 12.16).

(a)

(b)

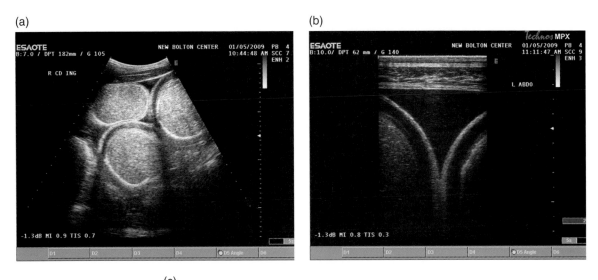

(c)

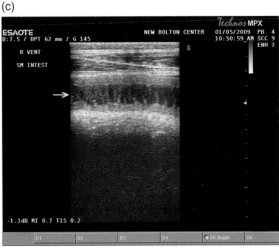

Figure 12.14   Small intestinal hypertrophy. Images are obtained from an adult horse with weight loss and a 2 day history of colic. (a) Dilated, stacked loops of small intestine with intraluminal fluid. Two populations are present: one dilated but compressible with normal wall thickness and one population of turgid, thick-walled small intestine. (b) High-frequency image of the thickened small intestinal walls and hypoechoic peritoneal fluid. (c) High-frequency image demonstrating the hypertrophied muscular layer of the small intestine (arrow).

In normal neonatal foals, the stomach can occasionally be seen from both the ventral and right side of the abdomen. Heteroechoic fluid due to milk clot formation is normally present within the stomach although gaseous distension with little to no fluid can also be normal if the foal has not recently nursed. Gastric distension in foals should prompt evaluation of the duodenum for ulceration or stricture. Uncommonly, foals with hypoxic ischemic injury may hemorrhage into the stomach and blood clots may be seen sonographically (Figure 12.17).

Peritoneal fluid, peritonitis, and gastrointestinal rupture

Characterization of the peritoneal fluid is best performed with a high-frequency transducer. Typical sonographic findings in cases of peritonitis (p. 169) include an increased volume of anechoic, hypoechoic, heteroechoic, or echogenic fluid. There may be hypoechoic fibrin strands long the peritoneum, abdominal organs, or gastrointestinal viscera. In some cases there is thickening

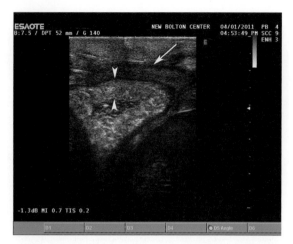

Figure 12.15   Adhesions. Two week postoperative image of a loop of small intestine adhered to ventral abdominal wall at the incision site. The intestinal wall is thickened (between arrowheads) and tethered to the body wall by a layer of hypoechoic fibrin (arrow). In real time, the adhesion was made apparent by the lack of normal gliding of the small intestine against the peritoneum.

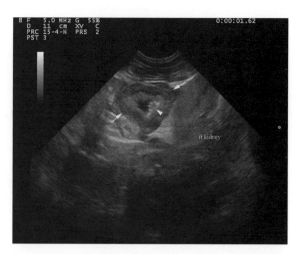

Figure 12.17   Duodenitis. Transcutaneous image obtained in right 16th intercostal space of neonatal foal. The caudal pole of the kidney is indistinctly seen dorsal to the thick-walled loop of duodenum (arrows). There is intraluminal gas (arrowhead) along the dorsal mucosal margin and the duodenum has a two-layered appearance consisting of an echogenic inner layer and hypoechoic outer layer. Dorsal is to the right of the image.

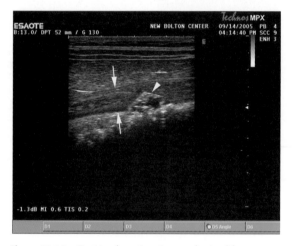

Figure 12.16   Gastric ulceration. Image obtained from yearling with chronic colic and weight loss. Serosal and mucosal margins of the wall of the stomach are noted by arrows. Hyperechoic gas can be seen dissecting into the wall of the stomach (arrowhead) consistent with ulceration. At postmortem, the stomach was massively enlarged and contained numerous ulcers secondary to duodenal stricture and chronic outflow obstruction.

and corrugation of the small and/or large intestinal walls. (Figure 12.18) The abdomen should be carefully evaluated for abnormalities of the gastrointestinal viscera (Figure 12.18) as well as for the presence of abscesses or neoplastic masses. Rarely, peritonitis may be secondary to hepatic disease such as with bile peritonitis or cirrhosis and sonographic evaluation of the liver should be considered (Figure 12.18). Rupture of a portion of the gastrointestinal tract (p. 171) will result in heteroechoic flocculent peritoneal fluid with dorsal accumulations of free gas (Figure 12.18). The site of rupture is often difficult to identify.

Hemoperitoneum

Horses with acute intra-abdominal hemorrhage may present for evaluation of colic.[8,9,39] Horses with hemoperitoneum also commonly have dull mentation, weakness, and concurrent signs of shock (tachycardia, pale mucous membranes, cool extremities). Hemoperitoneum is easily identified upon sonographic evaluation of the ventral abdomen as echogenic fluid that swirls either due to respiratory motion or active hemorrhage (Figure 12.19). Hematomas within the peritoneal

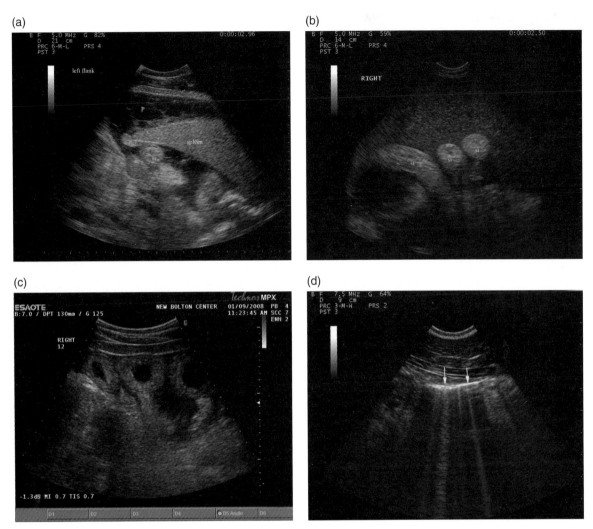

Figure 12.18   Peritonitis. (a) Transcutaneous image of chronic fibrinous peritonitis obtained from the left flank. Note tip of spleen surrounded hypoechoic fluid and the echogenic strands of fibrin within the fluid and coating the spleen. Small intestine (SI) can be seen floating in the peritoneal fluid (P). (b) Image of gastrointestinal rupture with echogenic peritoneal fluid and small intestine (SI) visible floating within the fluid. (c) Image from foal with peritonitis. Note echoic, thick-walled, distended but not turgid small intestinal loops within hypoechoic peritoneal fluid. (d) Image obtained from weanling with acute onset colic and endotoxemia. Free gas (arrows) is present in the dorsal aspect of the left paralumbar fossa, immediately adjacent to the peritoneum. The horse had ruptured a gastric ulcer. Dorsal is to the right of the image.

cavity will appear as relatively homogeneous, hypoechoic irregular masses that typically settle along the ventral abdominal wall (Figure 12.19). The spleen will be small in cases of acute hemorrhage due to splenic contraction. Complete evaluation of the abdomen should be performed in an attempt to identify the source of the hemorrhage. Common sources of hemorrhage include the spleen,

female reproductive tract, and mesenteric vessels.[8,9,39] The liver is a less frequent source. Both trauma and neoplastic processes should be considered as possible inciting causes.[8,9,39] Horses with hemoperitoneum are typically managed medically with conservative fluid therapy, plasma, whole blood transfusion, and procoagulants. Surgery is indicated in horses where a site of hemorrhage is

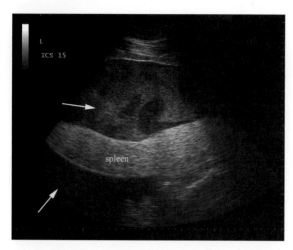

Figure 12.19   Large hemoabdomen in a gelding. Note the echoic peritoneal fluid (arrows) that surrounds the contracted spleen. In real time, the fluid has a swirling appearance. The cause of the hemoabdomen was not identified.

identified sonographically that can be approached surgically and in horses that are persistently painful. Often the site of hemorrhage is not identified.

Periparturient hemorrhage (p. 284) is an important cause of abdominal pain in the mare.[2] In peripartum mares with hypovolemic shock, transcutaneous sonographic evaluation of the ventral abdomen looking for hemoperitoneum, and/or hemorrhage into the uterine lumen or wall will allow a rapid, definitive diagnosis of hemorrhage in many cases without the added stress of a transrectal sonographic evaluation. Once the mare is stabilized a more complete sonographic evaluation of the broad ligament and uterus can be performed to determine the location and extent of hemorrhage. Bleeding from the uterine arteries may result in hemorrhage within the broad ligament, into the uterine wall, into the uterine lumen, and/or into the peritoneal cavity.[46] Broad ligament hematomas are best identified transrectally (p. 120) and often have a mixed echogenic sonographic appearance (Figure 12.20). The specific appearance will vary depending on the age of the hematoma and whether there is concurrent infection. Intraluminal uterine hemorrhage in the postpartum mare appears as swirling echogenic fluid and may have ventrally positioned hypoechoic clots (Figure 12.20).[46] Intramural uterine hemorrhage may be seen in either the late pregnant or postpartum mare.[46] It is characterized by the presence of a hypoechoic fluid layer within the uterine wall. The fluid is immediately beneath the serosal surface of the uterus in contrast to uteroplacental separation where fluid accumulates between the uterus and placenta (Figure 12.20). If intramural uterine hemorrhage is identified in a pregnant mare, complete uteroplacental and fetal sonographic assessment is indicated.[46]

Hernias

Diaphragmatic hernia

Diaphragmatic hernia is an uncommon cause of colic in the horse.[20,43] A diaphragmatic hernia should be considered as a differential diagnosis in a horse or foal showing signs of colic with a history of trauma (including birth) or a broodmare that has recently foaled particularly post dystocia. Clinical signs may be acute or chronic and the hernia may be congenital or acquired.[20,43] Displacement of gastrointestinal viscera into the thoracic cavity can usually be diagnosed via sonographic examination of the thorax and cranial abdomen although the diagnosis may be missed if the hernia is centrally located and the displaced gastrointestinal viscera are not against the thoracic wall. In some cases, the diagnosis may be missed if clinical signs such as tachypnea, muffled lung sounds, or borborygmi over the thorax are absent and specific sonographic examination of the thorax is not undertaken.[20,43] For this reason, evaluation of the ventral thorax and diaphragm is recommended when performing a complete abdominal sonographic examination in horses with colic.

Left-sided hernias appear more commonly than right-sided hernias.[20,43] Single or multiple abdominal organs may be herniated into the thorax including large and small colon, small intestine, spleen, stomach, pancreas, and/or liver.[20,43] Increased wall thickness of displaced intestine may indicate compromised bowel (Figure 12.21). With acute tears of the diaphragm, there is usually increased fluid in both the abdomen and thorax. The fluid may be echogenic and swirling consistent with hemorrhage. Pneumothorax, when present, is identified as a hyperechoic, nonmoving linear echo that casts an acoustic shadow similar to aerated lung along the dorsal aspect of the thorax. Once identified, the size of a diaphragmatic hernia can be estimated by carefully scanning the diaphragm from dorsal to ventral in all intercostal spaces.

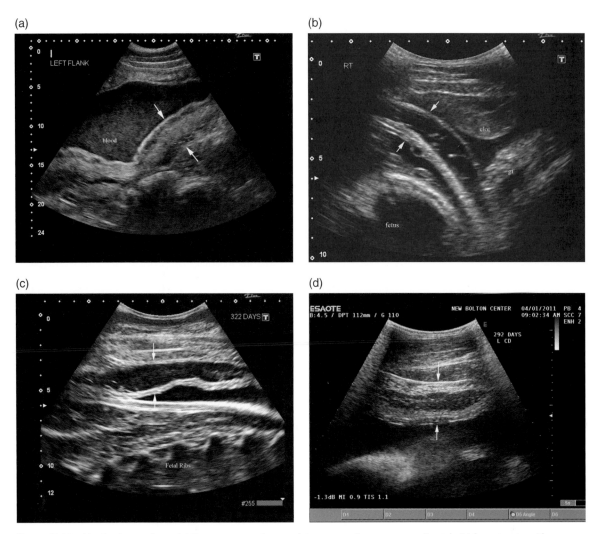

Figure 12.20   Uterine hemorrhage. (a) Transcutaneous image of the uterus of a mare approximately 36 h postpartum. The mare presented for mild abdominal discomfort immediately post foaling. The echoic swirling fluid in the uterine lumen is blood. (b and c) Transcutaneous images of the gravid uterus of a mare at 322 days of gestation. Mare was presented for abdominal pain and hemorrhagic shock. A moderate amount of swirling echoic fluid with clots was present in the peritoneal cavity. Extensive areas of the uteroplacental unit (between arrows) contained hypoechoic fluid within the uterine wall consistent with either marked intramural hemorrhage and/or edema. The location of the fluid within the uterine wall is in contrast to the location of fluid with uteroplacental separation in figure (d). Transcutaneous image of the uteroplacental unit (between arrows) of a mare at 297 days of gestation. Note marked thickening of uteroplacental unit with hypoechoic fluid accumulation between the uterus and placenta.

Peritoneopericardial hernia[35] and retrosternal (Morgagni) diaphragmatic hernias have been identified in horses[37] but their sonographic appearances have not been described.

Diaphragmatic hernias can be repaired surgically either by direct suturing or mesh herniorrhaphy via a ventral midline approach or through a rib resection made with guidance via a flank incision and thoracoscopy. Inaccessible hernias can be left unrepaired. The prognosis for survival is generally guarded to fair depending on the size and location of the hernia.

Other hernias

Inguinal or scrotal herniation (p. 285) is a consideration in cases of acute colic in the adult male horse. Transcutaneous sonographic evaluation

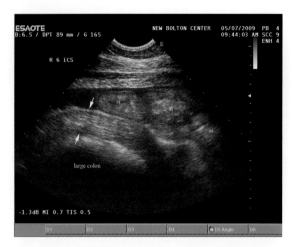

Figure 12.21 Diaphragmatic hernia. Image obtained from right 6th intercostal space; dorsal is to the right of the image. Small intestine (SI) and fluid is seen on the thoracic side of the diaphragm (between arrows) and large colon on the abdominal side.

of the inguinal canal and scrotum will reveal the presence of small intestine and/or omentum. The intestine will be thick-walled, dilated, and amotile if the vascular supply has been compromised. Echoic omentum may be seen herniated together with the small intestine or by itself. There can be variable amounts of fluid within the scrotum. The affected testicle may be increased in echogenicity suggesting obstruction of the testicular vascular supply.

Abdominal wall and umbilical hernias (p. 280) may also be a cause of abdominal pain. The hernias are usually readily apparent on physical examination, and sonography is used to determine the specific contents of the hernia and the viability of any herniated intestine. Compromised intestine will be thick-walled and may be distended and hypo- or amotile. Sonography may also be used to measure the size of the body wall defect and determine if adhesions are present.

Masses

Various types of masses may be the cause of either acute or chronic colic in the horse. As these can be located almost anywhere within the abdomen, complete transcutaneous and transrectal sonographic evaluation is indicated unless signalment, history, and/or physical examination findings can direct the sonographic evaluation. Masses may be obscured from sonographic view by the presence of a gas-filled viscus between the transducer and the mass.

Abscesses

Common locations for abscess formation include mesenteric lymph nodes, perirectal or perivaginal locations, within the spleen or liver or within intestinal walls. The sonographic appearance of an abscess depends on the location, chronicity, and presence or absence of anaerobic infection, but they generally appear as reasonably well circumscribed, ovoid masses containing heteroechoic fluid, and hypoechoic to echogenic capsules. Hyperechoic gas will be present in anaerobic infections or if centesis or drainage has been attempted prior to sonographic evaluation (Figure 12.22). With chronicity the abscess capsule becomes thickened and the contents may become less fluidy and more homogeneous and echoic. Lymphadenopathy and intestinal adhesions may be present in association with an abscess. When a perirectal or perivaginal abscess is detected, the urinary system should be closely evaluated to determine if there is involvement or obstruction of the ureters (Figure 12.22). Sonography is very useful for monitoring response to antimicrobial therapy. A resolving abscess may be seen as a collapsed mass with only the capsule and a small amount of fluid or fibrin within the abscess. The abscess may be sonographically visible for a period of time after resolution of clinicopathological signs. Often perirectal and perivaginal abscesses can be drained per rectum or per vagina, respectively. While intraabdominal abscess are typically treated medically with antimicrobial drugs, if signs of colic are persistent exploratory celiotomy may be indicated. It is usually not possible to resect the abscess. Drainage through the body wall may be achievable. Bypass of the bowel that is adhered to the abscess can be performed. More often horses are euthanized.

The specific sonographic characteristics of intraabdominal abscesses and lymphadenopathy in foals with *Rhodococcus equi* infections have been described.[42] Colic was a presenting clinical sign in some of the cases.[42] Abscesses were often along the

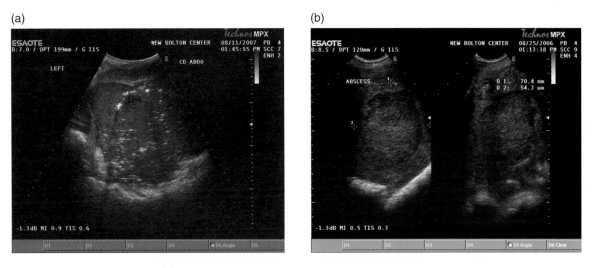

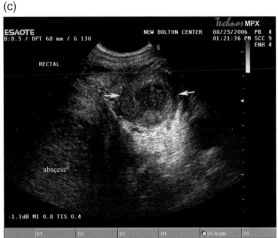

Figure 12.22   Abscesses. (a) Transcutaneous image of a large intra-abdominal abscess post castration. Note the hyperechoic flecks throughout the abscess, some of which cast acoustic shadows consistent with gas. Gas within the abscess may be due to anaerobic infection or the result of gas dissecting along the surgery site. The image was obtained from the caudal ventral abdominal window. The right side of the abdomen is to the right of the image. (b) Transrectal images of a perirectal abscess obtained from a broodmare, approximately 3 months post foaling. Note the large heterechoic mass consisting of heterechoic fluid surrounded by an hypoechoic capsule. The mass was located to the right of the bladder and immediately adjacent to the right ureter. (c) Image shows thick-walled right ureter (between arrows) containing heterechoic fluid adjacent to the abscess. The ureter could be followed to the bladder and urine was seen emptying into the bladder. The right kidney was evaluated for pyelonephritis or obstructive hydronephrosis and neither was found. Foaling trauma was the presumed cause of the abscess and ureteritis.

ventral abdomen but were also seen medial to the liver, spleen, or stomach[43] (Figure 12.23). The abscesses were of mixed echogenicity without hyperechoic gas echoes and were often well circumscribed but occasionally poorly marginated.[42] Capsule thickness varied. There was often an associated lymphadenopathy with single or clustered enlarged lymph nodes of mixed echogenicity (Figure 12.23).[42] There were adhesions of various portions of the intestinal tract to some abscesses.[42] Increased peritoneal fluid was not typical.

The sonographic findings associated with metastatic *Streptococcus equi* subspecies *equi* infections have also been described in a small number of

(a)

(b)

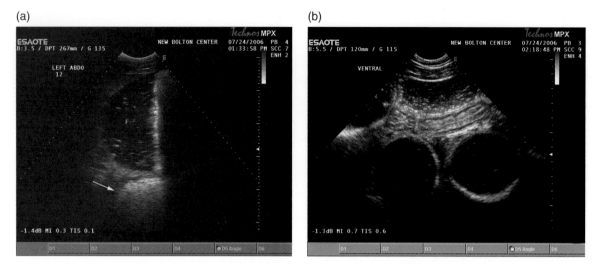

Figure 12.23   Rhodococcus equi intra-abdominal abscess. (a) Transcutaneous image of a *Rhodococcus equi* intra-abdominal abscess axial to the stomach of a foal (arrow). There is marked fluid distension of the stomach (F). The foal presented because of acute colic with fever and large volume reflux. Dorsal is to the right of the image. (b) Multiple populations of small intestine were identified in this foal, including amotile, dilated and turgid loops, collapsed amotile loops, and distended but compressible loops that were hypomotile to amotile. At postmortem, the small intestine was obstructed by adhesions of the small intestine to the abscess.

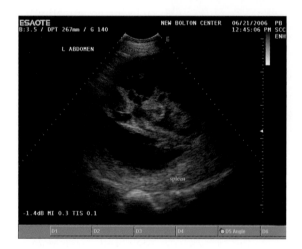

Figure 12.24   Large hematoma within the splenic parenchyma. The hematoma consists of anechoic fluid (serum) and echoic material (clots). Only a small amount of splenic parenchyma can be seen. Image obtained in the left 14th intercostal space. Dorsal is to the right of the image.

cases.[40] The abscesses were of variable size, typically circular to spherical in shape with a smooth or nodular surface, and an echogenic capsule. The echogenicity was homogeneous and hypoechoic or of mixed echogenicity.[40] Hyperechoic

gas echoes were not present. The locations of the abscesses were variable although mesenteric lymph node involvement was common.[40] Lymphadenopathy and thickening of adjacent intestine was present in some cases.[40]

Hematomas

Splenic hematomas may be seen in horses with and without a history of trauma and in horses with hemangiosarcoma.[47] Splenic hematomas may occur with or without concurrent hemoperitoneum. They may be loculated mostly anechoic masses within otherwise normal splenic parenchyma or they may contain echogenic to hyperechoic strands or masses representing clot formation within seroma fluid (Figure 12.24). If the hematoma is recent the fluid within the hematoma may be hypoechoic. The remaining splenic architecture should be normal in appearance although the overall size of the spleen will be small if hemorrhage was recent. Maturing hematomas may be difficult to definitively distinguish from splenic abscess and clinical examination findings should guide the diagnosis. Aspiration or drainage of splenic hematomas may lead to infection and abscess formation.

(a)

(b)

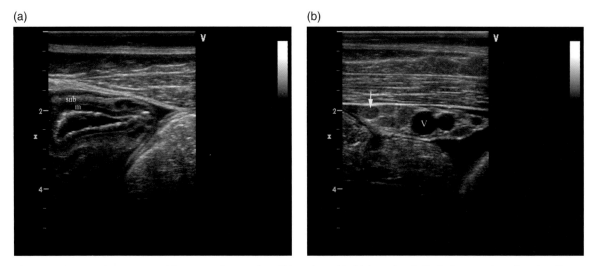

Figure 12.25 Lymphosarcoma. (a) Transverse image of small intestine with thickened wall displaying prominent layering. The submucosal layer is increased in echogenicity consistent with cellular infiltrate. (b) Mesenteric lymphadenopathy from the same horse. Multiple "pea-sized" hypoechoic, homogenous lymph nodes (arrow) adjacent to mesenteric vessels (V) are present in the cecal mesentery.

Enterolithiasis

Sonography in not the diagnostic method of choice for identifying enteroliths, because they are frequently positioned in areas of the intestinal tract that are sonographically inaccessible. When suitably located, enteroliths will appear as spherical intraluminal structures that cast strong acoustic shadows.

Neoplasia

Neoplasia (p. 223) can be found anywhere within the abdominal cavity and can have a variety of sonographic appearances.[22,48] A complete description of all possible sonographic findings in the various types of neoplastic processes is beyond the scope of this chapter. However, certain types of neoplasia are more frequently encountered in the workup of acute or chronic colic. Prognosis for survival is generally poor unless a discrete area of bowel that is surgically accessible for resection is affected.

Alimentary lymphoma

Both alimentary and multicentric lymphoma can cause abdominal pain in the horse although weight loss, lethargy, and ventral edema are more commonly observed.[48] Because alimentary lymphoma can cause a protein losing enteropathy, the primary differentials are inflammatory bowel disease and right dorsal colitis. The sonographic findings in the alimentary form of lymphoma include increased thickness and echogenic infiltrate usually within the submucosal layer of the intestine (Figure 12.25).[22] Other subtle findings may include folding of the mucosal layer of the small intestine without obvious infiltrate. There is often an increase in anechoic or hypoechoic peritoneal fluid and mesenteric lymphadenopathy may be present.[22] Alimentary lymphoma can affect multiple areas of the small and/or large intestine or result in focal infiltrate of the intestinal wall.[22] Discrete intra-abdominal masses may be seen although intraluminal masses are more suggestive of adenocarcinoma.[48] Involvement of other abdominal organs is not uncommon and the line between the alimentary and multicentric forms becomes blurred. Both splenic and hepatic involvement is common.[48] The spleen becomes enlarged and may be seen along the right ventral or even right ventrolateral aspect of the abdomen. Discrete masses may be scattered throughout the spleen or densely packed and bulging from the capsular surface.[22] The masses may be homogenous and hypoechoic or may take on a more complex appearance with

(a)

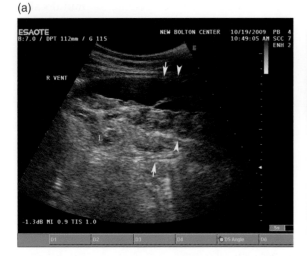

(b)

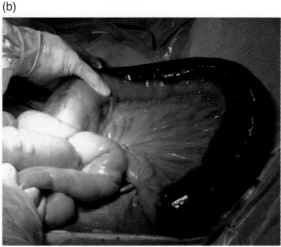

Figure 12.26   Small intestinal hemangiosarcoma. (a) Longitudinal image of a loop of small intestine with an intramural hematoma. Anechoic fluid (serum) and hypoechoic material (clot) are present within the wall of the small intestine (between arrowheads). The serosal surfaces are marked by arrows and the lumen by an "L." In real time, the lumen was identified by movement of ingesta. (b) Intraoperative photograph of the small intestine of the same horse. A diagnosis of hemangiosarcoma was made at postmortem.

areas of calcification that cast acoustic shadows (Figure 12.25). In contrast to the spleen, discrete masses are uncommon in the liver.[22] Instead, the liver becomes enlarged with rounded margins and may extend below the costochondral junction on the right side of the abdomen. The liver becomes diffusely increased in echogenicity with loss of architectural detail.[22] When masses are present they may have a complex pattern of echogenicity. In the absence of involvement of other abdominal organs or discrete masses, the alimentary form of lymphoma is sonographically similar to inflammatory bowel disease (Figure 12.25). Sonographic features that definitively differentiate these two diseases have not been described.

Hemangiosarcoma

Hemangiosarcoma is a malignant neoplasm originating from the vascular endothelium and an important differential for horses that present with acute abdominal pain and intra-abdominal hemorrhage. In reviewing 35 cases of disseminated hemangiosarcoma, intraperitoneal hemorrhage was present in 26% of the cases.[47] Masses within the spleen were common, but the kidneys, liver, mesentery, gastrointestinal viscera, diaphragm, ovaries, adrenal glands, and lymph nodes were affected in some cases.[47] Specific sonographic

findings have not been described for disseminated hemangiosarcoma. A large loculated, heteroechoic mass suggestive of a hematoma within the wall of the small intestine has been seen in the right caudoventral abdomen of a Standardbred stallion with acute abdominal pain and gastric reflux (Figure 12.26). The length of the hematoma was estimated to be at least 30 cm and the small intestinal lumen was decreased in size compared to unaffected small intestine. At postmortem, the horse was diagnosed with hemangiosarcoma affecting the duodenum from the duodenocolic ligament to 66 cm aborally. There was no dissemination to other abdominal organs or the thorax. The sonographic findings in this case are similar to those described for a jejunal intramural hematoma[3] and therefore not specific to hemangiosarcoma.

Gastric neoplasia

Gastric masses are uncommonly identified on sonographic evaluation of the horse with chronic colic. Horses with gastric neoplasms typically have a history of weight loss, anorexia, and anemia without specific mention of abdominal pain.[48] Gastric squamous cell carcinoma appears as a large, heterogeneous mural mass associated with the greater curvature of the stomach although

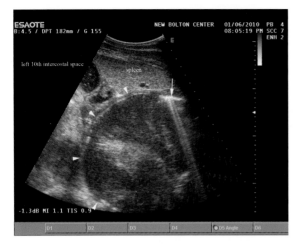

Figure 12.27   Gastric myxoma. Transcutaneous image of a mass (arrowheads) within the stomach of miniature horse with history of recurrent choke. The hyperechoic echoes (arrow) are due to gas accumulation in the dorsal portion of the stomach. The stomach was imaged over 7 intercostal spaces. Gastric leiomyosarcoma, myxoid variant, was diagnosed postmortem. Dorsal is to the right of the image.

homogeneous masses or abscessed masses have been observed.[49] Because metastatic spread is common with carcinoma, numerous masses may be present throughout the peritoneal cavity, within the omentum, along the serosal surfaces of the intestinal tract, or within the liver and spleen.[49] Large peritoneal effusions are common with widespread metastasis.

A large slightly heterogenous, intraluminal gastric mass was imaged in one horse with a history of weight loss, diarrhea, and melena (Figure 12.27). Because the mass was adjacent to the body wall, a transcutaneous sonographic-guided biopsy was performed and histopathology revealed gastric myxosarcoma.[14] Myxosarcoma is a very rare and poorly described neoplasm affecting the equine gastrointestinal tract.[14] Other differentials for gastric masses should include lymphoma, adenocarcinoma, leiomyoma, mesothelioma, and gastrointestinal stromal cell tumor.[49]

Gastrointestinal stromal cell tumors (GIST)

Gastrointestinal stromal cell tumors are of myogenic, neurogenic, or undifferentiated mesenchymal cell origin and can arise from the stomach, small intestine, cecum, or large colon, although cecum and ileum are the most commonly reported

sites.[11,32] Masses may be solitary or multifocal.[11] Sonographically, they appear as heteroechoic round to multilobular masses that are often well demarcated, arising from the serosal or mural regions of the gastrointestinal tract (Figure 12.28). The mass can be quite large and have extensive vascular attachments.[11] Colic with hemoabdomen may be the presenting problems. Metastasis has not been reported in the horse.

Ovarian tumors

Ovarian tumors are occasionally the cause of colic in the mare. If large, these may be identified on transcutaneous sonographic evaluation of the caudal paralumbar fossa region. Granulosa cell tumors are the most common ovarian tumors. Sonographically they appear as large multiloculated masses that may be difficult to differentiate from a transitional ovary that contains numerous anechoic follicles or from an ovarian hematoma. Differentiation is made based on the lack of a palpable ovulation fossa with granulosa cell tumors. Less commonly these tumors may occasionally appear as large multiloculated masses or as solid echoic heterogeneous or homogeneous masses.

Ovarian adenocarcinoma[31] and teratoma[28] are less commonly reported. The sonographic appearance of a teratoma has been described as a follicle-like structure containing echoic masses.[28] Ovarian carcinoma may appear as a large heteroechoic mass within the right paralumbar fossa or flank region and may become large enough to compress the right kidney (Figure 12.29). As with other carcinomas, metastasis to other organs may be present as well as peritoneal or thoracic effusions.[31] The sublumbar lymph nodes may be enlarged.

Other

Urolithiasis

Uroliths may be the cause of chronic low-grade colic and renal sonographic examination should be part of the complete abdominal evaluation.[12,27] Uroliths may be identified on transcutaneous evaluation of the kidneys or transrectal evaluation of the lower urinary tract and left kidney. Nephroliths are hyperechoic structures within the renal parenchyma

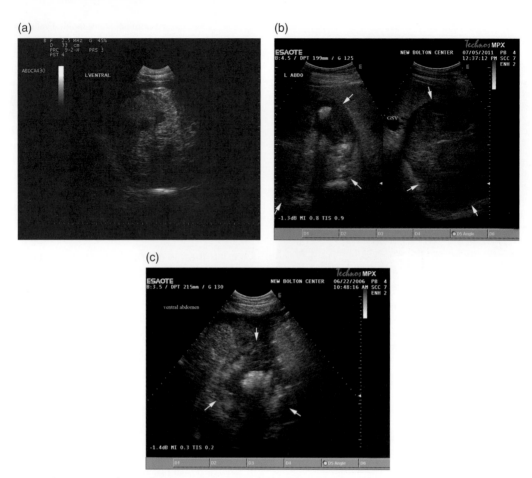

Figure 12.28 Gastrointestinal stromal tumor (GIST). Images obtained from horses with acute colic of varying severity. (a) Large well-circumscribed heterechoic GIST along left ventral abdomen. Horse presented with hemoabdomen (not shown) and hemorrhagic shock. Mass was successfully removed at surgery. (b) Large well-circumscribed heterechoic GIST located in left cranioventrolateral abdomen between the spleen (GSV, gastrosplenic vein) and stomach (not shown). Horse also had a right dorsal displacement of the large colon and the contribution of the GIST to colic signs is unknown. Gastric origin of GIST identified at postmortem. (c) Image of an heterechoic GIST along right ventral abdomen in aged gelding.

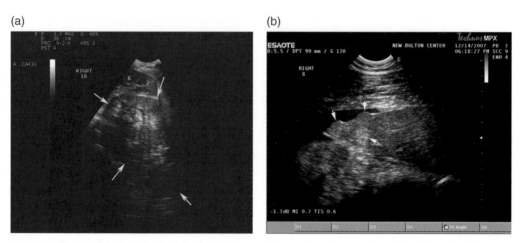

Figure 12.29 Ovarian neoplasia. (a) Large heterechoic mass medial to and compressing the right kidney (K). (b) Metastatic masses within liver (arrows) are hyperechoic relative to the normal liver parenchyma, oval to round, and bulge from the surface. There is an hypoechoic peritoneal effusion visible at the ventral tip of the liver. Ovarian carcinoma with metastasis to the liver was confirmed at postmortem. Dorsal is to the right of the image.

(a)

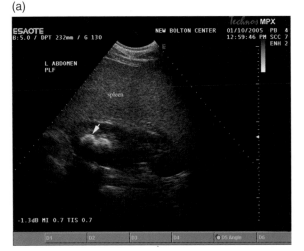

(b)

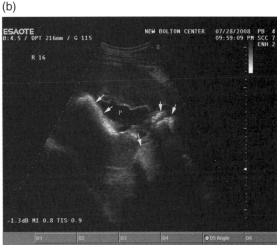

Figure 12.30   Nephrolithiasis. (a) Transcutaneous image of left kidney with nephrolith that casts an acoustic shadow. There is no evidence of hydronephrosis. Dorsal is to the right of the image. (b) Transcutaneous image of right kidney showing multiple nephroliths of varying echogenicities and degrees of calcification. The renal pelvis is also dilated (P). There is also loss of the normal corticomedullary distinction. Dorsal is to the right of the image.

and cast acoustic shadows (Figure 12.30). The more calcified nephroliths cast an acoustic shadow from the side of the nephrolith nearest the transducer whereas those with a more proteinaceous content cast acoustic shadows from the far side of the nephrolith. Nephroliths may be obstructive resulting in concurrent hydronephrosis with marked renal pelvic dilatation and cortical thinning in severe cases.[27] Nephroliths are occasionally found in horses without a history of colic or renal disease.[27]

Transrectal evaluation of the ureters should be performed if nephroliths are identified or if hydronephrosis without nephrolithiasis is identified. The normal sonographic appearance of the ureters has been described.[12] Ureteroliths are hyperechoic structures that cast acoustic shadows and result in hydroureter proximal to the obstruction. If the obstruction is complete there will be hydronephrosis and an inability to see urine empty into the bladder from the affected ureter (Figure 12.31).

Cholelithiasis

Fever, icterus, and mild intermittent colic are common signs of horses with cholangiohepatitis and cholelithiasis.[23] Sonographic evaluation of these horses will aid in determining the degree of biliary distension, ruling in or out other hepatic

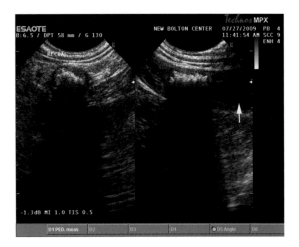

Figure 12.31   Obstructive ureterolithiasis. Transrectal sonogram of ureter with echogenic material in the lumen. The material casts an acoustic shadow consistent with calcification and is obstructing the ureter as evidenced by distension of the ureter proximal to the ureterolith (arrow).

diseases such as hepatitis or neoplasia, and guiding the selection of a site to biopsy. The liver should be scanned from both the right and left sides of the abdomen and followed to its ventral margin on each side. Common sonographic findings of cholangiohepatitis include hepatic enlargement and increased echogenicity. Biliary distension is

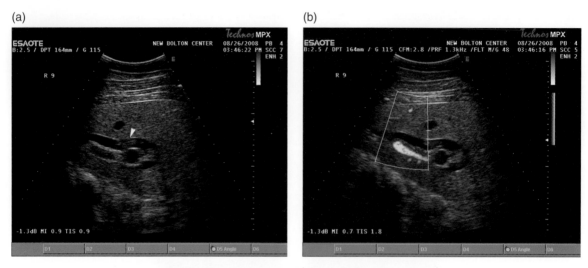

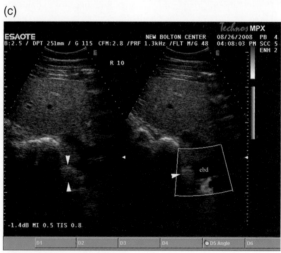

Figure 12.32   Biliary obstruction. All images are of the right liver lobe of a horse with chronic colic and fever. Dorsal is to the right of all images. (a) Image of right liver lobe showing marked biliary distension and hypoechoic material within an intrahepatic bile duct (arrow). (b) Power Doppler of same image in (a). Note color signal indicating blood flow in the hepatic vein that is running parallel to the bile duct. (c) Images of porta hepatis showing hypoechoic material (arrowheads) within common bile duct, dilation of the common bile duct (CBC), and color signal within the adjacent portal vein.

identified as a parallel channel sign consistent with dilated bile ducts adjacent to the branches of the portal vein. Choleliths are most often hyperechoic and may or may not cast acoustic shadows. Evaluation of the porta hepatis is important for identifying large biliary stones within the common bile duct as these can cause significant biliary obstruction and colic pain. Visibility of the porta hepatis may require 28 cm or more depth of penetration in some adult horses (Figure 12.32).

Foreign bodies have been reported to occur in the common bile duct and act as a nidus for stone formation and obstruction.[17]

References

1. Albanese, V., Credille, B., Ellis, A., Baldwin, L., Mueller, P.O.E. & Woolums, A. (2011) A case of a colocolic intussusception in a horse. *Equine Veterinary Education*, **23**, 281–285.

2. Arnold, C.E., Payne, M., Thompson, J.A., Slovis, N.M. & Bain, F.T. (2008) Periparturient hemorrhage in mares: 73 cases (1998–2005). *Journal of the American Veterinary Medical Association*, **232**, 1345–1351.

3. Beckman, K.E., Del Piero, F., Donaldson, M.T., Seco, O. & Reef, V. (2008) Imaging diagnosis—Intramural hematoma, jejunal diverticulum and colic in a horse. *Veterinary Radiology & Ultrasound*, **49**, 81–84.

4. Bell, R.J. & Textor, J.A. (2010) Caecal intussusceptions in horses: A New Zealand perspective. *Australian Veterinary Journal*, **88**, 272–276.

5. Bernard, W.V., Reef, V.B., Reimer, J.M., Humber, K.A. & Orsini, J.A. (1989) Ultrasonographic diagnosis of small-intestinal intussusception in three foals. *Journal of the American Veterinary Medical Association*, **194**, 395–397.

6. Busoni, V., Busscher, V.D., Lopez, D., Verwilghen, D. & Cassart, D. (2010) Evaluation of a protocol for fast localised abdominal sonography of horses (FLASH) admitted for colic. *Veterinary Journal*, **188**, 77–82.

7. Chaffin, M.K., Fuenteabla, I.C., Schumacher, J., Welch, R.D. & Edwards, J.F. (1992) Idiopathic muscular hypertrophy of the equine small intestine: 11 cases (1980–1991). *Equine Veterinary Journal*, **24**, 372–378.

8. Conwell, R.C., Hillyer, M.H., Mair, T.S., Pirie, R.S. & Clegg, P.D. (2010) Haemoperitoneum in horses: A retrospective review of 54 cases. *Veterinary Record*, **167**, 514–518.

9. Dechant, J.E., Nieto, J.E. & Le Jeune, S.S. (2006) Hemoperitoneum in horses: 67 cases (1989–2004). *Journal of the American Veterinary Medical Association*, **229**, 253–258.

10. Dechant, J.E., Whitcomb, M.B. & Magdesian, K.G. (2008) Ultrasonographic diagnosis—Idiopathic muscular hypertrophy of the small intestine in a miniature horse. *Veterinary Radiology & Ultrasound*, **49**, 300–302.

11. Del Piero, F., Summers, B.A., Cumings, J.F., Mandelli, G. & Blomm, E.A. (2001) Gastrointestinal stromal tumors in equids. *Veterinary Pathology*, **38**, 689–697.

12. Diaz, O.S., Smith, G. & Reef, V.B. (2007) Ultrasonographic appearance of the lower urinary tract in fifteen normal horses. *Veterinary Radiology & Ultrasound*, **48**, 560–564.

13. Dowling, P.M. & Todhunter, P. (1994) What is your diagnosis? Chronic ileocecal intussusception. *Journal of the American Veterinary Medical Association*, **205**, 39–40.

14. Edens, L.M., Taylor, D.D., Murray, M.J., Spurlock, G.H. & Anver, M.R. (1992) Intestinal myxosarcoma in a thoroughbred mare. *Cornell Veterinarian*, **82**, 163–167.

15. Epstein, K., Short, D., Parente, E., Reef, V. & Southwood, L. (2008) Serial gastrointestinal ultrasonography following exploratory celiotomy in normal adult ponies. *Veterinary Radiology & Ultrasound*, **49**, 584–588.

16. Fontaine-Rodgerson, G. & Rodgerson, D.H. (2001) Diagnosis of small intestinal intussusception by transabdominal ultrasonography in 2 adult horses. *Canadian Veterinary Journal*, **42**, 378–380.

17. Gerros, T.C., McGuirk, S.M., Biller, D.S., Stone, W.C. & Ryan, J. (1993) Choledocholithiasis attributable to a foreign body in a horse. *Journal of the American Veterinary Medical Association*, **202**, 301–303.

18. Gomaa, N., Uhlig, A. & Schusser, G.F. (2011) Effect of buscopan compositum on the motility of the duodenum, cecum and left ventral colon in healthy conscious horses. *Berliner und Munchener Tierarztliche Wochenschrift*, **124**, 168–174.

19. Gorvy, D.A., Edwards, G.B. & Proudman, C.J. (2008) Intra-abdominal adhesions in horses: A retrospective evaluation of repeat laparotomy in 99 horses with acute gastrointestinal disease. *Veterinary Journal*, **175**, 194–201.

20. Hart, S.K. & Brown, J.A. (2009) Diaphragmatic hernia in horses: 44 cases (1986–2006). *Journal of Veterinary Emergency and Critical Care*, **19**, 357–362.

21. Hendrickson, E.H., Malone, E.D. & Sage, A.M. (2007) Identification of normal parameters for ultrasonographic examination of the equine large colon and cecum. *Canadian Veterinary Journal*, **48**, 289–291.

22. Hillyer, M.H. (1994) The use of ultrasonography in the diagnosis of abdominal tumors in the horse. *Equine Veterinary Education*, **6**, 273–278.

23. Johnston, J.K., Divers, T.J., Reef, V.B. & Acland, H. (1989) Cholelithiasis in horses: Ten cases (1982–1986). *Journal of the American Veterinary Medical Association*, **194**, 405–409.

24. Jones, S.L., Davis, J. & Rowlingson, K. (2003) Ultrasonographic findings in horses with right dorsal colitis: Five cases (2000–2001). *Journal of the American Veterinary Medical Association*, **222**, 1248–1251.

25. Kihurani, D.O., Carstens, A., Saulez, M.N. & Donnellan, C.M. (2009) Transcutaneous ultrasonographic evaluation of the air-filled equine stomach and duodenum following gastroscopy. *Veterinary Radiology & Ultrasound*, **50**, 429–435.

26. Korolainen, R. & Ruohoniemi, M. (2002) Reliability of ultrasonography compared to radiography in revealing intestinal sand accumulations in horses. *Equine Veterinary Journal*, **34**, 499–504.

27. Laverty, S., Pascoe, J.R., Ling, G.V., Lavoie, J.P. & Ruby, A.L. (1992) Urolithiasis in 68 horses. *Veterinary Surgery*, **21**, 56–62.

28. Lefebvre, R., Theoret, C., Dore, M., Girard, C., Laverty, S. & Vaillancourt, D. (2005) Ovarian teratoma and endometritis in a mare. *Canadian Veterinary Journal*, **46**, 1029–1033.

29. Mitchell, C.F., Malone, E.D., Sage, A.M. & Niksich, K. (2005) Evaluation of gastrointestinal activity patterns in healthy horses using B mode and Doppler ultrasonography. *Canadian Veterinary Journal*, **46**, 134–140.

30. Moll, H.D., Schumacher, J., Dabareiner, R.M. & Slone, D.E. (1993) Left dorsal displacement of the colon with splenic adhesions in three horses. *Journal of the American Veterinary Medical Association*, **203**, 425–427.

31. Morris, D.D., Acland, H.M. & Hodge, T.G. (1985) Pleural effusion secondary to metastasis of an ovarian adenocarcinoma in a horse. *Journal of the American Veterinary Medical Association*, **187**, 272–274.

32. Muravnick, K.B., Parente, E.J. & Del Piero, F. (2009) An atypical equine gastrointestinal stromal tumor. *Journal of Veterinary Diagnostic Investigation*, **21**, 387–390.

33. Navas de Solis, C., Palmer, J.E., Boston, R.C. & Reef, V.B. (2012). The importance of ultrasonographic pneumatosis intestinalis in equine neonatal gastrointestinal disease. *Equine Veterinary Journal*, **44** (Suppl 41), 64–68.

34. Ness, S.L., Bain, F.T., Zantingh, A.J., *et al.* (2011) Ultrasonographic visualization of colonic mesenteric vasculature as an indicator of large colon right dorsal displacement and/or 180 degree volvulus in horses. In: *Proceedings of the 10th Equine Colic Research Symposium*, Indianapolis, Indiana, pp. 128–129.

35. Orsini, J.A., Koch, C. & Stewart, B. (1981) Peritoneopericardial hernia in a horse. *Journal of the American Veterinary Medical Association*, **179**, 907–910.

36. Parker, R.A., Barr, E.D. & Dixon, P.M. (2011) Treatment of equine gastric impaction by gastrotomy. *Equine Veterinary Education*, **23**, 169–173.

37. Pauwels, F.F., Hawkins, J.F., MacHarg, M.A., Rothenbuhler, R.D., Baird, D.K. & Moulton, J.S. (2007) Congenital retrosternal (Morgagni) diaphragmatic hernias in three horses. *Journal of the American Veterinary Medical Association*, **231**, 427–432.

38. Pease, A.P., Scrivani, P.V., Erb, H.N. & Cook, V.L. (2004) Accuracy of increased large-intestine wall thickness during ultrasonography for diagnosing large-colon torsion in 42 horses. *Veterinary Radiology & Ultrasound*, **45**, 220–224.

39. Pusterla, N., Fecteau, M.E., Madigan, J.E., Wilson, W.D. & Magdesian K.G. (2005) Acute hemoperitoneum in horses: A review of 19 cases (1992–2003). *Journal of Veterinary Internal Medicine*, **19**, 344–347.

40. Pusterla, N., Whitcomb, M.B. & Wilson, W.D. (2007) Internal abdominal abscesses caused by streptococcus equi subspecies equi in 10 horses in California between 1989 and 2004. *Veterinary Record*, **160**, 589–592.

41. Reef, V.B. (1998) Adult abdominal ultrasonography. In: *Equine Diagnostic Ultrasound* (ed V.B. Reef), pp. 295–335. W.B. Saunders, Philadelphia, Pennsylvania.

42. Reuss, S.M., Chaffin, M.K., Schmitz, D.G. & Norman, T.E. (2011) Sonographic characteristics of intraabdominal abscessation and lymphadenopathy attributable to rhodococcus equi infections in foals. *Veterinary Radiology & Ultrasound*, **52**, 462–465.

43. Romero, A.E. & Rodgerson, D.H. (2010) Diaphragmatic herniation in the horse: 31 cases from 2001–2006. *Canadian Veterinary Journal*, **51**, 1247–1250.

44. Ross, M.W., Stephens, P.R. & Reimer, J.M. (1988) Small colon intussusception in a broodmare. *Journal of the American Veterinary Medical Association*, **192**, 372–374.

45. Santschi, E.M., Slone, D.E., Jr, Frank, W.M., 2nd. (1993) Use of ultrasound in horses for diagnosis of left dorsal displacement of the large colon and monitoring its nonsurgical correction. *Veterinary Surgery*, **22**, 281–284.

46. Sertich, P.L. (1998) Ultrasonography of the genital tract of the mare. In: *Equine Diagnostic Ultrasound* (ed V.B. Reef), pp. 417–418. W.B. Saunders Company, Philadelphia, Pennsylvania.

47. Southwood, L.L., Schott, H.C., 2nd, Henry, C.J., *et al.* (2000) Disseminated hemangiosarcoma in the horse: 35 cases. *Journal of Veterinary Internal Medicine*, **14**, 105–109.

48. Taylor, S.D., Pusterla, N., Vaughan, B., Whitcomb, M.B. & Wilson, W.D. (2006) Intestinal neoplasia in horses. *Journal of Veterinary Internal Medicine*, **20**, 1429–1436.

49. Taylor, S.D., Haldorson, G.J., Vaughan, B. & Pusterla, N. (2009) Gastric neoplasia in horses. *Journal of Veterinary Internal Medicine*, **23**, 1097–1102.

50. Vainio, K., Sykes, B.W. & Blikslager, A.T. (2011) Primary gastric impaction in horses: A retrospective study of 20 cases (2005–2008). *Equine Veterinary Education*, **23**, 186–190.

51. Valdes-Martinez, A. & Waguespack, R.W. (2006) What is your diagnosis? Cecocolic intussusception. *Journal of the American Veterinary Medical Association*, **228**, 847–848.

13 Abdominal Radiographic Examination

Sarah M. Puchalski

Department of Surgical and Radiological Sciences, School of Veterinary Medicine, University of California, Davis, CA, USA

Chapter Outline

Indications	**149**	**Procedure**	**152**
Preparation	**150**	Adult horse	153
Equipment	150	Foals	155
X-ray generator	150	**Application of abdominal radiography**	
Cassettes/detector and cassette holder	150	**to the colic patient**	**155**
Markers	151	Enterolithiasis	155
Safety equipment	151	Sand accumulation	156
Patient	152	Metallic foreign material	157
Sedation/restraint	152	Diaphragmatic hernia	157
Gut fill	152	Foal	157

Indications

Abdominal radiography in the horse is a useful ancillary diagnostic test for colic workup. This noninvasive test can be utilized to aid in the identification of the underlying cause and therefore expedite the development of a therapeutic plan, medical or surgical, in horses presenting with clinical signs of colic. Radiography is of particular import in horses that have been housed in geographic regions where either sand enteropathy (p. 217) or enterolithiasis (p. 218) is a differential diagnosis for colic. In smaller equids including foals, donkeys, and miniature horses, abdominal radiography provides a more complete evaluation. In general, radiography should be considered a complementary diagnostic imaging test to abdominal sonography (p. 116).

The size of the adult horse continues to challenge the clinical utility of abdominal radiography. While the advent and more common use of digital radiography has improved the value of radiographs in general, the facts remain that in most adult horses the X-ray generator is near its maximum capacity, multiple projections are needed, and orthogonal projections are not possible. Even with these difficulties, radiography remains a highly sensitive and specific test for the diagnosis of enterolithiasis (Figure 13.1)[5,7,8,11] and highly sensitive test for the presence of sand (Figure 13.2).[4,9] In smaller horses and foals, a more detailed evaluation of the abdomen can be performed, including contrast gastrointestinal studies, thereby augmenting this diagnostic test's clinical utility (Figure 13.3).[1,2]

Few contraindications to radiography exist per se. The use of sedation and restraint for the acquisition of radiographs is a clinical decision based on the patient's status. Abdominal radiography in the horse uses the highest ionizing radiation dose in veterinary diagnostic radiography. This results in the highest scatter radiation doses to personnel. Care should be taken to keep the radiation dose to the staff and associated personnel as low as reasonably achievable (ALARA). Abdominal radiography is generally reserved for use at large referral hospitals.

Preparation

Equipment

X-ray generator

The generator should be capable of 100–120 kVp and 100–200 mAs. Settings will depend on the detector system.

Cassettes/detector and cassette holder

Large size cassettes (14" × 17") or a large detector are recommended. A grid is optional with most

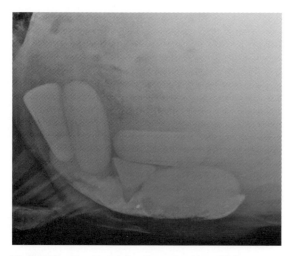

Figure 13.1 Cranioventral radiograph with multiple enteroliths in the large colon. At necropsy, there were six enteroliths retrieved. One enterolith was in the small colon, likely causing obstruction and clinical signs of colic.

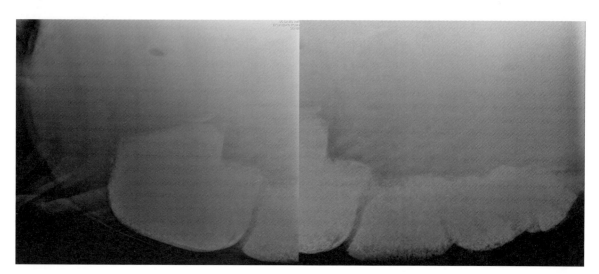

Figure 13.2 Overlapping ventral radiographs with sand in the ventral colon. The mineral opaque sand is moderately opaque, heterogeneous, and has an irregular dorsal margin. Note that the ventral sacculations are outlined by the radiopaque sand.

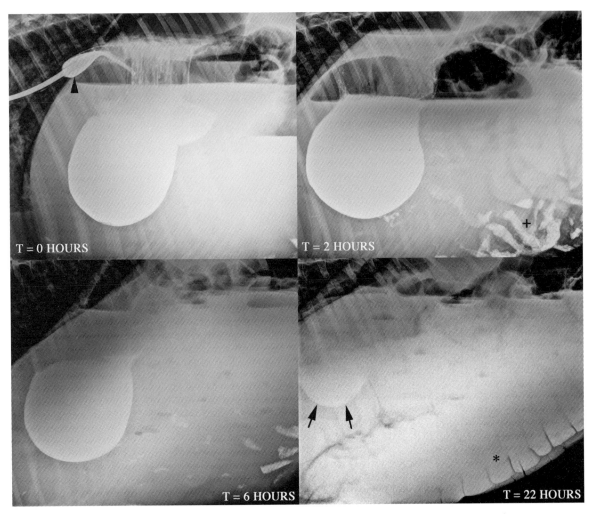

Figure 13.3 Gastrointestinal contrast study in a 5-year-old miniature horse with small intestinal (duodenal) muscular hypertrophy. At the beginning of the study, barium sulfate suspension (2% weight/volume) is seen in the nasogastric tube and distal esophagus (arrowhead). At 2 h after administration, barium is present within the stomach and the small bowel (+). At 6 h, barium is present within the stomach. At 22 h, barium is present within the large intestine (*) but also within the stomach (arrows). This represents delayed gastric emptying.

digital systems. A freestanding cassette holder or a linked overhead radiography system is recommended (Figure 13.4). Never hand-hold cassettes for abdominal radiographs.

Markers

Radiolucent markers on the skin surface aid in obtaining complete coverage of the abdomen.

Safety equipment

Radiation safety is critical. Limit the number of personnel to as few people as possible and preferably those with low or no occupational exposure. Appropriate shielding includes lead aprons, thyroid protection, and cornea protection. All personnel with occupational exposure should wear radiation dosimeters on the outside of their leaded aprons.

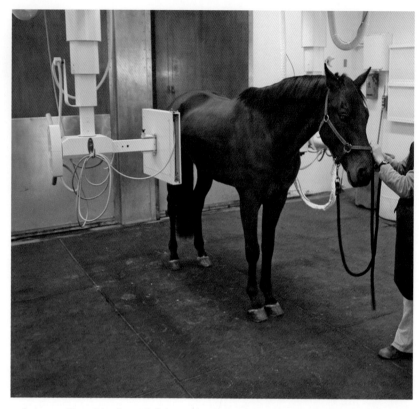

Figure 13.4   A horse being positioned for the mid-abdominal radiograph using a linking overhead radiography system.

Patient

Sedation/restraint

Sedation should be used judiciously to maintain immobility while the radiography equipment moves around the horse. This can usually be achieved with an alpha-2 agonist (p. 54).

Gut fill

Excess gut fill will result in underexposure of the abdomen. Underexposure is easily detected on analogue film screen radiographs as excessive whiteness in the image. Underexposure is more difficult to detect on digital radiographs. Underexposure manifests as a lack of contrast between intra-abdominal structures within the abdomen. If there is underexposure as the result of excess gut fill, radiographic reexamination after fasting may be prudent.

Procedure

The accuracy of abdominal radiography as a diagnostic test is dependent on the provision of a high-quality diagnostic examination that includes an adequate number of views and appropriate interpretation. The radiographic identification of sand or enteroliths is relatively straightforward. The diagnosis of many other disease processes, such as mechanical or functional ileus, can only be supported by radiographic findings. Furthermore, the identification of many radiographic abnormalities is subjective. For example, while distension of small bowel is characteristic of obstruction in other species, no guidelines for pathological distension of small or large bowel in the horse exist (Figure 13.5). The presence of bowel distension or feed impaction should be considered with other findings and is often supportive of a clinical diagnosis (Figures 13.6 and 13.7).

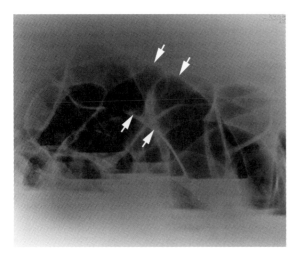

Figure 13.5   Caudodorsal radiograph showing severe small intestinal gas distension (arrows). At surgery, this horse had a small intestinal strangulating lipoma.

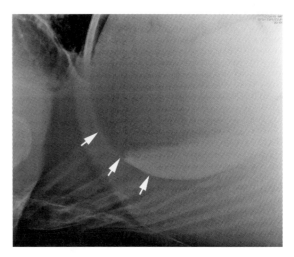

Figure 13.7   Cranioventral radiograph showing mottled opacity feed material within the gastric lumen. The mineral opaque material accumulating in the ventral stomach outlines the wall of the stomach (arrows). This horse had peritonitis. An exploratory celiotomy was performed to identify a gastric impaction with devitalized small bowel secondary to a strangulating lipoma.

(2)   Mid-abdomen (Figure 13.10): Using a line from the point of the hip to the ventral body wall, just caudal to the elbow, center the beam at the costochondral junctions, halfway between the views made at the limits of the line.

(3)   Cranioventral (Figure 13.11): The cranioventral corner should be positioned at the limits of the line drawn from the point of the hip to the ventral body wall caudal to the elbow. Center the collimator light on the cranioventral abdomen at the level of chondral portion of the last rib. The collimator light should include the ventral body wall.

(4)   Caudoventral (Figure 13.12): Center the beam in the middle of the flank, ventral to the first view.

Figure 13.6   Cranioventral radiograph showing mottled opacity feed material in the ventral colon. This horse had an impaction colic that was managed successfully with medical therapy.

Adult horse

A complete examination of an adult horse usually requires four views when taken on 14 × 17 cassettes (Figure 13.8).

(1)   Caudodorsal (Figure 13.9): Center the beam 45° forward and ventral from the point of the hip in the flank.

Note that geometric magnification is an important and inevitable factor in abdominal radiography. Generally, abdominal radiographs are made with the beam entering on the left and exiting the right or vice versa. Lateralized lesions will be projected as markedly size discrepant on the radiographs. In absence of the orthogonal projection, magnification cannot be corrected for. Producing radiographs from both sides when a specific lesion arises can partially mitigate this problem; the lesion will be most accurately depicted when it is closest to the detector.

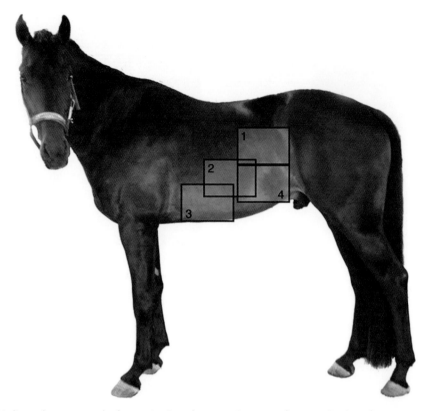

Figure 13.8   This figure demonstrates the four projections that comprise a complete examination of an average, adult horse abdomen.

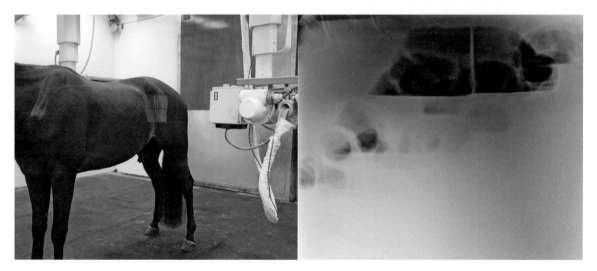

Figure 13.9   The normal caudodorsal radiograph (see Figure 13.12). This image is made with the beam center in the flank 45° ventral and cranial to the point of the hip.

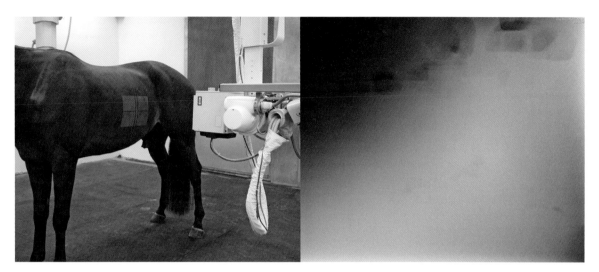

Figure 13.10   The normal mid-abdominal radiograph. This radiograph is made by dividing the distance between the caudodorsal and cranioventral projections.

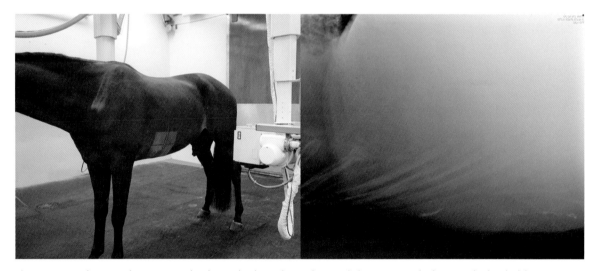

Figure 13.11   The normal cranioventral radiograph. This radiograph is made by centering the beam at the level of the costochondral junctions caudal to the point of the elbow.

Foals

The procedure will depend on the patient size. Radiographs of larger foals, miniature horses, and donkeys are best made standing. Smaller or sicker patients can be imaged in lateral recumbency, lying on a cassette or detector. Ventral dorsal radiographs remain difficult to obtain and often radiographs made from both sides of the abdomen can be helpful.

Application of abdominal radiography to the colic patient

Enterolithiasis

Abdominal radiography is highly sensitive and specific for diagnosing enterolithiasis (p. 218).[11] The use of computed radiography has slightly increased overall sensitivity and specificity, and of

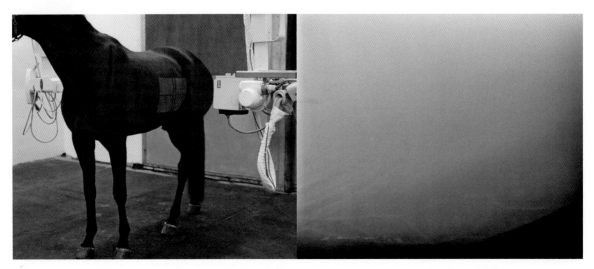

Figure 13.12 The normal caudoventral radiograph. This is made by moving the beam center, within the flank, ventral from the caudodorsal radiograph.

(a)   (b)

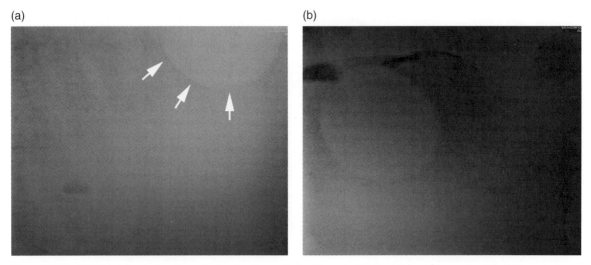

Figure 13.13 (a) Mid-abdominal radiograph showing the ventral outline of a faintly visible, solitary enterolith. (b) In order to better visualize the enterolith, the beam center was moved caudal and dorsal. The enterolith was present in the small colon and was removed via colon enterotomy.

particular importance, improved the ability to detect enteroliths in the small colon (Figure 13.13).[6] Occasionally, clinical importance is assigned to the size of an enterolith. Geometric magnification is a factor in the accurate measurement of any radiographic finding, particularly large anatomic structures, such as the equine abdomen. The most accurate, and smallest, measurement will be made when the object is closest to the detector.

Sand accumulation

Abdominal radiographs are very useful for the identification of intestinal sand accumulation.[3,9] Unfortunately, the identification of sand does not indicate its clinical importance. Recent efforts have been directed at the development of scoring systems to increase the predictive value of

Table 13.1   Radiographic scoring sheet for sand accumulation.

Radiographic feature	Score*
Location	
Cranioventral	1
Other	0
Number of accumulations	
0	0
1–2	1
≥3	3
Opacity (compared to rib or vertebral body)	
Much less opaque	0
Mixed	1
More or as opaque	2
Homogeneity	
Heterogeneous	0
Mixed	1
Homogeneous	2
Thickness of sand: width of rib	
1–3×	0
4–5×	1
>5×	2
Thickness of sand: width of rib	
<10	0
10–20	1
>20	2

*Radiographic score 7/12 (83%) likelihood of being associated with a positive diagnosis of sand colic.
Source: Keppie et al. (2008).

Table 13.2   Radiographic scoring sheet for sand accumulation.

Radiographic feature	Score*
No sand	0
<5 × 5 cm	1
≤5 × 15 cm or ≤15 × 5 cm	2
≤5 × 15 cm or ≤15 × 5 cm close to the ventral abdominal wall	3
>5 × 15 cm or >15 × 5 cm. If an accumulation was thin (<5 cm) but longer than 15 cm it was graded as a 4.	4

*Horses without clinical signs referable to the gastrointestinal tract had a score ≤2 whereas horses with a sand impaction had scores >2. Sand impaction was associated with accumulations that were more dense than the rib and homogeneous.
Source: Kendall et al. (2008).

radiographs for diagnosing sand colic (p. 217)[3,4] (Tables 13.1 and 13.2) and to increase the value of this test as a monitoring technique for the medical management of this condition.[3,9] Keppie et al.[4] developed a scoring system based on the location, number of accumulations, opacity, homogeneity, thickness, and length of the accumulation. This scoring system improved consistency between observers and diagnostic accuracy when compared to subjective evaluation alone.[4] In general, increased size and number of sand accumulations, increased opacity, homogeneity, and more distinct margins are associated with sand colic and diminish over time with medical management (Figure 13.2).

Metallic foreign material

Radiography can be used to identify ingested metallic foreign objects in adult horses.[10] Horses with metallic foreign material often present with peritonitis. It is recommended to focus the radiographic examination on the cranial abdomen when a metallic wire is suspected to be the cause of peritonitis.[10]

Diaphragmatic hernia

Thoracic radiography can be used to diagnose a diaphragmatic hernia with identification of abdominal viscera within the thoracic cavity. Abdominal sonography, however, is used more commonly for this type of diagnosis (see Chapter 12 on Abdominal Sonographic Evaluation [p. 136]).

Foal

In foals a more complete evaluation of the gastrointestinal tract can be performed using standing lateral radiographs.[1,2] In the normal foal, a small amount of gas is expected in the stomach, small intestine, small colon, and less frequently in the cecum and rectum (Figure 13.14). Furthermore, the length of the first lumbar vertebra can give an indication of pathological distension of small intestine, whereby, the diameter of small intestine should be less than the length of L1.[2] These guidelines predate the common use of abdominal sonography. Currently, abdominal sonography provides a complete evaluation of the abdominal viscera and radiography should be considered complementary. Radiographs can be particularly useful when gas distension of the intestinal tract precludes sonographic examination of the abdomen or bowel (Figures 13.15 and 13.16).

Contrast radiography can also be used to evaluate gastric emptying (Figure 13.17) in foals with suspected gastric outflow obstruction.[12] After gastric decompression by nasogastric tube, barium (10 mL/kg) is administered and standing lateral radiographs are obtained immediately and 5, 15, 30, 60, and 90 min after administration. A diagnosis of gastric outflow obstruction is made based on minimal or no contrast material being observed aboral to the stomach or the duodenum after 30–90 min.

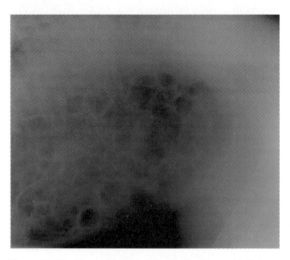

Figure 13.14 Normal lateral abdominal radiograph of a 10-day-old foal. There is mild gas accumulation in the stomach, small intestine, and colon.

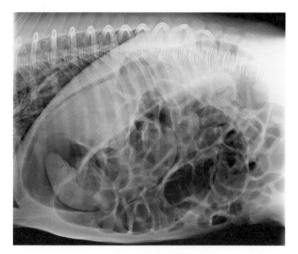

Figure 13.15 Lateral abdominal radiograph of a 2-day-old foal with moderate to severe gas distension of small and large bowel. This foal had a severe meconium impaction that needed surgery to resolve. An enterotomy was performed at the sternal flexure to remove the impaction.

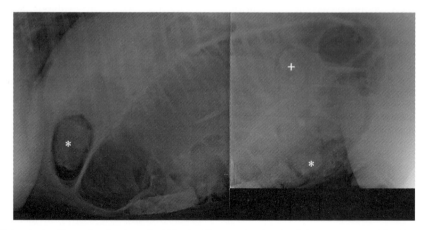

Figure 13.16 Abdominal radiographs of a 4-week-old foal with a small colon fecalith (+). Inspissated fecal material is present in the large colon (*).

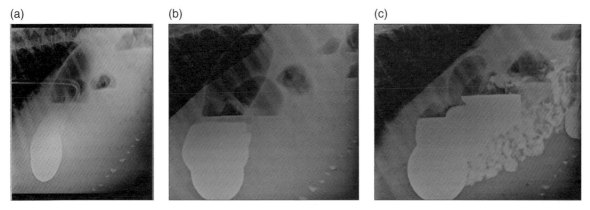

Figure 13.17   Contrast radiographic series of a 4-month-old foal with a duodenal stricture (a) immediately following barium administration, (b) 50 min, and (c) 90 min post-barium.

References

1. Campbell, M.L., Ackerman, N. & Peyton, L.C. (1984) Radiographic gastrointestinal anatomy of the foal. *Veterinary Radiology & Ultrasound*, **25**, 194–204.
2. Fischer, A.T., Kerr, L.Y. & O'Brien, T.R. (1987) Radiographic diagnosis of gastrointestinal disorders in the foal. *Veterinary Radiology & Ultrasound*, **28**, 42–48.
3. Kendall, A., Ley, C., Egenvall, A. & Bröjer, J. (2008) Radiographic parameters for diagnosing sand colic in horses. *Acta Veterinaria Scandinavica*, **50**, 17.
4. Keppie, N.J., Rosenstein, D.S., Holcombe, S.J. & Schott, H.C., 2nd. (2008) Objective radiographic assessment of abdominal sand accumulation in horses. *Veterinary Radiology & Ultrasound*, **49**, 122–128.
5. Lloyd, K., Hintz, H.F., Wheat, J.D. & Schryver, H.F. (1987) Enteroliths in horses. *Cornell Veterinarian*, **77**, 172–186.
6. Maher, O., Puchalski, S.M., Drake, C. & le Jeune, S.S. (2011) Abdominal computed radiography for diagnosis of enterolithiasis in horses: 142 cases (2003–2007). *Journal of the American Veterinary Medical Association*, **239**, 1483–1485.
7. Murray, R.C., Constantinescu, G.M. & Green, E.M. (1992) Equine enterolithiasis. *Compendium on Continuing Education: Equine Practices*, **14**, 1104–1112.
8. Rose, J.A., Rose, E.M. & Sande, R.D. (1980) Radiography in the diagnosis of equine enterolithiasis. In: *Proceedings 26th Annual Meeting of the American Association of Equine Practitioners*, Anaheim, CA, pp. 211–219.
9. Ruohoniemi, M., Kaikkonen, R., Raekallio, M. & Luukkanen, L. (2001) Abdominal radiography in monitoring the resolution of sand accumulations from the large colon of horses treated medically. *Equine Veterinary Journal*, **33**, 59–64.
10. Soffler, C. & Hackett, E.S. (2011) Ingested wires in the equine abdomen: 13 cases (2003–2010). In: *Proceedings 10th Equine Colic Research Symposium*, Indianapolis, Indiana, p. 189.
11. Yarbrough, T.B., Langer, D.L., Snyder, J.R., Gardner, I.A. & O'Brien, T.R. (1994) Abdominal radiography for diagnosis of enterolithiasis in horses: 141 cases (1990–1992). *Journal of the American Veterinary Medical Association*, **205**, 592–595.
12. Zedler, S.T., Embertson, R.M., Bernard, W.V., Barr, B.S. & Boston, R.C. (2009) Surgical treatment of gastric outflow obstruction in 40 foals. *Veterinary Surgery*, **38**, 623–630.

14 Trocharization

Joanne Fehr

Equine Emergency Department, Pilchuck Animal Hospital, Snohomish, WA, USA

Chapter Outline

Indications	160	Paralumbar approach	161
Preparation	161	Transrectal approach	162
Procedure	161	**Complications**	162

Indications

Trocharization involves the placement of a needle-like instrument equipped with a cannula through the body wall to withdraw or release gas or fluid. In the horse, trocharization is most frequently performed into the cecal base in the right paralumbar fossa. Trocharization is used in the treatment of colic on rare occasions when clinical signs, physical examination, and treatment options dictate. In the horse, due to the susceptibility to peritonitis and intraperitoneal adhesion formation, trocharization may be performed in cases of severe large colon distention when either surgical intervention is not an option or when there is respiratory compromise and transportation to the surgical facility is needed.

Cecal trocharization is indicated if a considerable amount of gas distention is present in the right ventral colon and cecum suggestive of a primary large intestinal lesion, and surgical intervention is not an immediate option. Cecal trocharization may be performed to provide more time for medical treatment and resolution in a nonsurgical case. Examples of such lesions include nephrosplenic ligament entrapment, right dorsal displacement, small colon impaction, and colitis. Note that the base of the cecum may not be within the right paralumbar fossa in a horse with a right dorsal displacement; therefore, there may not be a good window for trocar placement and substantial gas release.

Severe large colon gas distention can lead to the demise of a horse being transported to a referral hospital, not usually due to rupture, but due to cardiovascular collapse from poor venous return and insufficient ventilation. These effects are exacerbated

Practical Guide to Equine Colic, First Edition. Edited by Louise L. Southwood.
© 2013 John Wiley & Sons, Inc. Published 2013 by John Wiley & Sons, Inc.

in the animal which becomes recumbent in the trailer due to excessive pain. Therefore, trocharization prior to transportation or anesthesia in a severely distended patient may be necessary. A horse with a large colon volvulus is an example of a type of case that may require trocharization and decompression as part of the cardiovascular and respiratory stabilization.

Preparation

A list of things that you will need to perform trocharization is provided in Table 14.1. Patient selection for this procedure is very important to minimize the risk of potential complications. Abdominal auscultation with percussion ("pinging") and palpation of the left and right paralumbar fossa as well as palpation per rectum (p. 22) is used to determine if there is a sufficiently large pocket of gas within the base of the cecum. Palpation per rectum should be performed with the use of sedation (p. 54) and/or Buscopan® (p. 58) to improve the assessment of colonic distention and location. Sonographic examination (p. 116) can also be used to help identify an ideal location for trocharization.

Trocharization is best approached through the dorsal aspect of the right paralumbar fossa, whereby the catheter should consistently enter the base of the cecum if performed in an area with a strong "ping" on auscultation (Figure 14.1). Trocharization through the left paralumbar fossa can be considered following cecal trocharization in the horse that still has excessive abdominal distention, pain, and a strong "ping" in the left dorsal paralumbar fossa. Before this procedure is performed on the left side, it is strongly recommended to sonographically evaluate this area and determine the location of the caudal aspect of the spleen as well as the presence of any small colon or jejunum. Trocharization on the left side inherently carries more risk of complications due to the normal location of other abdominal structures.

Once the location for trocharization has been identified, the hair should be clipped and a surgical preparation performed. A bleb of 2% lidocaine is placed under the skin and into the abdominal musculature for local analgesia. The patient should be sedated with xylazine and butorphanol for

Table 14.1   What you will need to perform trocharization for decompression of the colic patient.

- Stethoscope
- Rectal sleeve and lubrication
- ± Sonography equipment
- Clippers and preparation
- Sedation (xylazine and butorphanol)
- ± Buscopan®
- 6–8 mL of 2% lidocaine in syringe with 20-gauge needle
- Sterile gloves
- 18-Gauge 5 in. intravenous catheter
- ± Extension set and cup with water
- 5 mL of gentamicin or procaine penicillin G
- Broad-spectrum systemic antimicrobial drugs

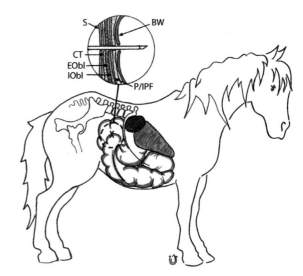

Figure 14.1   Right lateral and cross-sectional view of placement of an 18-gauge catheter into the gas-filled cecum. S, skin; CT, cutaneous trunci muscle; EObl, external abdominal oblique muscle; IObl, internal abdominal oblique muscle; P, peritoneum; IPF, intraperitoneal fat; BW, bowel wall.

the procedure to minimize movement while the gas is released.

Procedure

Paralumbar approach

Trocharization is performed using a 14-gauge 6 in. intravenous catheter inserted at a 90° angle to the skin and directed toward the opposite paralumbar fossa

(a)
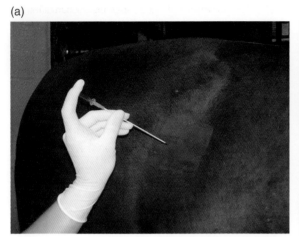

(b)
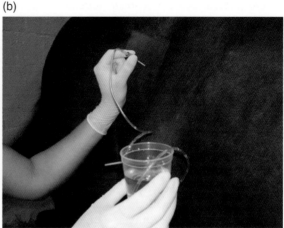

Figure 14.2   (a) Trocharization is performed in the upper right paralumbar fossa using an 18-gauge 6 in. intravenous catheter. (b) An intravenous extension set can be attached to the end of the catheter once the stylet is removed and the unattached end placed in a cup of water. Bubble formation in the water indicates that gas is still being retrieved, and when the bubbling ceases there is no more gas and the catheter can be removed.

(Figure 14.2). Once the catheter has passed through the skin and the abdominal musculature, a "pop" will be felt as it enters the base of the cecum, and at this point gas can be heard and felt through the catheter. When the gas is released the colon may pull away from the abdominal wall; therefore, it is important to set the catheter in a few centimeters and to monitor it closely during the procedure. Once the catheter is seated well into the gas pocket, the stylet should be removed to minimize damage to the colon from patient movement. The catheter is held in place until gas stops flowing (1–10 min). An intravenous extension set can be placed on the end of the catheter with the unattached end of the extension set placed in a small cup of water (Figure 14.2). While gas is being expelled bubbles are observed in the water, and when the bubbling ceases there is no more gas and the catheter can be carefully removed. Gentamicin or procaine penicillin G (5 mL) is injected into the tract as the catheter is removed from the abdominal cavity. Horses that undergo trocharization should be treated with broad-spectrum parenteral antimicrobial drugs before or immediately following trocharization.

Transrectal approach

Per rectum trocharization of the large colon has been performed in cases of severe large colon gas distention that could not be treated with trochariza-

tion through a paralumbar fossa approach. This procedure carries considerable risks and is not recommended unless there are absolutely no other treatment options. The patient is placed in stocks, sedated, and given intravenous Buscopan® (p. 58) for rectal relaxation. Then the rectum is evacuated of feces and a 1.5 in. 19-gauge needle attached to an extension set is passed into the rectum while cupped in the palm of the hand. Once the gas-filled colon is felt at the tip of the fingers, the needle is carefully rotated within the palm and inserted through the rectal mucosa and into the gas-filled viscera. Alternatively, the needle can be protected by placing the bevel against the index or middle finger during positioning. A 60 mL syringe is attached to the extension set and gas is suctioned out while the needle is held in place with the hand or gas can be relieved as for the paralumbar fossa approach. The amount of gas removal is variable and multiple insertions are not recommended. Gentamicin or procaine penicillin G (5 mL) is infiltrated into the colonic and rectal walls as the needle is withdrawn and again protected in the palm of the hand for removal.

Complications

The risk of perforation of the wall of the cecal base or right ventral colon causing acute peritonitis is inherent with this procedure but with good pre-procedural assessment and patient selection as well as appropriate sedation this can be minimized. Intraabdominal hemorrhage secondary to laceration of colonic vasculature or the spleen is also a complication that may not be determined until sometime after the procedure. The formation of an intraabdominal, intramural, or extraabdominal abscess secondary to fecal contamination from catheter placement and removal can also occur. Horses should be monitored closely for fever, tachycardia, tachypnea, dull mentation, inappetence, and colic, possibly indicating the development of a complication following the procedure.

While trocharization can be a life-saving procedure, complications should be considered and it should be reserved for horses with severe abdominal distention or during medical management of horses (or foals) for which surgery is not a treatment option. It is also important to recognize that if the primary lesion is not corrected, the gas distention will typically recur. Depending on the underlying cause or progress being made with medical treatment, repeat trocharization may be necessary.

15 Medical versus Surgical Treatment of the Horse with Colic

Louise L. Southwood

Department of Clinical Studies, New Bolton Center, School of Veterinary Medicine, University of Pennsylvania, Kennett Square, PA, USA

Chapter Outline

General indications for surgery	**164**	Proximal enteritis	167
Persistent or severe abdominal pain	165	Ileal impaction	167
Lack of response to medical management	165	Large colon impaction	167
		Cecal impaction	168
Signs of complete or partial intestinal obstruction	165	Small colon impaction	168
		Colitis	169
Ancillary tests	166	Right dorsal colitis	169
Sonographic examination	166	Peritonitis	169
Abdominocentesis and peritoneal fluid analysis	166	Postpartum hemorrhage	170
Indications for specific lesions	**166**	**The decision for euthanasia without surgical treatment**	**170**
Small intestinal lesions	166	Prognostic indices	170
Strangulating obstruction	166	Gastrointestinal tract perforation	171

General indications for surgery

Medical management with enteral fluids, laxatives and lubricants; anti-inflammatory analgesia; and sedative analgesia is performed initially on most horses/foals with colic (see Chapter 5 on Management of Mild Colic [p. 45]). Intravenous (IV) fluids are necessary in some horses that do not respond to initial treatment with analgesic drugs and enteral fluids. There is a positive response to medical management in the vast majority (~95%) of patients. The decision regarding whether or not to undergo an abdominal exploration on a horse with colic can be challenging. While some horses are severely painful and emergency surgery or euthanasia is indicated, other horses may respond

---

Practical Guide to Equine Colic, First Edition. Edited by Louise L. Southwood.
© 2013 John Wiley & Sons, Inc. Published 2013 by John Wiley & Sons, Inc.

temporarily to analgesia and the need for surgery may not be so apparent. Care should be taken with the use of analgesics in horses with colic that are not particularly painful and for which a diagnosis has not been made so as to not treat signs of pain that can indicate the need for surgery. It is also often necessary to feed these horses small and then increasing amounts to assess gastrointestinal tract function and allow signs of colic to be manifest.

It is important to keep in mind that exploratory surgery is a diagnostic as well as a therapeutic procedure. The earlier a horse with a surgical lesion is treated, the better the prognosis and the fewer and less severe are the postoperative complications. Therefore, the decision to undergo exploratory surgery should be made as early as possible during the course of treatment. On the other hand, colic surgery is expensive and obviously considered an invasive procedure that should not be performed without careful consideration of several factors not the least of which is the financial resources and expectations of the client (see Chapter 8 on Referral of the Horse with Colic [p. 71]). Careful patient assessment is necessary to make the optimum decision. Emphasis on the criteria used in decision-making for horses/foals with abdominal pain will also vary somewhat in different geographical regions based on the typical lesions seen at a particular practice. Modifications to general criteria for surgery are also made for horses/foals with a specific diagnosis for the cause of colic.

Persistent or severe abdominal pain

The most important indication for exploratory celiotomy, particularly on an emergency basis, is severe or persistent abdominal pain and lack of response to treatment with analgesic drugs.[14,24] Recurrence of abdominal pain when analgesic drug effects have worn off is also an indication for surgery.[24]

Most horses with colic signs have been treated with flunixin meglumine at least once. Flunixin meglumine should not be administered at the high dose rate more frequently than every 12 h. A sedative-analgesic drug is usually selected if the horse remains painful during this time period. As a guideline, if a horse with an undiagnosed cause of colic that has been administered flunixin meglumine requires sedation with

- xylazine with or without butorphanol every 1–2 h for several doses and/or
- pain recurs within 1–2 h following treatment with detomidine, exploratory surgery is likely indicated.

Horses with strangulating lesions are usually unresponsive to such an analgesic regimen. Additional diagnostic tests can also be performed including sonographic evaluation (p. 116) and abdominocentesis with peritoneal fluid analysis (p. 87) to support the diagnosis of a strangulating obstruction.

Lack of response to medical management

Indications that a horse is responding to medical management include resolution of signs of pain; bright, alert, and responsive demeanor; heart rate decreasing to within normal limits; improved intestinal borborygmi; resolution of abdominal distention; and defecation. The horse should have a good appetite and willingly graze. Palpation per rectum findings should return to within normal limits. The response to medical management should occur over a 6–36 h period and is often gradual. Either a lack of improvement or worsening of clinical signs including pain, mentation, tachycardia, tachypnea, hypomotile to absent gastrointestinal signs, worsening abdominal distention, and apparent intestinal obstruction are indications for surgery.

Signs of complete or partial intestinal obstruction

In addition to persistent or recurrent abdominal pain, nasogastric reflux (NGR), worsening abdominal distention, lack of fecal output, and deteriorating intestinal borborygmi are indications of a complete intestinal obstruction. Occasionally a horse's signs of pain will abate with flunixin meglumine administration, but if there is no improvement in gastrointestinal tract function surgery may also be indicated.

Reflux following nasogastric intubation can be an indication of a small intestinal obstruction (although some horses with colonic displacements can also have NGR). Horses with a mechanical obstruction, particularly involving the distal jejunum and ileum, tend to have volumes of NGR that are initially low (<2 L) and then gradually increase over time as fluid builds up in an aboral to oral direction. Ancillary diagnostic tests are generally indicated to differentiate strangulating from non-strangulating small intestinal obstruction.

Unresolving or worsening abdominal distention is an indication of large intestinal obstruction. Right-sided distention may indicate cecal disease, and horses with a nephrosplenic ligament entrapment often have left-sided distention. Generalized distention can be observed associated with large (ascending) or small (descending) colonic obstruction. Lack of fecal output particularly with initiation of treatment can indicate an obstruction or generalized ileus often associated with serious disease. An absence of intestinal borborygmi, particularly if persistent, is associated with the need for surgery.[24]

Partial obstruction can include intramural hematoma, colonic displacement, foreign body obstruction, and neoplasia. Clinical signs consistent with a partial obstruction include mild to moderate pain that is responsive to treatment with flunixin meglumine but recurs; scant soft to liquid feces; and reduced appetite; and decreased intestinal borborygmi.

Ancillary tests

Sonographic examination

Sonography (p. 116) can be used to evaluate the volume and character of the peritoneal fluid, intestinal distention and thickness, and anatomical aberrations. Diagnosis of the cause of colic can direct medical versus surgical treatment. Some lesions for which sonography can be as useful for diagnosing include the following:

(1) Peritonitis (p. 130)
(2) Hemoperitoneum (p. 134)
(3) Small intestinal distention (p. 128)
   (a) Proximal enteritis versus strangulating obstruction
(4) Nephrosplenic ligament entrapment (p. 121)
(5) Right dorsal displacement (p. 120)
(6) Large colon volvulus (p. 122)
(7) Cecal versus colonic impaction (p. 123)
(8) Sand colic (p. 124)

(9)   Typhlocolitis (p. 215)
(10) Abdominal and perirectal masses (p. 137)

Abdominocentesis and peritoneal fluid analysis

Peritoneal fluid analysis (p. 87) is most useful for distinguishing strangulating from nonstrangulating obstructions, diagnosing peritonitis and hemoabdomen, and rarely identifying neoplastic cells. Peritoneal fluid color, total protein concentration, nucleated cell count, and lactate concentration (initial and change over time) are used to help distinguish between some types of lesions and the need for surgical treatment. Surgery is indicated for horses with serosanguinous fluid. The ratio of total protein concentration and nucleated cell count can be used to differentiate strangulating from inflammatory lesions (see below). High ratio of peritoneal fluid to plasma lactate concentration or increase in peritoneal fluid lactate concentration with serial measurement is an indication for surgery.[15]

Indications for specific lesions

Small intestinal lesions

It can be particularly challenging to determine when surgery is necessary for horses with small intestinal lesions. (See Clinical scenarios 5, 8, and 10, located in Appendix A) Strangulating lesions and simple (e.g., ileal impaction) or functional obstructions (e.g., proximal enteritis) occur with different frequencies in different geographical regions and can, at least initially, present similarly with mild to moderate signs of colic that are often responsive to analgesia; tachycardia; distended loops of small intestine on palpation per rectum; and NGR. Therefore, other diagnostic tools are often necessary:

- Sonographic evaluation (p. 128)
- Peritoneal fluid analysis (p. 87)
- Laboratory data (p. 78)

Strangulating obstruction

Horses with small intestinal strangulating lesions tend to have persistent pain that is only temporarily responsive to analgesic drugs; tachycardia (>52 beats/min); intestinal borborygmi that are markedly decreased or absent; increasing volume of NGR with failure of gastric decompression to resolve signs of pain; and variable palpation per rectum findings with often none or only 1–2 loops of distended small intestine palpable. Serosanguinous peritoneal fluid is generally indicative of a strangulating obstruction and the need for surgery. Horses with strangulating lesions tend to have moderate to marked increase in both peritoneal fluid total protein concentration (3-5 g/dL) and nucleated cell count (15,000–60,000 cells/uL). Peritoneal fluid lactate concentration is higher than plasma lactate concentration. Abdominal sonography can reveal an increase in volume of peritoneal fluid and amotile distended small intestine of variable thickness.

Proximal enteritis

Horses with proximal enteritis (p. 207) are typically managed medically. Briefly, clinical signs include pain progressing to quiet demeanor, large volumes of NGR,[18] multiple loops of distended small intestine on palpation per rectum (p. 27) and transcutaneous sonographic examination (p. 128), yellow to orange peritoneal fluid with high total protein (>4 mg/dL), and nucleated cell count typically within normal limits (<10000 cells/μL).[11] Horses may be pyrexic (rectal temperature >101.5°F[38.5°C]). Horses with proximal enteritis or ileus typically have a large volume of NGR (>7 L) at the initial evaluation and these patients often begin to decrease in NGR volume with treatment. Signs of pain and tachycardia improve with gastric decompression. Horses are treated with IV fluid therapy (p. 99). Care should be taken with use of analgesic and motility modifying drugs during the initial 24 h or until a definitive diagnosis of proximal enteritis is obtained. Exploratory celiotomy is indicated in horses that have persistent signs of pain, clinical deterioration, and with reflux rates consistently ≥4 L/h for a 24–48 h period.[23] Surgery is primarily a diagnostic procedure for horses suspected of having proximal enteritis. Although surgical decompression was generally not shown to be beneficial for horses with proximal enteritis, 25% of horses did cease refluxing postoperatively.[23]

Ileal impaction

Horses with ileal impaction (p. 208) initially present with intermittent, moderate to severe abdominal pain that is responsive to treatment with analgesics.[7,10,13] The pain is thought to be associated with intestinal spasm in the region of the impaction. The temperature, pulse, and respiratory rate are within normal limits and intestinal borborygmi are present. There is usually no reflux following nasogastric tube passage at this point in the disease process. Small intestinal distention develops in cases that are not resolved with medical management within 8–10 h of obstruction. With the progression of small intestinal distention, abdominal pain becomes persistent, intestinal borborygmi decrease, and the horse becomes nonresponsive to analgesia administration. NGR develops in 15–20% of cases.

Medical treatment can be pursued initially when a diagnosis is made based on history and palpation per rectum findings, and when the abdominal pain and small intestinal distention have not progressed or in cases where economics preclude surgical management. Surgery is indicated in patients that are persistently or moderately to severely painful, have small intestinal distention, and/or show any signs of cardiovascular deterioration. The impacted material can be massaged into the cecum. If the intestinal wall is edematous and hemorrhagic, an enterotomy may be necessary; however, this should be reserved for severe cases.[7]

Large colon impaction

Horses with a large colon impaction (p. 217) are usually managed successfully with enteral fluids (p. 62) and analgesia (p. 51). See Clinical scenario 6 (located in Appendix A). The prognosis for survival of horses with a large colon impaction undergoing exploratory celiotomy was reported to be only 58%.[3] The main reason for nonsurvival was colonic rupture at surgery. Horses with large colon impactions often get extremely painful when the impacted ingesta is rehydrated and may even begin refluxing; therefore, signs of pain may not be an indication for surgery in these cases and other clinical findings should be used.

Horses with large colon impaction should be either taken to surgery early in the course of treatment if it is clear they are not responding to treatment or medical management should be pursued until the impaction resolves. Some of the clinical features that should be considered when deciding on medical or surgical treatment of the horse with a large colon impaction include the following:

- abdominal distention;
- intestinal borborygmi;
- fecal output;
- heart rate;
- NGR; and
- abdominal palpation per rectum findings.

Horses with an impaction that are responding to medical management do not have obvious abdominal distention and have intestinal borborygmi that are within normal limits or hypermotile. Horses will generally be passing even small volumes of feces and have feces in the rectum upon palpation. Depending on the frequency and volume of enteral fluid administration, an impaction should resolve within 24–72 h[9] and should be checked for improvement on palpation per rectum.

Horses may develop a right dorsal displacement (p. 220) during treatment for an impaction and this will be apparent based on persistent or worsening abdominal pain, palpation per rectum, lack of defecation, and increasing abdominal distention. Surgery is indicated if this occurs. Surgical correction of large colon impactions can be challenging. A large celiotomy incision should be made to avoid rupture of the heavy, distended, friable colon during exteriorization. The pelvic flexure enterotomy can also be performed prior to complete exteriorization of the colon to reduce the tension on the colonic wall.

Cecal impaction

While somewhat controversial, many surgeons recommend managing horses with cecal impactions (p. 214) surgically because of the risk of cecal perforation even with minimal preemptive clinical signs. Of horses presenting to a referral hospital with a cecal impaction, about 25% result in cecal perforation: 10/114 (9%) had ruptured at admission; 7/54 (13%) of horses treated medically ruptured; and 12/49 (24%) of horses were euthanized at surgery because of cecal rupture.[16] In earlier reports of cecal impaction, 40–60% of horses had cecal rupture.[1,2] The lower incidence of cecal rupture in the more recent study was attributed to early recognition and treatment of cecal impaction. However, the

challenge still remains regarding whether or not to take a horse with a cecal impaction to surgery. Owners must be provided with sufficient information to make an informed decision:

- Horses with cecal impaction can be successfully managed medically with a good (80%) survival rate; however, impaction resolution may take several days.[16]
- There is a risk of cecal rupture which is fatal and can occur with little warning.
- Prognosis for survival with surgery is excellent (96%).[16]

The only difference between horses managed medically compared with those managed surgically was that horses treated surgically were significantly more likely to have signs of moderate or severe pain than were horses treated medically.[16]

There were no significant differences in peritoneal fluid total protein concentration or nucleated count between medically and surgically treated horses, indicating that evaluation of abdominal fluid was seldom useful in assessing whether surgery is necessary.[16] There may also be geographical differences in causes of cecal impaction which may influence the success with medical management.

Surgery is, therefore, strongly recommended in horses with a cecal impaction with the following:

- signs of pain;
- moderate to marked cecal distention;
- tachycardia;
- lack of feces; and/or
- high packed cell volume (PCV) or blood lactate concentration.

Surgery involves evacuation of the cecum through a typhlotomy only or typhlotomy combined with bypass via an ileo-/jejuno-colostomy. There was no difference in survival between horses treated using the two surgical techniques.[16] Cecal perforation can occur with little preemptive indication during medical management. Tachycardia, tachypnea, injected oral mucous membranes, and fever are signs consistent with cecal perforation (see below).

Small colon impaction

Horses with small colon impaction (p. 221) can respond to medical management. However, because of the distal location of the small colon along the gastrointestinal tract and its function being water resorption and formation of fecal balls, it can be extremely difficult to provide sufficient water per os to hydrate the impacted material. The average length of time for resolution of small colon impaction was 8 days compared to 5 days for horses with a large colon impaction.[6]

Horses with small colon impaction are predisposed to reimpaction suggesting either an intestinal motility disturbance causing the impaction or as a result of the associated inflammation. Diarrhea and salmonellosis have been associated with small colon impaction and may either be a cause or a consequence of the small colon impaction.

Similar to horses with a large colon impaction, signs of persistent pain, a lack of feces, absent intestinal borborygmi, and abdominal distention are indications of the need for surgery. Surgical correction most commonly involves a high enema. Some horses may require a small colon enterotomy. A pelvic flexure enterotomy is recommended to prevent reimpaction.

Colitis

Colitis (p. 215) refers to colonic inflammation and is considered a medical condition. A typical presentation of a horse with colitis is colic signs progressing to dull mentation, fever, leukopenia/neutropenia, hypoproteinemia/hypoalbuminemia, hyponatremia, and diarrhea. Horses may have only a few of these clinical features. Horses suspected of having colitis should be isolated from other hospitalized patients because it can be associated with infectious causes. Treatment includes IV fluid therapy (p. 99), antiendoxic drugs (p. 246), analgesia (p. 51), and laminitis prevention (typically applying ice to the hooves). Occasionally a horse with colitis needs to undergo surgery. Indications for surgery in horses with colitis include persistent pain, moderate to severe abdominal distention, cessation of diarrhea with lack of fecal production, and/or severe clinical deterioration with signs of shock. Reasons include colonic infarction, small colon impaction, or colonic displacement or volvulus. Horses with colitis may benefit from enterotomy and intraluminal treatment with Equine Bio-sponge® (DTO-smectite) or psyllium HCl during surgery.

Right dorsal colitis

Right dorsal colitis (p. 216) is a manifestation of nonsteroidal anti-inflammatory drug (NSAID) toxicity and is diagnosed based on a history of NSAID use, clinical signs of colic/diarrhea, hypoalbuminemia, and identification of thickened right dorsal colon sonographically. The majority of horses with right dorsal colitis are managed successfully with medical treatment (avoiding NSAIDs, corn oil, psyllium, sucralfate, dietary modifications). However, surgery is indicated in horses with right dorsal colitis that are painful despite attempts to provide analgesia. Surgical management includes bypass of the right dorsal colon, right dorsal colon resection and anastomosis, or resection with bypass.

Peritonitis

Peritonitis is defined as a peritoneal fluid-nucleated cell count >10 000/μL.[5] There are numerous causes of peritonitis. See Clinical scenario 9 (located in Appendix A). Peritonitis associated with *Actinobacillus equuli* respond favorably to medical management.[8] However, peritonitis can also be caused by ischemic intestine, which requires surgical resection and anastomosis for the patient to survive; the earlier the surgery is undertaken the more likely a better the outcome. Several clinical features have been identified to determine which equine cases with peritonitis respond to medical treatment and cases that require surgery:[19]

- Absence of colic signs, normal intestinal borborygmi, normal feces during hospitalization, no NGR, and yellow/orange peritoneal fluid are associated with survival to discharge without surgery.
- Moderate to severe pain, fever during hospitalization, absent intestinal borborygmi, less than normal or no feces during hospitalization, and distended small intestine on palpation per rectum were associated with a concurrent abnormality.

Transcutaneous sonographic examination (p. 133) may provide useful information in horses with peritonitis to determine the necessity for surgery. The usefulness of peritoneal fluid lactate in horses/

foals with peritonitis is unlikely to be useful and considerably more research into markers of ischemic intestine in horses with peritonitis is necessary.

Postpartum hemorrhage

Mares with postpartum hemorrhage (p. 283) often present with signs of colic. Mares with postpartum hemorrhage should be managed medically. However, the primary differential diagnosis for colic in a postpartum mare is a large colon volvulus[4] requiring immediate surgical correction. Palpation per rectum (p. 34) and sonography (p. 134, 138) can be used to differentiate the two lesions. Key distinguishing clinical features include the following: mares with postpartum hemorrhage tend to be slightly older; are admitted to the hospital closer to parturition; and are more likely to have anemia, hypoproteinemia, and hypofibrinogenemia compared to mares admitted for other reasons.[4]

The decision for euthanasia without surgical treatment

Unfortunately there are still some horses and foals with colic that are euthanized without treatment. The most common reasons for euthanasia are (1) financial limitations to treatment imposed by the owner and (2) the perception that the horse would not do well with surgery.

With the increasing expense associated with veterinary care, clinicians need to be fiscally responsible when managing complicated colic cases. Keeping expenses associated with medical and surgical treatment of horses with colic to a minimum without compromising patient care may allow more owners to pursue treatment of their horses. Careful consideration of several aspects of treatment can keep expenses reasonable

- necessity, duration, and rate of IV fluid therapy;
- duration of perioperative antimicrobial drugs;
- use of plasma as a colloid and antiendotoxin; therapy;
- duration of general anesthesia and surgery; and
- early referral and surgical treatment when necessary prior to the patient being critically ill.

Some horses are euthanized because of a history of recurrent colic, particularly recurrent colic that has been managed with multiple surgical procedures. The age of the horse is also another reason for owners deciding to euthanize their horse rather than pursuing surgical treatment. Recently, however, it was shown that geriatric horses with strangulating small intestinal lesions do as well as younger mature horses.[21] While geriatric horses with large intestinal simple obstructions had a lower survival than younger mature horses, the prognosis was still good to excellent for the geriatric horses (p. 286).

Prognostic indices

There are several prognostic indices that can be used to predict, with modest accuracy, the survival and likelihood of a complicated recovery. While these clinical findings may provide owners with some indication of outcome and cost of treatment, there are many cases that require surgery to determine lesion severity and the likelihood of a favorable outcome (Clinical scenario 4, located in Appendix A). It is, therefore, strongly recommended to determine the prognosis for survival at surgery. These clinical measurements, however, can be very useful when used in combination and in conjunction with mean arterial pressure and changes in plasma lactate concentration, PCV, total plasma protein during anesthesia, and surgery to help the owner make an informed decision regarding whether or not to complete the procedure and recover the horse or foal.

The most notable prognostic indices are heart rate, PCV, and plasma lactate, creatinine, and glucose concentrations.[16,20] These indices reflect the level of pain and the patient's cardiovascular status which are related to the extent of intestinal damage and likely the duration of illness.

Plasma lactate concentration has most recently received attention with regard to prognosis. Horses admitted on an emergency basis with a high plasma lactate concentration had a worse prognosis compared to horses with a lower lactate concentration.[22] Plasma lactate was particularly useful for predicting survival in horses with serious disease such as colitis or large colon volvulus.[22] Plasma lactate concentration was significantly lower in survivors (2.98 ± 2.53 mmol/L) compared with nonsurvivors (9.48 ± 5.22 mmol/L) with large colon volvulus and lower in horses with a viable colon (3.30 ± 2.85 mmol/L) compared with horses with a nonviable colon (9.1 ± 6.09 mmol/L).[12] Plasma lactate concentration <6.0 mmol/L had a sensitivity of 84% and a specificity 83% for predicting horse survival.[12] See Chapter 9 on Clinical Laboratory Data (p. 78).

Gastrointestinal tract perforation

See Clinical scenario 7 (located in Appendix A). The prognosis for survival of horses with gastrointestinal tract perforation is grave.[17] Euthanasia is indicated in almost all cases and can be performed prior to surgery if the diagnosis can be confirmed. The classic presentation of a horse with gastrointestinal perforation is that of severe signs of pain followed by subsidence of pain with progression to dull mentation, profuse sweating, endotoxemia (injected to red to purple mucous membranes, injected sclera, fever), shock (tachycardia, tachypnea, cool extremities, poor jugular refill), and death. Horses with gastrointestinal perforation are often reluctant to walk, have a frantic appearance, and may become recalcitrant as signs of shock progress. Perforation leads to severe leukopenia and progressively increasing PCV despite IV fluid therapy and worsening hypoproteinemia/hypoalbuminemia. Plasma lactate and creatinine concentrations are usually high and increases with progression of shock.

Palpation per rectum findings consistent with perforation include collapsing of the rectum around the arm and a floating sensation associated with loss of negative intra-abdominal pressure. A roughened serosal surface may also be appreciated in some horses associated with severe peritoneal contamination.

Perforation is usually suspected based on history as well as clinical and laboratory findings. Confirmation of the diagnosis is made using peritoneal fluid analysis (p. 87) with or without transcutaneous sonographic examination (p. 133). Abdominocentesis reveals green-brown peritoneal fluid with particulate matter particularly if performed using the teat cannula method (p. 89). Cytological analysis of the fluid is necessary to differentiate peritoneal contamination from enterocentesis. Key cytological findings in horses with a perforated gastrointestinal tract are large numbers mixed intracellular bacteria and damaged or lysed nucleated cells (cells are often damaged almost beyond recognition). It is important to keep in mind that peritoneal fluid-nucleated cell count and total protein are often within normal limits in horses with gastrointestinal perforation, most likely because of dilution but also because of nucleated cell lysis.

Abdominal sonographic examination may reveal a moderate to marked increase in intraperitoneal fluid volume. Particulate matter may be visible. Bowel is also seen to be thickened in response to severe peritonitis. Sonography is also an important tool to guide abdominocentesis.

Exploratory celiotomy is necessary in some cases to confirm the diagnosis of gastrointestinal perforation. Except in rare cases where peritoneal contamination is minimal, euthanasia is indicated for humane reasons.

References

1. Campbell, M.L., Colahan, P.C., Brown, M.M., Grandstedt, M.E. & Peyton, L.C. (1984) Cecal impaction in the horse. *Journal of the American Veterinary Medical Association*, **184**, 950–952.
2. Collatos, C. & Romano, S. (1993) Cecal impaction in horses: Causes, diagnosis and medical treatment. *Compendium on Continuing Education for the Practicing Veterinarian*, **15**, 976–981.
3. Dabareiner, R.M. & White, N.A. (1995) Large colon impaction in horses: 147 cases (1985–1991). *Journal of the American Veterinary Medical Association*, **206**, 679–685.
4. Dolente, B.A., Sullivan, E.K., Boston, R. & Johnston, J.K. (2005) Mares admitted to a referral hospital for postpartum emergencies: 163 cases (1992–2002). *Journal of Veterinary Emergency and Critical Care*, **15**, 193–200.
5. Dyson, S. (1983) Review of 30 cases of peritonitis in the horse. *Equine Veterinary Journal*, **15**, 25–30.
6. Frederico, L.M., Jones, S.L. & Blikslager, A.T. (2006) Predisposing factors for small colon impaction in horses and outcome of medical and surgical treatment: 44 cases (1999–2004). *Journal of the American Veterinary Medical Association*, **229**, 1612–1616.
7. Freeman, D.E. (1999) Small intestine. In: *Equine Surgery* (eds J.A. Auer & J.A. Stick), 2nd edn., pp. 232–257. WB Saunders Co, Philadelphia, Pennsylvania.
8. Gollard, L.C., Hodgson, D.R., Hodgson, J.L., *et al.* (1994) Peritonitis associated with *Actinobacillus equuli* in horses: 15 cases (1982–1992). *Journal of the American Veterinary Medical Association*, **205**, 340–343.

9. Hallowell, G.D. (2008) Retrospective study assessing efficacy of treatment of large colonic impactions. *Equine Veterinary Journal*, **40**, 411–413.

10. Hanson, R.R., Schumacher, J., Humburg, J. & Dunkerley, S.C. (1996) Medical treatment of horses with ileal impactions: 10 cases (1990–1994). *Journal of the American Veterinary Medical Association*, **208**, 898–900.

11. Johnston, J.K. & Morris, D.D. (1987) Comparison of duodenitis/proximal jejunitis and small intestinal obstruction in horses: 68 cases (1977–1985). *Journal of the American Veterinary Medical Association*, **191**, 849–854.

12. Johnston, K., Holcombe, S.J. & Hauptman, J.G. (2007) Plasma lactate as a predictor of colonic viability and survival after 360 degrees volvulus of the ascending colon in horses. *Veterinary Surgery*, **36**, 563–567.

13. Little, D. & Blikslager, A.T. (2002) Factors associated with development of ileal impaction in horses with surgical colic: 78 cases (1986–2000). *Equine Veterinary Journal*, **34**, 464–468.

14. Peloso, J.G. (1996) When to send a horse with signs of colic: Is it surgical, or is it referable? A survey of the opinions of 117 equine veterinary specialists. In: *Proceedings of the 42nd Annual Convention of the American Association of Equine Practitioners*, Denver, Colorado, pp. 250–253.

15. Peloso, J.G. & Cohen, N.D. (2010) Using serial peritoneal fluid lactate concentrations in referred horses with signs of colic to identify strangulating intestinal lesions. In: *Proceedings of the American College of Veterinary Surgeons Symposium*, Seattle, Washington.

16. Plummer, A.E., Rakestraw, P.C., Hardy, J. & Lee, R.M. (2007) Outcome of medical and surgical treatment of cecal impaction in horses: 114 cases (1994–2004). *Journal of the American Veterinary Medical Association*, **231**, 1378–1385.

17. Pratt, S.M., Hassel, D.M., Drake, C. & Snyder, J.R. (2003) Clinical characteristics of horses with gastrointestinal ruptures revealed during initial diagnostic evaluation: 149 cases (1990–2002). In: *Proceedings 49th Annual Convention of the American Association of Equine Practitioners*, New Orleans, Louisiana, pp. 366–370.

18. Seahorn, T.L., Cornick, J.L. & Cohen, N.D. (1992) Prognostic indicators for horses with duodenitis-proximal jejunitis. 75 horses (1985–1989). *Journal of Veterinary Internal Medicine*, **6**, 307–311.

19. Southwood, L.L. & Russell, G. (2007) The use of clinical findings in the identification of equine peritonitis cases that respond favorably to medical therapy. *Journal of Veterinary Emergency and Critical Care*, **17**, 382–390.

20. Southwood, L.L., Gassert, T. & Lindborg, S. (2010) Colic in geriatric compared to mature nongeriatric horses. Part 1: Retrospective review of clinical and laboratory data. *Equine Veterinary Journal*, **42**, 621–627.

21. Southwood, L.L., Gassert, T. & Lindborg, S. (2010) Colic in geriatric compared to mature nongeriatric horses. Part 2: Treatment, diagnosis and short-term survival. *Equine Veterinary Journal*, **42**, 628–635.

22. Tennent-Brown, B.S., Wilkins, P.A., Lindborg, S., Russell, G. & Boston, R.C. (2010) Sequential plasma lactate concentrations as prognostic indicators in adult equine emergencies. *Journal of Veterinary Internal Medicine*, **24**, 198–205.

23. Underwood, C., Southwood, L.L., McKeown, K.P. & Knight, D. (2008) Complications and survival associated with surgical compared with medical management of horses with duodenitis-proximal jejunitis. *Equine Veterinary Journal*, **40**, 373–378.

24. White, N.A., Elward, A., Moga, K.S., Ward, D.L. & Sampson, D.M. (2005) Use of web-based data collection to evaluate analgesic administration and the decision for surgery in horses with colic. *Equine Veterinary Journal*, **37**, 347–350.

16 Colic Surgery

Kira L. Epstein[1] and Joanne Fehr[2]

[1]Department of Large Animal Medicine, College of Veterinary Medicine, University of Georgia, Athens, GA, USA
[2]Equine Emergency Department, Pilchuck Animal Hospital, Snohomish, WA, USA

Chapter Outline

Indications	**174**
Preparation	**174**
Cardiovascular stabilization	174
Analgesic drugs	174
Antimicrobial drugs	175
General anesthesia	175
Surgical site preparation	176
Exploratory procedures	**176**
Ventral approaches	177
Incision	177
Anatomy of the ventral exploratory celiotomy	178
Cecum	178
Small intestine	179
Large colon	181
Transverse colon	182
Small colon	182
Other abdominal organs	182
Body wall closure	183
Lateral approaches	185
Incision	185
Anatomy of the lateral exploratory celiotomy	186
Body wall closure	186
Laparoscopy	187
Laparoscope and instrumental portals	187
Laparoscopic anatomy	188
Closure	188
Selected surgical procedures	**189**
Needle decompression	189
Overview of the enterotomy procedure	190
Pelvic flexure enterotomy	190
Typhlotomy	190
Small intestinal enterotomy	191
Small colon enterotomy	191
Partial typhlectomy	191
Overview of the intestinal resection and anastomosis procedure	192
Jejunojejunostomy and jejunoileostomy	193
Jejunocecostomy	193
Ileocecostomy and ileocolostomy	194
Large colon resection and anastomosis	195
End-to-end technique	195
Side-to-side anastomosis	197
Small colon resection and anastomosis	197
Colopexy	202
Diagnosis and correction of selected specific conditions	202

Practical Guide to Equine Colic, First Edition. Edited by Louise L. Southwood.
© 2013 John Wiley & Sons, Inc. Published 2013 by John Wiley & Sons, Inc.

Indications

Abdominal surgery is used for the diagnosis and treatment of horses with signs of acute or chronic intermittent colic. The decision to pursue exploratory surgery is based on clinical signs, diagnostic tests, and response to therapy (see Chapter 15 on Medical versus Surgical Treatment of the Horse with Colic [p. 164]). The most consistent and reliable indicator for surgery in horses with colic is pain. The level of pain, persistence or recurrence of pain, and response to analgesics should be considered. Any horse with diagnostic findings consistent with a strangulating lesion of the gastrointestinal tract, such as serosanguinous peritoneal fluid (p. 90) or thickened, amotile, distended small intestine on sonographic evaluation of the abdomen (p. 128), should be taken to surgery immediately. Surgery is also indicated for horses with diagnostic findings consistent with a nonstrangulating lesion of the gastrointestinal tract that are not responding to medical management. Some diseases of nongastrointestinal organs that also cause signs of colic, such as uterine torsion, within the abdomen may require surgical treatment. Complications can occur following colic surgery (see Chapter 19 on Postoperative Complications [p. 244]); however, early surgical intervention is critical for a favorable outcome with fewer complications.

Preparation

Cardiovascular stabilization

Horses and foals with signs of colic often have signs of cardiovascular instability or shock. Signs include tachycardia, tachypnea, dry, injected/toxic oral mucous membranes, prolonged capillary and jugular refill time, cool extremities, dull mentation, and high blood or plasma lactate concentration. Intravenous fluid therapy is necessary to improve cardiovascular stability prior to general anesthesia and surgery (see Chapter 11 on Intravenous Catheterization and Fluid Therapy [p. 99]):

- Hypertonic (7%) saline can be given at 4 mL/kg (2 L/500 kg) initially to rapidly increase the intravascular fluid volume in patients with signs of shock and should be followed with isotonic fluids.
- Intravenous polyionic isotonic fluids can be administered as 20 mL/kg (10 L/500 kg horse) boluses until clinical signs improve.
- Hetastarch or pentastarch up to 10 mL/kg (5 L/500 kg horse) can be administered to increase the intravascular volume and can provide colloidal support for patients at risk of hypoproteinemia/hypoalbuminemia.

It is unlikely that horses with strangulating lesions will be completely cardiovascularly stable prior to general anesthesia and surgery should not be delayed. Occasionally antiendotoxin therapy (e.g., polymixin B) may also be indicated prior to surgery (p. 246).

Some horses will have severe abdominal distension necessitating decompression prior to surgery. Cecal and colonic decompression is achieved with trocharization (p. 160). Gastric decompression with nasogastric intubation (p. 38) should also be performed prior to surgery to prevent gastric rupture on induction of general anesthesia. It is recommended to anesthetize the horse with the nasogastric tube in place when the horse has had a large volume of reflux to allow gastric decompression during surgery; care should be taken to avoid corneal injury from the tube or gastric contents. The tube can be removed when the horse is positioned in lateral recumbency for recovery; caution should be taken during removal to avoid trauma to the ethmoid turbinates and hemorrhage.

Analgesic drugs

Flunixin meglumine should be administered to horses for analgesia and as an anti-inflammatory drug prior to surgery. It is important to not administer flunixin meglumine if it has been given within the previous 8–12 h because of its potential renal and gastrointestinal toxic effects. In this instance either a half-dose can be given preoperatively or a whole dose can be given during surgery or recovery from general anesthesia. Horses requiring surgery are often painful and additional analgesia with xylazine/butorphanol or detomidine may become necessary (see Chapter 6 on Analgesia [p. 51]).

Antimicrobial drugs

Antimicrobial drugs are administered immediately prior to surgery and preferably within 30–60 min of making the body wall incision. It is important to be familiar with preparation time for surgery (assembling staff, induction of general anesthesia, positioning on the surgical table, and skin preparation) so that antimicrobial drugs are not administered too early before surgery. Intravenous potassium penicillin and gentamicin are the most common prophylactic antimicrobial drugs used for colic surgery. Care should be taken with gentamicin administration in horses with a high admission plasma creatinine concentration (>2.5 mg/dL) because of its potential for nephrotoxicity. Alternative antimicrobial drugs that can be used for gram negative spectrum include ceftiofur and enrofloxacin. Routine use of enrofloxacin should be avoided, however, because of the risk of antimicrobial drug resistance. Enrofloxacin should not be used in young horses (<2 years old) because of the potential to cause an arthropathy. Antimicrobial drugs with a short half-life (i.e., potassium penicillin) should be readministered during surgery every 2–3 h.

General anesthesia

General anesthesia protocols vary between hospitals. In preparation for general anesthesia, the horse should (ideally) be cleaned; hooves picked and shoes removed if the horse is not trying to lie down and roll; and the mouth rinsed in preparation for orotracheal intubation. The hair on the ventral abdomen can be clipped and the skin cleaned prior to induction of general anesthesia if it is safe to do so. The hooves can be wrapped with elastic adhesive bandage material to protect the horse and padded floor during recovery from general anesthesia. In many hospitals the leather or nylon halter is replaced with a rope halter for recovery to prevent facial nerve injury.

The patient usually has a jugular vein catheter placed upon hospital arrival for drug and fluid administration. Preanesthetic drugs commonly used are xylazine and butorphanol. General anesthesia is usually induced with a combination of diazepam and ketamine or guaifenesin and ketamine. Adult Thoroughbred horses are intubated with a 26–30 mm internal diameter (ID) orotracheal tube. The orotracheal tube for a foal will typically be 9–14 mm ID, small pony 14–16 mm ID, and adult draft horse 30–36 mm ID. General anesthesia is maintained with isoflurane or sevofluorane in 100% oxygen.

Electrodes for electrocardiogram monitoring are connected using a base-apex lead configuration and a facial or transverse facial artery catheter placed to measure the arterial blood pressure and collect arterial blood samples for blood gas analysis.

Horses undergoing abdominal surgery usually require intermittent positive pressure ventilation with respiratory rate (6–12 breaths/min) and tidal volume (12–15 mL/kg) based on body weight. The inspiratory:expiratory (I:E) ratio should be 1:2 at the most.[20] The minute volume is varied by adjusting respiratory rate, tidal volume, or inspiratory pressure as indicated by blood gas analysis.[20] The peak inspiratory pressure should be 35–45 cmH$_2$O; however, if alveolar recruitment maneuvers are necessary a higher pressure may be tolerated.[14]

Polyionic isotonic fluids are administered at 10 mL/kg/h.[20] Horses are monitored closely during the procedure. Routinely used monitoring includes heart rate; mucous membrane color; electrocardiogram; end tidal carbon dioxide; and mean arterial blood pressure (MAP).

Mean arterial pressure should be maintained >70 mmHg to ensure adequate tissue perfusion. Mean arterial pressure is maintained >70 mmHg using a dobutamine constant rate infusion.[20] If dobutamine is insufficient to maintain mean arterial pressure in a satisfactory range, norepinephrine or phenylephrine can be used as part of the regimen.

Arterial blood gas analysis is performed throughout the procedure depending on the critical illness of the patient; arterial oxygen tension should be maintained >100 mmHg and carbon dioxide tension <50 mmHg.

(a)   (b)   (c)

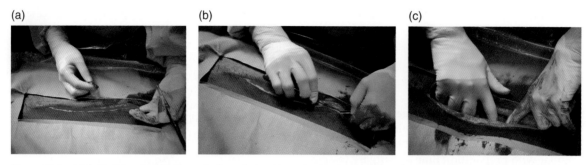

Figure 16.1   (a) A 20–35 cm incision is made through the skin and subcutaneous tissue beginning at the umbilicus and extending in a cranial direction. The scar is associated with a previous colic surgery. (b) The midline incision is extended through the linea alba using a fresh #10 scalpel blade. Forceps are used to elevate the body wall and guard the abdominal contents. It is important to not cut on but between the two arms of the forceps. (c) The peritoneum is penetrated and the peritoneal cavity opened using digital pressure. Note that there is an adhesive around the fenestration in the drape alleviating the need for towel clamps in the surgical field. There is also a plastic pocket associated with the drape to assist with keeping the intestine on the horse's ventral abdomen during surgery. Cranial is to the left. The surgeon is standing on the left side of the horse.

Surgical site preparation

The horse is moved to the surgical table usually using a hoist-monorail system or mobile surgical table, and positioned in dorsal or lateral recumbency for the ventral and lateral approaches, respectively. The horse should be adequately padded to prevent neuromuscular complications. The horse's limbs are usually attached to the table or poles to prevent movement if the depth of anesthesia is inadequate.

The hair on the ventral abdomen is clipped and not shaved. The skin is scrubbed clean often using either a povidone-iodine or chlorhexidine-based scrub. Once the skin is clean, the skin is aseptically prepared using either povidone-iodine and alcohol or chlorhexidine and sterile water. The surgical site is draped. There are several different methods for draping but most involve quarter drapes and a large fenestrated drape. Fenestrated drapes are available with adhesive around the edge of the fenestration to avoid the necessity of towel clamps within the surgical field and a large plastic pocket to help keep the bowel on the horse's abdomen during surgery (Figure 16.1). Some surgeons also use an iodine-impregnated adhesive drape.

Exploratory procedures

The equine abdomen can be approached from the ventral abdomen (midline or paramedian) or from either side laterally. Abdominal exploration can be performed with traditional or, less commonly, laparoscopic surgical techniques.

A ventral approach using a traditional surgical technique is the most appropriate for the vast majority of horses with acute colic. This approach provides the best access for assessment and treatment of the gastrointestinal tract. Disadvantages of the approach include that it is invasive, requires general anesthesia and recovery, and provides limited access to structures in the dorsal abdomen. The abdominal cavity is usually explored through a ventral midline approach. However, some surgeons prefer a ventral paramedian approach and one study indicated that incisional herniation is less common than following a midline approach.[1] The ventral paramedian approach can also be used in horses with a ventral midline incisional infection; when adhesions between bowel and the body wall at the previous midline incision are anticipated; or at a stage in healing when it may not be ideal to re-enter the abdomen through the previous surgical site. Within the first week, wounds are in the acute inflammatory and proliferative phases of healing and are not gaining much tensile strength (collagen deposition). The most rapid increase in tensile strength (collagen deposition) occurs between 7 and 14 days as the proliferative phase ends and the remodeling phase begins.[32] Some surgeons prefer not to disrupt the incision once the strength begins to increase and, therefore, will use a paramedian incision.

Although a lateral approach using a traditional surgical technique has limited application in horses with colic, it can provide access to structures in the

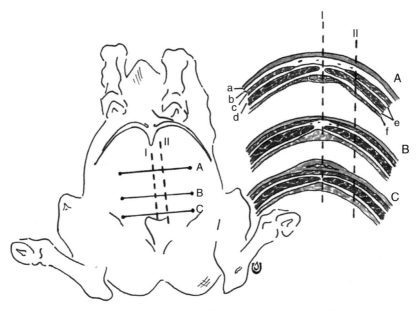

Figure 16.2 Schematic illustration of the ventral approaches to the equine abdomen. I, midline incision; II, paramedian incision; a, skin; b, subcutaneous layer; c, cutaneous trunci muscle; d, rectus abdominus muscle; e, rectus sheath; f, retroperitoneal fat.

dorsal abdomen that are not possible from the ventral abdomen (e.g., nephrosplenic space, right dorsal colon, ovaries). Additionally, a flank incision can provide good access to the uterus, particularly in pregnant mares with a uterine torsion. The approach can be made through the flank or using a rib resection to access the cranial aspect of the abdomen. The procedure can be performed with the horse standing and sedated or in lateral recumbency under general anesthesia. The standing approach is not feasible in horses with uncontrollable pain and not indicated if there is a risk of entering the thorax during a rib resection. Once the incision is made, access is limited to the structures directly adjacent to the incision (e.g., uterus for uterine torsion, right dorsal colon in horses with right dorsal colitis) because of the thick body wall and short flank length in the horse combined with the large abdominal cavity. Therefore, the surgeon must have a definitive diagnosis before deciding on this approach.

Laparoscopic approaches are used most frequently in horses with chronic intermittent colic signs or postoperatively in horses developing complications referable to the gastrointestinal tract or peritoneal cavity (e.g., adhesions). Specific portions of the abdomen are seen depending upon the portal placement. Lateral portals can be used in standing horses to view the dorsal abdomen while ventral portals can be used in dorsally recumbent horses to view the ventral abdomen.[10] As a minimally invasive technique, laparoscopy decreases recovery time and potential for incisional complications. The application of laparoscopy to horses with acute colic is limited due to restricted access and risk of complications from intestinal wall perforation when there is intestinal distension. Additionally, there are very few lesions that can be treated laparoscopically (e.g., selected nephrosplenic entrapments, some intraabdominal adhesions, uterine or bladder tears).[2,12,21] The combination of a traditional with a laparoscopic surgical technique (i.e., hand-assisted laparoscopy) may expand the number of techniques available for treatment (e.g., diaphragmatic hernia repair, mass removal, abscess removal).

Ventral approaches

Incision

The abdominal cavity is accessed ventrally through a midline or paramedian approach for colic (Figures 16.1 and 16.2). The ventral midline approach is started at or 1-cm cranial to the umbilicus and extended 20–35 cm (15 cm in a foal) in a cranial direction. For a midline incision, the umbilicus or just cranial to the umbilicus is the best

(a)

(b)

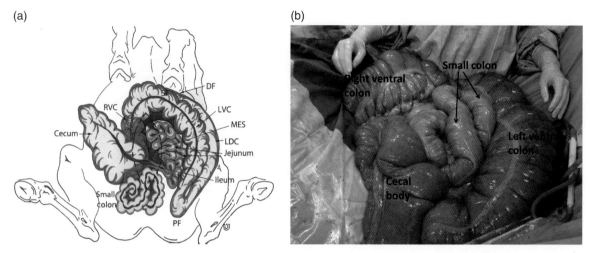

Figure 16.3 (a) Schematic illustration identifying portions of the gastrointestinal tract accessible from the ventral midline incision. C, cecum; RVC, right ventral colon; SF, sternal flexure; LVC, left ventral colon; PF, pelvic flexure; LDC, left dorsal colon; DF, diaphragmatic flexure; SC, small colon; MES, mesentery of the jejunum with arcuate vessels. (b) Photograph of exteriorized intestine. The surgeon is standing on the left side of the horse.

location to begin the incision because it is the easiest place to identify the linea alba. The paramedian incision is made in a similar location but approximately 5 cm to the left or right of midline depending on the expected lesion site. The paramedian incision can also be made in a more cranial or caudal direction based on the tentative diagnosis.

Once the skin and subcutaneous tissues are incised, the incision for a ventral midline approach is made through the linea alba whereas the incision for a paramedian approach is made to either side of the midline through the external rectus sheath, rectus abdominis muscle, and the internal rectus sheath. When making a paramedian incision, the surgeon must take care to control hemorrhage from the rectus abdominis muscle using electrocautery or ligation with 3-0 synthetic absorbable suture material. Because the linea alba is fibrous, hemorrhage from a midline incision is minimal and is usually controlled by temporarily applying hemostats or using electrocautery. After the body wall is incised, the surgeon bluntly enters the peritoneum with digital pressure.

The incision can be extended in a cranial or caudal direction, if necessary, to assess or correct the lesion. A midline incision can be extended in a cranial direction whereas the caudal extent of the incision is limited by the prepuce in male or castrated male horses. The ribs limit the cranial extent

of a paramedian incision; however, a paramedian incision can be extended further in a caudal direction in male or castrated male horses.

Anatomy of ventral exploratory celiotomy

A systematic approach is developed by each surgeon to ensure complete abdominal exploration. The order in which the abdomen is explored is not as important as the consistency of the approach. Although differences in surgeon preference exist, in general, evaluation of the gastrointestinal tract is performed first followed by evaluation of non-gastrointestinal tract organs including diaphragm, liver, spleen, reproductive tract, and urinary tract. The portions of the gastrointestinal tract accessible from a ventral approach are shown in Figure 16.3.

Cecum

In a normal horse, the first part of the gastrointestinal tract identified from a ventral abdominal approach is the cecum. The cecum is located on the right side of the abdomen with the apex oriented in a cranial and ventral direction (Figure 16.4). The cecum is easily identified because it is a large blind sac with an average volume of 30 L and length of over 1 m in an adult horse.[6] The cecal apex and a portion of the body can be exteriorized through a ventral approach. However, the remainder of the cecal body and the

(a)

(b)

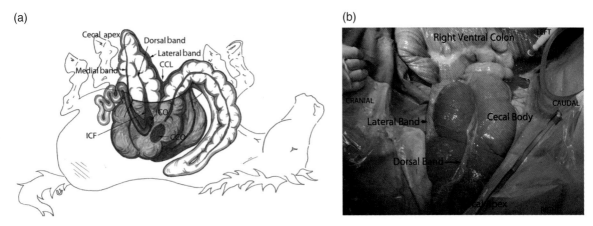

Figure 16.4 (a) Schematic illustration depicting cecal orientation. Lighter colored parts of the intestine are able to be exteriorized. ICO, ileocecal orifice; CCO, cecocolic orifice; ICF, ileocecal fold; CCL, cecocolic ligament. (b) Photograph of exteriorized cecum showing the apex and body and the cecal bands. Note that the cecum has been reflected backward toward the caudal aspect of the horse and the ventral cecal band is not visible.

cecal base (cranial part or cupula and caudal part) can only be palpated. There are four bands on the cecum: dorsal, ventral, medial, and lateral (Figure 16.4). The medial and lateral cecal artery and vein course in the medial and lateral cecal bands. Common lesions affecting the cecum include cecal impaction (p. 214), cecal tympany, and cecocolic intussusception (p. 214), and cecal perforation (p. 215). The cecum can also be affected in horses with a large colon volvulus (p. 220).

Because the cecum is located at the junction of the small and large intestines, it is an important anatomic landmark during exploration of the abdomen. Depending upon the lesion, distension, and surgeon preference, following identification and evaluation of the cecum exploration can continue with the small or large intestine.

Small intestine

To locate the small intestine, the surgeon follows the ileocecal fold arising from the dorsal cecal band to the ileum where it becomes the antimesenteric band of the ileum (Figure 16.5). The dorsal cecal band is distinguished from the other bands by a thin, freely moveable portion. The ileocecal orifice and the distal portion of the ileum are palpable, but cannot be exteriorized. The ileum is approximately 0.7 m in length.[9] Once the ileum is located, it is traced in an oral direction to the jejunum. The ileum can be differentiated from the jejunum by several anatomic characteristics. The ileum has a thin antimesenteric fold, is

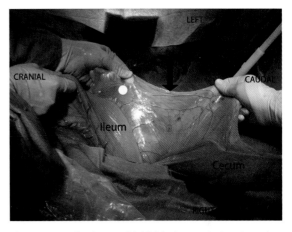

Figure 16.5 The ileocecal fold (black arrow) arises from the dorsal band of the cecum and can be followed to the ileum. The ileum should be followed in an aboral direction to the ileocecal orifice which cannot be exteriorized.

thicker due to a more developed muscular layer, and is fed by a singular vessel in the mesentery (ileal artery) compared to the arcuate vessels in the mesentery of the jejunum (Figure 16.6). The ileal artery is a branch of the ileocolic artery which branches from the cranial mesenteric artery. The arcuate arteries of the jejunum connect adjacent jejunal arteries which are also branches of the cranial mesenteric artery.[3,9]

The jejunum is the longest portion of the small intestine (17–28 m in an adult horse)[7] and all but a short oral segment can be exteriorized from a

(a)   (b)

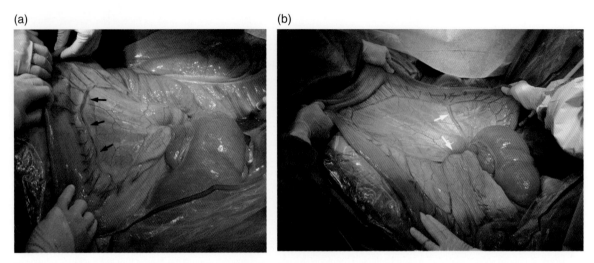

Figure 16.6   The ileal vessels (black arrows) are parallel to the mesenteric border of the ileum (a) whereas the jejunal vessels (white arrows) have an arcuate pattern with branches from the cranial mesenteric artery (b).

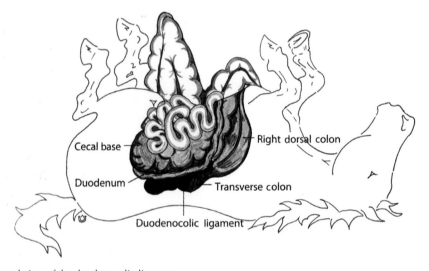

Cecal base

Duodenum

Right dorsal colon

Transverse colon

Duodenocolic ligament

Figure 16.7   Lateral view of the duodenocolic ligament.

ventral approach. The surgeon exteriorizes the jejunum in an oral direction until the duodenocolic ligament is palpated on the left side of the dorsal abdomen. The duodenocolic ligament attaches the antimesenteric aspect of the duodenum to the transverse colon at the junction of the duodenum and jejunum (Figure 16.7).

The duodenum has a very short mesentery and cannot be exteriorized. It can be traced in an oral direction from the duodenocolic ligament to the pylorus. The duodenum courses orad from left to right caudal to the base of the cecum, then from the caudal flexure it courses in a cranial direction on the right side of the abdomen to the cranial flexure, and then from right to left to end at the pylorus of the stomach. The cranial flexure and ampulla where the bile and pancreatic ducts enter the duodenum create a duodenal sigmoid flexure (Figure 16.8). The duodenum is approximately 1 m in length.[9]

Lesions affecting the small intestine include pedunculated lipoma (p. 209), epiploic foramen entrapment (p. 211), segmental or mesenteric

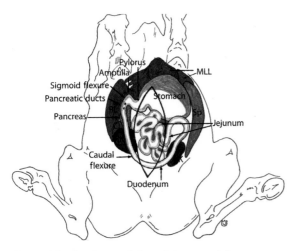

Figure 16.8 Cranioventral view of the open abdomen through a midline incision with the large colon and cecum removed. Shown is the stomach, pylorus, ampulla, duodenal sigmoid flexure, pancreas, pancreatic ducts, and pathway of the duodenum along the dorsal body wall. LK, left kidney; RK, right kidney; Sp, spleen; MLL, medial and lateral left liver lobe; RL, right lateral lobe; CL, caudate lobe.

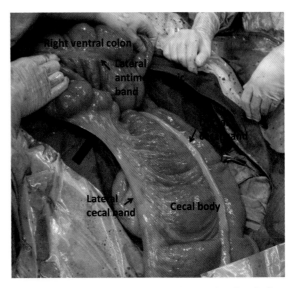

Figure 16.9 The large (ascending) colon can be identified by following the lateral cecal band to the cecocolic ligament (large black arrow) that attaches to the lateral mesenteric (free) band of the right ventral colon. Cranial is at the top left of the photograph.

volvulus (p. 212), inguinal hernia (p. 284), ileocecal intussusception (p. 213), ileal impaction (p. 208), and ileal hypertrophy (p. 130).

Large colon
The large, or ascending, colon is located by following the lateral cecal band to the cecocolic ligament which attaches the cecum to the lateral antimesenteric (free) band of the right ventral colon (Figure 16.9). From oral to aboral, the large colon has four parts and three flexures: right ventral colon → sternal flexure → left ventral colon → pelvic flexure → left dorsal colon → diaphragmatic flexure → right dorsal colon (Figure 16.10). The large colon is 3–3.7 m long and has a capacity of 50–60 L in an adult horse.[26] The colic branch of the ileocolic artery supplies the ventral colons and the right colic artery, a branch of the cranial mesenteric artery, supplies the dorsal colons.[3,26] Most of the large colon is freely moveable within the abdomen and can be exteriorized from a ventral approach because it is only attached on the right side (i.e., the ventral colon is attached to the cecum and dorsal colon, and the dorsal colon is attached to the body wall). The ventral and dorsal colons are connected by a mesocolon. The right and left ventral colons and sternal flexure have haustra (sacculations) and

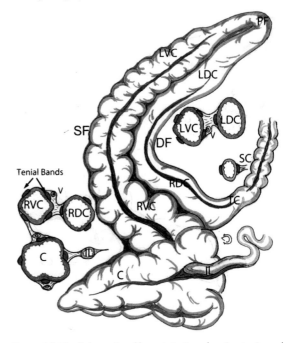

Figure 16.10 Schematic of large intestine showing tenia and sacculations, with cross-sectional view. IL, ileum; C, cecum; RVC, right ventral colon; SF, sterna flexure; LVC, right ventral colon; PF, pelvic flexure; LDC, left dorsal colon; DF, diaphragmatic flexure; RDC, right dorsal colon; TC, transverse colon; SC, small colon; V, vessels.

thick fibrous tenia (bands) whereas the right and left dorsal colons and pelvic and diaphragmatic flexures do not have any sacculations (Figure 16.10). The dorsal colon has tenia (bands) but they are less obvious and appear more muscular. The pelvic flexure and left dorsal colon have one tenial band and the right dorsal colon has three tenial bands.

The first step in evaluating the large colon is determining the orientation. In the normal large colon, the pelvic flexure is in the left caudal abdomen, the sternal and diaphragmatic flexures in the cranial abdomen and the ventral and dorsal colons are ventral and dorsal, respectively. The right dorsal colon can be palpated as it empties into the transverse colon. The cecocolic ligament should be straight. The orientation is assessed by tracing the ventral colons (using the bands for guidance) until the pelvic flexure is identified and followed to the dorsal colons which are traced back to the right side and the beginning of the transverse colon.

Common lesions affecting the large colon include intraluminal obstructions (ingesta [p. 217], sand [p. 217], enteroliths [p. 218]), large colon displacement (right dorsal [p. 220]; left dorsal or nephrosplenic ligament entrapment [p. 219]), and large colon volvulus (p. 220).

Transverse colon
The transverse colon is evaluated solely by palpation because it cannot be exteriorized and lies close to the dorsal body wall due to the short mesocolon (Figure 16.10). It travels in an aboral direction from right to left cranial to the cecal base connecting the right dorsal colon to the small colon. It is located by tracing either the right dorsal colon aborad or the small colon orad. The transverse colon can be obstructed by enteroliths or sand.

Small colon
The small, or descending, colon is easily identified by palpation within the caudal abdomen. It is not abnormal for the small colon to be identified in other areas of the abdomen. The small colon often contains fecal balls which are readily palpated. The diameter of the normal small colon is approximately 7–10 cm, which is slightly larger than the normal small intestine.[26] The small colon is approximately 3.5 m long in an adult horse.[26] The small colon has a wide, muscular antimesenteric band, sacculations, and a fatty mesocolon (Figure 16.11). The left colic

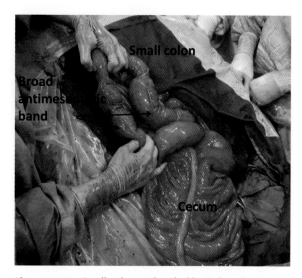

Figure 16.11 Small colon is identified by its broad antimesenteric band and sacculations. The oral and aboral aspects of the small colon cannot be exteriorized. The small colon can be palpated in an oral direction toward the transverse colon and then in an aboral direction toward the rectum. Fecal balls can often be palpated within the small colon particularly in the aboral aspect.

artery and cranial rectal artery, branches of the caudal mesenteric artery, provide the blood supply to the small colon. These vessels have multiple anastomosing branches that create an arcuate pattern within the mesentery.

The small colon is evaluated by identifying a loop by palpation and which is then exteriorized. The loop is then traced orad to the transverse colon (left side) and in an aboral direction to the rectum. The most oral and aboral parts cannot be exteriorized.

The small colon is most commonly affected by impaction (p. 220) and other intraluminal obstructions such as fecaliths and enteroliths or sand. Rarely strangulating lesions occur, most commonly a strangulating pedunculated lipoma.

Other abdominal organs
The stomach is usually evaluated solely by palpation. However, the greater curvature can sometimes be seen if the stomach is distended and/or the incision is extended in a cranial direction. The stomach is located in the left cranial abdomen caudal to the liver. The greater curvature can be palpated, often through omentum, and traced from left to right to the pylorus. The pylorus is muscular

and conical and can be traced to the duodenum (Figure 16.8). Gastric lesions requiring surgical treatment are rare. Gastric outflow obstruction in foals (p. 280), thought to occur as a sequela to gastroduodenal ulceration and inflammation, can be managed by performing a gastrojejunostomy with or without duodenojejunostomy.[34]

The diaphragm separates the abdomen from the thorax and serves as the cranial border of the abdominal cavity. The equine diaphragm inserts on the thoracic wall from the 8th and 9th costral cartilages then along the costochodral junctions of the 9th–15th ribs to the middle of the 18th rib and then ends at the dorsal/vertebral aspect of the 17th intercostal space.[3] It should be palpated for any irregularities or defects (hernias). Herniation of abdominal contents through a diaphragmatic defect can cause colic; however, this is relatively uncommon.

The liver is located in the cranial abdomen just caudal to the diaphragm. The right lobe of the liver is much larger than the left, especially in younger animals. The liver has a sharp border, smooth surface and a firm, spongy texture. Horses have left, quadrate, right, and caudate lobes.[6] Horses with liver disease may show signs of colic. Colic associated with obstruction of the biliary tract (cholelithiasis within the common bile duct) can be diagnosed and, in some cases, treated surgically.

The spleen is located immediately adjacent to the left body wall. The size is variable depending upon the degree of splenic contraction. The spleen usually spans most of the craniocaudal length of the left abdomen. It can extend from the dorsal aspect of the abdominal cavity to midline or even just to the right of midline. The spleen has an irregular surface and firm, muscular texture. The spleen is used to locate the nephrosplenic ligament by tracing the caudal aspect of the spleen dorsally and then cranially along its visceral aspect until the ligament is encountered (Figure 16.12).

The left kidney is medial to the dorsal aspect of the spleen and the right kidney is slightly more cranial on the right side of the aorta. The kidneys are firm and rounded. They are retroperitoneal and frequently covered by a substantial layer of fat. Ureters are usually not evaluated in horses because they are not normally palpable and rarely affected by disease. The bladder is located in the caudal abdomen. It is supported by the round ligaments

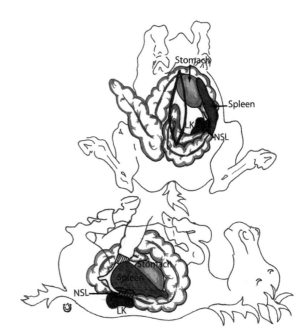

Figure 16.12 The nephrosplenic ligament from the ventral and left lateral view with the colon entrapped. LK, left kidney; NSL, nephrosplenic ligament.

of the bladder. When empty, the bladder lies within the pelvic cavity. As it becomes distended it extends further into the abdomen and the round ligaments become taught.

In males, most of the reproductive tract is not within the abdomen. However, the inguinal rings should be evaluated for size and intestinal herniation. The testicular vessels and vas deferens are also examined as they exit the abdomen through the rings. Herniation is primarily a concern in intact males. The inguinal rings are located on either side of midline at the cranial aspect of the ventral pelvis.

In females, the uterus and ovaries are within the abdominal cavity. The body of the uterus is located dorsal to the bladder on midline. Once identified, it can be traced caudally to the cervix within the pelvic cavity and cranially to each horn and associated ovary. Problems causing colic and requiring surgery affecting the urogenital system include inguinal hernia (p. 284), and uterine torsion (p. 282) and rarely urolithiasis.

Body wall closure

The holding layer for body wall closure of a midline incision is the linea alba and for a paramedian incision the external rectus sheath. The body wall is typically closed with #2 or #3 absorbable suture material, primarily polyglactin 910. In the linea alba, a simple continuous pattern is used most frequently (Figure 16.13). When a paramedian approach has been made, the external rectus sheath is apposed more often using interrupted patterns such as cruciate or near-far-far-near. However, continuous or interrupted patterns are likely suitable for both midline and paramedian incisions. Some surgeons close the peritoneum when performing a paramedian approach and suggest that the complication rate is decreased.[18]

After body wall closure, the overlying tissues can be closed in one or two layers (Figures 16.13 and 16.14). Closure of the subcutaneous tissue is performed with 2-0 absorbable suture in a simple continuous pattern. Some surgeons prefer not to close the subcutaneous layer to minimize suture material in the incision and decrease time for closure. Closure of the subcutaneous tissue does not appear to affect the security of the closure or alter postoperative wound drainage.[4]

Skin can be closed with 2-0 or 0 suture material or staples. Sutured closure may be accomplished with absorbable suture material in a buried subcuticular suture pattern (Figures 16.13 and 16.14) or absorbable suture material in a simple continuous pattern. In one study, staples increased the risk for incisional infection compared to a simple continuous suture for skin closure.[33] Although no studies have compared incisional

complications associated with the subcuticular suture pattern to the alternatives in horses, evaluation in other species and clinical experience has been favorable.[8,27,31] The skin can also be apposed using cyanoacrylate adhesive glue (Figure 16.14).

Following closure, some surgeons elect to cover the incision for recovery and/or a period of time after surgery. Prior to recovery, the incision can be covered with an iodine-impregnated adhesive (or

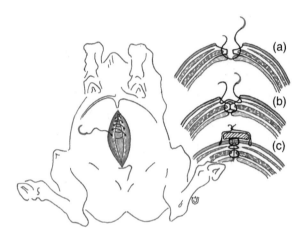

Figure 16.13 Body wall closure, three layers. (a) Linea closure placing bites 1.2–1.5 cm from the edge through the linea or external sheath of the rectus abdominis muscle in a simple continuous pattern using a #3 absorbable suture material. (b) Closure of the subcutaneous layer using a simple continuous pattern with 2–0 monofilament absorbable suture material. (c) Skin closure using wide stainless steel staples placed at least 1 cm apart and oversewn with a stent.

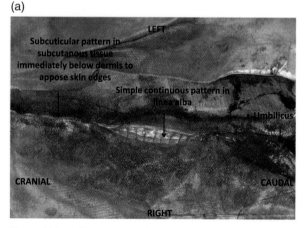

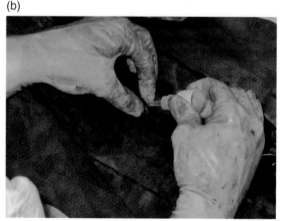

Figure 16.14 There are several methods to appose the subcutaneous tissue and skin. Illustrated is a subcuticular pattern in the subcutaneous tissue immediately below the dermis to appose the skin (a) with cyanoacrylate adhesive to seal the skin wound (b).

(a)

(b)

(c)

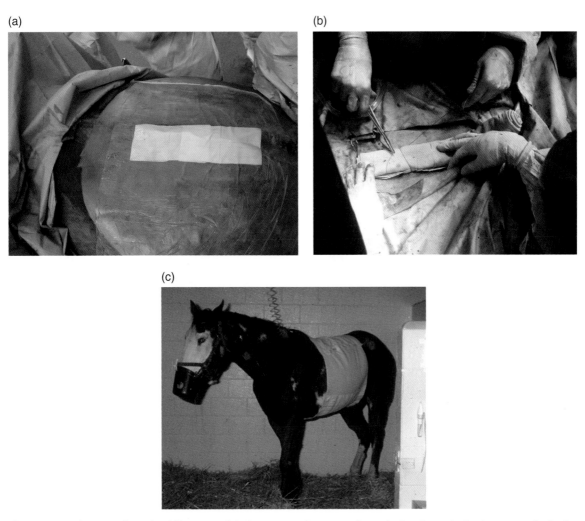

Figure 16.15 The surgical site should be covered during recovery from general anesthesia using an iodine-impregnated adhesive drape (a), stent bandage (b). An abdominal bandage can be used to decrease postoperative incisional complications (c).

incise) drape or a stent bandage (Figure 16.15). Additionally or alternatively, the entire abdomen can be bandaged postoperatively. A decrease in incisional infections was associated with the iodine-impregnated adhesive bandage and an increase in incisional infection with a stent bandage was identified in one study.[22] Regardless of type of wound protection used, it should be removed and skin cleaned immediately following recovery from general anesthesia. Placement of an elastic abdominal bandage immediately after surgery and maintenance for 2 weeks decreased incisional complications.[30] A reusable abdominal bandage

made for horses has been used to treat incisional complications (Figure 16.15).[19]

Lateral approaches

Incision

A modified grid approach (Figures 16.16 and 16.17) is used to achieve the best access from a flank approach. The flank is the area between the tuber coxae and the last rib. If the surgery is being performed with the horse standing, local anesthetic is

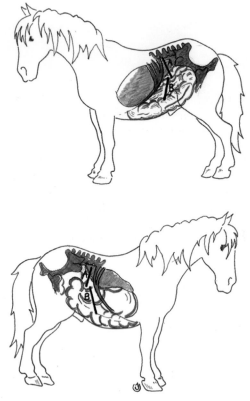

Figure 16.16 Schematic illustration of left and right paralumbar and flank incisions.

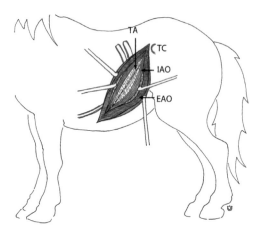

Figure 16.17 Modified grid approach to a flank incision. TC, tuber coxae. The incision is made through the skin and subcutaneous layer, followed by sharp incision through external abdominal oblique muscle (EAO). The fibers of the internal abdominal oblique muscle (IAO) are bluntly separated. Sharp incision through the transversus abdominis (TA) is made to expose the peritoneum.

infused in a line block. The skin incision is made caudodorsally to cranioventrally parallel to the internal abdominal oblique muscle. After the skin and subcutaneous tissues are incised, the external abdominal oblique muscle is incised and then the fibers of the internal abdominal oblique muscles are separated. Then the transversus abdominis muscle is incised. The surgeon must then bluntly dissect through any retroperitoneal fat and use quick blunt pressure to penetrate the peritoneum and enter the abdomen. The peritoneum will be sensitive and the surgeon should use appropriate caution when opening this layer.

Access to the more cranial abdomen can be achieved through a rib resection. The surgeon should be aware and prepared for the risk of entering the thorax and if the risk is considered high, general anesthesia should be considered. If surgery is being performed with the horse standing, local anesthetic is infused in a line block. The skin, subcutaneous tissues, and musculature are incised over the selected rib. The periosteum is incised over the center of the rib and elevated circumferentially. Obstetric wire is used to transect the rib dorsally and ventrally to allow removal. The periosteum on the medial aspect of the rib is incised.

Anatomy of lateral exploratory celiotomy

Access to abdominal organs is limited from a lateral approach. From the right flank, portions of the small colon, small intestine, uterus, right ovary, and right inguinal ring can be accessed. Rib resections performed on the right can provide access to the base of the cecum, duodenum, and right dorsal colon. From the left flank, the left dorsal and ventral colons, pelvic flexure, small colon, left kidney, nephrosplenic ligament, caudal border of the spleen, uterus, left ovary, and left inguinal ring can be accessed. Rib resection performed on the left can increase access to the left kidney, spleen, and nephrosplenic ligament.

Body wall closure

If a modified grid approach has been used, the incision is closed in four layers. It is unnecessary, and often impossible, to close the peritoneum and transversus abdominis muscle. The internal abdominal oblique and external abdominal oblique muscles are closed separately with #2 absorbable suture material in a simple continuous pattern. The holding layer for the body wall is the external abdominal oblique muscle. The subcutaneous layer is closed with 2-0 absorbable suture material in a simple continuous pattern. The skin can be closed with 0 or 2-0 absorbable suture material in a simple continuous pattern combined with a simple interrupted pattern or skin staples. Seroma formation is not uncommon. Removal of several staples will provide easy drainage, if necessary. If a continuous pattern is used, several interrupted sutures should be placed at the ventral aspect of the incision to allow drainage if needed.

If a rib resection has been performed, the incision is closed in three layers. Note that if the thoracic cavity was opened, the diaphragm should be sutured to the body wall at the beginning of surgery to minimize contamination of the thoracic cavity during surgery. The peritoneum and periosteum are closed with absorbable suture in a continuous or interrupted suture pattern. Closure of the subcutaneous tissue and skin is similar to the modified grid approach. Placement of a drain between the periosteum and subcutaneous tissues may help reduce seroma formation and associated wound complications.

Laparoscopy

Laparoscope and instrument portals

A rigid videoendoscope is used for visual assessment during laparoscopy. Interventions are performed with laparoscopic instruments through instrument portals or a surgeon's hand through a traditional incision or specialized portals. Intra-abdominal pressure is negative in the normal horse. Insufflation with carbon dioxide using a pump can be used to separate the body wall and organs from one another and provide more space for the laparoscope and instruments to be used. The location of the structure being accessed determines how much, if any, insufflations is required.

The first portal that is placed is for the laparoscope (Figure 16.18). The other portals can then be placed under visual guidance. The location and number of portals required is determined by the procedure being performed. It is possible to injure intra-abdominal organs or vessels within the

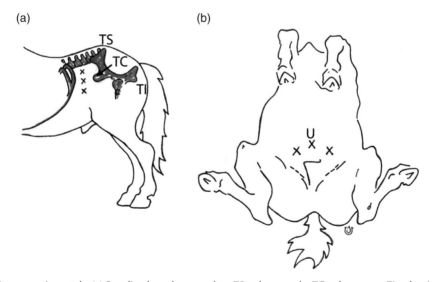

Figure 16.18 Laproscopic portals. (a) Standing lateral approaches. TS, tuber sacrale; TC, tuber coxae; TI, tuber ischii; F, greater trochanter of the femur; X, portals for camera and instruments. Central portal placed midway between the last rib and the TC, instrument portals placed 10 cm proximally and distally based on procedure and surgeon preference. (b) Dorsal recumbency portals. Arthroscope portal over umbilicus (U), instrument portals placed 10–15 cm cranial to the external inguinal rings (EIR) and 10 cm lateral to midline.

Table 16.1 Laparoscopic anatomy and diagnoses in horses with colic.

Portal location	Structures visible	Lesions associated with colic that can be diagnosed laparoscopically
Right lateral	Left lateral, quadrate, and right liver lobes, stomach (pyloric region), gastrosplenic ligament, spleen (apex), duodenum, common bile duct, cecum, right kidney, epiploic foramen, diaphragmatic flexure, right dorsal and ventral large colons, transverse colon, jejunum, small colon, rectum, bladder, vaginal ring, diaphragm Female: right ovary, right uterus, mesovarium, broad ligament Male: mesorchium, vas deferens ± Pelvic flexure	Cholelith in common bile duct, right dorsal colitis, uterine tear, rupture of mesocolon and small colon ischemia, diaphragmatic hernia, inguinal hernia, adhesions
Left lateral	Left liver lobe, stomach (caudal blind sac), gastrosplenic ligament, spleen, nephrosplenic ligament, left kidney, small colon, duodenocolic ligament, bladder, vaginal ring, diaphragm Female: left ovary, left uterus, mesovarium, broad ligament Male: mesorchium, vas deferens ± Rectum, jejunum, left dorsal and ventral large colons, pelvic flexure	Nephrosplenic entrapment, uterine tear, rupture of mesocolon and small colon ischemia, diaphragmatic hernia, inguinal hernia, adhesions
Ventral	Ventral liver lobes, ventral spleen, apex and body of cecum, cecocolic fold, right and left ventral large colons, sternal and pelvic flexures, jejunum, small colon, prepubic tendon, bladder, inguinal rings, diaphragm Female: vaginal wall, cervix Male: mesorchium, vas deferens, cremaster muscle ± Stomach, gastrosplenic ligament	Diaphragmatic hernia, inguinal hernia, adhesions

body wall during portal placement.[5,13] To minimize risk of injury to intra-abdominal structures during placement of the portal for the videoendoscope, the surgeon can insufflate the abdomen first through a blunt catheter or specialized needle. The specialized needle retracts the sharp portion when pressure drops (i.e., with the negative intraperitoneal pressure). Specialized portals that have sharp trocars that retract when pressure drops can also be used. If hand-assisted laparoscopy is being performed, the incision for the hand can be made first and surgeon's hand can protect the intra-abdominal structures during portal placement.

Laparoscopic anatomy

Different intra-abdominal structures are visible and accessible depending upon the approach used. Table 16.1 includes information on the structures that are seen from right and left lateral and ventral portal placement. Additionally, examples of conditions associated with colic that can be diagnosed laparoscopically are given.[10]

Regardless of the approach, the amount of each structure that can be seen varies with gastrointestinal distension/fill and insufflation. Instruments can be used to manipulate the intestine, particularly the small intestine and small colon, to allow visibility of additional loops of intestine and other structures.

Closure

Laparoscopic portals are closed in two layers—the external abdominal oblique or ventral body wall and the skin. Absorbable suture in a simple interrupted or cruciate pattern is used in the external abdominal oblique muscle or ventral body wall. The skin can be closed with interrupted suture or staples. Larger incisions used for hand-assisted

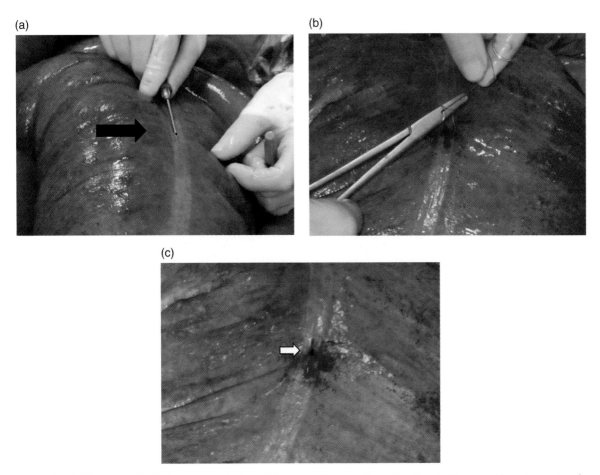

Figure 16.19 The large colon is decompressed using a 14-gauge 1 1/2 in. needle and suction. (a) The serosal layer is penetrated with the needle (black arrow) and tunneled in the submucosa before being passed through the mucosa and into the intestinal lumen. (b) The needle hole can be closed using 3-0 synthetic absorbable suture material in an interrupted (c, white arrow) or cruciate suture pattern.

laparoscopy are closed as described for the lateral or ventral abdominal approaches.

Selected surgical procedures

Needle decompression

Needle decompression is performed with a 14 gauge 1 1/2-in. needle in adult horses (18 gauge 1 1/2 in. needle for foals and small intestine) attached to tubing connected to suction (Figure 16.19). Needle decompression is most commonly performed in the large colon and cecum, but can be used in other intestinal structures if indicated. The site selected for decompression should be grasped and exteriorized if possible. The needle should penetrate the serosa, tunneled through the submucosa, and then passed through the mucosa into the intestinal lumen. When all of the gas is removed, the site of needle penetration should be grasped with a moistened 4 × 4 gauze sponge and the needle removed. The 4 × 4 gauze sponge is discarded and the site inspected for feed material, leakage, and/or hemorrhage. A partial thickness (serosa, muscle layers, submucosa) single cruciate or interrupted suture using 2-0 or 3-0 synthetic absorbable suture material can be used based on surgeon preference and the presence of leakage or hemorrhage (Figure 16.19).

Overview of enterotomy procedure

An enterotomy is most often performed to evacuate impacted ingesta or other material causing an obstruction (e.g., sand, enterolith, fecalith, foreign body), remove ingesta oral to a lesion, or obtain an intestinal biopsy sample. An intestinal biopsy can also be obtained using an 8 mm skin biopsy punch.

Prior to performing an enterotomy, the region of bowel to be opened is exteriorized from the abdomen and appropriate draping is used to contain contamination. Sodium carboxymethyl cellulose can be applied to the serosal surface of the intestine to form a coating which can facilitate removal of contamination at the completion of the enterotomy procedure. A stab incision is used to start an enterotomy. The mucosa tends to separate from the other layers if the stab incision is not made properly. Care should be taken, however, to ensure that the stab incision does not penetrate through the bowel wall on the opposite side of the lumen. Once the blade has entered the lumen of the bowel, the incision is extended.

When the surgeon is ready to close the enterotomy, the region is lavaged with polyionic isotonic fluids to remove any gross contamination. An enterotomy is typically closed using a full thickness simple continuous pattern oversewn with a Cushing or Lembert pattern. Care should be taken to avoid stenosis of the intestinal lumen during enterotomy site closure. The holding layer in all intestine is the submucosa and care must be taken to include this layer in any pattern that is not full thickness, such as Cushing and Lembert patterns. Lavage is repeated as necessary during the closure and at the end of the procedure.

Pelvic flexure enterotomy

The most common location for a large colon enterotomy is at the pelvic flexure (Figure 16.20) because of the ease with which this part of the large colon can be exteriorized from the abdomen. However, an enterotomy can be performed at any site that can be exteriorized well enough to prevent abdominal contamination. An enterotomy at a site other than the pelvic flexure is generally used for removal of a specific obstructing objected (e.g., an enterolith that cannot be manipulated to the pelvic flexure), procedure (e.g., right ventral colon enterotomy for correction of cecocolic

intussusception[15]), or biopsy of the affected colon. A pelvic flexure enterotomy is performed on the antimesenteric aspect of the bowel and the incision is oriented longitudinally. A large colon enterotomy is performed with the large colon placed on a tilted table (colon tray) that is draped and abutted to the flank of the horse (generally on the left side). If the enterotomy is performed at a location closer to the abdomen additional draping as for typhlotomy and small intestinal enterotomy is necessary.

Ingesta is removed through a pelvic flexure enterotomy by placing a hose with warm tap water within the lumen to hydrate the ingesta. The ingesta is massaged toward the enterotomy site. An enterolith or other foreign body can also be "floated" toward the pelvic flexure enterotomy site by distending the colon with water through the enterotomy.

A large colon enterotomy is closed using 2-0 synthetic absorbable suture material in a full thickness simple continuous pattern oversewn with a Cushing pattern. Recently, staples (TA-90, US Surgical Corporation) have been reported to result in rapid and effective enterotomy closure.[28]

Typhlotomy

A typhlotomy incision is performed near the cecal apex and in a location that will allow gravity to help minimize contamination during removal of ingesta. After exteriorizing the cecum usually over the right side of the patient's abdomen, the cecum is isolated from the abdomen using a combination of laparotomy sponges and drapes (e.g., a split-sheet drape). Care needs to be taken during evacuation of cecal ingesta because of its close proximity to the abdomen. It is also important to evacuate the cecal cupula particularly in horses with a cecal impaction to prevent reimpaction. Complete evacuation of the cupula may involve insertion of the surgeon's hand though the typhlotomy to scoop out impacting ingesta.

A typhlotomy is closed with a full thickness simple continuous pattern oversewn with a Cushing or Lembert pattern; 2-0 or 0 absorbable suture material can be used. Occasionally serosal trauma and contamination at the apex during evacuation of the cecum is severe and a partial typhlectomy using stapling equipment (e.g., TA-90 or ILA-100, United States Surgical Corporation) and oversewing the staple line with a Cushing pattern.

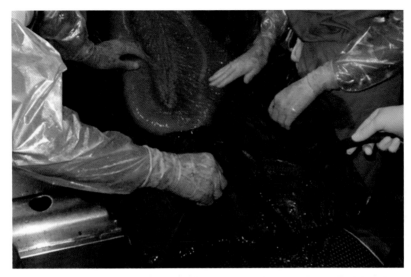

Figure 16.20   Pelvic flexure enterotomy being performed with the colon positioned on a tilted table (colon tray). There is a sterile plastic bag placed over the tray.

Small intestinal enterotomy

An enterotomy of the small intestine is performed on the antimesenteric aspect of the bowel and the incision is oriented longitudinally. If possible, the surgeon should select an area that can be easily exteriorized from the abdomen to minimize contamination without excessive tension on the mesentery. Once the region is selected, it should be isolated from the abdomen using a combination of laparotomy sponges and drapes (e.g., a split-sheet drape). A small intestinal enterotomy can be closed in several ways depending on the surgeon's preference; 2-0 or 3-0 absorbable suture can be used regardless of the pattern chosen. A two-layer closure can be performed with the first layer being a full thickness or mucosal/submucosal simple continuous pattern and the second layer being a simple continuous, Cushing or Lembert pattern in the seromuscular layer. Alternatively, a single layer closure with a Lembert pattern can be used. If the surgeon is concerned that the lumen size will be compromised, the incision can be closed transversely which results in the ends of the incision at the middle of the closure and increased intestinal circumference at the enterotomy site.

Small colon enterotomy

A small colon enterotomy is performed on the antimesenteric aspect of the bowel through the thick, muscular antimesenteric band (Figure 16.21). After the location is chosen, the region of small colon is isolated from the abdomen using a combination of laparotomy sponges and drapes (e.g., split-sheet drape). The incision is oriented longitudinally. A small colon enterotomy is closed with a full thickness simple continuous pattern oversewn with a Cushing or Lembert pattern; 2-0 synthetic absorbable suture material is used.

Partial typhlectomy

A partial typhlectomy is most commonly performed to resect nonviable or severely contaminated tissue. A partial typhlectomy is performed through a ventral midline incision and can involve the apex only or the body and the apex. The region selected for typhlectomy is isolated from the abdomen. Double ligation of the medial and lateral cecal vessels can be performed with 0 absorbable suture material except when only the apex is being resected in the area where the medial and lateral cecal vessels have arborized. Large, full-thickness stay sutures should be placed in the cecum laterally and medially because the cecum will tend to retract into the abdomen once the apex-body is transected. Typhlectomy can be hand sewn or stapled. For a hand sewn typhlectomy, atraumatic intestinal clamps are placed proximal to the resection site to minimize contamination.

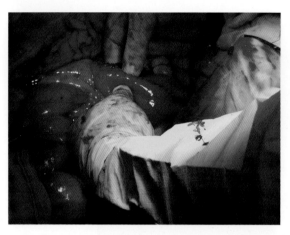

Figure 16.21 Small colon enterotomy used to remove an enterolith. The enterotomy was performed on the antimesenteric band of the small colon. The small colon enterotomy was closed using a full thickness simple continuous oversewn with a Lembert pattern.

The portion to be resected is sharply excised and the cecum is closed with 0 absorbable suture material in a full-thickness simple continuous or Parker Kerr pattern then oversewn with a Cushing's or Lembert pattern. Using a stapling technique, a double row of staples (e.g., TA-90 or ILA-100, US Surgical Corporation) serves as the first layer of the closure. The staples are oversewn with 0 or 2-0 absorbable suture material in a Cushing's or Lembert pattern. If a stapled typhlectomy is performed, the stapling device is placed prior to resection and serves to prevent contamination and stabilize the intestine during sharp excision. Depending on the width of the cecum at the resection site, multiple 90 or 100-mm staple cartridges may be required.

Overview of the resection and anastomosis procedure

A resection and anastomosis is most often performed to remove nonviable bowel. Assessment of intestinal viability is generally performed subjectively by assessment of the serosal (and mucosal if an enterotomy has been performed) surface of the bowel. Viability is based on color (grey and dark blue or green are associated with nonviability), motility, wall thickness (very thin wall is associated with nonviability), and palpation of a pulse. Note that assessment of serosal color is inherently unreliable for assessing colonic viability. Returning the affected part of bowel to the abdomen for a brief period and then reassessing can be useful. Other techniques have been reported including fluorescein dye, Doppler, pulse oximetry, and histology; however, they have not gained widespread clinical use.

The first step in any resection and anastomosis is selection and isolation of the region to be resected from the abdomen using laparotomy sponges or drapes. The lumen of the adjacent bowel is occluded using Penrose drains tied in single-throw knot and secured with hemostats or atraumatic intestinal clamps.

Ligation of mesenteric vessels supplying the section of bowel to be resected is then performed. For small intestinal and small colon resections, vessels are isolated from the mesentery using sharp and blunt dissection. While minimizing the amount of mesenteric fat in the ligature is important, care should be taken to avoid vessel trauma during dissection to isolate the vessel. Closure of the vessels can be performed using ligatures, staples, or vessel sealing devices.[29] If using ligatures, double ligation of the vessels with a proximal encircling and distal transfixation ligature is recommended; 0 or 2-0 absorbable suture is used based on size of the vessel. Staples are applied to the vessel using a Ligate-Divide Staple device (LDS, US Surgical Corporation), which applies two staples to the vessel and transects the vessel between the staples. Placement of a ligature proximal to the staple is recommended. Vessel sealing devices (e.g., LigaSure, Tyco Healthcare Inc, Mansfield, MA) can be used to cut and seal vessels up to and including 7 cm in diameter.[29] Again, to reinforce the closure, the surgeon may elect to place a proximal ligature. The vessels and associated mesentery are transected as the vessels are ligated or sealed.

For large colon resection and anastomosis, the right colic and colic branch of the ileocolic arteries and veins are double ligated using 0 absorbable suture material (Figure 16.22) or the vessels are occluded using a TA-90 (US Surgical Corporation).[16,17] When double ligation using suture material is performed, the proximal ligature should include a portion of the mesentery to serve as a transfixation ligature. While stapling the vessels is reported to be easier than ligation, it is more expensive and these devices are not designed for vessel ligation. Careful assessment of hemostasis and ligation of any vessels that continue to hemorrhage must be performed.

Jejunojejunostomy and jejunoileostomy

Jejunojejunostomy and jejunoileostomy are most commonly hand sewn end-to-end anastomoses. Once the region to be resected is selected and isolated and the vessels are ligated, atraumatic intestinal clamps, such as Doyens, or Penrose drains are placed 6–10 cm oral and aboral to the region to prevent the flow of ingesta. The intestine is transected using a fresh scalpel blade at a 60° angle so that the mesenteric side is longer than the antimesenteric side (Figure 16.23). The angle serves to increase the circumference of the bowel at the anastomosis to assure the adequate lumen diameter. Stay sutures are placed at the antimesenteric and mesenteric aspect and put under tension to maintain lumen size during anastomosis. Anastomosis for jejunojejunostomy and jejunoileostomy can be performed using 2-0 or 3-0 absorbable suture material in a one-layer Lembert pattern or in two layers with the first layer being a simple continuous pattern in the mucosa-submucosa only and the second layer being either a simple continuous appositional or continuous or interrupted inverting Lembert pattern. A full thickness simple continuous over-sewn with a Lembert pattern can also be used; however, is unnecessary to prevent leakage and likely causes stenosis.[23,24] Regardless of the method of closure, the continuous patterns must be interrupted at 180° to prevent a purse-string effect. The anastomosis is lavaged and checked for leakage. The mesentery is closed in a simple continuous pattern with 2-0 absorbable suture material.

Jejunocecostomy

Jejunocecostomy can be performed as an end-to-side or side-to-side anastomosis. With either method, the region to be resected is identified, draped, the vessels ligated, and the flow of ingesta restricted as described for jejunojejunostomy. If the surgeon is planning on performing a jejunocecostomy it is helpful to keep the cecum as empty as possible prior to the anastomosis (i.e., contents of the small intestine should be emptied through an enterotomy in the intestine that will be resected).

The portion of the ileum adjacent to the ileocecal orifice that will remain in the abdomen is blind ended (ileal "stump"). The ileal "stump" is closed

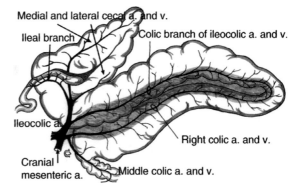

Figure 16.22 Vascular ligature placement for a large colon resection.

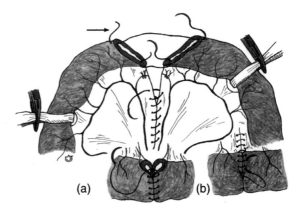

Figure 16.23 End-to-end jejunojejunostomy. Stay sutures placed on the mesenteric and antimesenteric jejunum (arrow). Penrose drains placed across the intestine to stop the flow of ingesta during the anostomosis. (a) First layer closure using #2-0 monofilament absorbable suture placed in a simple continuous full thickness pattern interrupted at 180°. (b) Second layer closure using #2-0 monofilament absorbable suture in a partial thickness Cushing pattern. Simple continuous closure of the mesentery.

in two layers. The first layer can be performed with a stapling device (TA-90, US Surgical Corporation) or full thickness simple continuous or Parker Kerr pattern oversewn with a Cushing or Lembert pattern using 2-0 absorbable suture material.

Regardless of the type of anastomosis being performed, the jejunum is attached to the cecum between the dorsal and medial band as close to the base of the cecum as possible (Figure 16.24). It is critical to make sure that the jejunal mesentery is dorsal and that the jejunum has not been rotated on its mesentery prior to performing a jejunocecostomy.

It is often helpful to begin mesenteric closure prior to performing the jejunocecostomy, particularly for a side-to-side technique.

An end-to-side jejunocecostomy is performed using a three-layer anastomosis technique using 2-0 absorbable suture material. Stay sutures are placed from the cecum to the antimesenteric (one stay suture) and mesenteric (another stay suture) aspect of the jejunum. One side of the jejunum 5 mm away from the cut edge is sutured to the cecum between the stay sutures using a Cushing or Lembert pattern. A typhlotomy is made between the stay sutures and the cut edges of the cecum and jejunum are sutured in a full thickness simple continuous pattern interrupted at the ends of the typhlotomy, which is also the mesenteric and antimesenteric aspect of the jejunum. The side of the jejunum that was not previously sutured to the cecum is oversewn with a Cushing or Lembert pattern. The stay sutures should be removed or left in place once the long ends are cut short.

A side-to-side jejunocecostomy is performed by blind ending the distal aspect of the viable jejunum as described for the ileum. Stay sutures are placed 12–14 cm apart between the antimesenteric border of the distal jejunum and the cecum with the blind end closest to the base of the cecum. The antimesenteric aspect of the jejunum is sutured to the cecum between the stay sutures with 2-0 absorbable suture in a Cushing's or Lembert pattern; this layer is often offset by about 1 cm from the antimesenteric aspect of the jejunum so that the anastomosis is precisely on the antimesenteric border. The anastomosis should end as close to the blind end of the jejunum as possible to prevent formation of a pocket. The anastomosis can be created using an ILA-100 stapling device (US Surgical Corporation) that is inserted into the lumen of the jejunum and cecum through stab incisions at one end of the proposed anastomosis site. The ILA-100 is applied creating two double rows of intestinal staples with an anastomosis in between the two rows (Figure 16.24). The anastomosis can also be created by making an 8 cm incision in the jejunum and cecum and suturing the cecum to the jejunum with a full thickness simple continuous pattern secured at each end of the incision using 2-0 absorbable suture material. Either anastomosis is oversewn with a Cushing or Lembert pattern between the cecum and jejunum on the side of the jejunum that was not previously sutured to the cecum. The anastomosis is lavaged and checked for leakage.

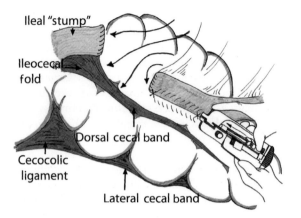

Figure 16.24   Schematic illustration of a side-to-side jejunocecostomy using an ILA-100 stapling device. Arrows indicate closure of the jejunal mesentery to the ileocecal mesentery and ileal stump.

Mesenteric closure can be challenging and should not result in tension on the jejunum adjacent to the jejunocecostomy because this can cause kinking, volvulus, and obstruction. Mesenteric closure can be performed with 2-0 absorbable suture material in a simple continuous pattern by suturing the mesentery adjacent to the ileum across the ileal "stump" to the ileocecal fold, then suturing the mesentery to the ileocecal fold to the level of the jejunocecostomy. The mesentery adjacent to the jejunum forming the anastomosis can be sutured across the blind end (side-to-side technique) to the cecum. The redundant mesentery can then be sutured together as for a jejunojejunostomy.

Ileocecostomy and ileocolostomy

Ileocecostomies are performed to bypass the distal ileum or ileocecal orifice without resection. The selected site is draped and the flow of ingesta is temporarily restricted. A side-to-side anastomosis is performed as described for the jejunocecostomy. Closure of the lumen of the ileum distal to the anastomosis with staples that do not interfere with mesenteric vessels to prevent accumulation of ingesta between the anastomosis and ileocecal orifice can be performed based on surgeon experience.

A jejuno- or ileocolostomy is performed to bypass the cecum. The procedure is performed similarly to a jejuno- or ileocecostomy with a stapled or handsewn side-to-side anastomosis created between the antimesenteric border of the jejunum or ileum and the right ventral colon between the medial and lateral free band. A complete or incomplete bypass can be performed. A complete bypass involves transecting the jejunum/ileum between the cecum and the anastomosis site. Transection should be performed adjacent to the anastomosis to prevent formation of a blind pocket.

Large colon resection and anastomosis

Large colon resection is performed most commonly to prevent recurrence of colonic displacements or volvulus and when colonic viability is in question in patients with a large colon volvulus. Importantly, when performing a colon resection in patients with a volvulus, the resection and anastomosis are often not performed in healthy tissue.

End-to-end or side-to-side large colon anastomosis can be performed and is based on surgeon preference. The colon should be exteriorized and emptied through a pelvic flexure enterotomy (p. 190) prior to resection and anastomosis. Care should be taken to avoid leaving excessive fluid in the right colons, because it can cause excessive contamination at the time of resection and anastomosis. Careful draping with laparotomy sponges and drapes should be performed to isolate the site of the resection and anastomosis from the abdomen because the surgeon is often resecting as much large colon as possible and will be very close to the abdominal incision. The right dorsal colon is anastomosed to the right ventral colon.

End-to-end technique
The most difficult aspect of performing an end-to-end anastomosis is the disparity of lumen size between the dorsal and ventral colons. The dorsal colon should be transected on an angle to minimize this disparity (Figure 16.25). An incision can be created along the antimesenteric aspect of the dorsal colon to further increase the circumference. The colon has a tendency to retract into the abdomen following resection and care should be taken to ensure that the colon remains exteriorized and abdominal contamination is avoided; it is advisable to perform the resection with ample colon remaining to avoid abdominal contamination. Closure of the anastomosis is with two layers using 0 synthetic absorbable suture material in a full thickness simple continuous pattern oversewn with a Cushing or Lembert pattern (Figure 16.26).

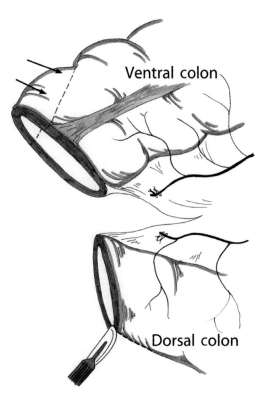

Figure 16.25 Schematic illustration of an end-to-end large colon anastomosis addressing disparity in size with either a fish-mouth incision along the antimesenteric aspect of the dorsal colon, or removal and closure of an antimesenteric section of the ventral colon (arrows).

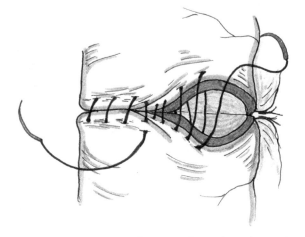

Figure 16.26 Schematic illustration of a two layer closure of large colon end-to-end anastomosis using a full thickness simple continuous pattern oversewn with a Cushing pattern interrupted at 180°.

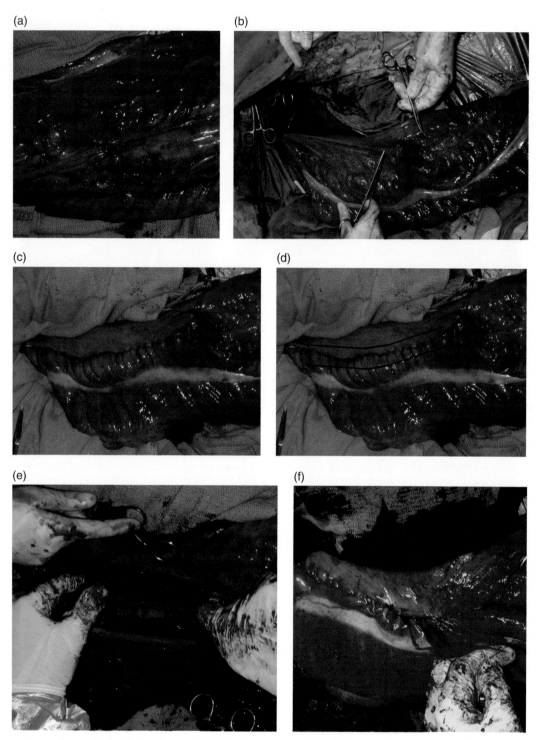

Figure 16.27   Side-to-side large colon resection and anastomosis showing (a) vessel ligation, (b) placement of stay sutures between the right dorsal and ventral colon, (c) suturing the first layer of the three-layer anastomosis, (d) site for stab incisions and placement of ILA-100 in the right dorsal and ventral colons, if a stapling technique is to be used, (e) creation of the enterotomy to form an anastomosis between the dorsal and ventral colons. Closure of this layer is by using a full-thickness simple continuous pattern interrupted at 180° at the proximal and distal aspects of the anastomosis. (f) suturing the third layer using a Cushing pattern (oversewing the full-thickness simple continuous layer),

(g)   (h)

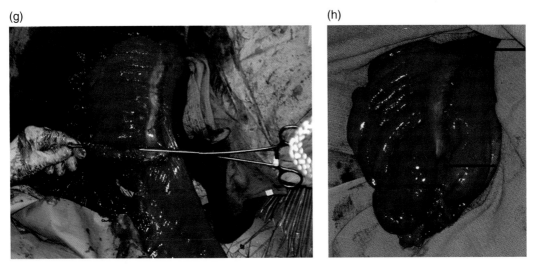

Figure 16.27 (cont'd)   (g) resection of the right ventral colon using noncrushing clamps and a simple continuous pattern on the cut edges that is oversewn with a Cushing pattern (the dorsal colon is similarly resected), and (h) completed large colon resection and anastomosis with arrows indicating site of anastomosis.

The two layers are interrupted at 180° to prevent a purse-string effect.[7,26] Suturing the mesocolic border of the colon can be challenging and it is critical to ensure that the intestinal wall and not the mesocolon is included in each suture placement; the mesocolic aspect of the Lembert or Cushing pattern should be performed initially followed by apposition of the cut edges of the dorsal and ventral colons. The antimesocolic border can then be oversewn. The main advantage of this technique is that the size of the anastomosis does not decrease with time; however, it can be more technically difficult to perform.

Side-to-side anastomosis

Performing the anastomosis prior to resection facilitates extensive large colon resection and anastomosis (Figure 16.27). Stay sutures are placed in the right ventral (RVC) and right dorsal colons (RDC) approximately 30–35 cm apart, immediately adjacent to the vessel ligation site. A 25–30 cm simple continuous suture line using #0 absorbable suture material is placed between the RDC and RVC, a 15–25 cm stoma is created using either hand-sewn or stapled (ILA-100, US Surgical Corporation) techniques and the anastomosis is completed by over sewing the suture or staple line with a simple continuous suture. If the colon is edematous, staples

cannot be used to perform the anastomosis. The resection is performed by occluding the lumen of the RVC and RDC using either Doyen or modified Sullins-Scudder intestinal clamps, and the RVC followed by RDC are resected either using staples (TA-90 or ILA-100, US Surgical Corporation) or sutures in two layers. A Parker-Kerr suture pattern can be used to reduce contamination during resection. The advantage of a side-to-side technique is that it is technically easier to perform and an extensive part of the colon can be resected; however, the size of the anastomosis can decrease with time and stenosis with recurrence of colic signs can occur.

Small colon resection and anastomosis

Hand sewn end-to-end anastomosis is performed for lesions of the small colon requiring resection. The site of resection is identified, draped, the flow of ingesta is restricted, and the vessels are ligated as described for jejunojejunostomy. Note that the vessels supplying the small colon are parallel to the mesenteric border and not the arcuate vessels of the jejunum. Small colon resections are generally performed in two layers although a one-layer closure has been reported. The first layer can be full thickness or mucosa-submucosa in a simple continuous pattern using 2-0 or 0 synthetic absorbable suture material. The second layer is most often

Table 16.2 Methods for diagnosis and correction of selected lesions.

Lesion	Diagnosis of lesion	Surgical correction of lesion	Procedure
Cecum			
Tympany	Marked gas distension without obstruction of aboral intestine	Remove gas	Needle decompression (p. 189)
Impaction (p. 214)	Fluid—fluidy ingesta within cecum marked cecal distension Ingesta—firm ingesta within cecum with moderate to marked distension	Remove ingesta	Typhlotomy (p. 190) ± Jejuno-/ileocolostomy (p. 194) (based on surgeon preference)
Cecocecal or cecocolic intussusception (p. 214)	Cecal apex cannot be identified or exteriorized during exploration Cecal apex palpable within cecum (cecocecal) or right ventral colon (cecocolic)	Reduction is attempted by messaging intussuscepted cecum while applying gentle traction	Reducible—typhlectomy, if necessary (p. 191) Nonreducible—cecocecal with just tip involved → typhlectomy without reduction; Cecocolic → right ventral colotomy for reduction ± typhlectomy (p. 190–191)
Small intestine			
Strangulating pedunculated lipoma (p. 209)	Trace small intestine in oral direction from ileum until encounter with thin band (stalk of lipoma) encircling the intestine	Isolate and transect stalk (under visual guidance if able to exteriorize) Empty small intestinal contents by milking into cecum or through an enterotomy (particularly if planning jejunocecostomy)	± Enterotomy (p. 191) ± Resection and anastomosis: jejunojejunostomy, jejunoileostomy, or jejunocecostomy (p. 193)
Epiploic foramen entrapment (p. 211)	Trace small intestine in oral direction from ileum until encounter loop going through epiploic foramen (almost always from left to right)	Identify segment on either side of foramen—feed entrapped segment through while applying gentle traction on nonentrapped segment Methods to make reduction easier: push fluid and gas from entrapped intestine through to nonentrapped intestine; squeeze edema out of entrapped intestine; push nonentrapped intestine back through foramen; transect entrapped intestine Avoid pulling up on intestine and tearing portal vein Empty small intestinal contents by milking into cecum or through an enterotomy (p. 191)	± Enterotomy (p. 191) ± Resection and anastomosis: jejunojejunostomy, jejunoileostomy, or jejunocecostomy (p. 193)
Jejunal volvulus (p. 212)	Trace small intestine in an oral direction from ileum until encounter area that is twisted on its mesenteric attachment	Rotate segment of twisted intestine Empty small intestinal contents by milking into cecum or through an enterotomy	± Enterotomy (p. 191) ± Resection and anastomosis: jejunojejunostomy, jejunoileostomy, or jejunocecostomy (p. 193)

Condition	Findings/Diagnosis	Procedure	Surgical options
Mesenteric rent (p. 284)	Trace small intestine orally from ileum until encounter loop going through a tear/rent in the mesentery of the small intestine or small colon	Identify segment on either side of rent—feed entrapped segment through while applying gentle traction on nonentrapped segment If necessary enlarge rent—stretching minimizes risk to mesenteric vessels, but scissors can be used if necessary Empty small intestinal contents by milking into cecum or through an enterotomy	± Enterotomy (p. 191) ± Resection and anastomosis: jejunojejunostomy, jejunoileostomy, or jejunocecostomy (p. 193)

Inguinal herniation (p. 285)	Diagnosis should be made preoperatively combining examination per rectum with scrotal palpation and sonographic evaluation	• Combined ventral and inguinal approach:
		  ○ Identify segment on either side of inguinal ring feed entrapped intestine into abdomen while applying gentle traction on nonentrapped intestine
		  ○ If necessary enlarge inguinal ring with stretching or careful use of scissors
		  ○ Perform abdominal exploration and empty small intestinal contents by milking into cecum or through an enterotomy
		• Inguinal approach can be performed alone if entrapped intestine appears viable and is easily reduced
		• Laparoscopic approach can be used if reduction is easy and intestine is viable
		• Castration is recommended, but testicle saving procedures have been described
			• Combined ventral and inguinal approach:
			  ○ Castration, closure of vaginal tunic, ± closure of external inguinal ring
			  ○ ± Enterotomy (p. 191)
			  ○ ± Resection and anastomosis: jejunojejunostomy (p. 193), jejunoileostomy (p. 193), jejunocecostomy (p. 193)
			• Inguinal approach:
			  ○ Castration, closure of vaginal tunic, ± closure of external inguinal ring
			• Laparoscopic:
			  ○ Castration can be performed with laparoscopic or traditional surgical technique
			  ○ Laparoscopic methods for inguinal ring closure have been described

Ileocecal intussusception (p. 231)	Ileum is found within the cecum when the ileocecal ligament is used to locate the ileum	Reduction is attempted by pushing on the intussuscepted portion of the ileum within the cecum while applying gentle traction to the nonentrapped ileum or jejunum
		
		The small intestine must be emptied either into the cecum (if reducible [not preferred if performing jejunocecostomy] or after bypass if nonreducible) or through an enterotomy
			• Reducible:
			  ○ ± Enterotomy (p. 191)
			  ○ ± Jejunocecostomy (p. 193)
			• Nonreducible:
			  ○ Bypass with jejunocecostomy or ileocecostomy (p. 193)
			  ○ ± Enterotomy (p. 191)

Ileal impaction (p. 208)	Ileum moderately to markedly distended with ingesta	Hydration of the impaction with fluid in the oral small intestine, fluid and/or carboxymethylcellulose injected into the small intestine with a needle, or fluid put in intestine through an enterotomy Hydrated ingesta is then milked into the cecum or emptied through an enterotomy (selected by surgeon's preference if feel manipulation required would be too harmful to ileum) Empty small intestinal contents by milking into cecum or through an enterotomy	± Enterotomy (p. 191)

(Continued)

Table 16.2 (Cont'd)

Lesion	Diagnosis of lesion	Surgical correction of lesion	Procedure
Ileal hypertrophy (p. 130)	Palpation of markedly thickened ileum combined with distension of the oral small intestine and inability to milk contents through the ileocecal orifice	Small intestinal contents should be emptied through an enterotomy prior to bypass or through the anastomosis into the cecum after bypass	Jejunocecostomy (p. 193) ± Enterotomy (p. 191)
Large colon			
Large colon volvulus (p. 220)	Distended large colon rather than cecum is generally the presenting organ Variable discoloration and/or thickening of the large colon A twist of the large colon is found when the large colon is traced from the pelvic flexure toward the dorsal body wall Most often the volvulus is at the level of the cecocolic ligament or base of the colon	Correction is by untwisting the colon (most often requires clockwise rotation) Distension with gas, fluid and ingesta can make untwisting difficult and risk rupture of the colon—needle decompression and/or enterotomy can be used as necessary	Needle decompression (p. 189) and/or enterotomy (p. 190) ± Large colon resection and anastomosis (p. 195)
Right dorsal displacement (p. 220)	Distended large colon rather than cecum is generally the presenting organ When the large colon is traced, a portion is lateral to the cecum and the pelvic flexure is frequently in the cranial abdomen rather than the left caudal abdomen	Correction is by replacing the colon in the correct orientation Distension with gas, fluid, and ingesta can make correction difficult and risk rupture of the colon—needle decompression and/or enterotomy (especially with concurrent right dorsal colon impaction) can be used as necessary	Needle decompression (p. 189) ± Enterotomy (p. 190)

Nephrosplenic or renosplenic entrapment (p. 219)	Distended cecum and large colon are identified upon opening the abdomen
	When the right ventral colon is traced toward the left ventral colon, the colon is found within the nephrosplenic space
		• Ventral approach:
		  ○ The colon is gently moved dorsal and lateral to the spleen until it is in the correct location
		  ○ Phenylephrine can be given intravenously to shrink the spleen and ease correction
		• Laparoscopic correction has been reported
			Needle decompression (p. 189) ± Enterotomy (p. 190)

Intraluminal obstruction (ingesta or sand impaction, enterolith, or fecalith) (p. 217–219)	Distended cecum and large colon are identified upon opening the abdomen
	Palpation of the colon reveals the obstructing material
	Note: enteroliths and fecaliths may not be palpable initially if feed is impacted around them
		• Feed and sand impaction—hydration and evacuation through pelvic flexure enterotomy
		• Enteroliths and fecaliths
		  ○ Surrounding ingesta is hydrated and removed through pelvic flexure enterotomy
		  ○ Lith is moved as far orad (out of abdomen) as possible and removed through a second enterotomy
			• Pelvic flexure enterotomy (p. 190)
			• Pelvic flexure and dorsal colon enterotomy (p. 190)

Transverse colon Intraluminal obstruction (ingesta or sand impaction, enterolith, or fecalith)	Same as intraluminal obstruction of the large colon	Same as intraluminal obstruction of the large colon	Same as intraluminal obstruction of the large colon
Small colon Intraluminal obstruction (ingesta or sand impaction, enterolith, trichophytobezoar, or fecalith) (p. 221)	Distention of the small colon oral to the lesion and progressive distension of the large colon and cecum are identified upon opening the abdomen Palpation of the small colon reveals the obstructing material Feed and sand impactions are long, firm tubes Fecaliths and bezoars may be solitary, rounded, hard obstructions, or hidden within ingesta	• Feed and sand—hydration and evacuation of the contents using a high enema and/or enterotomy • Fecaliths and bezoars—enterotomy over the lesion if can exteriorize; if unable to exteriorize must be moved orally or aborally to a safe location for an enterotomy • The large colon should always be evacuated via a pelvic flexure enterotomy to decrease the likelihood of re-obstruction of the small colon	• Feed and sand—high enema ± small colon enterotomy (p. 191) • Fecaliths and bezoars—enterotomy (p. 191) • ALL—pelvic flexure enterotomy (p. 190)
Pedunculated lipoma (p. 209)	Distension of the oral small colon and progressive distension of the large colon and cecum A thin band (stalk of lipoma) is found encircling a portion of the small colon	Isolate and transect stalk (under visual guidance if able to exteriorize) Consider evacuation of the large colon via a pelvic flexure enterotomy to decrease the likelihood of obstruction at site	± Small colon resection and anastomosis (p. 197) ± Pelvic flexure enterotomy (p. 190)
Urogenital tract Uterine torsion (p. 282)	Diagnosis can generally be made preoperatively based on examination per rectum At surgery, a twist in the uterine body and tightened broad ligaments of the uterus confirm the diagnosis	• Ventral approach—untwist the uterus using a rocking motion; fluid within the abdomen can help "float" the uterus and make untwisting easier • Lateral approach—enter abdomen on side uterus is twisting toward (right for clockwise from behind and left for counterclockwise from behind); untwist the uterus using a rocking motion	
Cystolith	Diagnosis made palpation per rectum of emptied bladder and cystoscopy	• Parainguinal approach or caudal midline—removal through cystotomy • Laparoscopic cystotomy has been described	Cystotomy

a Cushing or Lembert pattern.[25] Mesocolon defects should be closed with 2-0 absorbable suture in a simple continuous pattern.

Colopexy

Colopexy is performed to create an adhesion between the colon and the ventral body wall to prevent recurrence of large colon displacement and volvulus. It is most often performed in broodmares.[11] The lateral free tenial band of the left ventral colon (35 cm) is sutured to the ventral abdominal wall 6 cm to the left of midline using #2 polypropylene suture material in an interrupted or continuous pattern.[11] An incision is made through the parietal peritoneum and retroperitoneal fat to ensure appropriate suture placement to prevent breakdown during recovery from general anesthesia.[11] Care must be taken to avoid penetrating the bowel lumen. Complications include weight loss, abdominal pain, dehiscence, catastrophic colonic rupture, and fistulous tracts associated with suture penetration of the colonic lumen.[11]

Diagnosis and correction of selected specific conditions

A brief summary of methods for diagnosis and correction of selected conditions is shown in Table 16.2. Quizzes for each chapter, additional clinical scenarios, and video demonstrations of surgical procedures are available online at www.wiley.com/go/southwood.

References

1. Anderson, S.L., Vacek, J.R., Macharg, M.A. & Holtkamp, D.J. (2011) Occurrence of incisional complications and associated risk factors using a right ventral paramedian celiotomy incision in 159 horses. *Veterinary Surgery*, **40**, 82–89.
2. Busschers, E., Southwood, L.L. & Parente, E.J. (2007) Laparoscopic diagnosis and correction of a nephrosplenic entrapment of the large colon in a horse. *Equine Veterinary Education*, **19**, 60–63.
3. Budras, K., Sack, W.O. & Rock, S. (2003) *Anatomy of the Horse: An Illustrated Text*, 4th edn. Schlutersche, Hannover, Germany.
4. Coomer, R.P., Mair, T.S., Edwards, G.B. & Proudman, C.J. (2007) Do subcutaneous sutures increase risk of laparotomy wound suppuration? *Equine Veterinary Journal*, **39**, 396–399.
5. Desmaizieres, L.M., Martinot, S., Lepage, O.M., Bareiss, E. & Cadoré, J.L. (2003) Complications associated with cannula insertion techniques used for laparoscopy in standing horses. *Veterinary Surgery*, **32**, 501–506.
6. Dyce, K.M., Sack, W.O. & Wensing, C.J.G. (1996) *Textbook of Veterinary Anatomy*, 2nd edn. W.B. Saunders Company, Philadelphia, Pennsylvania.
7. Ellis, C.M., Lynch, T.M., Slone, D.E., Hughes, F.E. & Clark, C.K. (2008) Survival and complications after large colon resection and end-to-end anastomosis for strangulating large colon volvulus in seventy-three horses. *Veterinary Surgery*, **37**, 786–790.
8. Fick, J.L., Novo, R.E. & Kirchhof, N. (2005) Comparison of gross and histologic tissue responses of skin incisions closed by use of absorbable subcuticular staples, cutaneous metal staples, and polyglactin 910 suture in pigs. *American Journal of Veterinary Research*, **66**, 1975–1984.
9. Freeman, D.E. (2006) Small intestine. In: *Equine Surgery* (eds J.A. Auer & J.A. Stick), 3rd edn., pp. 401–436. Saunders Elsevier, St. Louis, Missouri.
10. Galuppo, L.D. (2002) Laparoscopic anatomy. In: *Equine Diagnostic and Surgical Laparoscopy* (ed A.T.J. Fischer). W.B. Saunders Company, Philadelphia, Pennsylvania.
11. Hance, S.R. & Embertson, R.M. (1992) Colopexy in broodmares: 44 cases (1986–1990). *Journal of the American Veterinary Medical Association*, **201**, 782–787.
12. Hassel, D.M. & Ragle, C.A. (1994) Laparoscopic diagnosis and conservative treatment of uterine tear in a mare. *Journal of the American Veterinary Medical Association*, **205**, 1531–1536.
13. Hendrickson, D.A. (2008) Complications of laparoscopic surgery. *Veterinary Clinics of North America: Equine Practice*, **24**, 557–571.
14. Hopster, K., Kastner, S.B.R., Rohn, K. & Ohnesorge, B. (2011) Intermittent positive pressure ventilation with constant positive end-expiratory pressure and alveolar recruitment manoeuvre during inhalation anaesthesia in horses undergoing surgery for colic, and its influence on the early recovery period. *Veterinary Anaesthesia and Analgesia*, **38**, 169–177.
15. Hubert, J.D., Hardy, J., Holcombe, S.J. & Moore, R.M. (2000) Cecal amputation within the right ventral colon for surgical treatment of nonreducible cecocolic intussusception in 8 horses. *Veterinary Surgery*, **29**, 317–325.
16. Hughes, F.E. & Slone, D. (1997) Large colon resection. *Veterinary Clinics of North America: Equine Practice*, **13**, 341–350.
17. Hughes, F.E. & Slone, D.E. (1998) A modified technique for extensive large colon resection and anastomosis in horses. *Veterinary Surgery*, **27**, 127–131.
18. Klohnen, A. & Panizzin, L. (2008) Incisional complications after right paramedian celiotomy in horses

with colic: 57 cases (2002–2005). In: *Proceedings of the 9th International Equine Colic Research Symposium*, Liverpool, U.K.

19. Klohnen, A., Lores, M. & Fischer, A.T.J. (2008) Management of post operative abdominal incisional complications with a hernia belt: 85 horses (2001–2005). In: *Proceedings of the 9th International Equine Colic Research Symposium*, Liverpool, U.K.

20. Koenig, J., McDonell, W. & Valverde, A. (2003) Accuracy of pulse oximetry and capnography in healthy and compromised horses during spontaneous and controlled ventilation. *Canadian Journal of Veterinary Research*, **67**, 169–174.

21. Lansdowne, J.L., Boure, L.P., Pearce, S.G., Kerr, C.L. & Caswell, J.L. (2004) Comparison of two laparoscopic treatments for experimentally induced abdominal adhesions in pony foals. *American Journal of Veterinary Research*, **65**, 681–686.

22. Mair, T.S. & Smith, L.J. (2005) Survival and complication rates in 300 horses undergoing surgical treatment of colic. Part 2: Short-term complications. *Equine Veterinary Journal*, **37**, 303–309.

23. Mendez-Angulo, J.L., Ernst, N.S. & Mudge, M.C. (2010) Clinical assessment and outcome of a single-layer technique for anastomosis of the small intestine in horses. *Veterinary Record*, **167**, 652–655.

24. Nieto, J.E., Dechant, J.E. & Snyder, J.R. (2006) Comparison of one-layer (continuous Lembert) versus two-layer (simple continuous/Cushing) hand-sewn end-to-end anastomosis in equine jejunum. *Veterinary Surgery*, **35**, 669–673.

25. Prange, T., Holcombe, S.J., Brown, J.A., *et al.* (2010) Resection and anastomosis of the descending colon in 43 horses. *Veterinary Surgery*, **39**, 748–753.

26. Rakestraw, P.C. & Hardy, J. (2006) Large intestine. In: *Equine Surgery* (eds J.A. Auer & J.A. Stick), 3rd edn., pp. 436–478. Saunders Elsevier, St. Louis, Missouri.

27. Ranaboldo, C.J. & Rowe-Jones, D.C. (1992) Closure of laparotomy wounds: Skin staples versus sutures. *British Journal of Surgery*, **79**, 1172–1173.

28. Rosser, J., Brounts, S., Slone, D., *et al.* (2011) Pelvic flexure enterotomy closure using a TA-90 stapling device: A retrospective study of 85 horses. In: *Proceedings of the 10th International Colic Research Symposium*, Indianapolis, Indiana, pp. 186–187.

29. Rumbaugh, M.L., Burba, D.J., Natalini, C., Hosgood, G. & Moore, R.M. (2003) Evaluation of a vessel-sealing device for small intestinal resection and anastomosis in normal horses. *Veterinary Surgery*, **32**, 574–579.

30. Smith, L.J., Mellor, D.J., Marr, C.M., Reid, S.W. & Mair, T.S. (2007) Incisional complications following exploratory celiotomy: Does an abdominal bandage reduce the risk? *Equine Veterinary Journal*, **39**, 277–283.

31. Sylvestre, A., Wilson, J. & Hare, J. (2002) A comparison of 2 different suture patterns for skin closure of canine ovariohysterectomy. *Canadian Veterinary Journal*, **43**, 699–702.

32. Theoret, C.L. (2006) Wound repair. In: *Equine Surgery* (eds J.A. Auer & J.A. Stick), 3rd edn. Elsevier, St. Louis, Missouri.

33. Torfs, S., Levet, T., Delesalle, C., *et al.* (2010) Risk factors for incisional complications after exploratory celiotomy in horses: Do skin staples increase the risk? *Veterinary Surgery*, **39**, 616–620.

34. Zedler, S.T., Embertson, R.M., Bernard, W.V., Barr, B.S. & Boston, R.C. (2009) Surgical treatment of gastric outflow obstruction in 40 foals. *Veterinary Surgery*, **38**, 623–630.

17

Specific Causes of Colic

Eileen S. Hackett

Department of Clinical Sciences, Colorado State University, Fort Collins, CO, USA

Chapter Outline

Gastric diseases	**205**	
Gastric ulceration	205	
Gastric impaction	205	
Gastric rupture	206	
Small intestinal disease	**207**	
Inflammatory disease	207	
Proximal enteritis	207	
Simple obstruction	208	
Ileal impaction	208	
Ascarid impaction	208	
Functional obstruction	209	
Equine grass sickness	209	
Strangulating obstruction	209	
Strangulating pedunculated lipoma	209	
Epiploic foramen entrapment	211	
Gastrosplenic ligament entrapment	211	
Jejunal volvulus	212	
Meckel's diverticulum	212	
Mesodiverticular band	213	
Jejunal intussusception	213	
Ileocecal intussusception	213	

Cecal disease	**214**
Cecal impaction	214
Cecocolic intussusception	214
Cecal perforation	215
Large (ascending) colon disease	**215**
Inflammatory disease	215
Colitis	215
Right dorsal colitis	216
Simple obstruction	217
Impaction	217
Sand enteropathy	217
Enterolithiasis	218
Nephrosplenic ligament entrapment	219
Right dorsal displacement	220
Strangulating obstruction	220
Large colon volvulus	220
Small (descending) colon disease	**221**
Impaction	221
Mesenteric rent	222
Meconium retention	222
Neoplasia	**223**

Practical Guide to Equine Colic, First Edition. Edited by Louise L. Southwood.
© 2013 John Wiley & Sons, Inc. Published 2013 by John Wiley & Sons, Inc.

Colic is a nonspecific term for abdominal pain. In horses, colic is most often caused by gastrointestinal disease and is often categorized by the affected region and whether the lesion results in intestinal ischemia. Familiarization with specific causes of colic and associated clinical signs allows the veterinarian to establish a coherent list of differential diagnoses and select the appropriate treatments. It should be recognized that the most common cause of colic is "gas or spasmodic colic" with the majority of horses responding to basic medical management (p. 45). Early recognition of the cause of colic and appropriate treatment will likely improve outcome. Several causes of colic can and should be managed medically. It is important to recognize that despite the inability to detect the specific cause of colic prior to surgery, the type of lesion and need for surgery can be identified (see Chapter 15 on Medical versus Surgical Treatment of the Horse with Colic [p. 164].

Gastric diseases

Gastric ulceration

Gastric ulceration is highly prevalent in mature horses, occurring in 60–90% of horses evaluated in some studies.[3,101] Gastric ulcer syndrome is most commonly reported in horses undergoing intense exercise such as racing and showing.[57,96,145] Gastric ulceration within the squamous epithelial regions is thought to be due to overexposure with gastric acid. Ulceration within the glandular mucosal regions is thought to be due to inadequate protective mechanisms. Ulcers are more commonly found in the squamous epithelium, adjacent to the margo plicatus and the lesser curvature, than the glandular mucosa.[32] Gastric ulceration can result in decreased performance, inappetence, and poor body condition.[32,100] Gastric ulceration can also be a primary source of colic signs, even if the degree of ulceration is not severe. Diets composed of alfalfa hay and grain have been associated with higher gastric pH and a lower number and severity of nonglandular squamous gastric lesions than diets composed of bromegrass hay.[102]

Secondary gastric ulceration has been documented in horses hospitalized for abdominal pain due to primary lesions of the intestinal tract;

the prevalence of gastric ulceration in horses presenting with abdominal pain was nearly 50%.[33] A second study indicated that gastric ulceration is a frequent occurrence in horses hospitalized both for colic and for other medical conditions.[110]

Gastric ulceration is diagnosed using a flexible videoendoscope. A 3 m endoscope will allow complete examination of the stomach and pyloric outflow in most adults and a shorter endoscope may be used in foals. Adult horses should be fasted for 8–12 h or longer to evacuate ingesta prior to examination. Endoscopy allows distention with room air and direct visibility of the gastric mucosal surface. Horses are typically sedated for ease of examination. Care should be taken to evacuate insufflated air following examination to prevent discomfort.

Treatment of gastric ulceration includes antacids, H_2-receptor antagonists, proton pump inhibitors, and surface binding agents. Daily oral dosing of omeprazole, a proton pump inhibitor, has been shown to effectively treat and prevent gastric ulceration in horses.[12] Prognosis is generally good to excellent. Rarely horses and foals will develop a perforating gastric ulcer (p. 206). Foals can also develop pyloric or duodenal stenosis creating a gastric outflow obstruction secondary to gastroduodenal ulceration and inflammation (p. 280).[151] Clinical signs with this syndrome typically include bruxism, ptyalism, colic, and spontaneous reflux.[151] Diagnosis based on clinical signs can be confirmed with contrast radiography (p. 158). Treatment is supportive and when medical treatment is unsuccessful, gastrojejunostomy is necessary to bypass the stenosed pylorus-duodenum.[151]

Gastric impaction

Gastric impaction is defined as excess feed material confined to the stomach. Feed may dehydrate with acute or chronic delayed gastric emptying and hypodypsea.[17] Type of feed, improper mastication, and eating behaviors are implicated in formation of gastric impactions.[28] In addition, gastric impaction can be composed of poorly digestible ingested material such as persimmon seeds, mesquite beans, or large quantities of beet pulp.[28,71,78,81] Gastric impaction secondary to consumption of *Senecio jacobaea* or ragwort has been reported.[98] Horses with gastric impaction may display moderate to severe signs of colic.[9] Concurrent gastric impaction can exacerbate colic severity in horses with another primary lesion. It may be difficult to completely place the tube in the stomach or confirm that the stomach has been reached upon nasogastric intubation in horses with gastric impaction (p. 43). Transcutaneous sonography (p. 130) is a noninvasive method to identify gastric distention when nasogastric intubation is unsuccessful.[91] Gastric impactions may be visible by endoscopy if the size of the impaction does not prevent passage of the endoscope through the cardia. Impactions due to persimmon phytobezoars have been documented via gastric endoscopy.[81]

Gastric impaction is often definitively diagnosed during exploratory celiotomy, although it is rarely the primary lesion in this instance. Gastric impactions can be easily palpated through the gastric wall at surgery and are often associated with gas distention due to fermentation and delayed emptying. Occasionally, intraoperative gastric decompression using a needle and suction (p. 189) is necessary to relieve distention of the stomach wall, especially if a prolonged anesthetic recovery is anticipated. During decompression, gastric vessels should be avoided and care should be taken to prevent leakage of gastric contents into the peritoneal cavity. Although reported, gastrotomy and evacuation are rarely necessary to resolve gastric impaction and should be avoided in most cases as the stomach is poorly accessible at surgery and risk of contamination is high.[81,103] Intraoperative gastric lavage via nasogastric tube combined with external gastric massage has also been used successfully to resolve impactions.[71] Intraoperative transmural injection of saline or water into the site of gastric impaction has been reported to be an effective treatment.[9]

Conservative treatment of gastric impaction confirmed at surgery or suspected based on physical examination consists of warm water gastric lavage every 2–3h for 8–12h in the standing horse with a large bore nasogastric tube. Resolution of the impaction is likely when feed material is no longer readily lavaged through the nasogastric tube. The veterinarian must decide in individual cases that are treated with gastric lavage, whether to leave the nasogastric tube indwelling or repeatedly pass the tube for each lavage. Risks associated with indwelling nasogastric tubes include pharyngeal trauma, esophageal rupture, and delayed gastric emptying (p. 44).[27,60] If the gastric impaction is left untreated, horses are at risk for gastric rupture. Successful resolution of gastric impaction may be confirmed endoscopically.[71]

Gastric rupture

Complete gastric rupture in mature horses is the most common source of gastrointestinal perforation and is typically fatal. Although occasionally horses develop spontaneous nasogastric reflux of fluid, most horses with severe gastric distention are at risk of gastric rupture. Gastric distention can be primary, as in cases of grain overload or gastric impaction, or secondary to reflux of fluid from the small intestinal tract due to obstruction, inflammatory conditions, or ileus. The latter is more common. Idiopathic gastric rupture can occur.[83,137] Horses may present for gastric rupture as a primary emergency, or develop gastric rupture in the postoperative recovery period following exploratory celiotomy. In postoperative colic patients receiving analgesia and supportive care, tachycardia, inappetence, dull mentation, and colic are the primary clinical signs of gastric distention which can result in gastric rupture without appropriate treatment. Therefore, in the postoperative period, care should be taken to maintain gastric decompression and monitor for signs of distention by transcutaneous sonography (p. 130) or periodic nasogastric intubation (p. 38) in horses at risk.

Clinical signs of gastric rupture include tachycardia, tachypnea, sweating, abdominal distention, and hyperemic or cyanotic mucous membranes. Horses with gastric rupture may have nasogastric reflux when intubated (p. 42).[137] Pneumoperitoneum is typically evident during examination per rectum (p. 36). Another sign of intestinal perforation is a gritty feel to the visceral serosal surfaces palpated per rectum. Horses with gastric rupture are typically hemoconcentrated and hypochloremic.[137] Trancutaneous abdominal sonographic examination will reveal excess free abdominal fluid consistent with peritoneal effusion (p. 133). Peritoneal fluid is exudative and

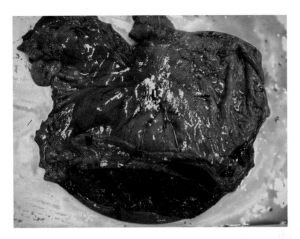

Figure 17.1 Postmortem image from an 18-year-old Quarter Horse mare with spontaneous gastric rupture secondary to gastric impaction. The site of rupture is along the greater curvature with marked reddening and hemorrhage evident from the site of perforation.

altered in appearance. Analysis reflects elevations in total protein, nucleated cell count, and neutrophil to mononuclear ratio. Peritoneal fluid cell counts may be lower than expected due to lysis upon exposure to gastric contents with low pH.[83] Plant material and intra- or extracellular bacteria may also be visible on peritoneal fluid evaluation (p. 90).

Gastric rupture typically occurs along the greater curvature of the stomach (Figure 17.1), although it can occur rarely between the greater and lesser curvature or on the lesser curvature.[137] Gross pathologic evidence of antemortem rupture, such as hemorrhage at the tear site and serosal inflammation of adjacent viscera, can assist in distinguishing this from postmortem rupture.

Humane euthanasia is indicated for adult horses with complete gastric perforation. Occasionally, exploratory celiotomy is performed to confirm gastric rupture prior to euthanasia. Although often fatal, a case report documenting the repair of complete gastric rupture in an adult horse opens the possibility of repair if surgery is attempted prior to gross contamination of the peritoneal cavity with ingesta and if the site of gastric tear is accessible.[70] Successful surgical treatment of a partial gastric rupture, affecting only the seromuscular portion of the gastric wall, has been reported.[14,130] In

foals, surgical repair for acute complete gastric perforation may be successful.[108]

Small intestinal disease

Inflammatory disease

Proximal enteritis

Proximal enteritis (PE), also known as anterior enteritis or duodenitis-proximal jejunitis (DPJ), is an inflammatory disorder of the small intestine. The specific etiology of PE is unknown. Multiple infectious (e.g., *Salmonella* spp. and *Clostridium* spp.) and toxic agents have been associated with some cases of PE, but diagnosis of a consistent causative agent has been elusive.[8,24] Incidence has been associated with feeding practices. In one study, horses with PE were more likely to consume a diet high in concentrates and pasture graze.[24]

Presenting signs include abdominal pain, dull mentation, endotoxemia, and fever or history of fever. PE is associated with copious nasogastric reflux. Compressible small intestinal loops are often palpable per rectum (p. 27). Abdominal sonographic examination (p. 128) may reveal variably distended small intestinal loops with normal wall thickness. Sixty-eight percent of horses with PE develop gastric ulceration within 24h of hospitalization.[33] Horses with PE can be distinguished from those with a mechanical small intestinal obstruction because they typically have a dull mentation rather than overt colic signs; greater quantity of nasogastric reflux particularly early in the course of the disease; lower degree of abdominal pain; and less tightly distended small intestinal loops palpable per rectum.[76] Peritoneal fluid of horses with PE tends to be yellow-orange with a very high total protein and relatively normal nucleated cell count. By contrast, a horse with a strangulating obstruction will often have serosanguinous peritoneal fluid with an increased total protein and nucleated cell count.

Treatment of PE involves frequent gastric decompression (p. 38), intravenous (IV) fluid therapy (p. 99), antiendotoxic therapy (p. 246), and supportive care. Food, water, and enteral medication should be restricted until intestinal function returns. See also Chapter 18 on Postoperative

Patient Care (p. 230) and Chapter 23 on Nutrition (p. 301).

Surgical treatment is occasionally pursued for this disease if the diagnosis is not definitive (Clinical scenario 10, located in Appendix A), if horses respond poorly to medical treatment, or if the attending veterinarian believes surgical decompression may shorten the course of disease. At surgery, the affected portions of the intestine appear grossly edematous, hemorrhagic, and may have yellow discoloration.[147] In a recent study comparing medical and surgical treatment of PE, 25% of horses ceased refluxing postoperatively. However, an overall benefit of surgery could not be demonstrated and horses undergoing surgical treatment for PE had a higher mortality most likely because surgical treatment was associated with more severe disease.[140]

Overall survival for horses suffering from PE is reported to be 66–87%.[124,140] Admission anion gap of ≥15.0 mEq/L and peritoneal fluid total protein ≥3.5 g/dL were associated with death in a study investigating prognostic indices for horses with PE.[124] Approximately one third of horses with PE developed laminitis in one report.[21] The presence of hemorrhagic nasogastric reflux and body weight ≥550 kg were risk factors for laminitis in this population.[21]

Simple obstruction

Ileal impaction

Ileal impaction occurs when coarse ingesta within the ileum causes a nonstrangulating obstruction. Feeding of Coastal Bermuda grass hay and tapeworm (*Anoplocephala perfoliata* [p. 318]) infection are identified risk factors for development of ileal impaction.[88]

Clinical signs in horses with ileal impaction initially include moderate colic pain, tachycardia, and decreased or absent ausculted gastrointestinal motility associated with intestinal spasm at the site of impaction.[88] The firm ileal impaction may be palpated on examination per rectum early in the disease process (p. 28).[58] With progression, generalized small intestinal distention becomes detectable on palpation per rectum (p. 27) and abdominal

sonographic examination (p. 128), and nasogastric reflux develops (p. 38).

Medical treatment of horses with ileal impaction includes IV analgesic (p. 51) and fluid therapy (p. 99). Laxatives (p. 47, 66) are administered via nasogastric tube if no reflux is present. If the horse has signs of nasogastric reflux, periodic gastric decompression may be needed.[58] Medical treatment should be pursued if the horse has, pain responsive to analgesia, no reflux, or if surgery is not a treatment option.[58] Surgical intervention may be recommended if the small intestine is persistently distended oral to the site of impaction rather than diminishing in size over time.[58] Surgical treatment most often involves manual external massage of the ileum in the area of the impaction and admixing of intestinal fluids oral to the impaction site prior to reduction of the small intestinal contents into the cecum.[59] Infiltration of the impaction site with saline, sodium carboxymethylcellulose, or dioctyl sodium succinate may be necessary to facilitate breakdown of the impaction. An enterotomy (p. 191) may be necessary. Rarely, horses with recurrent ileal impaction or ileal pathology, such as muscular hypertrophy or stricture, require a jejunocecostomy (p. 193) in addition to routine reduction of the impaction.[88] Prognosis following surgical reduction of ileal impaction is improved with early intervention and if intestinal bypass can be avoided.[37,59]

To aid in prevention of ileal impaction, treatment with praziquantel or pyrantel salts effective against *Anoplocephala perfoliata* infection is recommended (p. 318). Limiting feeding of Coastal Bermuda hay and poor quality hay high in lignin content may decrease the incidence of ileal impaction.[59]

Ascarid impaction

The gastrointestinal parasite *Parascaris equorum* (p. 321) has been associated with small intestinal luminal obstruction in foals. Impaction is usually seen in foals ages 3–4 months up to 1 year, prior to development of immunity to this parasite.[20] Affected foals are exposed at a young age. Risk of ascarid impaction is higher in foals with large worm burdens following anthelmintic administration. The site of ascarid impaction is typically the duodenum and proximal jejunum and is associated with clinical signs of proximal gastrointestinal obstruction such as small intestinal dilation and nasogastric reflux. Ascarids may be evident within the nasogastric reflux or feces. Ascarid impaction may obstruct the intestinal lumen, or may result in obstruction complicated by intussusception or volvulus.[26] Heavy worm burdens may predispose to intestinal rupture. Although the small intestine is most often affected by ascarid impaction, masses of ascarids can accumulate in the stomach and large intestine.[122]

Treatment of ascarid impaction may be medical if the obstruction is incomplete. If the ascarid impaction results in complete obstruction, surgical reduction can be attempted. Impactions are resolved with manual reduction with or without typhlotomy, small intestinal enterotomy at the site of impaction, or resection of devitalized intestinal segments. In most cases, prognosis following surgical correction is guarded particularly in foals < 1 year old.[122] A recent study, however, documented a 64% short-term and 27% long-term survival in surgically corrected simple and complicated obstructions, with death primarily due to development of abdominal adhesions and concurrent intestinal dysfunction.[26]

Prevention of ascariasis has become more difficult as regional resistance to macrocyclic lactones (ivermectin, moxidectin) and pyrimidine (pyrantel pamoate) has been recognized.[15,86,87,92] Benzimidazoles (oxybendazole, fenbendazole) and heterocyclic compounds (piperazine) are currently the most effective treatments against ascarids in young horses.[68,92,112] Fecal analysis of young horses may indicate whether their current deworming program is effective. Due to the poor prognosis associated with ascarid impaction, it is recommended that foals <1 year of age be treated with anthelmintics known to be regionally effective against *Parascaris equorum*. Along with regular deworming beginning at 6–8 weeks of age, foals should be enrolled in a fecal surveillance program.[26] See Chapter 24 on Gastrointestinal Parasitology and Anthelmintics (p. 321).

Functional obstruction

Equine grass sickness

Equine grass sickness (equine dysautonomia) is a polyneuropathy of the central and peripheral nervous systems with the most frequent occurrence in Great Britain and Western European countries.[149] It is not considered a cause of colic in the United States. The exact etiology is unknown; however, a toxicoinfectious form of botulism caused by *Clostridium botulinum* type C is thought to be the most likely cause.[149] Horses with acute grass sickness show signs of colic with rapid development of clinical signs. Gastric and small intestinal distention progresses to cecal and colonic obstruction with dehydrated ingesta.[149] At surgery, there is generalized small intestinal distention without a mechanical obstruction. Diagnosis of equine grass sickness is made based on histological finding of chromatolytic changes of autonomic neurons from an ileal biopsy obtained during exploratory celiotomy or at necropsy.[149] Acute equine grass sickness is most often fatal. Prevention includes (1) avoiding dietary changes during spring, (2) offering grazing animals supplementary forage, (3) avoiding disturbing pasture, and (4) tolerating low-level parasitism and avoiding overuse of anthelmintics.[149]

Strangulating obstruction

Strangulating pedunculated lipoma

Strangulating pedunculated lipomas are fatty tumors most commonly associated with the small intestinal mesentery. Lipomas are benign and slow growing, yet as they grow in size and weight, their mesenteric attachments elongate forming a stalk.[35] Lipomas on a stalk may then encircle adjacent segments of small intestine or small colon and result in strangulating obstruction. The risk of developing intestinal strangulation from a pedunculated lipoma increases as the horse ages, with most cases seen in horses >15 years old.[44]

Clinical signs are consistent with strangulating obstruction and include persistent signs of abdominal pain or dull demeanor, tachycardia, nasogastric reflux (p. 38), and decreased intestinal motility.

(a)

(b)

(c)

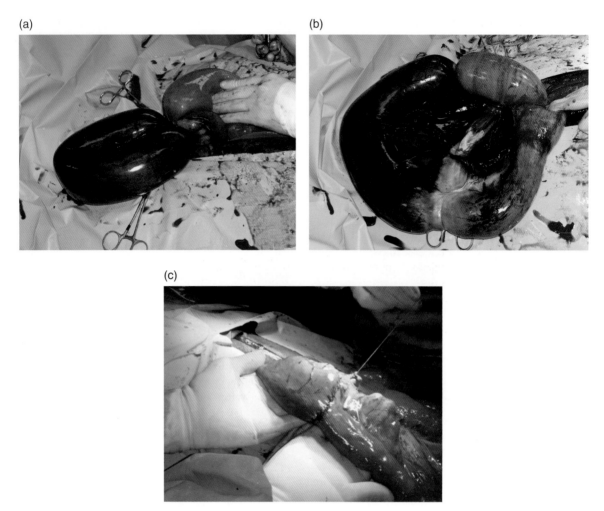

Figure 17.2   (a) Intraoperative photograph of a lipoma which has strangulated a short segment of jejunum. The affected jejunal segment has undergone hemorrhagic ischemia and is no longer viable. (b) Lipoma stalk has been transected. (c) The affected bowel is resected and a jejunojejunostomy performed.

Peritoneal fluid (p. 87) is typically serosanguinous, with elevations in nucleated cell count and total protein. Peritoneal fluid lactate higher than plasma lactate concentration at admission as well as an increase in peritoneal fluid over time may be useful for early identification of a strangulating obstruction.

Treatment consists of transection of the lipoma stalk using blunt dissection, Metzenbaum scissors, or an LDS stapling device (US Surgical Corporation) (Figure 17.2). The strangulating lipoma is often deep within the abdominal cavity necessitating blind transaction of the stalk, or if accessible, it may be exteriorized and the stalk transected.[13] Intestinal viability is assessed based on gross appearance of the strangulated segment. Rarely, the intestinal segment involved in the strangulation has limited vascular compromise and does not require resection. Jejunojejunostomy, jejunoileostomy, or jejuno-cecostomy (p. 193) is usually necessary. Horses with less severe illness and disease confined to the jejunal intestinal segment have a better prognosis following surgical correction.[48] Prognosis for survival is generally good (80–85%).

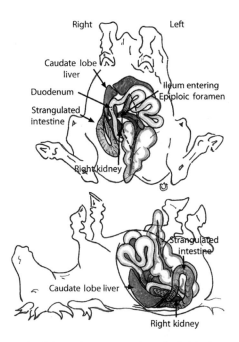

Figure 17.3 Schematic representation of epiploic foramen entrapment.

Epiploic foramen entrapment

The epiploic foramen is a 4–6 cm slit-shaped opening, separating the abdominal cavity from the omental bursa, through which small intestine can pass and become entrapped (Figure 17.3).[4] Incarceration of colonic intestinal segments within the epiploic foramen is rarely reported.[41,131] The anatomic boundaries of the epiploic foramen are the caudate lobe of the liver and caudal vena cava dorsally, and the right lobe of the pancreas, gastropancreatic fold, and portal vein ventrally.[4] A small intestinal segment can enter the epiploic foramen forming an epiploic foramen entrapment (EFE), with the vast majority occurring from left to right. Risk of EFE is higher in Thoroughbred or Thoroughbred-cross horses and in the winter months.[4] Crib biting and windsucking have been associated with development of EFE.[4–7]

Clinical signs include persistent abdominal pain of varying degrees. Abdominal sonography can be used to identify small intestinal distention and edema in the right cranial abdomen, allowing earlier diagnosis when examination per rectum is inconclusive (Clinical scenario 5, located in Appendix A).[141] Nasogastric reflux may be present.

Many lesions, however, involve the distal jejunum and ileum and reflux may not be a clinical feature early in the course of disease. Although surgical correction of EFE is the only effective treatment, indication for surgery based on clinical examination is not always clear. Persistent abdominal pain as well as high peritoneal fluid total protein and lactate concentrations predicts the need for surgery in most cases.[139,141]

Surgical treatment of EFE involves reduction by gentle traction combined with manual decompression of the incarcerated segment performed by massaging the intraluminal gas and liquid from the entrapped segment to the distal normal segment.[141] Sterile sodium carboxymethylcellulose can be used to facilitate reduction. Rupture of the bordering portal vein or caudal vena cava has been reported to occur during surgical reduction in a small number of cases resulting in fatal hemorrhage.[45,141] Following surgical reduction, the incarcerated intestinal segment is evaluated subjectively for viability and a resection is performed if the segment is judged to be nonviable. The majority of horses with EFE require intestinal resection.[45,141] The location of the nonviable incarcerated segment (jejunal versus ileal) will determine the type of anastomosis needed (jejunojejunostomy, jejunoileostomy, or jejunocecostomy [p. 193]). Ileal incarceration is common.[38]

Prognosis following surgical correction of EFE is reported to be up to 95% in the short term and up to 70% in the long term.[5,38,45,141] Factors affecting prognosis are preoperative peritoneal fluid protein concentration, degree of ileal involvement, and the necessity of jejunocecostomy.[45,141] Horses with EFE are more likely to have strangulating lesions affecting the ileum than other types of small intestinal strangulating obstruction.[45] Recurrence of EFE is rarely reported and the true prevalence of reentrapment is unknown.[4] Trauma associated with entrapment and surgical manipulation may result in adhesion and stricture of the foramen preventing reentrapment (Dr. Debbie Archer, University of Liverpool, Personal Communication).

Gastrosplenic ligament entrapment

The gastrosplenic ligament is a band of omentum extending from the hilus of the spleen to the left portion of the greater curvature of the stomach.[75] Most often entrapment of distal jejunal and ileal small intestinal segments through a rent in the gastrosplenic ligament results in strangulating obstruction. Incarceration of portions of both the large and small colon has also been reported.[113,138] Clinical signs consistent with strangulating obstruction of the small intestine are typically seen including persistent abdominal pain, nasogastric reflux (p. 38), small intestinal distention detected on examination per rectum (p. 27) or abdominal sonography (p. 128), and alterations in peritoneal fluid analysis (p. 87).[75]

Surgical treatment involves identification and reduction of the entrapped intestine via gentle traction. Incarcerated intestinal segments are detected lateral to the stomach and craniolateral to the spleen as the herniation through the ligament occurs in the caudal to cranial direction.[150] The entrapped intestinal segments are resected if nonviable (p. 193). The rent in the gastrosplenic ligament is not repaired from the ventral midline celiotomy incision due to limited surgical access, although standing laparoscopy may provide sufficient access for repair.[75] Long-term survival rate is reported to be 66–79%.[75,150]

Jejunal volvulus

Small intestinal volvulus occurs when the small intestine twists on the axis of the mesenteric attachment resulting in strangulating obstruction. The volvulus can occur at the root of the mesentery and involve >80% of the small intestine or affect only a segment of jejunum and/or ileum. The volvulus can be primary or secondary to other lesions of the small intestine. Small intestinal volvulus can occur at any age but is commonly seen in foals 2–4 months old[132,144] and horses <3 years old. Clinical signs include persistent and severe abdominal pain, tachycardia, abdominal distention (which is not typical for horses with small intestinal lesions), decreased intestinal motility, nasogastric reflux, and small intestinal distention on palpation per rectum.

Treatment for small intestinal volvulus is surgical.[132] The site of the volvulus is palpated, untwisted, decompressed, and evaluated. Need for resection and anastomosis (p. 192) of affected intestines is dependent on the degree of strangulation and subjective measures of viability (Figure 17.4).

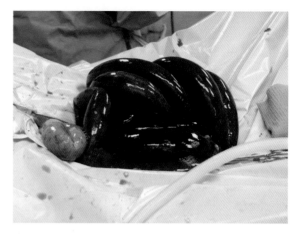

Figure 17.4 Intraoperative photograph of a 2-month-old colt with small intestinal volvulus. Note the extensive jejunal dilation and poor viability resulting from this strangulating obstruction.

Overall prognosis for horses with a jejunal volvulus treated surgically was 58% with 80% in horses that were recovered from general anesthesia surviving to hospital discharge, despite a high postoperative complication rate (48%).[132] Factors associated with nonsurvival were high presurgical peritoneal fluid protein concentration and nucleated cell count and need for jejunocecostomy as a surgical treatment.[133]

Meckel's diverticulum

Meckel's diverticulum is a remnant of the embryonic vitellointestinal duct that fails to atrophy completely.[129] The location of this remnant is in connection with the antimesenteric border in the region of the distal jejunum or ileum. Meckel's diverticulum can result in clinical illness by several mechanisms. The diverticulum can become a site of bacterial overgrowth and contribute to typhlitis and colitis. A Meckel's diverticulum can become distended with intestinal contents that can either protrude into the lumen of the intestinal tract resulting in obstruction or undergo necrosis and rupture.[146] Meckel's diverticulum can contribute to volvulus of the jejunum and ileum when these segments of the intestine twist around the vitelloumbilical band, a fibrous band extending from the distal end of the diverticulum to the umbilicus.[54] The diverticulum can also intussuscept into the lumen of the adjacent intestines and cause an obstruction, or it can loop around and strangulate adjacent intestine.[72] A vitelline cyst may form as a vitelline duct remnant connected to the intestinal mesentery, but not continuous with the antimesenteric border of the intestine.[31] The vitelline cyst may float freely in the abdomen or can potentially encircle and strangulate adjacent intestine.

The type of surgical correction is dependent on mechanism of injury. It is necessary to resect the diverticulum or cyst and associated intestine as well as other devitalized intestinal segments if present. Few reports of successful surgical treatment of Meckel's diverticulum exist.[54,72,146]

Mesodiverticular band

A mesodiverticular band is a congenital defect resulting from a persistent vitelline artery. Two vitelline arteries are associated with the vitelline duct during embryonic development.[31] In normal embryonic development, the left artery should completely regress, and the distal portion of the right artery will also regress, with the proximal portion persisting as the cranial mesenteric artery.[31] In cases of mesodiverticular band, a single band is typically present, although paired bands have been reported.[46] The mesodiverticular band extends from the cranial mesenteric artery or vein to the antimesenteric border of the intestine or to the site of Meckel's diverticulum. (Figure 17.5).[2]

Mesodiverticular bands can result in small intestinal strangulating obstruction when segments of bowel become entrapped within the space formed by the junction of the mesodiverticular band and the adjacent intestinal mesentery. The site of mesenteric attachment may develop a traumatic rent due to the weight of the entrapment, incarcerating the segments of intestine.[2] Mesodiverticular bands can also be incidental findings identified at surgery or necropsy.

Surgical resection of the mesodiverticular band and resection and anastomosis of the nonviable intestinal segments is the treatment for small intestinal strangulating obstruction caused by entrapment in a mesodiverticular band. Reported prognosis is good if the lesion is identified prior to intestinal rupture and septic peritonitis.[2,46] Surgeons should also consider resection of a mesodiverticu-

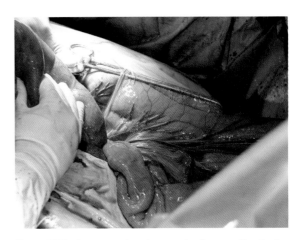

Figure 17.5   Intraoperative photograph of a mesodiverticular band identified as an incidental finding in a 7-year-old Arabian mare presenting with right dorsal colonic displacement. The instrument has been inserted into the pocket formed by the junction of the mesodiverticular band, jejunum, and jejunal mesentery.

lar band encountered as an incidental finding during exploratory celiotomy.

Jejunal intussusception

Jejunal intussusceptions occur when a segment of jejunum (intussusceptum) "telescopes" into an adjacent segment of jejunum (intussuscipiens). Jejunal intussusceptions are most commonly seen in neonates and young foals and often occur secondary to a motility disturbance (e.g., change in diet, enteritis, or ascariasis). Intussusceptions have also been associated with intestinal anastomoses, intramural masses, and PE in young mature horses and ponies and likely form and resolve spontaneously.

Treatment of a jejunal intussusception resulting in clinical signs of colic is abdominal surgery, reduction of the intussusception if possible, and if necessary, resection of the affected intestine, and jejunojejunostomy (p. 193). Prognosis is generally good.

Ileocecal intussusception

Ileocecal intussusception results from the passage or "telescoping" of a portion of the ileum (intussusceptum) into the cecum (intussuscipiens) through the ileocecal orifice. Young horses are often affected and tapeworms (*Anoplocephala perfoliata*) may be involved in the etiopathogenesis (Clinical scenario 2, located in Appendix A). Intussusceptions can be acute or chronic with variable length of the intussusceptum.[42] Luminal obstruction results from congestion and edema of the intussusceptum.[42] Loss of viability of the ileal segment contributes to signs consistent with a small intestinal strangulating obstruction. A firm, tubular mass may be palpable in the right dorsal abdomen on examination per rectum. The intussuscepted intestine can often be identified sonographically.

Surgical treatment involves reduction of the ileal intussusceptum and resection if nonviable. Jejunocecostomy (p. 193) is necessary following resection of the ileum. In cases where the ileal intussusceptum is not easily reducible and the intussusceptum is short in length, ileocecostomy (p. 194) has been described as an effective treatment.[11] When the ileal intussusceptum is long, resection of the intussusceptum through a typhlotomy is indicated to prevent obstruction of the cecocolic orifice and hemorrhage. Side-to-side jejunocecostomy to bypass the affected ileocecal region is then performed. Ileocecostomy (p. 194) may be indicated, even in cases with a reducible short ileocecal intussusception, to prevent recurrence. Deworming with an anthelmintic effective against tapeworms (i.e., praziquantel or pyrantel pamoate) is recommended (p. 318).

See Chapter 21 on Special Considerations for Umbilical hernia (p. 280), Inguinal hernia (p. 284), and Mesenteric rent (p. 284).

Cecal disease

Cecal impaction

Impaction of the cecum with ingesta is unique when compared to impactions in other regions of the gastrointestinal tract. Cecal impactions may consist of firm dehydrated ingesta or fluid ingesta that fails to empty due to cecal dysfunction. The clinical distinction, however, may not always be apparent.

Clinical signs of cecal impaction may be subtle, including reduced fecal output, altered fecal consistency, decreased intestinal motility on auscultation particularly in the right flank region, reduced appetite, dull demeanor, and mild abdominal pain.[117] Horses may also be exquisitely painful, especially upon palpation per rectum of the cecal

area. Nasogastric reflux may occur with compression of the duodenum by a markedly distended cecum. Adult and juvenile horses are predisposed to cecal impaction associated with concurrent medical conditions. These impactions may be accompanied by vague clinical signs of mild abdominal discomfort, despite the serious outcome if left untreated. Cecal impaction followed by perforation has recently been reported in foals undergoing anesthesia or nonsteroidal anti-inflammatory drug (NSAID) treatment for orthopedic procedures.[135]

Medical treatment of cecal impactions is used in horses considered to be at low risk of perforation based on examination per rectum and with mild signs of colic.[106] Treatment includes fasting, analgesia (p. 51), and laxatives (p. 47, 66), as well as IV (p. 99) and enteral fluid therapy (p. 62). The consequences of failure of medical therapy can be fatal; therefore, veterinarians responsible for treating horses with cecal impactions may often recommend surgical treatment. Spontaneous perforation is a risk, especially in cases where the cecum is tightly distended with fluid ingesta. Earlier surgical intervention could be lifesaving in foals showing classic signs of cecal impaction, in which monitoring with examination per rectum is not possible.[135] Surgical treatment for cecal impaction involves typhlotomy (p. 190) with evacuation of ingesta.[115] It is critical to ensure that the cecum is completely evacuated, including the cupula. In addition to typhlotomy, jejuno- or ileocolic anastomoses (p. 195) have been used to treat selected cases when recurrence is of concern (e.g., horses with a chronic impaction >7 days or other evidence of cecal dysfunction).[118] Complete bypass by jejunocolostomy or ileocolostomy is an effective treatment for horses with cecal impaction.[52] Incomplete bypass is not recommended, as it does not sufficiently decrease the flow of ingesta into the cecum.[25] Long-term prognosis for horses treated medically or surgically, via typhlotomy alone, was good in recent reports where low rates of recurrence were documented.[106,128] A slow postoperative refeeding regimen is recommended for horses with a cecal impaction managed by typhlotomy alone.

Cecocolic intussusception

Cecocecal intussusception is the passage or "telescoping" of the cecal apex into the cecal base.

Cecocolic intussusception is the passage of the cecum (intussusceptum) into the right ventral colon (intussuscipiens) through the cecocolic orifice. Affected horses are typically <3 years of age and Standardbred horses are overrepresented.[50,94] Tapeworms (*Anoplocephala perfoliata*) are likely important in the etiopathogenesis. Signs for both types of intussusception vary, with horses showing signs of either acute onset of abdominal pain or chronic pain, weight loss, and diminished fecal production dependent on the degree of luminal obstruction. A hard mass may be palpable in the right dorsal quadrant on examination per rectum.[18] Transcutaneous or transrectal sonographic examination (p. 127) may aid in diagnosis of cecal intussusception by identification of a "target" lesion indicating bowel within bowel.[11]

Surgical treatments may include reduction of the intussusception, and partial typhlectomy (p. 191) with or without colotomy. Reduction is often difficult particularly with a cecocolic intussusception; maintaining traction on the intussusceptum in combination with massage from outside of the right ventral colon can lead to successful reduction. Partial typhlectomy is often required following reduction due to loss of viability of the intussusceptum. When a reduction cannot be performed due to pronounced edema and thickening of the cecal apex, right ventral colotomy (p. 190) is necessary to reduce the cecal intussusception. Colotomy should be performed carefully with additional draping to limit risk of abdominal contamination and peritonitis with this procedure. Despite contamination concerns, horses undergoing partial typhlectomy via colotomy have a good prognosis.[73] Another treatment option for poorly reducible cecal intussusception is jejuno or ileocolostomy (p. 195) with or without oversew of the cecal base.[18,90]

Prognosis for surgically treated cecal intussusception in horses is good with early treatment.[94] If treatment is delayed, horses are at greater risk of peritonitis, intestinal perforation, or irreducible intussusception.[94] Deworming with an anthelmintic effective against tapeworms (i.e., praziquantel or pyrantel pamoate) is recommended (p. 320).

Cecal perforation

Cecal perforation has been associated with peripartum traumatic injury in mares and severe

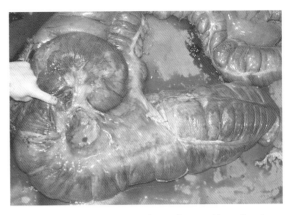

Figure 17.6   Necropsy image from a horse with perforation of the cecal base secondary to cecal impaction.

Anoplocephala perfoliata (tapeworm) infestation.[121] Cecal perforation may also be secondary to cecal impaction.[117] In these cases, the cecum will be dilated with ingesta at surgery or necropsy examination, and the colon may be relatively empty of ingesta. The site of perforation is variable within the cecal body or base (Figure 17.6).[117] Lesions within the mesentery of the cecal base may temporarily limit ingesta contamination of the peritoneal cavity, with these differences reflected in the peritoneal fluid analysis.

Clinical signs prior to perforation are variable and acute abdominal pain may not precede perforation.[117] Cecal perforation results in severe septic peritonitis and accompanying clinical signs (p. 171). Euthanasia is necessary upon suspicion or confirmation of cecal perforation.

Large (ascending) colon disease

Inflammatory disease

Colitis

Colitis refers to inflammatory disease of the large colon. Common causes include Potomac Horse Fever (*Neorickettsia risticii*), salmonellosis, and clostridiosis. However, in many cases the etiology is not determined. Clinical signs vary from mild self-limiting diarrhea to acute onset of shock and death. Horses can initially present with mild to moderate colic signs that progress to dull mentation and shock (tachycardia, hyperemic mucous membranes, prolonged capillary refill time, poor jugular refill, and cool extremities). Horses are often febrile and have diarrhea. Horses that are severely affected may have abdominal distention. Clinical laboratory findings include high PCV, hypoproteinemia/hypoalbuminemia, hyperlactatemia, azotemia, hyponatremia, hypochloremia, metabolic acidosis, and leukopenia/neutropenia. Palpation per rectum should be performed to confirm that horses do not have a different primary disease (e.g., small colon impaction) or a secondary lesion (e.g., colonic displacement or impaction). Abdominal sonographic examination can be used to confirm the diagnosis with the finding of a thick and fluid-filled cecum and colon without other abnormalities. Diagnosis of the etiological agent is based on isolation of the organism (Salmonella spp.) or toxins (clostridium spp.) from the feces, detection of the organism in the feces or blood using polymerase chain reaction (PCR) (Salmonella spp. or *Neorickettsia risticii*), or serology (*Neorickettsia risticii*).

Treatment of colitis is primarily supportive and involves IV fluid therapy (p. 99), colloidal support (p. 112), antiendotoxin treatment (p. 246), antidiarrheal medication (p. 248), and antimicrobial therapy in horses that are severely neutropenic. Because horses with colitis are at an increased risk of developing lamintis, preventive measures such as icing the feet and distal limbs are recommended. Horses suspected of having Potomac horse fever should be treated with oxytetracycline.

Complications associated with colitis include coagulopathy, colonic infarction, catheter-associated problems, laminitis, renal failure, and severe shock necessitating euthanasia. The prognosis is extremely variable depending on the disease severity, but overall is fair to good with prompt treatment.

Right dorsal colitis

Right dorsal colitis is inflammation and mucosal ulceration of the right dorsal colon. Right dorsal colitis is associated with administration of NSAIDs, in particular phenylbutazone. Risk of developing right dorsal colitis is thought to increase with high doses of phenylbutazone or when given in combination with water restriction or hypovolemia.[80] Experimentally, even moderate doses of phenylbutazone administered over weeks resulted in hypoalbuminemia, neutropenia, altered right dorsal colon arterial blood flow, and altered volatile fatty acid production.[97]

Clinical signs of right dorsal colitis include abdominal pain, fever, diarrhea, dull demeanor, anorexia, and hematochezia.[80] Hypoproteinemia and hypoalbuminemia are common sequelae to resultant colonic ulceration and inflammation. Peritoneal fluid protein and nucleated cell count are often high in acute disease. Transcutaneous abdominal sonography (p. 125) is useful in both diagnosis and monitoring treatment of horses with right dorsal colitis. Lesions consistent with right dorsal colitis are increased thickness and a hypoechoic layer corresponding to submucosal edema and inflammatory infiltrate.[79] Imaging of the right dorsal colon is best within the 11th, 12th, and 13th intercostal spaces caudal to the lung margin where it resides axial to the liver.[79] Radiolabeled white blood cell scintigraphy has been used to confirm right dorsal colitis via linear uptake in the right cranioventral abdomen at 20 h postinjection.[34]

Treatment of right dorsal colitis is varied. NSAIDs should be avoided. The use of cyclooxygenase-1 (COX-1) sparing NSAIDs has not been evaluated for managing horses with right dorsal colitis. If colic signs are present, dietary modification, analgesia, and fluid therapy are indicated. Dietary management consists of pelleted feed and restricted roughage.[22] Severely affected horses may require parenteral nutrition (p. 306). Corn oil, psyllium, and sucralfate can be used in an attempt to aid mucosal healing. Occasionally lesions in the right dorsal colon are so severe that intestinal perforation can occur. Injury and scarring resulting from the colonic lesions can predispose to stricture formation or functional obstruction. In these cases, surgical treatment is necessary. Surgical treatment includes bypass of the right dorsal colon, resection of the affected colon with anastomosis, or resection with bypass. Surgical bypass, in cases of stricture formation, can be completed by side-to-side anastomosis of the right dorsal colon oral to the lesion and the small colon.[22] With active disease nonresponsive to medical treatment, complete resection of the affected portion of the colon and end-to-end anastomosis between the remaining right dorsal colon and transverse colon may be necessary.[127] Alternatively, resection of the affected colon can be performed using an ILA-100 stapling device (US Surgical Corporation) leaving two blind ends, and then bypassing the resected colon by performing an anastomosis between the diaphragmatic flexure of the dorsal colon and the small colon. The prognosis is good with early recognition of right dorsal colitis achieved through monitoring total plasma protein in horses being treated with NSAIDs for longer than 2–3 days. The prognosis is guarded to poor for horses with severe disease.

Simple obstruction

Impaction

Large colon impaction is a common cause of colic in horses and results in nonstrangulating obstruction. Recent travel, stabling for 24 h per day, cribbing/windsucking, poor quality hay, inadequate water intake, infrequent dental care, recent orthopedic surgery and morphine use are risk factors for developing impaction of the large colon.[69,125] Other commonly used medications, such as NSAIDs and ocular atropine, decrease colonic motility and may predispose to impaction.[143,148]

The most common sites of colonic impaction are within anatomical areas of decreasing luminal diameter and upward flow of ingesta. Specifically, affected areas are the pelvic flexure at the junction of the left ventral and left dorsal colon (Figure 17.7), and the right dorsal colon at the junction of the right dorsal and transverse colons. Clinical signs of colonic impaction include abdominal pain, abdominal distention, and decreased intestinal motility. Abdominal pain may be cyclical, with episodes of moderate abdominal pain separated by hours of apparent comfort. Impactions at the pelvic flexure are easily palpated per rectum (p. 32); however, impactions within the right dorsal colon are often not palpated except in small horses or when the impaction is pushed toward the caudal abdomen.

Medical treatment of colonic impaction includes analgesia (p. 51), laxatives (p. 47, 66), IV (p. 99) and enteral fluid therapy (p. 62), and limiting feeding (Clinical scenario 6, located in Appendix A). Enteral fluid therapy with balanced electrolyte solution promotes hydration of colonic ingesta without risk of systemic electrolyte imbalance.[89] In a clinical study, horses with colonic impaction receiving enteral fluid therapy resolved more quickly than those receiving IV fluid therapy alone, with lower cost of treatment.[55] A theoretical added benefit of

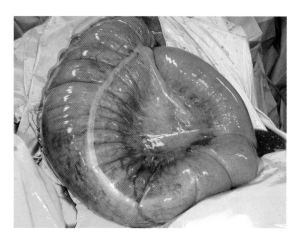

Figure 17.7 Intraoperative photograph of an impacted portion of the large colon which has been exteriorized from the abdomen. Note the serosal inflammation and ecchymosis associated with the impaction in the pelvic flexure.

enteral fluids administered as a bolus is stimulation of colonic motility via the gastro-colic reflex. Occasionally, surgery is necessary to resolve impactions that are not responsive to medical therapy (see Chapter 15 on Medical versus Surgical Treatment [p. 167]). In these cases, colonic contents are lavaged out with tap water through a pelvic flexure enterotomy (p. 190). Surgeons should exercise care when manipulating an impacted colon, as the heavy colonic contents increase risk of visceral perforation. A large body wall incision and beginning the pelvic flexure enterotomy prior to complete exteriorization of the impacted colon can help prevent perforation. Most cases of large colon impaction resolve with medical treatment, and the prognosis is excellent.[29]

Sand enteropathy

Sand ingested from the environment accumulates within the large colon and can result in mucosal irritation. Large amounts of sand accumulation can result in nonstrangulating obstruction (Figure 17.8). Horses consuming sand may have signs of diarrhea or poor body condition. Mucosal abrasion can result in signs of endotoxemia (p. 246). When a high sand burden results in obstruction, signs associated with colonic obstruction such as abdominal pain, tachycardia, and severe abdominal distention are observed. Auscultation of sand on the ventral

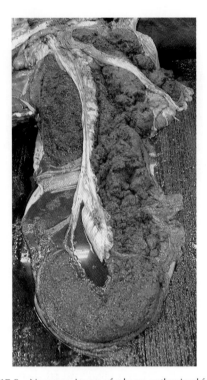

Figure 17.8   Necropsy image of a horse euthanized for clinical signs associated with severe sand enteropathy. The large intestines have been opened to reveal copious sand laden ingesta and large sand deposits in the pelvic flexure and right dorsal colon.

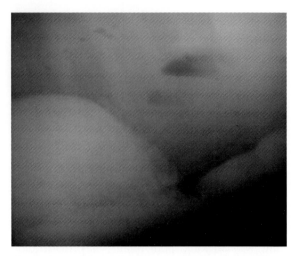

Figure 17.9   Abdominal radiograph of a horse with sand enteropathy. Note the accumulations of sand within the large and small colon.

abdomen is described as a useful tool in horses, although often when sand accumulation progresses to complete obstruction, a hypomotile gastrointestinal tract limits the usefulness of this technique. Floatation of feces to allow sedimentation can be a sensitive diagnostic test for sand exposure. Abdominal radiographic examination (p. 156) is useful to estimate sand burden in horses with sand exposure and clinical signs of sand enteropathy (Figure 17.9). Radiographically, the ventral aspect of the sand accumulation conforms to the shape of the colon and the dorsal aspect is flattened if the sand is settled out from the ingesta.[82] Transcutaneous abdominal sonography (p. 124) can be useful for detecting sand accumulations within portions of the intestinal tract adjacent to the ventral abdominal wall.[85]

Medical treatment includes IV (p. 99) and enteral fluids (p. 62) and laxative therapy (p. 47, 66). If the colon is not completely obstructed, continued feeding of small amounts of roughage or psyllium may hasten sand clearance. Although psyllium is often empirically recommended, its treatment efficacy is debated. Psyllium failed to facilitate sand elimination in an experimental study.[56] Abdominal radiographs can be useful to monitor sand clearance and response to medical treatment.[120] In cases of complete obstruction that fail to respond to analgesic therapy, surgical removal is possible via pelvic flexure enterotomy (p. 190). Horses oftentimes develop colonic displacement concurrently with sand obstruction, necessitating surgical correction.[53] Medical management of sand impaction associated with a complete obstruction is often unsuccessful and can result in colonic rupture.

Prognosis for surgical treatment of sand impaction is good.[111] Following successful treatment, horse owners should focus their efforts on prevention. Limiting access to sand is the main prevention strategy. This can be achieved by feeding horses off the ground and providing adequate good quality roughage feed sources. Periodic feeding of psyllium has also been recommended to aid in clearance of sand with continued environmental exposure.

Enterolithiasis

Enteroliths are struvite calculi that form within the right dorsal colon and can result in colonic obstruction of the right dorsal, transverse, and small colons.[63] Although enteroliths vary in shape, size, and texture, a distinct concentric ring appearance is consistently visible on cut section due to the formation around a central nidus of varying composition.[65] Breed and diet are risk factors for enterolithiasis. Arabians, Morgans, American Saddlebreds, and miniature breeds are at increased risk, as well as horses fed a diet rich in California- or Texas-grown alfalfa hay.[23,63]

Signs of enterolithiasis include mild abdominal pain, partial or complete colonic obstruction, and often normal peritoneal fluid. Despite limitations of this diagnostic technique in adult horses, enteroliths are radioopaque and often are visible on abdominal radiographs, especially when located within the right dorsal colon (p. 155). Enteroliths are rarely palpable on examination per rectum.[64] More often examination per rectum will simply confirm colonic obstruction. Enteroliths can also result in segmental pressure necrosis and perforation. In these cases, clinical signs of disease are more severe (p. 171).

Treatment of enterolithiasis involves surgical removal via an enterotomy (p. 190). Occasionally multiple enterotomies are necessary. Distending the colon with water can facilitate movement of enteroliths in the transverse colon region toward the pelvic flexure. Horses with enteroliths removed from the large colon require less complicated postoperative management than those with enteroliths removed from the small colon. This is because horses with small colon involvement may require slower return to full diet and short-term laxative treatment.[63] In a recent study, long-term survival did not differ between horses based on colonic location of enterolith obstruction; however, more horses were euthanized intraoperatively due to rupture or poor intestinal viability when the small colon was affected.[105] If an enterolith with flattened sides is encountered, there is likely to be multiple enteroliths whose close contact is responsible for the flattened appearance. Solitary enteroliths are spherical.

Colonic fluid from horses with enterolithiasis sampled at the time of surgical treatment has a higher pH and higher mineral concentrations than fluid from horses without enterolithiasis.[66] Feeding of concentrates and apple cider vinegar to acidify the colonic contents may aid in prevention.[63] In addition, grass hay diets have been shown to acidify the colonic environment and reduce mineral content of ingesta compared with alfalfa hay diets; therefore, feeding grass hay may also decrease the risk of enterolithiasis.[67]

Nephrosplenic ligament entrapment

Nephrosplenic ligament entrapment (NSLE), or left dorsal displacement of the large colon, occurs when the large colon migrates to the area dorsal to the nephrosplenic ligament and becomes entrapped between the spleen and left kidney. This entrapment results in a nonstrangulating large bowel obstruction. Horses with this lesion have mild to moderate signs of pain and may develop nasogastric reflux due to compression of the duodenum by the displaced colon.[61] Diagnosis is often obtained by examination per rectum of the nephrosplenic space (p. 29) (Clinical scenario 3, located in Appendix A). Transcutaneous abdominal sonographic imaging of the nephrosplenic orientation can also be used to aid in diagnosis and monitor correction (p. 121).[123]

Some horses with a NSLE will resolve the displacement spontaneously. There are several treatment options. Medical management with analgesic drugs (p. 51) as well as enteral (p. 62) and IV (p. 99) fluids is successful in many cases. Treatment with IV infusion of phenylephrine or etilefrine, potent α-1 adrenergic agonists, cause splenic contraction and is an important component of both medical and surgical correction. Jogging the horse for 5–10 min following phenylephrine treatment can result in correction. Colonic rupture has rarely been observed possibly associated with excessive jogging of chronicity of disease.

NSLE can also be corrected by rolling the horse under general anesthesia. The horse is positioned in right lateral recumbency, the hindlimbs are hoisted up and the horse rocked back and forth, then positioned into left lateral recumbency. Phenylephrine administration can assist with repositioning of the colon. Displacement correction is assessed using transcutaneous sonography or palpation per rectum.

Surgical correction is necessary for horses that do not respond to conservative management and is performed from a ventral midline or left paralumbar fossa celiotomy (Figure 16.12). Phenylephrine administration can also facilitate repositioning by decreasing the size of the spleen as can tilting the table or the horse to the right side. Correction via a standing laparoscopic approach can also been performed in horses that are showing minimal signs of pain and do not have colonic distention. Visceral penetration with surgical cannulas is a risk of this procedure with inappropriate patient selection.

Prognosis for medical and surgical correction is excellent, except in rare cases where horses develop additional gastrointestinal lesions.[61] NSLE has been known to recur in approximately 20% of horses.[116] Ablation of the nephrosplenic space via a standing laparoscopic approach can be used to prevent reincarceration. Nephrosplenic space ablation is achieved via approximation of the dorsal splenic capsule to the nephrosplenic ligament with suture or surgical mesh.[39,116] While usually staged, this procedure can be performed safely within days of ventral midline celiotomy when minimal insufflation pressure is used. Although nephrosplenic space ablation prevents left dorsal colonic displacement, other forms of colon malposition can occur.[40,116] Subtotal colonic resection (p. 195) or colopexy (p. 202) can be used as a nonspecific surgical procedure to prevent NSLE and other colonic displacements.

Right dorsal displacement

Displacement of the left colons to the right or cranial portions of the abdominal cavity is known as right dorsal displacement (RDD) and results in a nonstrangulating obstruction (Figure 17.10). Displacement can be accompanied by a 180° volvulus that does not result in vascular compromise. Clinical signs are consistent with colonic obstruction including moderate abdominal pain, abdominal distention, and large colon distention palpated per rectum (p. 28). Typically, horses do not have signs of endotoxemia. Serum gamma glutamyl transferase activity may be high due to acute extrahepatic compression of the bile duct by the displaced colon.[49]

Treatment for RDD is surgical repositioning via a ventral midline celiotomy. However, some horses with a colonic displacement may respond to medical treatment involving withholding feed, analgesia (p. 51) as well as enteral (p. 62) and IV fluid (p. 99) therapy.

Short-term prognosis for RDD is excellent, although a recent report suggests that horses with RDD are more likely to experience recurrent episodes of colic following surgical correction, than with other types of colonic displacement.[93]

Strangulating obstruction

Large colon volvulus

Large colon volvulus (LCV), sometimes referred to as colonic torsion, occurs when there is twisting of the intestines on the axis of the mesenteric attachment resulting in a strangulating obstruction (Figure 17.11). Most horses with LCV have severe abdominal pain and abdominal distention. The degree of abdominal pain is so severe that, in most cases, it is poorly controlled with analgesia. Large colon tympanic distention may be palpable on palpation per rectum (p. 32). Transcutaneous

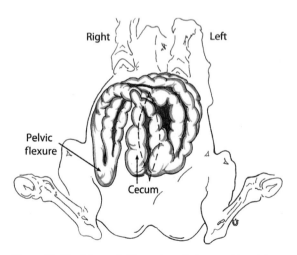

Figure 17.10   Schematic illustration of a horse with a right dorsal colonic displacement.

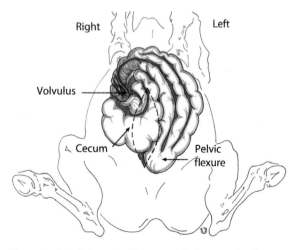

Figure 17.11   Schematic illustration of a horse with a large colon volvulus.

abdominal sonography (p. 122) has been used to identify nonsacculated large colon in the left ventral abdomen in horses with LCV and may be a useful diagnostic tool in horses where clinical signs are equivocal.[1] Colonic wall thickness ≥9 mm measured using transcutaneous sonography had a high specificity for LCV.[104]

Treatment is immediate surgical correction of the LCV (Figure 17.12). The volvulus predominantly occurs in a counterclockwise or ventromedial dorsolateral direction at the level of the cecocolic ligament or base of the colon. Occasionally the cecum will be involved in the volvulus. Needle decompression (p. 189) is necessary upon entering the peritoneal cavity. LCV correction can be challenging; however, manipulating the colon from the left side of the abdomen and tilting the table or horse slightly to the left can help with surgical derotation. The bowel should be kept moist. When the colon is heavy and the wall friable, performing a pelvic flexure enterotomy and evacuating the colonic contents may facilitate correction. Following correction, the attending surgeon must estimate if the colon is viable using subjective or objective criteria. Subjective criteria include color, pulse quality, motility, and degree of hemorrhage from an enterotomy site. Objective measures, such as analysis of intraoperative biopsy and colonic intraluminal pressure may not be practical or predictive in all situations.[95,142] If viability of the large colon is questionable, partial colonic resection may be recommended (p. 195).

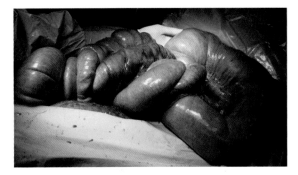

Figure 17.12 Intraoperative photograph of a horse with large colon volvulus. Note the serosal cyanosis typical of a colonic volvulus that has not yet been corrected. Upon correction, the colon color and other subjective parameters improved. This horse survived with minimal complications without the need for colonic resection.

Prognosis following surgical correction is linked to severity of illness and treatment. Admission of plasma lactate <6.0 mmol/L was predictive of survival in horses with LCV (Clinical scenario 4, located in Appendix A).[77] Postoperative transcutaneous sonographic evaluation of colonic wall thickness may be helpful for predicting viability and survival.[126] Assessment of lesion severity may not be as useful in predicting survival when the alternative surgical treatment of subtotal large colon resection and anastomosis is used.[95] Large colon resection in cases of LCV resulted in a short-term survival rate of 74%.[36] Horses did not have chronic problems related to the surgical procedure and most were able to return to their previous use.[36] Recurrence of LCV can occur in about 15% of affected horses. Colon resection (p. 195) or colopexy (p. 202) can be performed to prevent recurrence.

Small (descending) colon disease

Impaction

Small colon impaction, due to the intraluminal accumulation of dehydrated ingesta, results in a nonstrangulating obstruction (Figure 17.13). Ingestion of foreign material, such as trichophagia, has been associated with impaction. Enteroliths (p. 218) and fecaliths (p. 286) can also cause small colon obstruction. Fecal impaction is the most common disorder of this intestinal segment.[114] Clinical signs include abdominal pain and gas distention. Impaction is palpable per rectum (p. 33) in most cases.[43] Horses may have diarrhea at the time of initial examination. Diarrhea and impaction in this location are commonly seen together, indicating either joint risk factors or a complex dysfunction syndrome.[43] Fecal cultures may be positive for *Salmonella* spp. in these horses.[114]

Treatment of small colon impaction is analgesics (p. 51), laxatives (p. 47, 66), and enteral (p. 62) and IV fluid therapy (p. 99). Surgical treatment is an option for those horses that do not respond to medical treatment. Horses with pronounced abdominal distention are more likely to require surgical treatment.[43] Manual massage, surgical enema, or enterotomy are required to reduce impactions

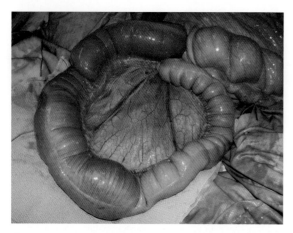

Figure 17.13   Segmental small colonic impaction in a yearling mixed breed filly. Note the junction of reddened and inflamed serosal and mesenteric surfaces of the oral small colon with the aboral segment that is normal in size and appearance.

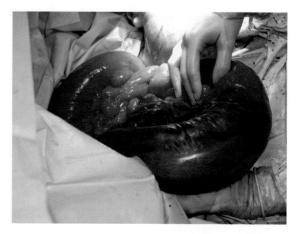

Figure 17.14   Segmental ischemia and necrosis of the small colon secondary to mesenteric rent which traumatically interrupted intestinal bloodflow. This injury occurred in a broodmare during parturition. The mare recovered well following resection and anastomosis of the small colon.

intraoperatively. Oftentimes, ingesta is evacuated from the large colon through a pelvic flexure enterotomy (p. 190) at the time of surgery to limit transit through the inflamed small colon during the immediate postoperative period. Prognosis for medical and surgical treatment of small colon impaction is good.[43]

Mesenteric rent

Traumatic rents in the intestinal mesentery may occur during foaling or the cause may be unknown. The pathologic opening that is formed may entrap adjacent intestines such as the jejunum, ileum, or small colon and result in strangulating obstruction.[16,51] Trauma to the mesentery may directly affect blood flow to the intestine (Figure 17.14). Hemorrhage resulting from mesenteric trauma may be reflected in peritoneal fluid analysis. Especially in mares post foaling, it is important to differentiate hemoabdomen due to a mesenteric rent from uterine artery bleeding because the treatments for these two conditions are different. Clinical signs include abdominal pain nonresponsive to analgesics, tachycardia, decreased intestinal motility, decreased fecal production, and alterations in peritoneal fluid.

Transrectal sonography may be more sensitive than transcutaneous abdominal sonography for diagnosing pathology associated with the small

colon.[47] Strangulation of a loop of small colon through a traumatic mesenteric rent may necessitate resection if viability of this loop is compromised. Resection of the bowel directly associated with the traumatized mesentery may also be necessary if this segment is nonviable.

Prognosis for horses undergoing surgical resection and end-to-end anastomosis of the small colon is good.[107] Closure of the mesenteric rent should be attempted during the initial surgical procedure to prevent reentrapment. If the site of the mesenteric rent is inaccessible from a ventral approach, laparoscopic repair in the standing horse may be an option.[134]

Meconium retention

Meconium retention is a disease of neonatal foals and a common source of colic pain in this age group.[19] Meconium is the first feces produced post birth and forms during fetal development. Foals unable to pass meconium within the first few hours of life may develop a meconium impaction, a nonstrangulating obstruction of the colon and rectum. Foals presenting with this disease are typically 24–48h old, with males overrepresented due to a relatively smaller pelvic inlet preventing passage of the impaction.[74] Clinical signs include straining to defecate, switching of the tail, and restlessness. Abdominal pain and distention may become severe with progression of this disease. Large bowel tympanic distention and small colon intraluminal obstruction may be visible with abdominal radiography (p. 157).

Treatment of meconium retention and impaction is primarily medical. Treatments include analgesics (p. 51), IV fluid therapy (p. 99), enemas, and laxatives administered via nasogastric tube (p. 38, 47, 62).[10] N-acetylcysteine retention enemas may dissolve impactions and facilitate passage, especially in foals where the site of impaction is within the pelvic inlet. Rarely surgical correction is required in foals refractory to medical treatment.[19] Manual surgical reduction or enterotomy is used in these cases. Foals undergoing surgical correction of meconium impaction are at risk for extensive serosal adhesions despite excellent short-term survival rates.[74] N-acetylcysteine enema treatment has improved medical outcomes and decreased the need for surgical intervention in foals with meconium impaction.[109] Meconium impaction may be prevented by early treatment with warm soapy water enemas if foals do not pass meconium within 3 h of birth. Care should be taken to prevent trauma to the rectal and colonic mucosa during enema administration. See Chapter 21 on Special Considerations (p. 278).

Neoplasia

Primary neoplasia of the equine intestinal tract resulting in colic is rare. Alimentary lymphoma is the most common intestinal neoplasia detected in horses.[136] Lymphoma within the lumen of the large colon has been reported to result in signs of non-strangulating obstruction.[30] Exfoliated neoplastic cells were not present in the peritoneal fluid of these cases to aid in preoperative diagnosis, though lymphoblastic peritoneal fluid has been described in other cases.[30,136] Outcome following surgical resection of alimentary lymphoma can be good unless the tumor has metastasized to the liver, spleen, and other sites.[30]

Large intestinal adenocarcinoma can result in recurrent abdominal pain, weight loss, chronic diarrhea, hematochezia, anorexia, and anemia.[62,84,119] Small intestinal adenocarcinomas are more likely to present with acute abdominal pain and nasogastric reflux.[99] Intestinal adenocarcinoma may result in clinical signs of disease prior to metastasis,

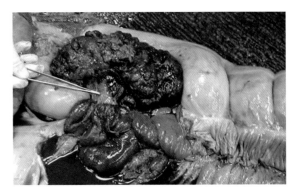

Figure 17.15 A 12-year-old Trakehner gelding presented with a history of chronic colic, weight loss, and hematochezia. A 22 cm diameter gastrointestinal stromal tumor was detected within the right ventral colon at necropsy.

improving the likelihood that surgical resection may result in a good outcome.[84,119]

Other tumor types, such as gastrointestinal stromal tumor (Figure 17.15), myxosarcoma, and smooth muscle tumors (lyomyoma and lyomyosarcoma) are rarely reported to occur in the equine intestinal tract resulting in abdominal pain.[136] Transcutaneous abdominal sonographic examination (p. 140–144) may detect abnormalities consistent with gastrointestinal neoplasia.[119] Definitive diagnosis of neoplasia is based on biopsy collected at surgery or necropsy examination. The largest retrospective study to date, evaluating 34 horses with intestinal neoplasia, documented a poor short-term survival and a median 1.9 month survival time from onset of clinical signs.[136]

References

1. Abutarbush, S.M. (2006) Use of ultrasonography to diagnose large colon volvulus in horses. *Journal of the American Veterinary Medical Association*, **228**, 409–413.
2. Abutarbush, S.M., Shoemaker, R.W. & Bailey, J.V. (2003) Strangulation of the small intestines by a meso-diverticular band in 3 adult horses. *Canadian Veterinary Journal*, **44**, 1005–1006.
3. Andrews, F.M. & Nadeau, J.A. (1999) Clinical syndromes of gastric ulceration in foals and mature horses. *Equine Veterinary Journal Supplement*, **29**, 30–33.
4. Archer, D.C., Proudman, C.J., Pinchbeck, G., Smith, J.E., French, N.P. & Edwards, G.B. (2004) Entrapment of the small intestine in the epiploic foramen in horses: A retrospective analysis of 71 cases recorded between 1991 and 2001. *Veterinary Record*, **155**, 793–797.

5. Archer, D.C., Freeman, D.E., Doyle, A.J., Proudman, C.J. & Edwards, G.B. (2004) Association between cribbing and entrapment of the small intestine in the epiploic foramen in horses: 68 cases (1991–2002). *Journal of the American Veterinary Medical Association*, **224**, 562–564.

6. Archer, D.C., Pinchbeck, G.L., French, N.P. & Proudman, C.J. (2008) Risk factors for epiploic foramen entrapment colic in a UK horse population: A prospective case-control study. *Equine Veterinary Journal*, **40**, 405–410.

7. Archer, D.C., Pinchbeck, G.K., French, N.P. & Proudman, C.J. (2008) Risk factors for epiploic foramen entrapment colic: An international study. *Equine Veterinary Journal*, **40**, 224–230.

8. Arroyo, L.G., Stampfli, H.R. & Weese, J.S. (2006) Potential role of *Clostridium difficile* as a cause of duodenitis-proximal jejunitis in horses. *Journal of Medical Microbiology*, **55**, 605–608.

9. Barclay, W.P., Foerner, J.J., Phillips, T.N. & MacHarg, M.A. (1982) Primary gastric impaction in the horse. *Journal of the American Veterinary Medical Association*, **181**, 682–683.

10. Bartmann, C.P., Freeman, D.E., Glitz, F., *et al.* (2002) Diagnosis and surgical management of colic in the foal: Literature review and a retrospective study. *Clinical Techniques in Equine Practice*, **1**, 125–142.

11. Bell, R.J. & Textor, J.A. (2010) Caecal intussusceptions in horses: A New Zealand perspective. *Australian Veterinary Journal*, **88**, 272–276.

12. Bell, R.J., Mogg, T.D. & Kingston, J.K. (2007) Equine gastric ulcer syndrome in adult horses: A review. *New Zealand Veterinary Journal*, **55**, 1–12.

13. Blikslager, A.T., Bowman, K.F., Haven, M.L., Tate, L.P., Jr. & Bristol, D.G. (1992) Pedunculated lipomas as a cause of intestinal obstruction in horses: 17 cases (1983–1990). *Journal of the American Veterinary Medical Association*, **201**, 1249–1252.

14. Boening Von, K.J. & Plocki, v.K.A. (1982) Uber die chirurgische versorgung einer partiellen, zirkulare magenruptur biem pferd. *Der Praktische Tierarzt*, **7**, 608–612.

15. Boersema, J.H., Eysker, M. & Nas, J.W.M. (2002) Apparent resistance of *Parascaris equorum* to macrocyclic lactones. *Veterinary Record*, **150**, 279–281.

16. Booth, T.M., Proudman, C.J. & Edwards, G.B. (2000) Entrapment of the small colon through a mesocolic rent in a mare. *Australian Veterinary Journal*, **78**, 603–604.

17. Borst, G.H., van der Weij, P.J. & Vos, J.H. (2004) Idiopathic gastric rupture in a Friesian foal. *Tijdschrift voor Diergeneeskunde*, **129**, 270–271.

18. Boussauw, B.H., Domingo, R., Wilderjans, H. & Picavet, T. (2001) Treatment of irreducible caecocolic intussusception in horses by jejuno(ileo)colostomy. *Veterinary Record*, **149**, 16–18.

19. Cable, C.S., Fubini, S.L., Erb, H.N. & Hakes, J.E. (1997) Abdominal surgery in foals: A review of 119 cases (1977–1994). *Equine Veterinary Journal*, **29**, 257–261.

20. Clayton, H.M. & Duncan, J.L. (1979) The development of immunity to *Parascaris equorum* infection in the foal. *Research in Veterinary Science*, **26**, 383–384.

21. Cohen, N.D., Parson, E.M., Seahorn, T.L. & Carter, G.K. (1994) Prevalence and factors associated with development of laminitis in horses with duodenitis/proximal jejunitis: 33 cases (1985–1991). *Journal of the American Veterinary Medical Association*, **204**, 250–254.

22. Cohen, N.D., Carter, G.K., Mealey, R.H. & Taylor, T.S. (1995) Medical management of right dorsal colitis in 5 horses: A retrospective study (1987–1993). *Journal of Veterinary Internal Medicine*, **9**, 272–276.

23. Cohen, N.D., Vontur, C.A. & Rakestraw, P.C. (2000) Risk factors for enterolithiasis among horses in Texas. *Journal of the American Veterinary Medical Association*, **216**, 1787–1794.

24. Cohen, N.D., Toby, E., Roussel, A.J., Murphey, E.L. & Wang, N. (2006) Are feeding practices associated with duodenitis-proximal jejunitis? *Equine Veterinary Journal*, **38**, 526–531.

25. Craig, D.R., Pankowski, R.L., Car, B.D., Hackett, R.P. & Erb, H.N. (1987) Ileocolostomy. A technique for surgical management of equine cecal impaction. *Veterinary Surgery*, **16**, 451–455.

26. Cribb, N.C., Cote, N.M., Boure, L.P. & Peregrine, A.S. (2006) Acute small intestinal obstruction associated with *Parascaris equorum* infection in young horses: 25 cases (1985–2004). *New Zealand Veterinary Journal*, **54**, 338–343.

27. Cruz, A.M., Li, R., Kenney, D.G. & Monteith, G. (2006) Effects of indwelling nasogastric intubation on gastric emptying of a liquid marker in horses. *American Journal of Veterinary Research*, **67**, 1100–1104.

28. Cummings, C.A., Copedge, K.J. & Confer, A.W. (1997) Equine gastric impaction, ulceration, and perforation due to persimmon (*Diospyros virginiana*) ingestion. *Journal of Veterinary Diagnostic Investigation*, **9**, 311–313.

29. Dabareiner, R.M. & White, N.A. (1995) Large colon impaction in horses: 147 cases (1985–1991). *Journal of the American Veterinary Medical Association*, **206**, 679–685.

30. Dabareiner, R.M., Sullins, K.E. & Goodrich, L.R. (1996) Large colon resection for treatment of lymphosarcoma in two horses. *Journal of the American Veterinary Medical Association*, **208**, 895–897.

31. De Bosschere, H., Simoens, P., Ducatelle, R. & Picavet, T. (1999) Persistent vitelline arteries in a foal. *Equine Veterinary Journal*, **31**, 542–544.

32. Dionne, R.M., Vrins, A., Doucet, M.Y. & Pare, J. (2003) Gastric ulcers in standardbred racehorses: Prevalence, lesion description, and risk factors. *Journal of Veterinary Internal Medicine*, **17**, 218–222.

33. Dukti, S.A., Perkins, S., Murphy, J., *et al.* (2006) Prevalence of gastric squamous ulceration in horses with abdominal pain. *Equine Veterinary Journal*, **38**, 347–349.

34. East, L.M., Trumble, T.N., Steyn, P.F., Savage, C.J., Dickinson, C.E. & Traub-Dargatz, J.L. (2000) The application of technetium-99 m hexamethylpropyle-neamine oxime (99mTc-HMPAO) labeled white blood cells for the diagnosis of right dorsal ulcerative colitis in two horses. *Veterinary Radiology & Ultrasound*, **41**, 360–364.

35. Edwards, G.B. & Proudman, C.J. (1994) An analysis of 75 cases of intestinal obstruction caused by pedunculated lipomas. *Equine Veterinary Journal*, **26**, 18–21.

36. Ellis, C.M., Lynch, T.M., Slone, D.E., Hughes, F.E. & Clark, C.K. (2008) Survival and complications after large colon resection and end-to-end anastomosis for strangulating large colon volvulus in seventy-three horses. *Veterinary Surgery*, **37**, 786–790.

37. Embertson, R.M., Colahan, P.T., Brown, M.P., Peyton, L.C., Schneider, R.K. & Granstedt, M.E. (1985) Ileal impaction in the horse. *Journal of the American Veterinary Medical Association*, **186**, 570–572.

38. Engelbert, T.A., Tate, L.P., Jr., Bowman, K.F. & Bristol, D.G. (1993) Incarceration of the small intestine in the epiploic foramen. Report of 19 cases (1983–1992). *Veterinary Surgery*, **22**, 57–61.

39. Epstein, K.L. & Parente, E.J. (2006) Laparoscopic obliteration of the nephrosplenic space using polypropylene mesh in five horses. *Veterinary Surgery*, **35**, 431–437.

40. Farstvedt, E. & Hendrickson, D. (2005) Laparoscopic closure of the nephrosplenic space for prevention of recurrent nephrosplenic entrapment of the ascending colon. *Veterinary Surgery*, **34**, 642–645.

41. Foerner, J.J., Ringle, M.J., Junkins, D.S., Fischer, A.T., MacHarg, M.A. & Phillips, T.N. (1993) Transection of the pelvic flexure to reduce incarceration of the large colon through the epiploic foramen in a horse. *Journal of the American Veterinary Medical Association*, **203**, 1312–1313.

42. Ford, T.S., Freeman, D.E., Ross, M.W., Richardson, D.W., Martin, B.B. & Madison, J.B. (1990) Ileocecal intussusception in horses: 26 cases (1981–1988). *Journal of the American Veterinary Medical Association*, **196**, 121–126.

43. Frederico, L.M., Jones, S.L. & Blikslager, A.T. (2006) Predisposing factors for small colon impaction in horses and outcome of medical and surgical treatment: 44 cases (1999–2004). *Journal of the American Veterinary Medical Association*, **229**, 1612–1616.

44. Freeman, D.E. & Schaeffer, D.J. (2001) Age distributions of horses with strangulation of the small intestine by a lipoma or in the epiploic foramen: 46 cases (1994–2000). *Journal of the American Veterinary Medical Association*, **219**, 87–89.

45. Freeman, D.E. & Schaeffer, D.J. (2005) Short-term survival after surgery for epiploic foramen entrapment compared with other strangulating diseases of the small intestine in horses. *Equine Veterinary Journal*, **37**, 292–295.

46. Freeman, D.E., Koch, D.B. & Boles, C.L. (1979) Mesodiverticular bands as a cause of small intestinal strangulation and volvulus in the horse. *Journal of the American Veterinary Medical Association*, **175**, 1089–1094.

47. Freeman, S.L., Boswell, J.C. & Smith, R.K. (2001) Use of transrectal ultrasonography to aid diagnosis of small colon strangulation in two horses. *Veterinary Record*, **148**, 812–813.

48. Garcia-Seco, E., Wilson, D.A., Kramer, J., *et al.* (2005) Prevalence and risk factors associated with outcome of surgical removal of pedunculated lipomas in horses: 102 cases (1987–2002). *Journal of the American Veterinary Medical Association*, **226**, 1529–1537.

49. Gardner, R.B., Nydam, D.V., Mohammed, H.O., Ducharme, N.G. & Divers, D.J. (2005) Serum gamma glutamyl transferase activity in horses with right or left dorsal displacements of the large colon. *Journal of Veterinary Internal Medicine*, **19**, 761–764.

50. Gaughan, E.M. & Hackett, R.P. (1990) Cecocolic intussusception in horses: 11 cases (1979–1989). *Journal of the American Veterinary Medical Association*, **197**, 1373–1375.

51. Gayle, J.M., Blikslager, A.T. & Bowman, K.F. (2000) Mesenteric rents as a source of small intestinal strangulation in horses: 15 cases (1990–1997). *Journal of the American Veterinary Medical Association*, **216**, 1446–1449.

52. Gerard, M.P., Bowman, K.F., Blikslager, A.T., Tate, L.P., Jr. & Bristol, D.G. (1996) Jejunocolostomy or ileocolostomy for treatment of cecal impaction in horses: Nine cases (1985–1995). *Journal of the American Veterinary Medical Association*, **209**, 1287–1290.

53. Granot, N., Milgram, J., Bdolah-Abram, T., Shemesh, I. & Steinman, A. (2008) Surgical management of sand colic impactions in horses: A retrospective study of 41 cases. *Australian Veterinary Journal*, **86**, 404–407.

54. Grant, B.D. & Tennant, B. (1973) Volvulus associated with Meckel's diverticulum in the horse. *Journal of the American Veterinary Medical Association*, **162**, 550–551.

55. Hallowell, G.D. (2008) Retrospective study assessing efficacy of treatment of large colonic impactions. *Equine Veterinary Journal*, **40**, 411–413.

56. Hammock, P.D., Freeman, D.E. & Baker, G.J. (1998) Failure of psyllium mucilloid to hasten evaluation of sand from the equine large intestine. *Veterinary Surgery*, **27**, 547–554.

57. Hammond, C.J., Mason, D.K. & Watkins, K.L. (1986) Gastric ulceration in mature thoroughbred horses. *Equine Veterinary Journal*, **18**, 284–287.

58. Hanson, R.R., Schumacher, J., Humburg, J. & Dunkerley, S.C. (1996) Medical treatment of horses with ileal impactions: 10 cases (1990–1994). *Journal of the American Veterinary Medical Association*, **208**, 898–900.

59. Hanson, R.R., Wright, J.C., Schumacher, J., Baird, A.N., Humburg, J. & Pugh, D.G. (1998) Surgical reduction of ileal impactions in the horse: 28 cases. *Veterinary Surgery*, **27**, 555–560.

60. Hardy, J., Stewart, R.H., Beard, W.L. & Yvorchuk-St-Jean, K. (1992) Complications of nasogastric intubation in horses: Nine cases (1987–1989). *Journal of the American Veterinary Medical Association*, **201**, 483–486.

61. Hardy, J., Minton, M., Robertson, J.T., Beard, W.L. & Beard, L.A. (2000) Nephrosplenic entrapment in the horse: A retrospective study of 174 cases. *Equine Veterinary Journal Supplement*, **32**, 95–97.

62. Harvey-Micay, J. (1999) Intestinal adenocarcinoma causing recurrent colic in the horse. *Canadian Veterinary Journal*, **40**, 729–730.

63. Hassel, D.M. (2002) Enterolithiasis. *Clinical Techniques in Equine Practice*, **1**, 143–147.

64. Hassel, D.M., Langer, D.L., Snyder, J.R., Drake, C.M., Goodell, M.L. & Wyle, A. (1999) Evaluation of enterolithiasis in equids: 900 cases (1973–1996). *Journal of the American Veterinary Medical Association*, **214**, 233–237.

65. Hassel, D.M., Schiffman, P.S. & Snyder, J.R. (2001) Petrographic and geochemic evaluation of equine enteroliths. *American Journal of Veterinary Research*, **62**, 350–358.

66. Hassel, D.M., Rakestraw, P.C., Gardner, I.A., Spier, S.J. & Snyder, J.R. (2004) Dietary risk factors and colonic pH and mineral concentrations in horses with enterolithiasis. *Journal of Veterinary Internal Medicine*, **18**, 346–349.

67. Hassel, D.M., Spier, S.J., Aldridge, B.M., Watnick, M., Argenzio, R.A. & Snyder, J.R. (2009) Influence of diet and water supply on mineral content and pH within the large intestine of horses with enterolithiasis. *Veterinary Journal*, **182**, 44–49.

68. Hearn, F.P. & Peregrine, A.S. (2003) Identification of foals infected with *Parascaris equorum* apparently resistant to ivermectin. *Journal of the American Veterinary Medical Association*, **223**, 482–485.

69. Hillyer, M.H., Taylor, F.G., Proudman, C.J., Edwards, G.B., Smith, J.E. & French, N.P. (2002) Case control study to identify risk factors for simple colonic obstruction and distension colic in horses. *Equine Veterinary Journal*, **34**, 455–463.

70. Hogan, P.M., Bramlage, L.R. & Pierce, S.W. (1995) Repair of a full-thickness gastric rupture in a horse. *Journal of the American Veterinary Medical Association*, **207**, 338–340.

71. Honnas, C.M. & Schumacher, J. (1985) Primary gastric impaction in a pony. *Journal of the American Veterinary Medical Association*, **187**, 501–502.

72. Hooper, R.N. (1989) Small intestinal strangulation caused by Meckel's diverticulum in a horse. *Journal of the American Veterinary Medical Association*, **194**, 943–944.

73. Hubert, J.D., Hardy, J., Holcombe, S.J. & Moore, R.M. (2000) Cecal amputation within the right ventral colon for surgical treatment of nonreducible cecocolic intussusception in 8 horses. *Veterinary Surgery*, **29**, 317–325.

74. Hughes, F.E., Moll, H.D. & Slone, D.E. (1996) Outcome of surgical correction of meconium impactions in 8 foals. *Journal of Equine Veterinary Science*, **16**, 172–175.

75. Jenei, T.M., Garcia-Lopez, J.M., Provost, P.J. & Kirker-Head, C.A. (2007) Surgical management of small intestinal incarceration through the gastrosplenic ligament: 14 cases (1994–2006). *Journal of the American Veterinary Medical Association*, **231**, 1221–1224.

76. Johnston, J.K. & Morris, D.D. (1987) Comparison of duodenitis/proximal jejunitis and small intestinal obstruction in horses: 68 cases (1977–1985). *Journal of the American Veterinary Medical Association*, **191**, 849–854.

77. Johnston, K., Holcombe, S.J. & Hauptman, J.G. (2007) Plasma lactate as a predictor of colonic viability and survival after 360 degrees volvulus of the ascending colon in horses. *Veterinary Surgery*, **36**, 563–567.

78. Jones, D.G., Greatorex, J.C., Stockman, M.J. & Harris, C.P. (1972) Gastric impaction in a pony: Relief via laparotomy. *Equine Veterinary Journal*, **4**, 98–99.

79. Jones, S.L., Davis, J. & Rowlingson, K. (2003) Ultrasonographic findings in horses with right dorsal colitis: Five cases (2000–2001). *Journal of the American Veterinary Medical Association*, **222**, 1248–1251.

80. Karcher, L.F., Dill, S.G., Anderson, W.I. & King, J.M. (1990) Right dorsal colitis. *Journal of Veterinary Internal Medicine*, **4**, 247–253.

81. Kellam, L.L., Johnson, P.J., Kramer, J. & Keegan, K.G. (2000) Gastric impaction and obstruction of the small intestine associated with persimmon phytobezoar in a horse. *Journal of the American Veterinary Medical Association*, **216**, 1279–1281.

82. Keppie, N.J., Rosenstein, D.S., Holcombe, S.J. & Schott, H.C., 2nd. (2008) Objective radiographic assessment of abdominal sand accumulation in horses. *Veterinary Radiology & Ultrasound*, **49**, 122–128.

83. Kiper, M.L., Traub-Dargatz, J. & Curtis, C.R. (1990) Gastric rupture in horses: 50 cases (1979–1987). *Journal of the American Veterinary Medical Association*, **196**, 333–336.

84. Kirchhof, N., Steinhauer, D. & Fey, K. (1996) Equine adenocarcinomas of the large intestine with osseous metaplasia. *Journal of Comparative Pathology*, **114**, 451–456.

85. Korolainen, R. & Ruohoniemi, M. (2002) Reliability of ultrasonography compared to radiography in revealing intestinal sand accumulations in horses. *Equine Veterinary Journal*, **34**, 499–504.

86. Lind, E.O. & Christensson, D. (2009) Anthelmintic efficacy on *Parascaris equorum* in foals on Swedish studs. *Acta Veterinaria Scandinavica*, **51**, 45.

87. Lindgren, K., Ljungvall, O., Nilsson, O., Ljungström, B.L. Lindahl, C. & Höglund, J. (2008) *Parascaris equorum* in foals and in their environment on a Swedish stud farm, with notes on treatment failure of ivermectin. *Veterinary Parasitology*, **151**, 337–343.

88. Little, D. & Blikslager, A.T. (2002) Factors associated with development of ileal impaction in horses with surgical colic: 78 cases (1986–2000). *Equine Veterinary Journal*, **34**, 464–468.

89. Lopes, M.A., White, N.A., 2nd, Donaldson, L., Crisman, M.V. & Ward, D.L. (2004) Effects of enteral and intravenous fluid therapy, magnesium sulfate, and sodium sulfate on colonic contents and feces in horses. *American Journal of Veterinary Research*, **65**, 695–704.

90. Lores, M. & Ortenburger, A.I. (2008) Use of cecal bypass via side-to-side ileocolic anastomosis without ileal transection for treatment of cecocolic intussusception in three horses. *Journal of the American Veterinary Medical Association*, **232**, 574–577.

91. Lores, M., Stryhn, H., McDuffee, L., Rose, P. & Muirhead, T. (2007) Transcutaneous ultrasonographic evaluation of gastric distension with fluid in horses. *American Journal of Veterinary Research*, **68**, 153–157.

92. Lyons, E.T., Tolliver, S.C., Ionita, M. & Collins, S.S. (2008) Evaluation of parasiticidal activity of fenbendazole, ivermectin, oxibendazole, and pyrantel pamoate in horse foals with emphasis on ascarids (*Parascaris equorum*) in field studies on five farms in Central Kentucky in 2007. *Parasitology Research*, **103**, 287–291.

93. Mair, T.S. & Smith, L.J. (2005) Survival and complication rates in 300 horses undergoing surgical treatment of colic. Part 1: Short-term survival following a single laparotomy. *Equine Veterinary Journal*, **37**, 296–302.

94. Martin, B.B., Jr., Freeman, D.E. & Ross, M.W. (1999) Cecocolic and cecocecal intussusception in horses: 30 cases (1976–1996). *Journal of the American Veterinary Medical Association*, **214**, 80–84.

95. Mathis, S.C., Slone, D.E., Lynch, T.M., Hughes, F.E. & Clarke, C.K. (2006) Use of colonic luminal pressure to predict outcome after surgical treatment of strangulating large colon volvulus in horses. *Veterinary Surgery*, **35**, 356–360.

96. McClure, S.R., Glickman, L.T. & Glickman, N.W. (1999) Prevalence of gastric ulcers in show horses. *Journal of the American Veterinary Medical Association*, **215**, 1130–1133.

97. McConnico, R.S., Morgan, T.W., Williams, C.C., Hubert, J.D. & Moore, R.M. (2008) Pathophysiologic effects of phenylbutazone on the right dorsal colon in horses. *American Journal of Veterinary Research*, **69**, 1496–1505.

98. Milne, E.M., Pogson, D.M. & Doxey, D.L. (1990) Secondary gastric impaction associated with ragwort poisoning in three ponies. *Veterinary Record*, **126**, 502–504.

99. Moran, J.A., Lemberger, K., Cadore, J.L. & Lepage, O.M. (2008) Small intestine adenocarcinoma in conjunction with multiple adenomas causing acute colic in a horse. *Journal of Veterinary Diagnostic Investigation*, **20**, 121–124.

100. Murray, M.J. (1992) Gastric ulceration in horses: 91 cases (1987–1990). *Journal of the American Veterinary Medical Association*, **201**, 117–120.

101. Murray, M.J., Schusser, G.F., Pipers, F.S. & Gross, S.J. (1996) Factors associated with gastric lesions in thoroughbred racehorses. *Equine Veterinary Journal*, **28**, 368–374.

102. Nadeau, J.A., Andrews, F.M., Mathew, A.G., *et al.* (2000) Evaluation of diet as a cause of gastric ulcers in horses. *American Journal of Veterinary Research*, **61**, 784–790.

103. Owen, R.A., Jagger, D.W. & Jagger, F. (1987) Two cases of equine primary gastric impaction. *Veterinary Record*, **121**, 102–105.

104. Pease, A.P., Scrivani, P.V., Erb, H.N. & Cook, V.L. (2004) Accuracy of increased large-intestine wall thickness during ultrasonography for diagnosing large-colon torsion in 42 horses. *Veterinary Radiology & Ultrasound*, **45**, 220–224.

105. Pierce, R.L., Fischer, A.T., Rohrbach, B.W. & Klohnen, A. (2010) Postoperative complications and survival after enterolith removal from the ascending or descending colon in horses. *Veterinary Surgery*, **39**, 609–615.

106. Plummer, A.E., Rakestraw, P.C., Hardy, J. & Lee, R.M. (2007) Outcome of medical and surgical treatment of cecal impaction in horses: 114 cases (1994–2004). *Journal of the American Veterinary Medical Association*, **231**, 1378–1385.

107. Prange, T., Holcombe, S.J., Brown, J.A., *et al.* (2010) Resection and anastomosis of the descending colon in 43 horses. *Veterinary Surgery*, **39**, 748–753.

108. Probst, C.W., Schneider, R.K., Hubbell, J.A. & Hart, E.C. (1983) Surgical repair of a perforated gastric ulcer in a foal. *Veterinary Surgery*, **12**, 93–95.

109. Pusterla, N., Magdesian, K.G. & Maleski, K. (2004) Retrospective evaluation of the use of acetylcysteine enemas in the treatment of meconium retention in foals: 44 cases (1987–2002). *Equine Veterinary Education*, **16**, 133–136.

110. Rabuffo, T.S., Hackett, E.S., Grenager, N., Boston, R. & Orsini, J.A. (2009) Prevalence of gastric ulcerations in horses. *Journal of Equine Veterinary Science*, **29**, 540–546.

111. Ragle, C.A., Meagher, D.M., Lacroix, C.A. & Honnas, C.M. (1989) Surgical treatment of sand colic. Results in 40 horses. *Veterinary Surgery*, **18**, 48–51.

112. Reinemeyer, C.R. (2009) Diagnosis and control of anthelmintic-resistant *Parascaris equorum*. *Parasites & Vectors*, **2**(Suppl 2), S8.

113. Rhoads, W.S. & Parks, A.H. (1999) Incarceration of the small colon through a rent in the gastrosplenic ligament in a pony. *Journal of the American Veterinary Medical Association*, **214**, 226–228.

114. Rhoads, W.S., Barton, M.H. & Parks, A.H. (1999) Comparison of medical and surgical treatment for impaction of the small colon in horses: 84 cases (1986–1996). *Journal of the American Veterinary Medical Association*, **214**, 1042–1047.

115. Roberts, C.T. & Slone, D.E. (2000) Caecal impactions managed surgically by typhlotomy in 10 cases (1988–1998). *Equine Veterinary Journal Supplement*, **32**, 74–76.

116. Rocken, M., Schubert, C., Mosel, G. & Litzke, L.F. (2005) Indications, surgical technique, and long-term experience with laparoscopic closure of the nephrosplenic space in standing horses. *Veterinary Surgery*, **34**, 637–641.

117. Ross, M.W., Martin, B.B. & Donawick, W.J. (1985) Cecal perforation in the horse. *Journal of the American Veterinary Medical Association*, **187**, 249–253.

118. Ross, M.W., Orsini, J.A. & Ehnen, S.J. (1987) Jejunocolic anastomosis for the surgical management of recurrent cecal impaction in a horse. *Veterinary Surgery*, **16**, 265–268.

119. Roy, M.F., Parente, E.J., Donaldson, M.T., Habecker, P. & Axon, J. (2002) Successful treatment of a colonic adenocarcinoma in a horse. *Equine Veterinary Journal*, **34**, 102–104.

120. Ruohoniemi, M., Kaikkonen, R., Raekallio, M. & Luukkanen, L. (2001) Abdominal radiography in monitoring the resolution of sand accumulations from the large colon of horses treated medically. *Equine Veterinary Journal*, **33**, 59–64.

121. Ryu, S.H., Bak, U.B., Kim, J.G., *et al.* (2001) Cecal rupture by Anoplocephala perfoliata infection in a thoroughbred horse in Seoul Race Park, South Korea. *Journal of Veterinary Science*, **2**, 189–193.

122. Ryu, S.H., Jang, J.D., Bak, U.B., Lee, C., Youn, H.J. & Lee, Y.L. (2004) Gastrointestinal impaction by *Parascaris equorum* in a Thoroughbred foal in Jeju, Korea. *Journal of Veterinary Science*, **5**, 181–182.

123. Santschi, E.M., Slone, D.E., Jr. & Frank, W.M., 2nd. (1993) Use of ultrasound in horses for diagnosis of left dorsal displacement of the large colon and monitoring its nonsurgical correction. *Veterinary Surgery*, **22**, 281–284.

124. Seahorn, T.L., Cornick, J.L. & Cohen, N.D. (1992) Prognostic indicators for horses with duodenitis-proximal jejunitis. 75 horses (1985–1989). *Journal of Veterinary Internal Medicine*, **6**, 307–311.

125. Senior, J.M., Pinchbeck, G.L., Dugdale, A.H. & Clegg, P.D. (2004) Retrospective study of the risk factors and prevalence of colic in horses after orthopaedic surgery. *Veterinary Record*, **155**, 321–325.

126. Sheats, M.K., Cook, V.L., Jones, S.L., Blikslager, A.T. & Pease, A.P. (2010) Use of ultrasound to evaluate outcome following colic surgery for equine large colon volvulus. *Equine Veterinary Journal*, **42**, 47–52.

127. Simmons, T.R., Gaughan, E.M., Ducharme, N.G., Dill, S.G., King, J.M. & Anderson, W.I. (1990) Treatment of right dorsal ulcerative colitis in a horse. *Journal of the American Veterinary Medical Association*, **196**, 455–458.

128. Smith, L.C.R., Payne, R.J., Boys Smith, S.J., Bathe, A.P. & Greet, T.R. (2010) Outcome and long-term follow-up of 20 horses undergoing surgery for caecal impaction: A retrospective study (2000–2008). *Equine Veterinary Journal*, **42**, 388–392.

129. Sprinkle, F.P., Swerczek, T.W. & Crowe, M.W. (1984) Meckel's diverticulum in the horse. *Equine Veterinary Science*, **4**, 175–176.

130. Steenhaut, M., Vlaminck, K. & Gasthuys, F. (1986) Surgical repair of a partial gastric rupture in a horse. *Equine Veterinary Journal*, **18**, 331–332.

131. Steenhaut, M., Vandenreyt, I. & Van Roy, M. (1993) Incarceration of the large colon through the epiploic foramen in a horse. *Equine Veterinary Journal*, **25**, 550–551.

132. Stephen, J.O., Corley, K.T., Johnston, J.K. & Pfeiffer, D. (2004) Small intestinal volvulus in 115 horses: 1988–2000. *Veterinary Surgery*, **33**, 333–339.

133. Stephen, J.O., Corley, K.T., Johnston, J.K. & Pfeiffer, D. (2004) Factors associated with mortality and morbidity in small intestinal volvulus in horses. *Veterinary Surgery*, **33**, 340–348.

134. Sutter, W.W. & Hardy, J. (2004) Laparoscopic repair of a small intestinal mesenteric rent in a broodmare. *Veterinary Surgery*, **33**, 92–95.

135. Tabar, J.J. & Cruz, A.M. (2009) Cecal rupture in foals: 7 cases (1996–2006). *Canadian Veterinary Journal*, **50**, 65–70.

136. Taylor, S.D., Pusterla, N., Vaughan, B., Whitcomb, M.B. & Wilson, W.D. (2006) Intestinal neoplasia in horses. *Journal of Veterinary Internal Medicine*, **20**, 1429–1436.

137. Todhunter, R.J., Erb, H.N. & Roth, L. (1986) Gastric rupture in horses: A review of 54 cases. *Equine Veterinary Journal*, **18**, 288–293.

138. Trostle, S.S. & Markel, M.D. (1993) Incarceration of the large colon in the gastrosplenic ligament of a horse. *Journal of the American Veterinary Medical Association*, **202**, 773–775.

139. Turner, T.A., Adams, S.B. & White, N.A. (1984) Small intestine incarceration through the epiploic foramen of the horse. *Journal of the American Veterinary Medical Association*, **184**, 731–734.

140. Underwood, C., Southwood, L.L., McKeown, L.P. & Knight, D. (2008) Complications and survival associated with surgical compared with medical management of horses with duodenitis-proximal jejunitis. *Equine Veterinary Journal*, **40**, 373–378.

141. Vachon, A.M. & Fischer, A.T. (1995) Small intestinal herniation through the epiploic foramen: 53 cases (1987–1993). *Equine Veterinary Journal*, **27**, 373–380.

142. Van Hoogmoed, L., Snyder, J.R., Pascoe, J.R. & Olander, H. (2000) Use of pelvic flexure biopsies to predict survival after large colon torsion in horses. *Veterinary Surgery*, **29**, 572–577.

143. Van Hoogmoed, L.M., Snyder, J.R. & Harmon, F. (2000) In vitro investigation of the effect of prostaglandins and nonsteroidal anti-inflammatory drugs on contractile activity of the equine smooth muscle of the dorsal colon, ventral colon, and pelvic flexure. *American Journal of Veterinary Research*, **61**, 1259–1266.

144. Vatistas, N.J., Snyder, J.R., Wilson, W.D., Drake, C. & Hildebrand, S. (1996) Surgical treatment for colic in the foal (67 cases): 1980–1992. *Equine Veterinary Journal*, **28**, 139–145.

145. Vatistas, N.J., Snyder, J.R., Carlson, G., et al. (1999) Cross-sectional study of gastric ulcers of the squamous mucosa in thoroughbred racehorses. *Equine Veterinary Journal Supplement*, **29**, 34–39.

146. Verwilghen, D., van Galen, G., Busoni, V., et al. (2010) Meckel's diverticulum as a cause of colic: 2 cases with different morphological features. *Tijdschrift voor Diergeneeskunde*, **135**, 452–455.

147. White, N.A., 2nd, Tyler, D.E., Blackwell, R.B. & Allen, D. (1987) Hemorrhagic fibrinonecrotic duodenitis-proximal jejunitis in horses: 20 cases (1977–1984). *Journal of the American Veterinary Medical Association*, **190**, 311–315.

148. Williams, M.M., Spiess, B.M., Pascoe, P.J. & O'Grady, M. (2000) Systemic effects of topical and subconjunctival ophthalmic atropine in the horse. *Veterinary Ophthalmology*, **3**, 193–199.

149. Wylie, C.E. & Proudman, C.J. (2009) Equine grass sickness: Epidemiology, diagnosis, and global distribution. *Veterinary Clinics of North America: Equine Practice*, **25**, 381–399.

150. Yovich, J.V., Stashak, T.S. & Bertone, A.L. (1985) Incarceration of small intestine through rents in the gastrosplenic ligament in the horse. *Veterinary Surgery*, **14**, 303–306.

151. Zedler, S.T., Embertson, R.M., Bernard, W.V., Barr, B.S. & Boston, R.C. (2009) Surgical treatment of gastric outflow obstruction in 40 foals. *Veterinary Surgery*, **38**, 623–630.

18

Postoperative Patient Care

Samantha K. Hart

Department of Clinical Studies, New Bolton Center, School of Veterinary Medicine, University of Pennsylvania, Kennett Square, PA, USA

Chapter Outline

Monitoring	**231**	Hydroxyethyl starch	236
Patient assessment	231	Formulating a fluid therapy plan	237
Physical examination	232	Anti-inflammatory and Analgesic drugs	238
Laboratory data	233	Nonsteroidal anti-inflammatory	
Central venous pressure	234	drugs (NSAID)	238
Arterial blood pressure	234	Intravenous lidocaine	239
Treatment	**235**	Butorphanol	239
Fluid therapy	235	Alpha-2 agonists	239
Crystalloids	235	Ketamine	239
Colloids	236	Antimicrobial drugs	239
Plasma	236	Feeding	241

Early referral and surgical treatment has improved the survival of colic patients, with most horses and foals undergoing surgery being recovered from general anesthesia. Postoperative management of colic patients is an important component in further improving outcome. General assessment and thorough physical examination play an important role in ensuring adequate treatment and that complications are addressed promptly. Having meticulous medical records to monitor trends over time is important. Use of a daily monitoring and treatment sheet can streamline patient care.

Most horses recovering from colic surgery are uncomplicated and require only routine management. Routine management typically includes short-term maintenance intravenous (IV) fluid therapy, analgesia, and perioperative antimicrobial drugs. Administration of adequate analgesia and the use of anti-inflammatory drugs are important in minimizing the negative effects of pain and inflammation on healing. Perioperative antimicrobial use is typically only indicated for up to 24h postoperatively; however, prolonged use may be indicated in individual cases when infection is present.

Practical Guide to Equine Colic, First Edition. Edited by Louise L. Southwood.
© 2013 John Wiley & Sons, Inc. Published 2013 by John Wiley & Sons, Inc.

More intensive monitoring such as laboratory data and the use of central venous and arterial blood pressure measurement may be indicated in more critical patients such as horses recovering from large colon volvulus or resection and anastomosis. Although isotonic crystalloid solutions are the mainstay IV fluid therapy, the use of colloid solutions may play an important role in maintaining tissue perfusion and oxygenation and ameliorating the effects of endotoxemia. See also Chapter 19 on Postoperative Complications (p. 244).

Monitoring

Patient assessment

The general assessment should begin from outside the patient's stall and should continue as the physical examination is performed. Questions that should be asked during the initial assessment include the following: Does the patient respond when approached? Does the patient come to the front of the stall, or does he/she remain at the back? Are the patient's ears forward and does the patient appear alert? Are there indications that the horse has been showing signs of distress, such as paw marks in shavings or straw?

Horses recovering from colic surgery should be closely monitored and observed for changes in attitude or reduced appetite. Although it is not uncommon for horses to be quiet in the immediate postoperative period, it should be expected that within 6 h of recovery from anesthesia the patient is bright and responsive. Subjectively it appears that horses in which there has been greater manipulation of the intestine, excessive tension on the mesentery (such as strangulating lesions of the small intestine or large colon), or resection and anastomosis performed tend to remain quiet for longer periods of time. Horses should be monitored closely for signs of colic which range in intensity from mild (inappetance, pawing intermittently, flank watching, flehmen) or moderate (pawing, kicking at abdomen, lying in sternal or lateral recumbency) to severe (violent thrashing, nonresponsiveness to sedation). Different horses respond differently to abdominal discomfort, although as a general rule older horses and draft breeds tend to be more stoic and mild signs of colic may be missed.

Nasogastric intubation (p. 38) is indicated in any postoperative colic patient showing signs of pain.

Postoperative colic patients should have a good appetite particularly for fresh grass. The most common reasons for inappetence following colic surgery are likely to be persistent pain either from gastric or intestinal dilatation or intestinal obstruction, development of enterocolitis (such as that associated with salmonellosis), the presence of nonviable intestine, or metabolic derangements such as hypertriglyceridemia.

Water intake should be closely monitored. Average water intake for an adult horse stalled and fed hay is approximately 50–65 mL/kg body weight/day; however, horses that are not eating or are receiving IV fluids may not drink nearly this volume. During the postoperative period, horses may be provided with a bucket of water containing electrolytes (in addition to a bucket of fresh plain water); a standard formula for this is 34.5 g sodium chloride (NaCl), 34.5 g sodium bicarbonate (NaHCO$_3$), and 14.2 g potassium chloride (KCl).

Although monitoring urine production (both volume and frequency) can be difficult, an adult horse is expected to produce between 5 and 15 L of urine per day. Adult horses should posture to urinate and produce a steady stream of clear (if on IV fluids) to cloudy yellow urine and several wet areas should be noted in the stall.

Fecal production and character should be closely monitored. A sudden decrease in fecal production may indicate alteration in gastrointestinal motility and potentially the development of an impaction. A 500 kg adult horse typically defecates five to seven times a day; however, if the horse is inappetant, held off feed, or if a pelvic flexure enterotomy or typhlotomy was performed at surgery, fecal production may be decreased. Additionally, horses placed on a low-bulk diet should also be expected to have decreased fecal production. If the feces passed are drier and firmer or less than expected, nasogastric intubation with water and electrolytes is warranted and the patient's hydration status assessed. Diarrhea in postoperative colics is of particular concern due to the increased risk of salmonellosis in these patients. Although loose feces or transient diarrhea may occur following colic surgery for large and small colon disease in particular, further investigation using fecal polymerase chain reaction (PCR) for *Salmonella* spp. should be performed. Enzyme-linked immunosorbent assay

(ELISA) for *Clostridium difficile* type A and *C. perfringens* toxins may also be performed, particularly if antimicrobials have been administered.

Physical examination

Horses should be examined every 2–6h in the postoperative period depending on how critical the patient is judged to be. Walk by or comfort checks should also be performed frequently to further monitor the horse. A minimum database that should be obtained at every examination is a TPR (temperature, pulse, respiration) as well as assessment of the mucous membranes. A complete physical examination consists of an overall assessment of the patient, mucous membranes, heart rate and peripheral pulse quality, respiratory rate and effort, lung auscultation, rectal temperature, and gastrointestinal auscultation.

The mucous membranes should be evaluated closely; tacky or dry mucous membranes may indicate dehydration while prolonged capillary refill time may indicate poor peripheral perfusion. The postoperative colic patient should have pink, moist mucous membranes with a capillary refill time < 2 seconds.

Tachycardia is most often due to either pain or shock; however, primary cardiac disease such as a tachyarrhythmia should also be considered if the heart rate is not consistent with the other clinical signs. Although horses may have a mild to moderate tachycardia in the immediate postoperative period (within the first 2–4h), persistent tachycardia (heart rate >50–60 beats/min) should be investigated and a nasogastric tube should always be passed to assess for the presence of reflux. Sources of pain in the postoperative colic patient include the gastrointestinal tract and the accumulation of gastric fluid, surgical site, and laminitis. Shock can be associated with endotoxemia, intestinal ischemia, and infection including salmonellosis.

Tachypnea can be associated with pain, shock, or respiratory tract disease. Tachypnea may be the only clinical sign associated with pain particularly in older horses. As such, it is recommended that a nasogastric tube be passed to assess for the presence of reflux in any tachypneic (or tachycardic) patient. Thoracic auscultation should be performed to monitor for any changes in pulmonic sounds, as postanesthetic pneumonia should be considered in patients with tachypnea particularly if associated with a fever.

Hypothermia is relatively uncommon in adult horses although it certainly is possible especially in the immediate postoperative period, and should be addressed if present. A more common cause of hypothermia is a spurious result due to pneumorectum, and is commonly encountered when an abdominal palpation per rectum is performed prior to obtaining the rectal temperature. Common causes of a fever which should be ruled out in adult horses in the postoperative period include endotoxemia, salmonellosis, incisional infection, catheter-associated infection, and postanesthetic pneumonia.[1] Septic peritonitis is an uncommon postoperative infection[1] and often occurs secondary to intestinal leakage, nonviable bowel, salmonellosis, and severe incisional infection. A fever developing after the second postoperative day appears to be more likely associated with an infection compared to a fever within the first 24–48 postoperative hours.[1] Fevers exceeding 102.5 °F (39 °C) and with a duration beyond 48h are also more likely to be associated with an infection than low-grade fevers of a short duration.[1]

Gastrointestinal motility may be subjectively assessed via auscultation in four quadrants: the left and right dorsal and ventral quadrants. Decreased gastrointestinal borborygmi are commonly heard in the immediate postoperative period and are typically associated with reduced motility and withholding feed.[2] Intestinal borborygmi should rapidly return to normal with the reintroduction of feed.[2] Hand walking and grazing appears to stimulate intestinal motility. Persistently absent intestinal borborygmi during the postoperative period should raise concerns regarding intestinal function and is often associated with other clinical signs consistent with poor bowel viability (tachycardia, fever, inappetence, lack of fecal output, abdominal distention).

Assessment of peripheral pulse quality and peripheral temperature (of the ears and distal limbs) is an important part of the physical examination of a postoperative patient. Studies in human critical care patients have shown that palpation of limb temperature is as useful as more quantitative measurements in characterizing tissue perfusion and oxygenation.[3,4] Cold ears and distal limbs in a postoperative colic patient may be an indication of poor peripheral perfusion, and close monitoring is warranted. Pulse quality may be used as a crude marker of cardiac output and peripheral tissue perfusion.[3] Common sites to assess peripheral pulses include the facial and transverse facial artery in the head, and the palmar and plantar digital arteries in the distal limbs. Digital pulses should also be closely monitored in postoperative colic patients, especially those which may be considered to be at increased risk of developing laminitis.

The incision and catheter site should also be examined. Horses should also be monitored for signs of laminitis by observing their stance and walking them in a circle in the stall, palpating the digital pulses, and feeling the hooves for warmth.

Laboratory data

Packed cell volume (PCV) and total plasma protein (TPP) concentration are typically monitored every 6–24h in postoperative colic patients. The frequency of monitoring will depend on how critical the case is and the use of IV fluid administration. Although it is not the gold standard to assess hydration status in horses, an elevation in PCV typically indicates hypovolemia and dehydration. Horses that are accumulating fluid in the gastrointestinal tract will often have a mild increase in their PCV prior to developing reflux or diarrhea. An elevation in TPP may be caused by several different factors, including dehydration. Hypoproteinemia leading to reduced colloid oncotic or osmotic pressure (COP) is of particular concern and potentially results in edema formation and exacerbation of hypovolemia and reduced tissue oxygenation. Protein, particularly albumin, as well as water and electrolytes are lost from the gastrointestinal tract in horses with severe mucosal injury and can also be lost from the vascular space during systemic inflammation and shock. An increase in PCV with concurrent decrease in TPP can be an indication that this is occurring and is generally associated with a poor prognosis. Hemorrhage is uncommon in the postoperative colic patient; however, a decrease in both PCV and TPP along with clinical signs of dull mentation, tachycardia, tachypnea, cool extremities, and abdominal pain is an indication that the horse may be hemorrhaging. PCV and

TPP can, therefore, be used as an initial guide to tailoring further diagnostic tests and IV fluid therapy in an individual colic patient.

COP is important in maintaining intravascular volume and is due to the osmotic force exerted by proteins within the vascular space (primarily albumin). Although measuring TPP is typically used as an assessment of COP, once a patient has received a synthetic colloid (such as hydroxyethyl starch) TPP read on a refractometer is no longer reliable. COP measured using a colloid osmometer can, therefore, be used to direct further therapy in horses receiving synthetic colloids. In all practicality, however, if the TPP is low, the COP is also likely to be low. Several formulae are available that allow calculation of COP from TPP (p. 100).[5]

Fibrinogen and serum amyloid A are used to evaluate the inflammatory response. An uncomplicated postoperative colic patient has a fibrinogen concentration of 500–800 mg/dL (5–8 g/L) and a site of infection should be considered in patients with concentrations exceeding these values. As a major acute phase protein, serum amyloid A may be a more sensitive and specific marker for postoperative inflammation and infection in colic patients compared to fibrinogen, which is considered a minor acute phase protein.[6]

Plasma creatinine concentrations can be used to assess tissue perfusion. Elevations in plasma creatinine concentration (azotemia, >1.5 mg/dL may be due to prerenal (dehydration and hypovolemia resulting in reduced tissue perfusion), renal (renal failure) or post-renal (obstruction or rupture of the lower urinary tract) causes. Differentiating between these causes is based on other diagnostic tests such as urinalysis and urinary fractional excretion of sodium. Most commonly in postoperative colic patients, azotemia is prerenal and should be addressed by adjusting the IV fluid therapy.

Lactate is produced as an end product of anaerobic glycolysis. Blood lactate concentrations can be used as a marker of peripheral tissue perfusion and oxygenation. The most common causes of hyperlactatemia (lactate concentration >1 mmol/L) in postoperative colic patients are hypovolemia, hypoxia, hypotension, and endotoxemia.

Blood glucose concentration should be assessed at least every 24h; however, if horses are receiving

IV dextrose supplementation, the blood glucose concentrations are typically measured every 4–6 h. Hyperglycemia has typically been permissible in postoperative colic patients due to factors such as stress and endotoxemia resulting in elevated blood glucose concentrations. Recently, however, it has been shown that hyperglycemia can worsen endotoxemia-induced gastrointestinal dysfunction and increase bacterial translocation, while insulin appears to have protective effects.[7-9] Horses with acute gastrointestinal disease with severe hyperglycemia (defined as blood glucose concentrations >200 mg/dL) are significantly more likely to die compared to those which are euglycemic or only mildly hyperglycemic.[10] Although the use of insulin either subcutaneously or as a constant rate infusion (CRI) requires more intensive monitoring, it may be warranted in persistently hyperglycemic patients. It is also important to closely monitor blood glucose concentrations in patients who are at risk of lipid derangements such as ponies, donkeys, miniature horses, horses with pituitary pars intermedia dysfunction (PPID) or metabolic syndrome, overweight and obese horses, and pregnant or lactating mares. Monitoring serum triglyceride concentrations is also indicated in these patients, or any horse which is held off feed for more than 24–48 h. Hypertriglyceridemia (>50 mg/dL) is common in postoperative colic patients. Almost all postoperative colic patients have a plasma triglyceride concentration between 100 and 300 mg/dL 24–36 h after surgery.[11] The triglyceride concentration should return to normal, however, within 72 h of surgery.[11] Marked or persistent hypertriglyceridemia should be addressed promptly with IV dextrose supplementation and insulin therapy if necessary, to prevent further fat mobilization and potential deterioration of the patient.

Urine-specific gravity (USG) is a useful parameter to assess hydration status in adult horses. Although the normal USG of adult horses is 1.025–1.050, horses receiving IV fluids may be isosthenuric (1.008–1.012). If a horse receiving IV fluids is hypersthenuric, this may indicate dehydration and the horse should be further evaluated. Typically a horse on IV fluids will have a USG of 1.013–1.020; if it is <1.013, the horse is likely being overhydrated, and if it is >1.020, the horse may benefit from a higher rate of IV fluid administration, particularly if indicated by other clinical signs. The USG may be monitored once a day while horses are receiving IV fluids or if there is concern about potential renal compromise such as in horses receiving potentially nephrotoxic drugs. Urine can also be assessed for the presence of glucose, which typically indicates hyperglycemia and overwhelming of the renal glucose transport mechanisms. The transport threshold for glucose in horses is 145–164 mg/dL and ideally blood glucose concentrations should be maintained below this level. Hyperglycemia resulting in glucosuria can result in diuresis due to the glucose in urine acting as an osmotic agent, emphasizing the importance of glucose control.

Central venous pressure

Central venous pressure (CVP) refers to the blood pressure within the intrathoracic portion of the cranial vena cava. It is used as a marker of central venous blood volume, vascular tone, and cardiac function and can be used to guide IV fluid therapy. CVP is particularly useful in hypoproteinemic, endotoxemic, and hypotensive horses. CVP is measured via a catheter placed into the intrathoracic portion of the cranial vena cava, which is attached to a water manometer positioned with zero at the point of the shoulder. All air bubbles should be removed from the line. Small oscillations in the fluid meniscus should be observed to confirm intrathoracic placement.[12] To ensure accuracy three readings are typically taken, with the average being used. Normal CVP in an adult horse is approximately 8–12 cm H_2O; however, in critically ill postoperative colic patients, the goal should be to achieve a CVP >5 cm H_2O.

Arterial blood pressure

Arterial blood pressure, and in particular mean arterial pressure (MAP), is used to assess the circulatory status in critically ill patients and provides an estimate of blood flow. Hypotension may be due to hypovolemia, hemorrhage, systemic inflammatory response syndrome (SIRS), or sepsis. Arterial blood pressure is either measured via direct or indirect methods; however indirect blood pressure monitoring is used most commonly. Direct arterial blood pressure measurements are obtained via an arterial catheter and are not often performed in conscious horses due to difficulty in maintaining a patent arterial catheter. However, horses under general anesthesia for colic surgery have an arterial catheter placed in the facial or transverse facial artery which can be secured in place using cyanoacrylate adhesive glue and suture material and used for several days postoperatively. Direct MAP in adult horses is 110–130 mmHg and should be maintained >60–70 mmHg.[13]

Indirect (noninvasive) arterial blood pressure is most often obtained via the oscillometric method using an occlusion cuff placed around the tail or limb. In adult horses, the base of the tail is most commonly used and appears to give more reliable results. The length of the internal inflatable bladder should be 80% of the tail base or limb circumference, and the bladder width should be 20–25% and 40–50% of the circumference of the tail and limb, respectively.[13] The oscillometric method provides systolic, diastolic, and mean arterial pressures as well as a pulse rate. Three readings should be performed with the average being used. It is also important to ensure that the pulse rate provided on the oscillometric monitor correlates with the actual heart rate of the horse. If the two do not correlate the blood pressure values may be spurious. Normal indirect MAP in adult horses is 85–95 mmHg.[14] It is important to recognize that arterial blood pressure is typically maintained until shock becomes decompensated, and earlier indicators of inadequate tissue perfusion should be monitored closely.

Treatment

Fluid therapy

IV fluid therapy is broadly categorized as crystalloid and colloid fluid therapy. Although crystalloid IV fluids are the mainstay of postoperative management of colic patients, colloidal support is often also important in the management of hypoproteinemic and persistently hypotensive patients. See also Chapter 11 on Intravenous Catheterization and Fluid Therapy (p. 99).

Crystalloids

Crystalloid fluids are used for the replacement of large volume deficits and also for maintenance of fluid requirements and ongoing losses such as diarrhea or reflux. Crystalloids contain water and electrolytes and may also contain glucose and a buffer such as lactate or acetate. They are classified as isotonic or hypertonic based on the concentration of solutes which determines the osmolality of the solution.

Isotonic crystalloid solutions may be categorized as balanced electrolyte solutions and isotonic saline (0.9%). Balanced electrolyte solutions have an electrolyte composition similar to that of plasma; they can be further classified as replacement or maintenance solutions. Replacement solutions are used for resuscitation and are relatively low in potassium, whereas maintenance solutions are higher in potassium and lower in sodium. Unfortunately, maintenance solutions are not available in 5 L bags and as such are often impractical to use in adult horses. Instead it is commonplace to supplement replacement fluids (such as Plasmalyte, Normosol-R, Lactated Ringer's Solution [LRS]) with 20 mEq/L of potassium chloride. Additional supplementation which may be used includes 23% calcium gluconate which is commonly added to isotonic fluids at approximately 100–125 mL/5 L bag of fluids, and magnesium sulfate which may be administered at 4–16 mg/kg body weight/day in IV fluids. Supplementation of magnesium sulfate is particularly useful in refractory hypocalcemia as this may be related to a magnesium deficiency. When administering crystalloid fluids supplemented with either potassium or calcium there are several precautions which should be noted. Administration of potassium containing fluids should be at rates which do not deliver >0.5 mEq/kg/h of potassium. Concurrent administration of calcium containing fluids and biologic colloids (plasma and whole blood) or bicarbonate containing solutions should be avoided due to the risk of precipitation.

Hypertonic solutions have an effective osmolality greater than that of plasma and act to draw water from the interstitium into the vascular space. Additionally, hypertonic saline may have anti-inflammatory and antiendotoxic properties.[15,16] Hypertonic saline is a 7.2% solution of sodium and chloride with an osmolality approximately nine times that of plasma. Hypertonic saline is more often used in the resuscitation of colic patients pre-operatively. It is important to note that when hypertonic solutions are administered, these should always be followed by administration of an isotonic fluid. The "rule of thumb" is 10 L of isotonic fluids should be given for every 1 L hypertonic solution.

Most crystalloid solutions are isotonic relative to plasma. Commonly administered isotonic poly-ionic fluids include 0.9% sodium chloride, LRS, Normosol-R, and Plasmalyte. It is expected that within 1 h of administration of crystalloid solutions, approximately 75% of the fluids will have redistributed to the interstitium. Crystalloids, therefore, primarily expand the interstitial space.

Colloids

Colloids are defined as fluids containing large molecular weight molecules which do not readily cross semipermeable membranes. Although crystalloid fluid therapy is key in managing postoperative colic patients, there is increasing interest in the use of colloid support. While crystalloid fluids are important in maintaining overall tissue hydration and vascular volume, colloids can be important in improving the hemodynamics and circulatory status of critical patients.

COP is determined by the presence of plasma proteins, primarily albumin, and the Gibbs–Donnan equilibrium. Loss of plasma COP can result in interstitial edema formation due to movement of fluid from the vascular space into the interstitium. Although peripheral edema is readily recognizable in the throat latch, pectoral, ventral, and preputial areas, of greater concern is edema formation within organs and tissues. This may result in potential negative effects on perfusion and tissue oxygenation as well as gastrointestinal tract function.

Colloids can be defined as either biologic or synthetic. The most commonly administered biologic colloid in horses is plasma; however, whole blood is also included in this category. The most commonly administered synthetic colloid is hydroxyethyl starch (hetastarch and pentastarch). Other synthetic colloids include dextrans and hemoglobin-based products; however, these are rarely used in adult horses.

Plasma

Albumin is the primary determinant of COP and plasma has a COP of approximately 25 mmHg. It is possible to have redistribution of albumin to the interstitium; additionally the high cost and large volumes required to provide adequate colloidal support mean that plasma is not typically used as the sole colloid in critical equine patients. However, plasma has several advantages compared to synthetic colloids as it is also a good source of globulin, fibronectin, clotting factors, and anticoagulants such as antithrombin. In addition, the use of hyperimmunized plasma may decrease the clinical signs associated with endotoxemia and improve short-term outcome.[17]

When administering plasma to horses it is important to closely monitor for the development of adverse reactions. Adverse reactions are typically mild and manifest as urticaria which may be fairly focal or diffuse. More severe anaphylactic reactions rarely occur. If an adverse reaction to plasma occurs, the infusion should be immediately discontinued and a physical examination should be performed. Diphenhydramine is typically used to treat mild hypersensitivity reactions. Further treatment such as administration of epinephrine or a corticosteroid will be dictated by the severity of the clinical signs. In an attempt to minimize the development of adverse reactions, several precautions should be taken. When initially administering plasma to a patient, the infusion is started at a slow rate while the patient's vital parameters are closely monitored for a minimum of 20 min. If the patient has not shown signs of an adverse effect at this time, the rate of infusion may be increased; however, monitoring should be continued at 30–60 min intervals during the infusion. It is also prudent to know the serial number of the plasma being administered and all bags of plasma administered to the patient should ideally have the same serial number. If this is not possible, when a bag of a different serial number is used the same protocol as for starting a plasma infusion should be repeated.

Hydroxyethyl starch

Hetastarch and pentastarch are the most commonly used synthetic colloid in adult horses in the United States and Europe/Australia, respectively.

Hetastarch is provided either as a 6% aqueous solution in saline or lactated electrolyte solution. Hetastarch has a wide range of molecular sizes (10–3000 kDa) with an average molecular mass of 450 kDa. The COP of hetastarch is 30 mmHg, and as such it is a more cost-effective colloid compared to plasma. The half life of Hetastarch in horses and foals with hypoproteinemia is approximately 24–36 h.[18] Pentastarch has a mean molecular weight of 200 kDa and a higher COP compared to that of hetastarch. Pentastarch can, therefore, expand the intravascular volume more effectively compared to hetastarch and has less profound effects on the coagulation system.[19]

Formulating a fluid therapy plan

When designing a fluid therapy plan for a patient, there are three fundamental questions which must be addressed: what volume of fluid is required, what type of fluid(s) is indicated, and what rate of fluids should be given.

To determine the volume of fluid required it is important to determine any fluid deficits that may exist, have an understanding of maintenance fluid requirements, and be able to estimate and anticipate ongoing losses. Determining fluid deficits that may be present is based on physical examination and routine laboratory data. It is important to note that 5% dehydration is thought to be the lower cutoff for what is possible to detect clinically.

To determine fluid deficits which may be present, the percentage dehydration is calculated as above and multiplied by the body weight in kilograms. For example, an adult horse weighing 500 kg which is estimated to be 5% dehydrated would have a fluid deficit of approximately 25 L. A general guide for fluid replacement rates is 10–20 mL/kg/h; however, rates of 20–45 mL/kg/h are tolerated in adult horses.[20] Maintenance fluid requirements in adult horses are estimated to be 2 mL/kg/h; however, this rate can be affected by several different factors including ambient temperature and humidity, and the presence of disease. Ongoing losses can be difficult to estimate depending on the disease process.

The presence of nasogastric reflux is easy to quantify. A simple way to monitor the reflux and estimate ongoing losses is to calculate the total volume of reflux produced in a 12 h period and then determine the average volume produced per hour. This is not only a useful way to monitor trends in nasogastric reflux production, but also allows the veterinarian to incorporate this average volume into a fluid therapy plan for the patient. When using this method, however, the actual fluid losses can be underestimated likely because of additional fluid loss into the gastrointestinal tract that is not quantified in the reflux. Therefore, use of other methods to evaluate adequacy of hydration, such as urine output, should also be used.

The presence of diarrhea is more difficult to quantify and as such we are often more reliant on other clinical parameters such as heart rate, urine output, laboratory data, and CVP and COP. Fluid loss in diarrhea can be upward of 200 mL/kg/day (100 L/500 kg/day or 4–5 L/500 kg/h), and also results in significant electrolyte loss.

For the uncomplicated postoperative colic patient (e.g, a horse recovering from surgery for a large colon displacement or impaction) the answers to the three fundamental questions of IV fluid therapy planning are fairly simple. IV fluids administered under general anesthesia will likely have resolved any hypovolemia and dehydration evident at presentation. These horses often require minimal intervention in the form of IV fluid therapy, and typically only require maintenance fluid rates for <24 h, if at all. It is advisable, however, to keep these horses on a low maintenance fluid rate (1–2 mL/kg/h) overnight after surgery in case they develop unforeseen complications. It is particularly important that these patients are provided with access to fresh water in the postoperative period. Enterally administered fluids (p. 62) can be used to supplement fluid therapy in these uncomplicated cases if water intake or fecal production is inadequate.

For more complicated cases such as horses with a large colon volvulus or those undergoing an extensive resection and anastomosis, IV fluid therapy becomes a more critical component of postoperative management. These horses are more likely to recover from general anesthesia with fluid, acid-base, and electrolyte imbalances present and, therefore, require more intense monitoring and management. Determination of fluid deficits should again be calculated based on results of thorough physical examination and routine laboratory work; however, this may be supplemented by measurement of CVP and COP. This is particularly important in hypoproteinemic, hypotensive, and endotoxemic horses where derangements in vascular endothelial function, vascular tone, and intestinal wall function can make management of fluid deficits with crystalloid therapy alone very difficult. In these cases, the use of crystalloid and colloid fluid therapy is indicated to provide adequate tissue hydration as well as to maintain vascular volume and adequate COP. Of particular concern in these patients is potential worsening of edema when high rates of crystalloid fluids are administered.

Colloidal support is typically indicated in hypoproteinemic patients to help improve the COP. Although plasma is widely used in hypoproteinemic patients, in an adult horse a total of at least 5–10 L of plasma would be required to raise the total protein by 0.5–1 g/dL. Additionally, approximately 60% of the albumin in plasma may redistribute from the vascular space resulting in loss of COP. This, therefore, makes plasma unsuitable as the sole colloid in hypoproteinemic adult horses due to the large volumes required and subsequent expense. A combination of hydroxyethyl starch and plasma has the advantage of improved COP from the hydroxyethyl starch combined with the antiendotoxic, anti-inflammatory, and hemostatic properties of plasma. Hydroxyethyl starch administered at a dose of 10 mL/kg/day has been shown to improve COP for 24 h and substantially expand plasma volume.[18] Doses >10 mL/kg/day should be avoided as this may result in significant effects on hemostasis with decreases in factor VIII, von Willebrand's factor, and platelet counts, and an increase in partial thromboplastin time (PTT).[21] Pentastarch is also administered at 10 mL/kg/day and because of its lower molecular weight and higher oncotic pressure, is more effective at expanding the intravascular space and also has fewer negative effects on coagulation.[19]

Further indications for the use of colloids in the management of postoperative colic include endotoxemia, hypotension, and persistent elevations in PCV. Hetastarch has been shown to modulate certain factors associated with endotoxemia,[22,23] and can be very useful in the management of hypo-

tensive patients and those in which there are persistent elevations in PCV despite presumably adequate fluid therapy. Hyperimmunized plasma is obtained from horses which have been immunized with a recombinant mutant *Escherichia coli* (J5) resulting in high levels of antibodies against LPS core antigen. This may be useful in the treatment of endotoxemia (p. 246).[17]

Anti-inflammatory and analgesic drugs

Although acute (surgical) pain is thought to have some protective effects, persistent pain can result in a catabolic state, immunosuppression, delayed wound healing, and adverse cardiovascular effects and ileus. Careful observation of the horse combined with physical examination will often allow even subtle signs of pain to be elucidated and can be used to determine the analgesic/anti-inflammatory requirements. Reduced locomotion and an elevated heart rate have been shown to be the most reliable indicators of pain in horses following exploratory celiotomy.[24]

The most commonly administered analgesic for postoperative colic patients is flunixin meglumine (see below). This is often the sole analgesic and appears to be adequate in most postoperative colic patients where only mild pain occurs. When horses continue to have evidence of discomfort despite the use of flunixin meglumine (tachycardia, signs of colic, inappetence), further analgesia is indicated. See also Chapter 6 on Analgesia (p. 51).

Nonsteroidal anti-inflammatory drugs (NSAID)

Administration of flunixin meglumine to postoperative colic patients is routinely done for its anti-inflammatory, analgesic, and antiendotoxic properties. Flunixin meglumine is typically administered at a dose of 0.5–1 mg/kg twice a day, and can be given either IV or orally. It results in excellent visceral analgesia, and at doses of 0.25 and 1 mg/kg results in attenuation of the clinical effects of endotoxemia.[25]

Flunixin meglumine acts in the arachidonic acid pathway by inhibiting the cyclooxygenase (COX) enzymes resulting in subsequent inhibition of production of prostaglandins and thromboxanes. Some of the analgesic and anti-inflammatory effects of NSAIDs occur via additional effects which are independent of COX inhibition.[26] Nonspecific inhibition of COX results in both homeostatic COX 1 and proinflammatory COX 2 enzymes being inhibited. There is some concern that administration may result in gastrointestinal ulceration and renal crest necrosis. Although the low dose of flunixin meglumine has been shown to be antiendotoxic, it is not an analgesic or anti-inflammatory dose. Postoperative colic patients in which there is persistent hypovolemia and endotoxemia may benefit from a low dose of flunixin meglumine in combination with other analgesic and anti-inflammatory drugs to preserve blood flow to the gastrointestinal mucosa and kidneys.

Recent studies have evaluated the effects of flunixin meglumine on ischemic injured intestine. These studies have shown that flunixin meglumine may impair recovery of ischemic injured small intestine[27] but not large colon.[28] The concurrent use of IV lidocaine[29] or misoprostol[30,31] may ameliorate these negative effects on the small intestine. The clinical relevance of these studies is unknown, as no prospective randomized clinical trials have been performed. There is much interest in the use of COX 1 sparing NSAIDs (e.g., firocoxib and meloxicam) to improve gastrointestinal repair following ischemic damage;[29,32] however use has to date been limited in postoperative colic patients.

Other NSAIDs that may be used in horses include phenylbutazone, ketoprofen, and carprofen. Phenylbutazone has previously been shown to be useful in attenuating the effects of endotoxin on the gastrointestinal tract.[33] There appears to be a greater risk of adverse effects which may be exacerbated by the presence of hypovolemia and dehydration.[34] Ketoprofen appears to be less nephrotoxic and ulcerogenic compared to flunixin meglumine and phenylbutazone.[35] It is rarely used in adult horses, however, due to the cost associated with administration.

Intravenous lidocaine

Lidocaine is a local anesthetic agent which acts to block sodium channels. Lidocaine may be useful as both an analgesic and anti-inflammatory; although it has previously been classified as a prokinetic, its likely effect is through ameliorating inflammation and the effects of ischemia and reperfusion in intestine.[36] It is administered as a CRI. Although several studies in normal horses have shown no positive effects on gastrointestinal motility,[37,38] it appears that in horses recovering from colic surgery the use of a lidocaine CRI may improve gastrointestinal motility and short-term survival.[39] Care should be taken when administering IV lidocaine because rapid administration can result in collapse and seizure. Horses rapidly improve once the lidocaine infusion is stopped; however, they can sustain injury during the episode.

Butorphanol

Butorphanol is an opioid which acts at both mu (antagonist) and kappa (agonist) receptors. Depending on the nature of the discomfort, butorphanol may be administered either as a single parenteral dose or as a CRI. Butorphanol may be beneficial in the postoperative period in decreasing cortisol levels and improving the behavior of horses; however, it does decrease gastrointestinal transit time.[40]

Alpha-2 agonists

Alpha-2 agonists such as xylazine and detomidine are commonly used for their sedative-analgesic effects in the management of postoperative signs of colic. Alpha-2 agonists are also excellent analgesics and lower doses may be used either alone or in combination with butorphanol. The use of CRI is also garnering much interest.[41] It is important to remember that the use of alpha -2 agonists will result in a temporary reduction of gastrointestinal motility.

Ketamine

Ketamine is a NMDA receptor antagonist, which is most commonly used in the induction and maintenance of general anesthesia. At subanesthetic doses, however, it can be useful in controlling sensitization and windup during pain.[42]

Antimicrobial drugs

The use of antimicrobial drugs in the postoperative period is somewhat controversial. In humans, there is substantial evidence that a single, appropriately timed, preoperative antimicrobial dose is as effective as multiple doses perioperatively.[43,44] Additionally, continuing antimicrobial prophylaxis beyond 24h appears to have no benefit and may increase development of antimicrobial resistance. Recently, guidelines for antimicrobial use in veterinary medicine have been published.[45] These guidelines recommend formulation of policies for antimicrobial drug use in an individual hospital and development of monitoring programs to detect emerging antimicrobial resistance patterns. Classification of antimicrobials as primary, secondary, or tertiary use is based on spectrum of activity, age of antimicrobial, risk of development of resistance, and level of threat to human health care. Monitoring and testing of infections via bacterial culture, pathogen identification, and susceptibility patterns by standardized methods allows an evidence-based approach to drug selection.

Use of postoperative antimicrobial drugs is dictated by the individual case. In patients undergoing procedures classified as clean or clean-contaminated (e.g., displacement correction, needle decompression, pelvic flexure enterotomy, jejunojejunostomy), all that is typically indicated is a single preoperative antimicrobial dose or antimicrobial prophylaxis for 24h. Cases in which there is pre-existing infection (e.g., abdominal abscess, intestinal leakage with septic peritonitis) or presence of nonviable intestine (e.g., large colon volvulus with severe mucosal damage) may require antimicrobials for longer than 24h; however, in these cases antimicrobial use is no longer prophylactic and should be guided by the likely microbial pathogens encountered and bacterial culture and sensitivity testing.

The most common antimicrobials used postoperatively in colic patients are a combination of penicillin and gentamicin. Penicillin is a time-dependent antimicrobial drug, whereby the tissue concentration should remain above the minimum inhibitory concentration of the target pathogen(s) (MIC) for as long as possible for effective pathogen killing. Potassium penicillin is typically used because it is administered IV; however, procaine penicillin administered IV is an alternative option. Some surgeons are reluctant to use procaine penicillin because of the potential risk of injury to the horse and staff associated with a procaine reaction.

It is also critical to educate staff that procaine penicillin cannot be administered IV because it may result in patient death. Potassium penicillin has been shown to stimulate myoelectric activity of the cecum and pelvic flexure in normal horses.[46] Clinically it may be associated with the passage of loose feces and signs of mild abdominal discomfort. Slow administration IV is warranted, and in some horses the dose may need to be diluted in 250–500mL of saline to a concentration of 22 000–44 000 U/mL for a 500kg horse.

Gentamicin is a concentration-dependent antimicrobial drug, with effective pathogen killing requiring peak concentrations to be at least 10–12 times MIC. Although the most widely used dose of gentamicin in adult horses is 6.6mg/kg IV every 24h, IV fluid therapy and endotoxemia can affect the pharmacokinetics of the drug.[47] It is recommended that peak (within 30–60min of a dose) and trough (8–23h after a dose) plasma gentamicin concentrations be assessed. The peak plasma concentration (ideal is 25–35μg/mL) will determine whether the dose is increased or decreased, and the trough plasma concentration (ideal is <2–3μg/mL) determines whether the dosing interval needs to be adjusted. Often dose rates of 8.8mg/kg are necessary to achieve adequate peak plasma concentrations. Gentamicin can result in acute renal tubular necrosis, and should be avoided in horses which may be at risk of renal hypoperfusion or are showing signs of renal failure. It is important to recognize that renal tubular damage is not associated with the peak, but rather the trough gentamicin concentration.

Alternative antimicrobials that may be administered include ceftiofur, ampicillin, and enrofloxacin. Ceftiofur may be administered as an alternative to penicillin and gentamicin as it is fairly broad spectrum. There is concern about the development of colitis and an increased risk of antimicrobial resistance. The routine use of enrofloxacin is not encouraged as this antimicrobial should be reserved for infections with documented sensitivity to fluoroquinolone antimicrobial drugs. Enrofloxacin should not be used in young horses because of the risk for developing an arthropathy.

Antimicrobial use is not without its risks. The primary risk in postoperative colic patients is antimicrobial-associated diarrhea. Typical clinical signs include dull mentation, inappetence, fever, and colic. Of most concern is the development of salmonellosis and clostridiosis. In these cases antimicrobial administration should be discontinued and further investigation undertaken including performing a complete blood count, clinical chemistry profile, and fecal analysis. Metronidazole may be effective for treating patients with clostridiosis. Isolation of these patients is important and often aggressive medical therapy with crystalloid and colloid fluid support is required.

Feeding

Details of postoperative feeding and nutrition are covered in Chapter 23 on Nutrition (p. 303). Feed can generally be reintroduced within 6 h of surgery in the uncomplicated colic patient. Hand walking with grazing is recommended initially when the patient has fully recovered from general anesthesia and is no longer ataxic. If the horse cannot be walked, fresh grass can be picked and offered. A typical refeeding regimen for an uncomplicated large colon displacement or volvulus or impaction would include a handful of grass or alfalfa hay every 3–4 h for 12 h, then a 1/4 flake of hay every 3–4 h for an additional 12 h, followed by a 1/2 flake of hay every 3–4 h, then free choice hay by 48 h (depending on the patient's caloric requirements). Many surgeons prefer to feed horses having undergone a small intestinal resection and anastomosis a pelleted complete feed which can be gradually introduced over about 72 h depending on the severity of disease and response to refeeding. Horses recovering from cecal and small colon impactions should have feed reintroduced very slowly and these horses may also benefit from a pelleted complete feed. If a pelleted complete feed is used, hay can be introduced days after surgery, gradually by the owner/caregiver following hospital discharge, or not at all.

Water can be offered ad libitum immediately after surgery, except for horses with small intestinal resection and anastomosis that appear likely to develop postoperative reflux (e.g., inflamed bowel at surgery, prolonged duration of colic prior to surgery). Horses that are refluxing often have the desire to consume large volumes of water. In postoperative colic patients in which postoperative reflux is anticipated, providing 2–3 L of water only and closely monitoring water intake and accumulation of gastric fluid accumulation is recommended.

References

1. Freeman, K.D., Southwood, L.L., Lane, J., Lindborg, S. & Aceto, H.W. (2012) Post operative infection, pyrexia, and perioperative antimicrobial drug use in surgical colic patients. *Equine Veterinary Journal*. **44**, 476–481.
2. Naylor, J.M., Poirier, K.L., Hamilton, D.L. & Dowling, P.M. (2006) The effects of feeding and fasting on gastrointestinal sounds in adult horses. *Journal of Veterinary Internal Medicine*, **20**, 1408–1413.
3. Lima, A., Jansen, T.C., van Bommel, M.D., Ince, C. & Bakker, J. (2009) The prognostic value of the subjective assessment of peripheral perfusion in critically ill patients. *Critical Care Medicine*, **37**, 934–938.
4. Schey, B.M., Williams, D.Y. & Bucknall, T. (2009) Skin temperature as a noninvasive marker of haemodynamic and perfusion status in adult cardiac surgical patients: An observational study. *Intensive and Critical Care Nursing*, **25**, 31–37.
5. Boscan, P. & Steffey, E.P. (2007) Plasma colloid osmotic pressure and total protein in horses during colic surgery. *Veterinary Anesthesia and Analgesia*, **34**, 408–415.
6. Jacobsen, S. & Andersen, P.H. (2007) The acute phase protein serum amyloid A (SAA) as a marker of inflammation in horses. *Equine Veterinary Education*, **19**, 38–46.
7. Brix-Christensen, V., Gjedsted, J., Andersen, S., *et al.* (2005) Inflammatory response during hyperglycemia and hyperinsulinemia in a porcine endotoxemic model: The contribution of essential organs. *Acta Anaesthesiologica Scandinavica*, **49**, 991–998.
8. Krogh-Madsen, R., Moller, K., Dela, F., Kronbrog, G., Jauffred, S. & Pedersen, B.K. (2004) Effect of hyperglycemia and hyperinsulinemia on the response of IL-6, TNF-α, and FFAs to low-dose endotoxemia in humans. *American Journal of Physiology: Endocrinology and Metabolism*, **286**, E766–E772.
9. Yajima, S., Morisaki, H., Serita, R., *et al.* (2009) Tumor necrosis factor-alpha mediates hyperglycemia-augmented gut barrier dysfunction in endotoxemia. *Critical Care Medicine*, **37**, 1024–1030.
10. Hassel, D.M., Hill, A.E. & Rorabeck, R.A. (2009) Association between hyperglycemia and survival in 228 horses with acute gastrointestinal disease. *Journal of Veterinary Internal Medicine*, **23**, 1261–1265.
11. Underwood, C., Southwood, L.L., Walton, R.M. & Johnson, A.L. (2010) Hepatic and metabolic

changes in surgical colic patients: A pilot study. *Journal of Veterinary Emergency and Critical Care*, **20**, 578–586.

12. Wilsterman, S., Hackett, E.S., Rao, S. & Hackett, T.B. (2009) A technique for central venous pressure measurement in normal horses. *Journal of Veterinary Emergency and Critical Care*, **19**, 241–246.

13. Marsh, P.S. (2010) Critical Care. In: *Equine Internal Medicine* (eds S.M. Reed, W.M. Bayly & D.C. Sellon), pp. 246–279. Saunders Elsevier, St. Louis, Missouri.

14. Parry, B.W., McCarthy, M.A. & Anderson, G.A. (1984) Survey of resting blood pressure values in clinically normal horses. *Equine Veterinary Journal*, **16**, 53–58.

15. Attuwaybi, B., Kozar, R., Gates, K., *et al.* (2004) Hypertonic saline prevents inflammation, injury, and impaired intestinal transit after gut ischemia/reperfusion by inducing heme oxygenase 1 enzyme. *Journal of Trauma*, **56**, 749–759.

16. van Haren, F.M.P., Sleigh, J., Cursons, R., La Pine, M., Pickkers, P. & van der Hoeven, J.G. (2011) The effects of hypertonic fluid administration on the gene expression of inflammatory mediators in circulating leucocytes in patients with septic shock: A preliminary study. *Annals of Intensive Care*, **1**, 2–8.

17. Spier, S.J., Lavoie, J.P., Cullor, J.S., Smith, B.P., Snyder, J.R. & Sischo, W.M. (1989) Protection against clinical endotoxemia in horses by using plasma containing antibody to an Rc mutant *E. coli (J5)*. *Circulatory Shock*, **28**, 235–248.

18. Jones, P.A., Bain, F.T., Byars, T.D., David, J.B. & Boston, R.C. (2001) Effect of hydroxyethyl starch infusion on colloid oncotic pressure in hypoproteinemic horses. *Journal of the American Veterinary Medical Association*, **218**, 1130–1135.

19. Strauss, R.G., Pennell, B.J. & Stump, D.C. (2002) A randomized, blinded trial comparing the hemostatic effects of pentastarch versus hetastarch. *Transfusion*, **42**, 27–36.

20. Seahorn, J.L. & Seahorn, T.L. (2003) Fluid therapy in horses with gastrointestinal disease. *Veterinary Clinic Equine*, **19**, 665–679.

21. Jones, P.A., Tomasic, M. & Gentry, P.A. (1997) Oncotic, hemodilutional, and hemostatic effects of isotonic saline and hydroxyethyl starch solutions in clinically normal ponies. *American Journal of Veterinary Research*, **58**, 541–548.

22. Hoffmann, J.N., Vollmar, B. & Laschke, M. (2002) Hydroxyethyl starch (130 kD), but not crystalloid volume support, improves microcirculation during normotensive endotoxemia. *Anesthesiology*, **97**, 460–470.

23. Lv, R., Zhou, Z.-Q., Wu, H.-W., Jin, Y., Zhou, W. & Xu, J.G. (2006) Hydroxyethyl starch exhibits antiinflammatory effects in the intestines of endotoxemic rats. *Anesthesia & Anagelsia*, **103**, 149–155.

24. Pritchett, L.C., Ulibarri, C., Roberts, M.C., Schneider, R.K. & Sellon, D.C. (2003) Identification of potential physiological and behavioral indicators of postoperative pain in horses after exploratory celiotomy for colic. *Applied Animal Behaviour Science*, **80**, 31–43.

25. Moore, J.N., Hardee, M.M. & Hardee, G.E. (1986) Modulation of arachidonic acid metabolism in endotoxic horses: Comparison of flunixin meglumine, phenylbutazone, and a selective thromboxane synthetase inhibitor. *American Journal of Veterinary Research*, **47**, 110–113.

26. Tegeder, I., Pfeilschifter, J. & Geisslinger, G. (2001) Cyclooxygenase-independent actions of cyclooxygenase inhibitors. *Journal of the Federation of American Societies for Experimental Biology*, **15**, 2057–2072.

27. Tomlinson, J.E. & Blikslager, A.T. (2004) Effects of ischemia and the cyclooxygenase inhibitor flunixin on in vitro passage of lipopolysaccharide across equine jejunum. *American Journal of Veterinary Research*, **65**, 1377–1383.

28. Matyjaszek, S.A., Morton, A.J., Freeman, D.E., Grosche, A., Polyak, M.M.R. & Kuck, H. (2009) Effects of flunixin meglumine on recovery of colonic mucosa from ischemic in horses. *American Journal of Veterinary Research*, **70**, 236–242.

29. Cook, V.L., Meyer, C.T., Campbell, N.B. & Blikslager, A.T. (2009) Effect of firocoxib or flunixin meglumine on recovery of ischemic-injured equine jejunum. *American Journal of Veterinary Research*, **70**, 992–1000.

30. Topcu, I., Vatansever, S., Var, A., Cavus, Z., Cilaker, S. & Sakarya, M. (2007) The effect of misoprostol, a prostaglandin E1 analog, on apoptosis in ischemia-reperfusion-induced intestinal injury. *Acta Histochemica*, **109**, 322–329.

31. Watanabe, T., Sugimori, S., Kameda, N., *et al.* (2008) Small bowel injury by low-dose enteric-coated aspirin and treatment with misoprostol: A pilot study. *Clinical Gastroenterology and Hepatology*, **6**, 1279–1282.

32. Little, D., Brown, A., Campbell, N.B., Moeser, A.J. Davis, J.L. & Blikslager, A.T. (2007) Effects of the cyclooxygenase inhibitor meloxicam on recovery of ischemia-injured equine jejunum. *American Journal of Veterinary Research*, **68**, 614–624.

33. King, J.N. & Gerring, E.L. (1989) Antagonism of endotoxin-induced disruption of equine bowel motility by flunixin and phenylbutazone. *Equine Veterinary Journal*, **21**, 38–42.

34. Reed, S.K., Messer, N.T., Tessman, R.K. & Keegan, K. (2006) Effects of phenylbutazone alone or in combination with flunixin meglumine on blood protein concentration in horses. *American Journal of Veterinary Research*, **67**, 398–402.

35. MacAllister, C.G., Morgan, S.J., Borne, A.T. & Pollet, R.A. (1993) Comparison of adverse effects of phenyl-

butazone, flunixin meglumine, and ketoprofen in horses. *Journal of the American Veterinary Medical Association*, **202**, 71–80.

36. Cook, V.L., Jones Shults, J., McDowell, M., Campbell, N.B., Davis, J.L. & Blikslager, A.T. (2008) Attenuation of ischaemic injury in the equine jejunum by administration of systemic lidocaine. *Equine Veterinary Journal*, **40**, 353–357.

37. Milligan, M., Beard, W., Kukanich, B., Sobering, T. & Waxman, S. (2007) The effect of lidocaine on postoperative jejunal motility in normal horses. *Veterinary Surgery*, **36**, 214–220.

38. Rusiecki, K.E., Nieto, J.E., Puchalski, S.M. & Snyder, J.R. (2008) Evaluation of continuous infusion of lidocaine on gastrointestinal tract function in normal horses. *Veterinary Surgery*, **37**, 564–570.

39. Malone, E., Ensink, J., Turner, T., *et al.* (2006) Intravenous continuous infusion of lidocaine for treatment of equine ileus. *Veterinary Surgery*, **35**, 60–66.

40. Sellon, D.C., Roberts, M.C., Blikslager, A.T., Ulibarri, C. & Papich, M.G. (2004) Effects of continuous rate intravenous infusion on butorphanol on physiologic and outcome variables in horses after celiotomy. *Journal of Veterinary Internal Medicine*, **18**, 555–563.

41. Wilson, D.V., Bohart, G.V., Evans, A.T., Robertson, S. & Rondenay, Y. (2002) Retrospective analysis of detomidine infusion for standing chemical restraint in 51 horses. *Veterinary Anesthesia and Analgesia*, **29**, 54–57.

42. Fielding, C.L., Brumbaugh, G.W., Matthews, N.S., Peck, K.E. & Roussel, A.J. (2006) Pharmacokinetics and clinical effects of a subanesthetic continuous rate infusion of ketamine in awake horses. *American Journal of Veterinary Research*, **67**, 1484–1490.

43. Bratzler, D.W. & Houck, P.M. (2004) Antimicrobial prophylaxis for surgery: An advisory statement from the National Surgical Infection Prevention Project. *Clinical Infectious Diseases*, **38**, 1706–1715.

44. McDonald, M., Grabsch, E., Marshall, C. & Forbes, A. (1998) Single versus multiple-dose antimicrobial prophylaxis for major surgery: A systematic review. *Australian and New Zealand Journal of Surgery*, **68**, 388–395.

45. Morley, P.S., Apley, M.D., Besser, T.E., *et al.* (2005) Antimicrobial drug use in veterinary medicine. *Journal of Veterinary Internal Medicine*, **19**, 617–629.

46. Roussel, A.J., Hooper, R.N., Cohen, N.D., Bye, A.D., Hicks, R.J. & Schulze, J.L. (2003) Evaluation of the effects of penicillin G potassium and potassium chloride on the motility of the large intestine in horses. *American Journal of Veterinary Research*, **64**, 1360–1363.

47. van der Harst, M.R., Bull, S., Laffont, C.M. & Klein, W.R. (2005) Influence of fluid therapy on gentamicin pharmacokinetics in colic horses. *Veterinary Research Communications*, **29**, 141–147.

19

Postoperative Complications

Diana M. Hassel

Department of Clinical Sciences, Colorado State University, Fort Collins, CO, USA

Chapter Outline

Fever	**244**	**Postoperative ileus**	**251**
Ischemia-reperfusion injury	**246**	Prevention	251
Endotoxemia and SIRS	**246**	Treatment	252
Prevention	246	**Septic peritonitis**	**253**
Treatment	247	Treatment	253
Diarrhea	**248**	**Postoperative intraperitoneal adhesions**	**255**
Prevention	248	Prevention	255
Treatment	248	Treatment	256
Recurrent colic	**249**	**Incisional complications**	**256**
Treatment	250	Treatment	258

Postoperative complications following ventral midline celiotomy for treatment of colic remain common despite many advances in surgical and postoperative management. Prevention, diagnosis, and treatment of the most commonly observed complications following ventral midline celiotomy will be discussed including fever, endotoxemia/ SIRS (systemic inflammatory response syndrome), diarrhea, recurrent colic, postoperative ileus (POI), peritonitis, adhesion formation, and body wall complications including incisional infection and herniation. Horses with strangulating obstructions appear to be particularly susceptible to many of these complications as a consequence of associated intestinal mucosal injury, absorption of endotoxin, and systemic compromise. See also Chapter 18 on Postoperative Patient Care (p. 230), Chapter 11 on Intravenous Catheterization and Fluid Therapy (p. 99), and Chapter 20 on Biosecurity (p. 262).

Fever

Fever following ventral midline celiotomy is a common entity and may be associated with many of the more common infectious and noninfectious

Practical Guide to Equine Colic, First Edition. Edited by Louise L. Southwood.
© 2013 John Wiley & Sons, Inc. Published 2013 by John Wiley & Sons, Inc.

postoperative complications. When fever is present, it is essential to attempt to determine a cause, as delays in the diagnosis of serious postoperative complications such as peritonitis or septic thrombophlebitis may have devastating consequences. A fever observed after the initial 48 h after surgery, lasting for longer than 48 h and >102.5 °F (39 °C), is more likely associated with an infection compared to a low-grade fever of short duration in the early postoperative period.[23]

If postoperative fever is observed, a complete blood count should be submitted to assist with diagnosis and to provide a baseline for future assessment of efficacy of therapy. The complete blood count should be normal in the postoperative colic patient. Leukopenia (neutropenia) can be observed in the early postoperative period in horses that had intestinal ischemia; however, persistent or severe leucopenia is often associated with compromised intestine, salmonellosis, or other severe infections. Similarly, the presence of immature (band) neutrophils (left shift) should raise concern that there is an infection. Fibrinogen concentration and serum amyloid A can also be used to provide some indication of whether the fever is associated with an infection. Uncomplicated postoperative colic patients typically have a fibrinogen concentration between 500 and 800 mg/dL.

Efforts to determine the cause of the fever should be performed. A table of common causes of postoperative fever and associated recommended initial diagnostic tests is provided in Table 19.1. Self-limiting fever following surgical treatment of extensive feed impactions involving the large or small colon can also be observed. These horses are more likely to be carriers of *Salmonella* sp.[37] and are believed to be febrile as a consequence of injury to the colonic mucosa. Treatment with nonsteroidal anti-inflammatory drugs (NSAIDs) and di-tri-octa-hedral (DTO) smectite per nasogastric tube is often successful in these cases.

Assessment, prevention, and treatment of endotoxemia (p. 246), colitis or diarrhea (p. 248), septic peritonitis (p. 253), and incisional infection (p. 256) as sources of fever will be discussed in depth.

Pneumonia or pleuropneumonia is a less common but potentially serious cause of fever, reported to occur in <1% of horses undergoing celiotomy for colic.[46] However, thoracic auscultation with rebreathing examination should be performed

Table 19.1 Common causes of fever following ventral midline celiotomy for treatment of colic with recommended initial diagnostic tests.

Common causes of fever	Recommended initial diagnostic tests
Endotoxemia/SIRS	Physical examination; CBC
Diarrhea/colitis	Physical examination; abdominal sonographic examination; CBC
Peritonitis	Abdominal sonographic examination; abdominocentesis/peritoneal fluid analysis
Thrombophlebitis	Remove IV catheter; physical examination; sonographic evaluation of affected vein
Bacterial pneumonia or pleuropneumonia	Auscultation of thorax with rebreathing examination; thoracic sonographic examination; TTW
Respiratory viral disease	Auscultation of thorax with rebreathing examination; nasal swabs for virus isolation
Incisional infection	Physical examination; sonographic evaluation of incision

CBC, complete blood count; IV, intravenous; TTW, transtracheal wash.

on any postoperative colic patient with a fever of unknown origin. If pneumonia is suspected, aerobic and anaerobic bacterial culture and sensitivity testing of a transtracheal wash sample is indicated with institution of appropriate antimicrobial therapy along with clinical monitoring facilitated by thoracic sonography and/or radiography.

Septic or nonseptic thrombophlebitis is another serious, but uncommon cause of fever in the postoperative colic patient, reported to occur in <1% of postoperative colic patients.[46] Daily evaluation of intravenous (IV) catheter sites for evidence of inflammation along with proper use of aseptic technique during catheter placement are important components of care in the postoperative colic patient. Short-term IV catheters and fluid lines should be changed every 72 h and the use of over-the-needle Teflon catheters avoided in horses considered at increased risk for thrombophlebitis. The tip of the IV catheter should be cultured when removed. Most horses respond favorably to IV catheter removal, hot packing the affected vein, and topical 1% diclofenac sodium (Surpass®) or dimethylsulfoxide (DMSO). Local or systemic antimicrobial drugs may be selected based on bacterial culture and sensitivity testing if the infection is severe. If refractory septic thrombophlebitis develops, surgical jugular vein thrombectomy should be considered.[64]

Ischemia-reperfusion injury

While most of the intestinal injury likely occurs during the ischemic phase necessitating resection of the affected bowel or euthanasia if it is too extensive or inaccessible, there is sufficient evidence that ongoing injury occurs following reperfusion that is beyond that associated with ischemia.[51] The areas of intestine in which this is primarily a concern are the large colon in horses with a volvulus and the distended segment of small intestine oral to a mechanical, usually strangulating, obstruction.[16,26] Occasionally the small intestine that has undergone ischemia appears potentially viable on initial examination only to develop a gray appearance within 30 min of reperfusion.

During ischemia, xanthine dehydrogenase is converted to xanthine oxidase. ATP is metabolized to hypoxanthine which accumulates. When oxygen is reintroduced into the tissues, hypoxanthine is metabolized by xanthine oxidase and the superoxide radical is generated. Superoxide is converted to hydrogen peroxide and then to a hydroxyl radical which ultimately is reduced to form water. These reactive oxygen species cause lipid membrane peroxidation leading to cell damage and generation of peroxyl radicals. Neutrophil chemotaxis and activation leads to formation of hypochlorite through myeloperoxidase and hydrogen peroxide creating extensive protein damage. Oxygen and nitrogen free radicals cause extensive DNA damage leading to apoptotic or necrotic cell death culminating in mucosal injury. Mucosal injury leads to endotoxin absorption, SIRS, and shock. Nonviable intestine is associated with signs of colic, fever, and septic peritonitis. The local intestinal inflammatory response likely contributes to POI and adhesion formation.

The most important measure for preventing the clinical impact of ischemia-reperfusion injury is early referral and surgical treatment. Use of cyclooxygenase-1 (COX-1) sparing NSAIDs, firocoxib and meloxicam, have been shown experimentally to lessen the impact of NSAIDs on restoration of the transepithelial barrier function following intestinal ischemia and reperfusion.[11,44,72] There have been several treatments including DMSO, IV lidocaine, and Carolina rinse that have been investigated to manage reperfusion injury;[9,10,17,18,77,81] however, none have really gained widespread clinical acceptance for prevention of reperfusion injury.

Endotoxemia and SIRS

Endotoxemia and the associated SIRS is a common clinical feature in horses with strangulating intestinal lesions and may also be observed with nonstrangulating obstructions. Lipopolysaccharide (LPS), also known as endotoxin, is found in abundance in the equine gastrointestinal lumen. Horses are exquisitely sensitive to even small amounts of endotoxin.[40] Normal intestinal mucosal function and intestinal motility prevent large amounts of LPS absorption from the intestinal lumen and the small amount that is absorbed is metabolized by the liver. Mucosal injury results in an increase in LPS absorption. When LPS is absorbed from the intestinal lumen it binds to LPS binding protein (LBP) which then binds to toll-like receptor-4 (TLR-4)-CD14 cell surface receptors. Intracellular signally results in transcription of inflammatory mediators, primarily interleukin-1 (IL-1) and tumor necrosis factor (TNF), via the NF-KB transcription factor. LPS absorption is also associated with other mediators of inflammation including prostaglandins, serotonin, histamine, kinins, platelet-activating factors, and others.[78] In horses with naturally occurring disease, signs of endotoxemia include hyperemic mucous membranes (Figure 19.1), POI and hypotensive shock.[40]

Prevention

Prevention of endotoxemia may be attempted by minimizing mucosal injury and eliminating the source of LPS. This may be accomplished through

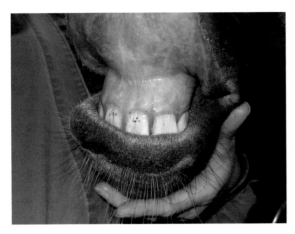

Figure 19.1 "Toxic" mucous membranes as demonstrated by generalized hyperemia with increased discoloration noted at the gum line. Mucous membrane color may vary from bright pink to blue/gray, with or without contrast at the gum line, depending on the stage and severity of endotoxemia.

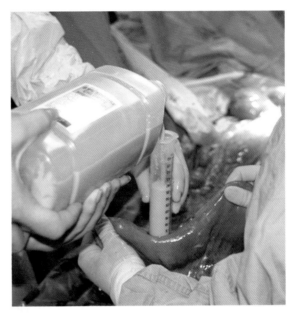

Figure 19.2 Intraoperative photograph demonstrating DTO smectite (Bio-Sponge®) administration into the lumen of the large colon via pelvic flexure enterotomy. Larger volumes may be infused via stomach pump with a nasogastric tube inserted to the origin of the right ventral colon. Typical dosages are 0.5–1 lb (250–500 g) DTO smectite in 1–1.5 L of water.

early recognition and treatment of strangulating obstructions, administration of endotoxin-binding agents such as polymyxin B in the early stages of disease, or direct binding of luminal endotoxin using orally or intraoperatively administered DTO smectite into the intestinal lumen to minimize availability of LPS for systemic absorption through a damaged intestinal wall (Figure 19.2). Pretreatment with NSAIDs has also been shown to be effective in preventing clinical signs related to endotoxemia.[50]

Treatment

Often, endotoxemia is an inevitable consequence of intestinal injury in the horse, so the focus is to minimize the consequences of endotoxin exposure through any or all of the following mechanisms. One of these is by providing a means of directly neutralizing LPS. This can be accomplished with the use of IV polymyxin B which acts through direct binding to the lipid A moiety of LPS, preventing its contact with receptor sites on mononuclear cells.[14] Other therapeutic avenues under investigation include the use of antibodies or other binding agents directed against receptors that play a key role in the inflammatory cascade initiated by LPS. These include antibodies directed

against the CD14 receptor on macrophages,[39] and inhibitors of TLR-4 signaling which are in the early phases of investigation for use in horses. Hyperimmune plasma containing antibodies directed against the LPS core antigen (J5 hyperimmune plasma) may also assist with neutralization of LPS while concurrently providing colloidal support.

A mainstay for treatment of endotoxemia has been the use of NSAIDs through their ability to inhibit the COX-mediated breakdown of arachidonic acid to prostaglandins. Flunixin meglumine has been the most commonly used nonspecific NSAID for horses with colic and has been shown to be effective in ameliorating the clinical signs of endotoxemia.[50] More recently, the use of COX-1 sparing inhibitors have been investigated in horses and have shown promise with regards to analgesic effects with a concurrent reduction in detrimental side effects of nonspecific COX inhibitors on epithelial recovery and intestinal permeability.[11,72,73] Low-dose aspirin therapy may be considered when hypercoagulable states are present, although efficacy of aspirin for platelet inhibition in horses is diminished.[35]

Broad-spectrum antimicrobial therapy may be indicated in horses with endotoxemia secondary to intestinal injury, as a profound neutropenia is a common feature of endotoxemia and bacteremia is likely to occur as a consequence of impaired mucosal barrier function.

IV fluid therapy (p. 99) remains as one of the most important treatments to combat the hemodynamic effects of LPS and associated SIRS. This consists of administration of balanced isotonic electrolyte solutions with or without concurrent use of colloids or hypertonic saline. Commonly used colloids in the horse with endotoxemia include hydroxyl ethyl starch (p. 113, 237) and fresh-frozen hyperimmune plasma (p. 112, 236).[39]

Ethyl pyruvate, a stable lipophilic derivative of pyruvate, has antioxidant properties through free-radical scavenging as well as anti-inflammatory effects through inhibition of NF-kB binding to nuclear DNA. Ethyl pyruvate decreased inflammatory mediator production following LPS stimulation both in vitro[12] and in vivo[66] and is safe to administer at 150 mg/kg as a continuous rate infusion (CRI).[36]

A table of commonly used drugs for the treatment of endotoxemia along with dosages and potential side effects is provided in Table 19.2.

Laminitis is an uncommon postoperative complication following colic surgery; however, is a common sequela of severe endotoxemia and SIRS. The pathophysiology of laminitis is complex and poorly understood and treatments are equally controversial.[2] A current recommendation, in addition to treatment of endotoxemia, is to apply ice to the hooves and distal limbs in any horse at risk for developing laminitis (e.g., patients with a high fever, colitis, and injected or toxic membranes).

Diarrhea

The prevalence of postoperative diarrhea in the colic patient varies widely, reportedly occurring in as little as 3.2%[46] of postoperative cases to as many as 53.2% with severe diarrhea (colitis) occurring in 27.5% in one study.[7] Prevalence appears to differ by geographic region or surgical facility, and these differences may, in part, be reflective of criteria used to define colitis.[28] Alternatively, the most common forms of surgically treated colic in various facilities may have an impact as well. Horses with sand and feed impactions of the large colon[58] and those with colonic volvulus[69] seem to be at higher risk for the development of postoperative diarrhea. It is likely that these horses experience more profound changes in the population of intestinal flora, enabling enteric pathogens to proliferate. The combination of perioperative broad-spectrum antimicrobial drugs, direct damage to the integrity of the colonic mucosa secondary to the primary condition and intraluminal lavage with hypotonic solutions, surgical evacuation of normal colonic content and its associated bacterial flora, and the stress of surgery, anesthesia, and the disease process itself places these horses at increased risk for the development of colitis.[28] See Chapter 20 on Biosecurity (p. 262).

Prevention

Effective prevention or early recognition and treatment are optimal for the management of postoperative colitis. An *in vivo* clinical trial investigating the use of DTO smectite for the prevention of diarrhea in horses following colic surgery revealed a marked reduction in the prevalence of postoperative diarrhea and improved clinical and hematologic parameters in the perioperative period compared with controls.[32] The author routinely administers DTO smectite intraoperatively in horses undergoing enterotomy of the pelvic flexure as a component of their surgical exploration (Figure 19.2). When risk for postoperative diarrhea is high, therapy with 1 lb DTO smectite (500 g) in 4 L water via nasogastric tube is continued twice daily for 1–4 days postoperatively in the average sized adult horse.

Treatment

Treatment for colic secondary to colitis and postoperative diarrhea in horses is primarily directed toward supportive therapy aimed at stabilizing hemodynamic parameters altered as a

Table 19.2   Commonly used drugs for the treatment of endotoxemia with dosages and potential adverse side effects.

Drug name	Dosage	Disadvantages
Polymyxin B sulfate	1 000–6 000 U/kg IV q8h	Nephrotoxic and neurotoxic
DTO smectite (Bio-Sponge®)	1–3 lb loading dose via NGT, then 1 lb PO q8–24h	Ineffective when ileus present as it tends to remain in the stomach
J5 hyperimmune plasma	4.4 mL/kg IV	Expensive
Flunixin meglumine	0.5 mg/kg IV q8h	Nephrotoxic; impairs GI mucosal healing
Aspirin	10 mg/kg PO q48h	Mucosal erosion/ulceration
Antimicrobials	K-penicillin: 22 000 IU/kg IV q6h Gentamicin: 6.6 mg/kg IV q24h	Antimicrobial-associated colitis Nephrotoxicity

IV, intravenous; PO, per os (orally)

consequence of profound fluid and electrolyte losses. Close monitoring via serial physical examinations, serial packed cell volume (PCV) and total plasma protein (TPP) measurements, and serum electrolyte, acid-base, and colloid oncotic pressure (COP) monitoring are often required in horses with moderate to severe colitis (see Chapter 18 on Postoperative Patient Care [p. 230]). Synthetic colloid solutions such as hydroxyl ethyl starch (5–10 mL/kg) or equine hyperimmune plasma are often necessary to assist with maintenance of COP to combat hypovolemia induced by fluid losses and increased vascular permeability. Other therapies are primarily directly toward combating the effects of endotoxemia and SIRS (Table 19.2). A universally accepted treatment is the use of NSAIDs; however, current investigations into newer COX-1 sparing NSAIDs, such as firocoxib, show promise in combating inflammation without compromising intestinal integrity or repair.[11] Use caution with nephrotoxic drugs such as the NSAIDs, polymyxin B, and gentamicin sulfate in hypovolemic horses. Monitoring of serum creatinine is indicated in horses with hypovolemia. The use of oral anti-diarrheal agents such as bismuth subsalicylate or DTO smectite is recommended as long as gastric and small intestinal motility is not impaired as a consequence of SIRS.

Systemic antimicrobial use in horses with colitis is controversial with the exception of the use of oral metronidazole in cases of Clostridial diarrhea. Considering their potential detrimental effects on gastrointestinal flora, the author restricts the use of antimicrobials to those horses with profound neutropenia (<2000 neutrophils/µL) which encompasses the majority of postoperative colitis cases. The reasoning for use of broad-spectrum antimicrobials in these cases is to protect against bacterial seeding of distant organs from intermittent bacteremia that may occur with intestinal barrier dysfunction.

There is scant evidence to promote the use of probiotics; however, administration of *Saccharomyces boulardii* has shown some promise in reducing the severity and duration of diarrhea.[19]

Recurrent colic

Postoperative colic is the most commonly reported complication in horses undergoing celiotomy for treatment of gastrointestinal disease, estimated to occur in approximately 29% of cases.[46,59] Signs of abdominal pain most commonly consist of pawing, rolling, stretching, turning the head toward the flank, kicking at the abdomen, curling of the upper lip, trembling, dog sitting, and repeatedly getting up and down. More subtle signs may consist of a dull mentation or poor appetite, recumbency, tachycardia, or tachypnea. It is unusual for adult horses to routinely lie down in the postoperative period and it is also of concern as it may lead to contamination of the surgical incision and subsequent incisional infection. If pain is observed in the postoperative period, an effort must be made to determine the underlying cause in order to implement effective management strategies.

Timing and nature of the onset of postoperative pain may provide important clues as to the causes

Table 19.3   Dosages and mechanisms of action of the most commonly used analgesic medications for the treatment of postoperative pain in horses.

Drug name	Dosage	Mechanism of action
Lidocaine	1.3 mg/kg IV bolus, then 0.05 mg/kg/min IV as a CRI	Anti-inflammatory, sympathoadrenal inhibition, analgesic
Flunixin meglumine	0.25–1.0 mg/kg IV q8–12h	NSAID—nonspecific cyclooxygenase inhibitor
Firocoxib	0.27 mg/kg (loading dose) then 0.09 mg/kg IV q24h	NSAID—COX-1 sparing inhibitor
Meloxicam	0.6 mg/kg IV q24h	NSAID—COX-1 sparing inhibitor
Xylazine	0.25–1.0 mg/kg IV as needed	Alpha-2 agonist
Detomidine	0.01–0.02 mg/kg IV or IM as needed	Alpha-2 agonist
Romifidine	0.04 mg/kg IV as needed	Alpha-2 agonist
Butorphanol	0.01–0.02 mg/kg IV or IM; 13 µg/kg/h as a CRI for 24h	Opioid agonist-antagonist
Fentanyl	1–2 10mg transdermal patches q48–72h	Opioid agonist
Ketamine	0.4–1.2 mg/kg/h CRI	Dissociative anesthetic

CRI, continuous rate infusion; IV, intravenous; PO, per os (orally); IM, intramuscular; q, every.

of pain. Pain observed in the immediate postoperative period may more likely represent surgical and incisional pain, rather than a new secondary lesion requiring further surgical intervention. Progressive resolution of signs of pain and good response to analgesics should occur if this is the case. Other sources of abdominal pain typically arise from bowel distention, spasm, mesenteric tension, ischemia, inflammation, peritonitis, or a combination of these factors.[33] Efforts to determine the underlying cause play an important role in response to therapy and in avoiding detrimental delays when relaparotomy is indicated. Poor or short-lived responses to potent analgesics such as alpha-2 agonists may indicate a need for relaparotomy.

Treatment

A multimodal approach to management of postoperative pain is likely the most effective, as it minimizes adverse side effects of high doses of any given drug. The most commonly used drugs for management of postoperative pain include NSAIDs, alpha-2 agonists, IV lidocaine, and opioid analgesics. A list of these drugs, their dosages, and mechanisms of action are provided in Table 19.3.

In selecting the optimal therapeutic agent for management of postoperative pain, keep in mind that both opioids and alpha-2 agonists will have a negative impact on propulsive motility in the equine gastrointestinal tract.[48] Although alpha-2 agonists and the opioid agonist-antagonist, butorphanol, have an impact on gastrointestinal motility, the duration of effect is short-lived in comparison to pure opioid agonists. Butorphanol administered as a CRI (13 µg/kg/h IV for 24h) in postoperative colic patients has been shown to decrease plasma cortisol and improve recovery characteristics of postoperative colic patients.[67] However, it also induced a delay in time to passage of first feces in the postoperative period,[68] so it should be used with discretion in horses at risk for POI (see below).

The most commonly used NSAID in horses with colic is the nonspecific COX inhibitor, flunixin meglumine. It provides good visceral analgesia in a dose-dependent fashion and helps to reduce inflammation as a consequence of exposure to endotoxin. Its disadvantages are the potentiation of gastric and intestinal ulceration, delayed mucosal healing in models of jejunal ischemia,[11] and nephrotoxicity. The use of COX-1 sparing NSAIDs has shown promise for providing visceral analgesia with fewer known adverse side effects.[11]

Repeat laparotomy may be indicated as part of the management for horses with colic signs that are unresponsive to analgesic drugs. As a guideline, horses that are unresponsive to two doses of detomidine are likely to have a lesion that requires surgical intervention. Types of lesions that cause these signs include intestinal ischemia, volvulus and other strangulating lesion, and obstruction at an anastomosis. Horses with recurrent intermittent signs of mild colic also often require a repeat laparotomy and causes include POI, obstruction at an anastomosis, (re)impaction, and adhesion formation.

Postoperative ileus

POI is a serious and sometimes fatal complication that is most prevalent following surgical management of small intestinal disease, but may occasionally be observed following correction of large colon disease. It occurs in 10–21% of postoperative colic patients, but has been reported to occur in as many as 50% of postoperative cases with small intestinal involvement.[8] The small intestine is most commonly affected and it is clinically characterized by fluid sequestration and loss of motility within the duodenum and jejunum with subsequent gastric fluid accumulation accompanied by a need to decompress the stomach every few hours via nasogastric intubation. POI is most often a clinical diagnosis and has been defined as >20 L of reflux following nasogastric tube passage during a 24 h period after surgery or >8 L at any single sampling time after surgery.[8,62] Failure to decompress the stomach results in signs of colic and the potential for gastric rupture. Sonographic evaluation of the ventral abdomen typically reveals fluid-filled, amotile loops of small intestine (Figures 19.3 and 19.4). Imaging of the stomach on the left mid-abdomen caudal to the 13th intercostal space also indicates presence of gastric distention (Figures 19.5 and 19.6).

Consistently reported risk factors for small intestinal POI include prolonged surgical and anesthetic time, presence of small intestinal lesions, and high admission PCV.[4,8,24] Additional proposed risk factors include intestinal ischemia, distention, peritonitis, electrolyte imbalances, endotoxemia, traumatic handling of the intestine, resection and anastomosis, and general anesthesia.[29]

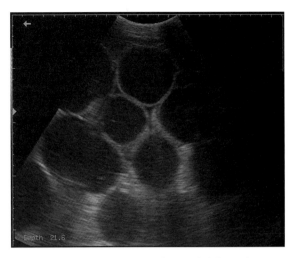

Figure 19.3 Transcutaneous caudoventral abdominal sonographic image demonstrating multiple fluid-filled distended loops of small intestine.

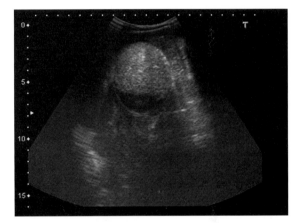

Figure 19.4 Sonographic image from the cranioventral abdomen of a horse with ileus and sedimentation of ingesta within the bowel lumen.

Prevention

Identification of horses at increased risk for POI is essential, as early treatment will likely have a greater positive impact than once adynamic ileus has been fully established. There is modest evidence that intraoperative administration of IV lidocaine and decompression of the large colon via pelvic flexure enterotomy may decrease the risk of small intestinal POI.[8,64] Attentiveness to good surgical technique and minimizing trauma through

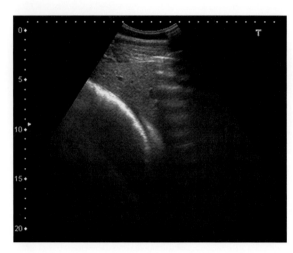

Figure 19.5 Transcutaneous sonographic image of a gas-distended stomach as viewed from the left 15th intercostal space. The spleen is evident adjacent to the stomach. Dorsal is to the left on the image.

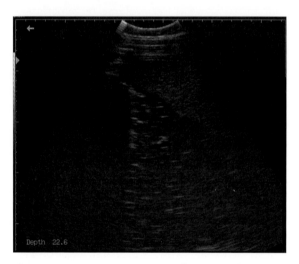

Figure 19.6 Transcutaneous sonographic image of a fluid-distended stomach with a gas cap dorsally as viewed from the left 16th intercostal space. In horses with ileus, swirling fluid of mixed echogenicity may be identified within the stomach lumen as is seen here. Dorsal is to the left.

the use of sterile carboxymethylcellulose while manipulating and decompressing distended small bowel may help to minimize bowel wall inflammation induced by handling. Similarly, minimizing surgical anesthetic time, adopting methods to combat endotoxemia, and closely monitoring the

patient for electrolyte or acid-base imbalances will likely contribute to an improved outcome.

Treatment

Prompt recognition of the onset of POI is an important component of postoperative monitoring. The hallmark of treatment for POI is supportive care, as evidence for efficacy of available prokinetic agents is limited. Supportive care consists primarily of gastric decompression, blood volume support through use of IV fluids and colloids when necessary, electrolyte support, acid-base monitoring, anti-inflammatory therapy, and antimicrobials when indicated. Administration of partial parenteral nutrition (p. 306) should be considered in horses with POI extending beyond 24–48h.

Passage of a nasogastric tube with siphoning (p. 38) should be performed upon any indication of the development of POI. This may consist of subtle abnormalities such as tachycardia, dull mentation, lack of interest in food, or mild colic. If copious amounts of reflux are obtained, the nasogastric tube may remain indwelling to allow routine decompression every 2–4h. Keep in mind that maintenance of an indwelling nasogastric tube has been associated with serious comorbidities such as pharyngeal trauma and esophageal rupture.[30,31] Experimentally, the presence of an indwelling nasogastric tube has been shown to contribute to a delay in gastric emptying in normal horses.[15]

Beyond application of appropriate supportive therapy, prokinetic agents are often utilized. IV lidocaine is the most commonly administered prokinetic[76] and its use has been associated with improved outcomes, reduced risk of POI, and reduced diameter of jejunum postoperatively as determined via transcutaneous sonographic evaluation.[5,74] However, in normal horses, IV lidocaine administration increases fecal transit time.[63] Its beneficial effects on motility in clinical cases are believed to be in part due to its anti-inflammatory effects.[10] Concurrent use of IV lidocaine with highly protein-bound drugs may increase the risk of toxicity, commonly manifest as tremors, muscle fasciculations, ataxia, or collapse.[49] If these signs are observed, discontinuing the CRI allows for rapid resolution due to the short half-life of lidocaine.

Table 19.4 Dosages and mechanisms of action of the most commonly used prokinetic drugs used for the treatment of postoperative ileus.

Drug name	Dosage	Mechanism of action
Lidocaine	1.3 mg/kg IV bolus, then 0.05 mg/kg/min IV as a CRI	Anti-inflammatory, sympathoadrenal inhibition, analgesic
Metoclopramide	0.25 mg/kg IV in 500 mL saline over 30–60 min q6–8h OR CRI at 0.01–0.05 mg/kg/h	Dopamine receptor antagonist; 5-HT$_4$ receptor agonist
Erythromycin	1.0 mg/kg in 1 L saline over 1 h q6h	Motilin agonist
Cisapride	0.1 mg/kg IM or IV q8h (compounding required due to poor oral bioavailability)	Cholinergic agonist; 5-HT$_4$ receptor agonist; 5-HT$_3$ receptor antagonist
Neostigmine	0.0044–0.022 mg/kg IM or SQ q20–60 min	Cholinesterase inhibitor

CRI, continuous rate infusion; IV, intravenous; IM, intramuscular; SQ, subcutaneous; q, every.

A list of the most commonly used prokinetic drugs, their dosages and mechanisms of action are provided in Table 19.4. Erythromycin or metoclopramide are the most commonly used prokinetic agents after IV lidocaine, and neostigmine is reserved for instances of POI involving the large colon. Most prokinetic agents have not been shown to improve motility in clinical cases of POI and are associated with adverse side effects such as colic, colitis (erythromycin), or CNS excitement (metoclopramide). Other agents described with questionable efficacy in horses with POI include bethanechol (muscarinic cholinergic agonist), as well as acepromazine and yohimbine (alpha-adrenergic antagonists).

The main differential diagnosis for POI is obstruction at an anastomosis site caused by stenosis or kinking of the bowel. These horses are unlikely to respond to medical treatment and early repeat laparotomy with revision of the anastomosis is advocated. Indications for repeat laparotomy in these cases include persistence of large volumes of reflux (i.e., >4 L/h) and duration of reflux beyond 48–72 h.

Septic peritonitis

Septic peritonitis in the postoperative colic patient is a serious complication with a fatality rate of 50–60%[32] necessitating early diagnosis and treatment whenever possible. While peritonitis occurs in all postoperative colic patients, septic peritonitis is an uncommon postoperative complication and often associated with another complication such as anastomosis leakage, nonvi-able intestine, salmonellosis, and severe incisional infection, or preexisting septic peritonitis.[22] Clinical signs of septic peritonitis include fever, colic, diarrhea, tachycardia, decreased borborygmi, and ileus.[32,47] Transcutaneous sonographic evaluation will reveal an increased volume of hyperechoic fluid or fluid mixed with hyperechoic debris (fibrin tags) (p. 133) and diagnosis may be confirmed via abdominocentesis with fluid analysis (p. 87). Exploratory celiotomy alone results in marked increases in nucleated cell counts (200 000 cells/μL) and total protein (6 g/dL) in the first postoperative week and, therefore, may complicate the diagnosis.[65] However, the presence of increased peritoneal fluid volume combined with evidence of degenerate neutrophils, intracellular or extracellular bacteria, low pH of peritoneal fluid (<7.3), and low glucose concentration in peritoneal fluid compared with systemic blood glucose concentration (>50 mg/dL difference) allows confirmation of a septic peritoneal process.[61] Potential causes of septic peritonitis in the postoperative period include necrosis of a segment of gastrointestinal tract either prior to or following surgical intervention, contamination at surgery, or leakage from the site of anastomosis.[29]

Treatment

Treatment for septic peritonitis in the postoperative colic patient must often include relaparotomy once the patient is hemodynamically stabilized. Determination and repair of the inciting cause via

(a)

(b)

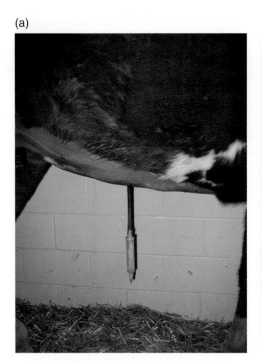
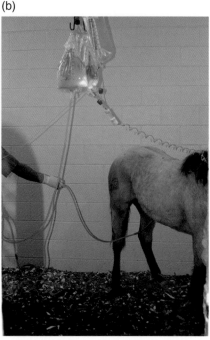

Figure 19.7 (a) Intraabdominal drain (30 French Argyle trocar catheter with additional fenestrations) with a one-way Heimlich valve attached to allow for passive drainage of peritoneal fluid. (b) Intraabdominal lavage performed in the standing patient. The Heimlich valve is aseptically removed and stored during peritoneal lavage. Five to ten liters of warmed isotonic fluids are administered via sterile argyle tubing, the horse is walked for 5–10 min, and the fluid is drained directly back into the IV fluid bags using gravity. The remaining peritoneal fluid drains passively through the Heimlich valve.

relaparotomy followed by aggressive peritoneal cavity lavage is essential to successful treatment. Placement of an indwelling peritoneal drain may be indicated at the time of relaparotomy to allow for continued peritoneal lavage in the postoperative period, or a drain may also be placed in the standing sedated patient. If placement of an abdominal drain is anticipated, omentectomy may be appropriate to reduce drain occlusion by omentum during postoperative lavage. A variety of options are available for drain placement in the equine abdomen, but careful adherence to principles of aseptic technique is essential with all drain systems. The system most commonly utilized at the author's hospital includes a 28–30 French Argyle trocar catheter (Covidien, Mansfield, MA) modified with addition of 4–6 fenestrations near the tip and fitted with a Heimlich one-way chest valve (BD, Franklin Lakes, NJ) secured with 18 gauge wire (Figure 19.7). Intraabdominal lavage may be performed several times daily via aseptic removal of the Heimlich valve and

application of a sterile tube system connected to a 5L bag of isotonic warmed fluids (Figure 19.7). Heparin is an optional additive (20–40IU/kg SQ q8h or added to lavage fluid) to help reduce peritoneal fibrin formation. Determination of when to discontinue peritoneal lavage may be dictated by subsequent fluid analyses to indicate progressive resolution of septic peritonitis.

Additional therapy for septic peritonitis includes antimicrobial therapy directed ideally toward pathogens isolated via peritoneal fluid culture and sensitivity. As absence of bacterial growth is common from peritoneal fluid and if gastrointestinal origin bacteria are suspected, broad-spectrum coverage including extended anaerobic coverage with metronidazole is appropriate. In addition, aggressive supportive therapy for treatment of hypovolemia, endotoxemia, and hypoproteinemia are often necessary. This may include IV fluid therapy, colloid supplementation, flunixin meglumine, and polymyxin B sulfate.

Postoperative intraperitoneal adhesions

Adhesions are the second most common reasons for relaparotomy in horses with colic.[56,57] Adhesions appear to occur most commonly in foals and in horses with lesions involving the small intestine. The combination of trauma to normal mesothelial surfaces, ischemia-reperfusion injury, disrupted fibrinolytic activity, and presence of peritoneal inflammation likely contribute to the development of adhesions, estimated to occur in 22% of horses undergoing surgery for disease of the small intestine.[1] POI of the small intestine is expected to increase risk for adhesion formation, as it is characterized by multiple amotile distended loops of small intestine with seromuscular inflammation in contact with one another. Colic with or without nasogastric reflux is the most common clinical sign associated with postoperative intraperitoneal adhesion formation. Diagnosis of adhesions of bowel to the ventral abdomen can be made sonographically; however, adhesions are most often diagnosed during repeat laparotomy, laparoscopy, or at necropsy.

Prevention

Table 19.5 lists multiple treatments and methods currently being utilized to prevent intraperitoneal adhesion formation in colic patients. Perhaps the most important of these is minimizing trauma during surgery. Good surgical practices such as timely decision making to undergo surgery, keeping the bowel moist at all times, providing adequate hemostasis, minimizing exposure of suture material, removing injured tissue, and gentle tissue handling, all likely result in reducing seromuscular injury and subsequent adhesion formation.[29] Omentectomy has been advocated by some surgeons for prevention of omental adhesions;[43] however, often adhesions associated with clinical signs of colic are not omental adhesions but rather bowel to bowel, bowel to mesentery, or bowel to body wall. Other methods described to prevent adhesions include anti-inflammatory therapy, alteration of the coagulation cascade, and use of mechanical barriers to prevent direct contact of injured surfaces.

Perioperative NSAIDs and antimicrobial drugs are routinely used during abdominal surgery and are known to reduce adhesion formation as inflammation and infection both predispose to adhesions. DMSO may also be used as an anti-inflammatory agent and at low doses has been shown to reduce adhesion formation in a model of ischemia-induced adhesion formation in foals.[71] The author routinely uses low-dose DMSO beginning intraoperatively and continuing for 2–3 days postoperatively in colic patients perceived to be at increased risk for adhesion formation. In addition to its effect on adhesion formation demonstrated in the foal model, this low dose has also been shown to reduce edema and neutrophil infiltration in the jejunum in a model of jejunal ischemia and reperfusion in adult horses.[18] In the same study, Carolina rinse, a tissue perfusate used for organ preservation, was also shown to be beneficial in reducing ischemia-induced inflammation. A second study using Carolina rinse applied topically and intraluminally also demonstrated protection against inflammation from ischemic insult,[81] thus making it a possible therapeutic agent to prevent adhesion formation in horses with ischemic injury of the small intestine. Carolina Rinse is not commercially available, but may be produced with readily available compounds.[20,21]

There is modest evidence that heparin therapy is effective in reducing adhesion formation in an ischemic bowel model in ponies.[55] Heparin acts as a cofactor to antithrombin, and markedly increases its efficacy in suppressing thrombin-mediated conversion of fibrinogen to fibrin. Use of low molecular weight heparin in horses has been shown to have fewer side effects on RBC agglutination-induced anemia and clotting times compared with unfractionated heparin.[22] Heparin therapy has also shown some promise in prevention of laminitis in horses with colic.[60]

Other methods reported for preventing adhesions are based on creation of a lubricating barrier and consist of intraoperative use of sterile 1% sodium carboxymethylcellulose (SCMC), intraperitoneal hyaluronic acid (HA), fucoidan solution (Peridan™, Bioniche Animal Health), peritoneal lavage with crystalloid solutions, and application of bioresorbable SCMC-HA acid membranes (Seprafilm®, Genzyme). SCMC may be applied directly onto bowel and gloved hands to minimize trauma to the bowel during handling, and also has

Table 19.5 Therapeutic agents or techniques utilized for prevention or minimizing adhesion formation and proposed mechanisms of action.

Agent or technique	Dosage	Mechanism of action
Minimize surgical trauma and suture exposure intraoperatively		
Omentectomy		Prevention of omental adhesions
NSAID (e.g., flunixin meglumine)	0.25–0.5 mg/kg IV q8h; 1.0 mg/kg IV q12h	Anti-inflammatory
Antimicrobial drugs	Variable	Reduces infection rates
DMSO (dimethylsulfoxide)	20 mg/kg IV q12h for 72 h	Anti-inflammatory
1% Sodium carboxymethylcellulose (SCMC)	Applied to bowel surfaces during handling and over anastomotic sites	Mechanical lubricating barrier
Heparin	40 IU/kg IV or SQ q8–12h	Enhances antithrombin activity
Sodium hyaluronate (HA)	Direct application of 0.4% HA solution	Mechanical lubricating barrier
Seprafilm® (SCMC + HA membrane)	Apply membrane over anastomosis or site of trauma	Mechanical lubricating barrier
Peritoneal lavage	5–10 L sterile isotonic polyionic solution intraoperatively and q6–12h postoperatively via abdominal drain	Removal of inflammatory mediators and fibrin; hydroflotation
Peridan™ (Fucoidan solution)	50 mL Peridan® in 5 L LRS (adults) 5 mL Peridan® in 500 mL LRS (foals)	Mechanical barrier when applied intraperitoneally at the completion of surgery

IV, intravenous; SQ, subcutaneous; q, every LRS, lactated Ringer's solution.

been instilled into the peritoneal cavity just prior to closure of the linea alba. Several experimental studies have demonstrated reduced adhesion formation in horses treated with 1% SCMC[34,54] and the SCMC-HA membrane.[53] Recently, a fucoidan-based solution (Peridan™, Bioniche Animal Health) was found to be effective in a foal jejunal abrasion model[80] and safe in an adult horse jejunojejunostomy model.[52]

Treatment

Horses that acquire adhesions resulting in clinical disease most often develop either a nonstrangulating or strangulating obstruction of bowel, and will present with signs of colic. Nonstrangulating obstructions might be observed with multiple hairpin turns or stricture due to bowel to bowel or bowel to mesentery adhesions, and this may be manifest as recurrent mild colic episodes. Once mature fibrous adhesions develop resulting in

bowel obstruction, resolution will require relaparotomy. Sites of adhesiolysis at relaparotomy will be prone to further adhesion formation, so use of prophylactic methods such as application of a SCMC-HA membrane to the site of adhesiolysis or other preventative therapy is recommended.

Laparoscopy can be used for diagnosis and treatment of postoperative intraperitoneal adhesions. Exploratory laparoscopy with the horse under general anesthesia in dorsal recumbency performed early in the postoperative period in patients at high risk for adhesion formation (e.g., foals, horses with preexisting adhesions and small colon impactions) can be used to identify adhesions and to perform adhesiolysis.

Incisional complications

The most commonly encountered complications involving the incision in postoperative colic patients include dehiscence (Figure 19.8), infection, and

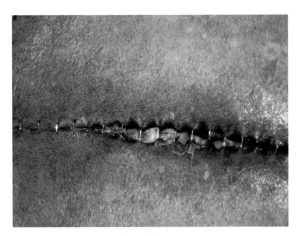

Figure 19.8   Abdominal wall dehiscence 4 days postoperatively in a horse demonstrating exposure of bowel retained only via skin staples.

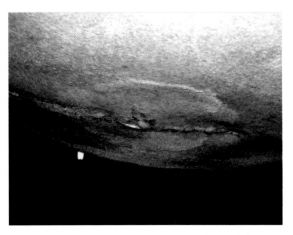

Figure 19.9   Incisional drainage from an infected abdominal incision 7 days postoperatively. Skin staples have been removed at the drainage site to facilitate ventral drainage. Note the presence of edema extending directly across the ventral midline.

herniation. Incisional dehiscence occurs in <3% of postoperative colic patients,[42,70,79] but is the most serious acute incisional problem and may be fatal. Dehiscence usually occurs within the first 8 days postoperatively and is best managed by immediate repair, incisional debridement, and abdominal lavage under general anesthesia. It is often preceded by serosanguinous discharge from the incision.[70] Predisposing factors are believed to be violent recovery from anesthesia, postoperative abdominal pain, and prolonged surgery time.[42,70] Technical error may also be an important component. Activities that contribute to increased intraabdominal pressure such as straining, excessive exercise, or whinnying also may play a role.

Incisional infection is a common complication, reported to occur in 7.4–37% of postoperative colic patients,[22,23,25,42,45,46,58,59,79] with infection rates increasing to as high as 87.5% following repeat celiotomy.[43] Known risk factors for incisional infection include repeat celiotomy, increased duration of surgery, leukopenia, postoperative pain, body weight >300 kg, older age (>1 year), use of a near-far-far-near pattern, application of a stent bandage for 3 days postoperatively, use of staples versus suture material in the skin, preexisting dermatitis and shaving the hair, and increased bacterial contamination of the skin immediately following anesthetic recovery.[25,27,42,46,75,79] Use of antibacterial-coated suture material for body wall closure was not protective.[3] Drainage most commonly develops

between 3 and 14 days postoperatively and may be preceded by fever and localized edema directly over the ventral midline incision (Figure 19.9). Although incisional edema is common, it typically is most prominent on either side of the incision, sparing the central region when infection is not present. Sonographic evaluation of the incisional site can facilitate diagnosis of infection and help identify sites to promote ventral drainage.

Methods reported to help prevent incisional infection include application of a protective iodine-impregnated adhesive (or incise) drape during anesthetic recovery,[38,42] application of an abdominal bandage during the postoperative period,[68] lavage of the linea alba with sterile saline after closure,[74] and application of topical antimicrobial drugs to the surgical wound during closure.[46] Body wall hernia formation is a common consequence of incisional infection with a 62.5-fold higher risk with the presence of incisional drainage.[38] Small incisional hernias often do not require treatment, but large hernias may be objectionable to owners cosmetically as well as being subject to trauma and, therefore, require treatment. Most recently, use of a specially designed hernia belt (CM Equine Products, Norco, CA) reduced the prevalence of hernia formation to 6% of horses with incisional complications and 0.5% of all horses undergoing surgery for colic during the study period.[41] Figure 19.10 demonstrates the equine hernia belt in place in a horse with a repaired incisional dehiscence.

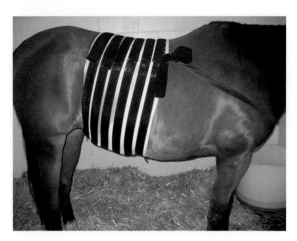

Figure 19.10 CM Equine hernia belt applied to a horse with dehiscence of the abdominal wall 4 days postoperatively. When applied properly, these belts may also be useful for the prevention and treatment of incisional hernias.

Treatment

Acute dehiscence requires general anesthesia, lavage, and debridement of the dehisced incision, and the body wall should be repaired with 18 gauge stainless steel wire in an interrupted vertical mattress pattern with stents. The linea alba can also be apposed with #2 or #3 polyglactin 910 in a simple continuous pattern and the subcutaneous tissue and skin routinely apposed (p. 183). Wires can be removed after 10–14 days.

Treatment for incisional infection should consist of establishing ventral drainage which often requires removal of selected skin staples or sutures. Following aseptic preparation, sampling of material for culture and sensitivity is recommended as it will facilitate directed antimicrobial therapy if indicated. Not all incisional infections require systemic antimicrobial therapy, but if the infection is extensive or the horse is systemically affected by the infection, antimicrobial use is justified. Culture and sensitivity testing is also helpful for monitoring trends in hospital antimicrobial drug resistance. Abdominal support may be applied if frequent changes can be provided to allow removal of exudate. Use of an equine hernia belt appears to hold promise for reducing the prevalence of incisional hernia formation postinfection.[41]

Treatment for incisional hernias may initially be conservative. The author has successfully utilized the CM Equine hernia belt for treatment of incisional hernias with or without the presence of infection. It is important to recognize that hernias do not necessarily require repair and horses can have normal functional lives with a hernia. Large hernias may require more aggressive surgical treatment, but repair should not be attempted until all infection has resolved and a firm, fibrous hernial ring is present (at least 3 months postsurgery). Preparation for surgery should include fasting and feeding of a complete pelleted feed for 2 weeks preoperatively to reduce abdominal weight.[29] Options for herniorrhaphy include primary closure, mesh implantation, mesh implantation with fascial overlay,[29] and laparoscopic mesh hernioplasty.[6]

References

1. Baxter, G.M., Broome, T.E. & Moore, J.N. (1989) Abdominal adhesions after small intestinal surgery in the horse. *Veterinary Surgery*, **18**, 409–414.
2. Belknap, J.K. (2010) The pharmacologic basis for the treatment of developmental and acute laminitis. *Veterinary Clinics of North America: Equine Practice*, **26**, 115–124.
3. Bischofberger, A.S., Brauer, T., Gugelchuk, G. & Klohnen, A. (2010) Difference in incisional complications following exploratory celiotomies using antibacterial-coated suture material for subcutaneous closure: Prospective randomised study in 100 horses. *Equine Veterinary Journal*, **42**, 304–309.
4. Blikslager, A.T., Bowman, K.F., Levine, J.F., Bristol, D.G. & Roberts, M.C. (1994) Evaluation of factors associated with postoperative ileus in horses: 31 cases (1990–1992). *Journal of the American Veterinary Medical Association*, **205**, 1748–1752.
5. Brianceau, P., Chevalier, H., Karas, A., *et al.* (2002) Intravenous lidocaine and small-intestinal size, abdominal fluid, and outcome after colic surgery in horses. *Journal of Veterinary Internal Medicine*, **16**, 736–741.
6. Caron, J.P. & Mehler, S.J. (2009) Laparoscopic mesh incisional hernioplasty in five horses. *Veterinary Surgery*, **38**, 318–325.
7. Cohen, N.D. & Honnas, C.M. (1996) Risk factors associated with development of diarrhea in horses after celiotomy for colic: 190 cases (1990–1994). *Journal of the American Veterinary Medical Association*, **209**, 810–813.

8. Cohen, N.D., Lester, G.D., Sanchez, L.C., Merritt, A.M. & Roussel, A.J., Jr. (2004) Evaluation of risk factors associated with development of postoperative ileus in horses. *Journal of the American Veterinary Medical Association*, **225**, 1070–1078.

9. Cook, V.L., Jones Shults, J., McDowell, M., Campbell, N.B., Davis, J.L. & Blikslager, A.T. (2008) Attenuation of ischaemic injury in the equine jejunum by administration of systemic lidocaine. *Equine Veterinary Journal*, **40**, 353–357.

10. Cook, V.L., Jones Shults, J., McDowell, M.R., *et al.* (2009a) Anti-inflammatory effects of intravenously administered lidocaine hydrochloride on ischemia-injured jejunum in horses. *American Journal of Veterinary Research*, **70**, 1259–1268.

11. Cook, V.L., Meyer, C.T., Campbell, N.B. & Blikslager, A.T. (2009b) Effect of firocoxib or flunixin meglumine on recovery of ischemic-injured equine jejunum. *American Journal of Veterinary Research*, **70**, 992–1000.

12. Cook, V.L., Holcombe, S.J., Gandy, J.C., Corl, C.M. & Sordillo, L.M. (2011) Ethyl pyruvate decreases proinflammatory gene expression in lipopolysaccharide-stimulated equine monocytes. *Veterinary Immunology and Immunopathology*, **141**, 92–99.

13. Cook, V.L., Holcombe, S.J., Fuller, K.A., *et al.* (2011) Ethyl pyruvate improves hemodynamic parameters in anesthetized horses. In: *Proceedings of the 10th Equine Colic Research Symposium*, Indianapolis, Indiana, p. 29.

14. Coyne, C.P. & Fenwick, B.W. (1993) Inhibition of lipopolysaccharide-induced macrophage tumor necrosis factor-alpha synthesis by polymyxin B sulfate. *American Journal of Veterinary Research*, **54**, 305–314.

15. Cruz, A.M., Li, R., Kenney, D.G. & Monteith, G. (2006) Effects of indwelling nasogastric intubation on gastric emptying of a liquid marker in horses. *American Journal of Veterinary Research*, **67**, 1100–1104.

16. Dabareiner, R.M., Sullins, K.E., White, N.A. & Snyder, J.R. (2001) Serosal injury in the equine jejunum and ascending colon after ischemia-reperfusion or intraluminal distention and decompression. *Veterinary Surgery*, **30**, 114–125.

17. Dabareiner, R.M., White, N.A., 2nd & Donaldson, L. (2003) Evaluation of Carolina Rinse solution as a treatment for ischemia reperfusion of the equine jejunum. *Equine Veterinary Journal*, **35**, 642–646.

18. Dabareiner, R.M., White, N.A., Snyder, J.R., Feldman, B.F. & Donaldson, L.L. (2005) Effects of Carolina rinse solution, dimethyl sulfoxide, and the 21-aminosteroid, U-74389G, on microvascular permeability and morphology of the equine jejunum after low-flow ischemia and reperfusion. *American Journal of Veterinary Research*, **66**, 525–536.

19. Desrochers, A.M., Dolente, B.A., Roy, M.F., Boston, R. & Carlisle, S. (2005) Efficacy of *Saccharomyces boulardii* for treatment of horses with acute enterocolitis. *Journal of the American Veterinary Medical Association*, **227**, 954–959.

20. Dukti, S. & White, N. (2008) Surgical complications of colic surgery. *Veterinary Clinics of North America: Equine Practice*, **24**, 515–534.

21. Feige, K., Schwarzwald, C.C. & Bombeli, T. (2003) Comparison of unfractioned and low molecular weight heparin for prophylaxis of coagulopathies in 52 horses with colic: A randomised double-blind clinical trial. *Equine Veterinary Journal*, **35**, 506–513.

22. Freeman, D.E., Hammock, P., Baker, G.J., *et al.* (2000) Short- and long-term survival and prevalence of postoperative ileus after small intestinal surgery in the horse. *Equine Veterinary Journal Supplement*, **(32)**, 42–51.

23. Freeman, K.D., Southwood, L.L., Lane, J., Lindborg, S. & Aceto, H.W. (2012) Post operative infection, pyrexia, and perioperative antimicrobial drug use in surgical colic patients. *Equine Veterinary Journal*. **44**, 476–481.

24. French, N.P., Smith, J., Edwards, G.B. & Proudman, C.J. (2002) Equine surgical colic: Risk factors for postoperative complications. *Equine Veterinary Journal*, **34**, 444–449.

25. Galuppo, L.D., Pascoe, J.R., Jang, S.S., Willits, N.H. & Greenman, S.L. (1999) Evaluation of iodophor skin preparation techniques and factors influencing drainage from ventral midline incisions in horses. *Journal of the American Veterinary Medical Association*, **215**, 963–969.

26. Gerard, M.P., Blikslager, A.T., Roberts, M.C., Tate, L.P., Jr. & Argenzio, R.A. (1999) The characteristics of intestinal injury peripheral to strangulating obstruction lesions in the equine small intestine. *Equine Veterinary Journal*, **31**, 331–335.

27. Gibson, K.T., Curtis, C.R., Turner, A.S., McIlwraith, C.W., Aanes, W.A. & Stashak, T.S. (1989) Incisional hernias in the horse. Incidence and predisposing factors. *Veterinary Surgery*, **18**, 360–366.

28. Hackett, E.S. & Hassel, D.M. (2008) Colic: Nonsurgical complications. *Veterinary Clinics of North America: Equine Practice*, **24**, 535–555.

29. Hardy, J. & Rakestraw, P.C. (2006) Postoperative care and complications associated with abdominal surgery. In: *Equine Surgery* (eds J.A. Auer & J.A. Stick), 3rd edn., pp. 499–515. Saunders Elsevier, St. Louis, Missouri.

30. Hardy, J., Stewart, R.H., Beard, W.L. & Yvorchuk-St-Jean, K. (1992) Complications of nasogastric intubation in horses: Nine cases (1987–1989). *Journal of the American Veterinary Medical Association*, **201**, 483–486.

31. Hassel, D.M., Smith, P.A., Nieto, J.E., Beldomenico, P. & Spier, S.J. (2009) Di-tri-octahedral smectite for the prevention of post-operative diarrhea in equids with surgical disease of the large intestine: Results of a randomized clinical trial. *Veterinary Journal*, **182**, 210–214.

32. Hawkins, J.F., Bowman, K.F., Roberts, M.C. & Cowen, P. (1993) Peritonitis in horses: 67 cases (1985–1990). *Journal of the American Veterinary Medical Association*, **203**, 284–288.

33. Hay, W.P. & Moore, J.N. (1997) Management of pain in horses with colic. *Compendium on Continuing Education for the Practicing Veterinarian*, **19**, 987–990.

34. Hay, W.P., Mueller, P.O., Harmon, B. & Amoroso, L. (2001) One percent sodium carboxymethylcellulose prevents experimentally induced abdominal adhesions in horses. *Veterinary Surgery*, **30**, 223–227.

35. Heath, M.F., Evans, R.J., Poole, A.W., Hayes, L.J., McEvoy, R.J. & Littler, R.M. (1994) The effects of aspirin and paracetamol on the aggregation of equine blood-platelets. *Journal of Veterinary Pharmacology and Therapeutics*, **17**, 374–378.

36. Holcombe, S.J., Cook, V.L., Jacobs, C.C., *et al.* (2011) Ethyl pyruvate and flunixin meglumine diminish clinical effects and proinflammatory gene expression following LPS challenge in horses. In: *Proceedings of the 10th Equine Colic Research Symposium*, Indianapolis, Indiana, p. 14.

37. House, J.K., Mainar-Jaime, R.C., Smith, B.P., House, A.M. & Kamiya, D.Y. (1999) Risk factors for nosocomial *Salmonella* infection among hospitalized horses. *Journal of the American Veterinary Medical Association*, **214**, 1511–1516.

38. Ingle-Fehr, J.E., Baxter, G.M., Howard, R.D., Trotter, G.W. & Stashak, T.S. (1997) Bacterial culturing of ventral median celiotomies for prediction of postoperative incisional complications in horses. *Veterinary Surgery*, **26**, 7–13.

39. Kelmer, G. (2009) Update on treatments for endotoxemia. *Veterinary Clinics of North America: Equine Practice*, **25**, 259–270.

40. King, J.N. & Gerring, E.L. (1991) The action of low dose endotoxin on equine bowel motility. *Equine Veterinary Journal*, **23**, 11–17.

41. Klohnen, A. (2009) New perspectives in postoperative complications after abdominal surgery. *Veterinary Clinics of North America: Equine Practice*, **25**, 341–350.

42. Kobluk, C.N., Ducharme, N.G., Lumsden, J.H., *et al.* (1989) Factors affecting incisional complication rates associated with colic surgery in horses: 78 cases (1983–1985). *Journal of the American Veterinary Medical Association*, **195**, 639–642.

43. Kuebelbeck, K.L., Slone, D.E. & May, K.A. (1998) Effect of omentectomy on adhesion formation in horses. *Veterinary Surgery*, **27**, 132–137.

44. Little, D., Brown, S.A., Campbell, N.B., Moeser, A.J., Davis, J.L. & Blikslager, A.T. (2007) Effects of the cyclooxygenase inhibitor meloxicam on recovery of ischemia-injured equine jejunum. *American Journal of Veterinary Research*, **68**, 614–624.

45. MacDonald, M.H., Pascoe, J.R., Stover, S.M. & Meagher, D.M. (1989) Survival after small intestine resection and anastomosis in horses. *Veterinary Surgery*, **18**, 415–423.

46. Mair, T.S. & Smith, L.J. (2005) Survival and complication rates in 300 horses undergoing surgical treatment of colic. Part 2: Short-term complications. *Equine Veterinary Journal*, **37**, 303–309.

47. Mair, T.S., Hillyer, M.H. & Taylor, F.G. (1990) Peritonitis in adult horses: A review of 21 cases. *Veterinary Record*, **126**, 567–570.

48. Merritt, A.M., Burrow, J.A. & Hartless, C.S. (1998) Effect of xylazine, detomidine, and a combination of xylazine and butorphanol on equine duodenal motility. *American Journal of Veterinary Research*, **59**, 619–623.

49. Milligan, M., Kukanich, B., Beard, W. & Waxman, S. (2006) The disposition of lidocaine during a 12-hour intravenous infusion to postoperative horses. *Journal of Veterinary Pharmacology and Therapeutics*, **29**, 495–499.

50. Moore, J.N., Garner, H.E., Shapland, J.E. & Hatfield, D.G. (1981) Prevention of endotoxin-induced arterial hypoxaemia and lactic acidosis with flunixin meglumine in the conscious pony. *Equine Veterinary Journal*, **13**, 95–98.

51. Moore, R.M., Bertone, A.L., Muir, W.W., Stromberg, P.C. & Beard, W.L. (1994) Histopathologic evidence of reperfusion injury in the large colon of horses after low-flow ischemia. *American Journal of Veterinary Research*, **55**, 1434–1443.

52. Morello, S., Southwood, L.L., Engiles, J.E., *et al.* (2012) Effect of intraperitoneal PERIDAN™ Concentrate Adhesion Reduction Device on clinical findings, infection, and tissue healing in an adult horse jejuno-jejunostomy model. *Veterinary Surgery*, doi: 10.1111/j.1532-950X.2012.00951.x. [Epub ahead of print].

53. Mueller, P.O., Hay, W.P., Harmon, B. & Amoroso, L. (2000) Evaluation of a bioresorbable hyaluronate-carboxymethylcellulose membrane for prevention of experimentally induced abdominal adhesions in horses. *Veterinary Surgery*, **29**, 48–53.

54. Murphy, D.J., Peck, L.S., Detrisac, C.J., Widenhouse, C.W. & Goldberg, E.P. (2002) Use of a high-molecular-weight carboxymethylcellulose in a tissue protective solution for prevention of postoperative abdominal adhesions in ponies. *American Journal of Veterinary Research*, **63**, 1448–1454.

55. Parker, J.E., Fibini, S.L., Car, B.D. & Erb, H.N. (1987) Prevention of intraabdominal adhesions in ponies by low-dose heparin therapy. *Veterinary Surgery*, **16**, 459–462.

56. Parker, J.E., Fubini, S.L. & Todhunter, R.J. (1989) Retrospective evaluation of repeat celiotomy in 53

horses with acute gastrointestinal disease. *Veterinary Surgery*, **18**, 424–431.

57. Parraga, M.E., Spier, S.J., Thurmond, M. & Hirsh, D. (1997) A clinical trial of probiotic administration for prevention of *Salmonella* shedding in the postoperative period in horses with colic. *Journal of Veterinary Internal Medicine*, **11**, 36–41.

58. Phillips, T.J. & Walmsley, J.P. (1993) Retrospective analysis of the results of 151 exploratory laparotomies in horses with gastrointestinal disease. *Equine Veterinary Journal*, **25**, 427–431.

59. Proudman, C.J., Smith, J.E., Edwards, G.B. & French, N.P. (2002) Long-term survival of equine surgical colic cases. Part 1: Patterns of mortality and morbidity. *Equine Veterinary Journal*, **34**, 432–437.

60. de la Rebiere de Pouyade, G., Grulke, S., Detilleux, J., *et al.* (2009) Evaluation of low-molecular-weight heparin for the prevention of equine laminitis after colic surgery. *Journal of Veterinary Emergency and Critical Care*, **19**, 113–119.

61. Rodgers, L. (1994) Evaluation of peritoneal pH, glucose, and lactate dehydrogenase levels as an indicator of intra-abdominal sepsis. *Proceedings of the American College of Veterinary Internal Medicine*, **12**, 173.

62. Roussel, A.J., Jr., Cohen, N.D., Hooper, R.N. & Rakestraw, P.C. (2001) Risk factors associated with development of postoperative ileus in horses. *Journal of the American Veterinary Medical Association*, **219**, 72–78.

63. Rusiecki, K.E., Nieto, J.E., Puchalski, S.M. & Snyder, J.R. (2008) Evaluation of continuous infusion of lidocaine on gastrointestinal tract function in normal horses. *Veterinary Surgery*, **37**, 564–570.

64. Russell, T.M., Kearney, C. & Pollock, P.J. (2010) Surgical treatment of septic jugular thrombophlebitis in nine horses. *Veterinary Surgery*, **39**, 627–630.

65. Santschi, E.M., Grindem, C.B., Tate, L.P., Jr. & Corbett, W.T. (1988) Peritoneal fluid analysis in ponies after abdominal surgery. *Veterinary Surgery*, **17**, 6–9.

66. Schroeder, E.L., Holcombe, S.J., Cook, V.L., *et al.* (2011) Preliminary safety and biological efficacy studies of ethyl pyruvate in normal mature horses. *Equine Veterinary Journal*, **43**, 341–347.

67. Sellon, D.C., Roberts, M.C., Blikslager, A.T., Ulibarri, C. & Papich, M.G. (2004) Effects of continuous rate intravenous infusion of butorphanol on physiologic and outcome variables in horses after celiotomy. *Journal of Veterinary Internal Medicine*, **18**, 555–563.

68. Smith, L.J., Mellor, D.J., Marr, C.M., Reid, S.W. & Mair, T.S. (2007) Incisional complications following exploratory celiotomy: Does an abdominal bandage reduce the risk? *Equine Veterinary Journal*, **39**, 277–283.

69. Southwood, L.L. (2004) Postoperative management of the large colon volvulus patient. *Veterinary Clinics of North America: Equine Practice*, **20**, 167–197.

70. Stone, W.C., Lindsay, W.A., Mason, E.D., *et al.* 1991. Factors associated with acute wound dehiscence following equine abdominal surgery. In: *Proceedings of 4th Equine Colic Research Symposium*, Athens, Georgia, p. 52.

71. Sullins, K.E., White, N.A., Lundin, C.S., Dabareiner, R. & Gaulin, G. (2004) Prevention of ischaemia-induced small intestinal adhesions in foals. *Equine Veterinary Journal*, **36**, 370–375.

72. Tomlinson, J.E. & Blikslager, A.T. (2005) Effects of cyclooxygenase inhibitors flunixin and deracoxib on permeability of ischaemic-injured equine jejunum. *Equine Veterinary Journal*, **37**, 75–80.

73. Tomlinson, J.E., Wilder, B.O., Young, K.M. & Blikslager, A.T. (2004) Effects of flunixin meglumine or etodolac treatment on mucosal recovery of equine jejunum after ischemia. *American Journal of Veterinary Research*, **65**, 761–769.

74. Torfs, S., Delesalle, C., Dewulf, J., Devisscher, L. & Deprez, P. (2009) Risk factors for equine postoperative ileus and effectiveness of prophylactic lidocaine. *Journal of Veterinary Internal Medicine*, **23**, 606–611.

75. Torfs, S., Levet, T., Delesalle, C., *et al.* (2010) Risk factors for incisional complications after exploratory celiotomy in horses: Do skin staples increase the risk? *Veterinary Surgery*, **39**, 616–620.

76. Van Hoogmoed, L.M., Nieto, J.E., Snyder, J.R. & Harmon, F.A. (2004) Survey of prokinetic use in horses with gastrointestinal injury. *Veterinary Surgery*, **33**, 279–285.

77. Van Hoogmoed, L.M., Nieto, J.E., Spier, S.J. & Snyder, J.R. (2004) In vivo investigation of the efficacy of a customized solution to attenuate injury following low-flow ischemia and reperfusion injury in the jejunum of horses. *American Journal of Veterinary Research*, **65**, 485–490.

78. Werners, A.H., Bull, S. & Fink-Gremmels, J. (2005) Endotoxaemia: A review with implications for the horse. *Equine Veterinary Journal*, **37**, 371–383.

79. Wilson, D.A., Baker, G.J. & Boero, M.J. (1995) Complications of celiotomy incisions in horses. *Veterinary Surgery*, **24**, 506–514.

80. Yamout, S., Bouré, L. & Theoret, C., *et al.* (2007) Evaluation of abdominal instillation of 0.03% fucoidan solution for the prevention of experimentally induced abdominal adhesions in healthy pony foals. In: *Proceedings of the European College of Veterinary Surgeons 16th Annual Meeting*, Dublin, Ireland.

81. Young, B.L., White, N.A., Donaldson, L.L. & Dabareiner, R.M. (2002) Treatment of ischaemic jejunum with topical and intraluminal Carolina Rinse. *Equine Veterinary Journal*, **34**, 469–474.

20 Biosecurity

Helen W. Aceto

Department of Clinical Studies, New Bolton Center, School of Veterinary Medicine, University of Pennsylvania, Kennett Square, PA, USA

Chapter Outline

Importance of biosecurity	**262**	Environment	268
Purpose of this chapter	262	"Global"	268
What is biosecurity?	263	**Biosecurity for the hospitalized equine**	
Why do we need biosecurity?	263	**colic patient**	**268**
Components of a biosecurity program	**264**	Specific concerns	268
Preventive measures	265	Patient management	269
Segregation by risk	265	Preventive measures	269
Cleaning and disinfection	265	Monitoring and surveillance	269
Hand hygiene	266	**Biosecurity for the equine colic patient**	
Barrier precautions and protective clothing	266	**at home**	**270**
Waste disposal	266	General recommendations for isolating	
Antimicrobial use	267	a horse at home	270
Other considerations	267	Recommendations for cleaning and disinfection	271
Oversight and reporting	267	Salmonella	272
Education	267	Preventive measures	272
Monitoring and surveillance	267	Monitoring shedding status	272
Patient	267	MRSA	273

Importance of biosecurity

Purpose of this chapter

It is not the purpose of this chapter to enumerate in great detail all aspects of biosecurity pertaining to veterinary medical facilities. Rather, the intent is to provide an overview of biosecurity plus specific practical recommendations for the management of infection risk among equine colic patients during hospitalization and after discharge (Sections 20.3 and 20.4).

What is biosecurity?

When originally coined, the term "biosecurity" meant preventing the introduction of a disease agent into a population whereas "biocontainment" referred to controlling the spread of an introduced agent. In a veterinary context, use of these terms was most commonly associated with livestock industries. In recent years, this terminology has increasingly been applied to practices put in place to control the spread of disease agents in veterinary hospitals. However, the situation in veterinary hospitals is generally more dynamic than many livestock operations. Moreover, the nature of medicine and the mission of veterinary hospitals is such that animals clinically affected by the very agents that have the potential to spread among the hospital population, as well as subclinical carriers that may go unrecognized, are always likely to be present. Because of this, the distinction between biosecurity and biocontainment has become ill-defined and a more broad definition of biosecurity, used interchangeably with infection control, is warranted. To this end, Dunowska et al.[27] suggest that biosecurity "encompasses all practices intended to prevent (limit) the introduction and spread of infectious diseases within a group of equine patients and their human caregivers," thereby protecting human, animal, and environmental health against biological threats.[55]

Why do we need biosecurity?

Biosecurity/infection control is an essential function at all health-care facilities including veterinary hospitals. While achieving excellence in veterinary care is a multifaceted process, it is impossible to reach that goal without employing logical infection control procedures. The standard of care at every veterinary hospital should include procedures that ensure a high standard of hygiene, awareness of the dangers of animal-to-animal, animal-to-person, and person-to-animal transfer of infectious agents, and reduce infection risk wherever possible. The aim of a biosecurity program is to establish those policies and procedures necessary to accomplish the objective of effectively managing and/or reducing infection risks, including infections that are hospital associated.

In human medicine, there is an extensive literature describing formal definitions for hospital-associated (as opposed to community associated) infections (HAIs).[23,37,44] The characterization of HAI is markedly less well-developed in veterinary medicine. Indeed, determining whether or not a particular infection is truly hospital associated may not be as simple as that described for human patients. Characteristics of the infectious organism may be important in developing a definition for veterinary patients. For example, Salmonella is the most important cause of nosocomial infections in large animal hospitals.[9,12,16,19,20,30,41,66,70,75,76] In human salmonellosis, the US Centers for Disease Control and Prevention (CDC) defines the time from infection to shedding of organisms and onset of diarrhea to be typically 1–3 days, although it is sometimes longer.[17] Little research has been done to measure the same parameters for salmonellosis in animals, nevertheless referral veterinary hospitals often assume that fecal shedding of Salmonella 72 h or later after admission is evidence of nosocomial infection.[32,33] However, a meta-analysis of experimental studies in large animals[4] indicates that differentiating between nosocomial and community-associated infection based on something crude like day of detection is extremely problematic. The time course of fecal shedding in experimental studies (and our own findings from surveillance of hospitalized patients) suggests it is far from certain that detection of Salmonella positive samples at ≥3 days is indicative of a HAI in large animal patients and a much longer period should be considered before a community-associated, hospital-expressed infection can be ruled less likely.[4] Just as importantly, even when Salmonella positive fecal samples are collected between 10 and 72 h after admission, the time course data from experimental studies indicate that these cases could be hospital-associated,[4] an example of which can be seen in a 1996 report of Salmonella Krefeld infections in a veterinary intensive care unit where 25% of infected horses had been in the unit for only 1 day when detected as infected.[62]

In addition to the lack of appropriate definitions, there is a paucity of published information regarding rates of HAI in either individual veterinary hospitals or comparative data across multiple centers. As a result, it can be difficult for veterinary hospitals to assess and manage infection risks or determine how well they may be performing. Such difficulties notwithstanding, it should be obvious that veterinary facilities caring for hospitalized animals are places where contagious disease-causing organisms, a greater proportion of which will be multidrug resistant (MDR) than is found in the general community, are present in high numbers and able to contact susceptible patients[19,20,29,41,47,58,59,76,78]. Consequently, all veterinary facilities that provide medical care to patients should be obliged to implement infection control practices. Over recent years, the number of large veterinary referral hospitals has increased as has our ability to treat more critical cases. In addition, advances in veterinary medicine in general and the methods used to manage equine colic cases in particular, have increased survival rates among these patients. Inevitable consequences of which are an increase in the potential vulnerability of our patient population and a concomitant increase in hospital exposure time; facts that mean HAI will undoubtedly continue to gain in importance in veterinary hospitals. The occurrence of HAI has both medical and economic consequences. The latter includes increased length of hospital stay, increased treatment costs, possible indemnification and legal costs, loss of future business, etc. Just as importantly, reports of nosocomial outbreaks of infectious disease in large animal veterinary teaching hospitals are abundant in the literature and only serve to underscore the need for an effective biosecurity program.[9,10,12,16,19,20,32,41,52,62,66,70,75,76,78] Veterinarians must therefore be proactive in developing infection control strategies that protect the hospitalized patient, the personnel who take care of them, and the entire veterinary facility. Appropriate infection control programs (ICPs) are integral to providing optimal patient care, ensuring a safe working environment for hospital employees, and protecting the hospital from financial loss and possible litigation, but the defensibility of this position is predicated on the following concepts:

(1) All reasonable precautions were taken.
(2) All reasonable expectations of risk were fully communicated to the client (with appropriate documentary evidence by way of confirmation).
(3) At the very least the minimal expected standard of care was delivered to the patient.

Nosocomial infections are an inherent risk of any hospitalization and are listed among the principle reasons for malpractice claims against human hospitals.[39] Such claims are also more likely to yield decisions in favor of the patient than are other types of claim.[39] Although currently less prevalent, the frequency of such legal claims is increasing in veterinary medicine. It is important to appreciate that even in hospitals with the highest standards of care and most-well-managed ICPs, not all nosocomial infections are preventable (and this should always be communicated to the client). However, any and all occurrences of nosocomial infection are indefensible when a properly implemented, comprehensive ICP is lacking. As a result, in addition to the obligation to provide the patient with the best possible care and protect public health, the increasing likelihood of significant monetary and professional cost of infection control failures means that the need for an appropriate ICP is only likely to increase.[8,51,53]

Implementation and, more importantly, long-term maintenance of an ICP is not problem free.[19] Some level of commitment is required to finance the program, to ensure its acceptance across all constituencies, and to rationally collect and use data to optimize the cost:benefit ratio of the program. Even in a relatively short period, it is, however, possible to effect major changes in attitude and behavior with respect to biosecurity that are ultimately to the benefit of patients, hospital, and personnel alike.

Components of a biosecurity program

At the outset it is important to appreciate that there is no "one-size-fits-all" program that can be used interchangeably for all veterinary facilities. Although the areas and functions that must be considered when developing and implementing an ICP will be broadly similar across facilities, details vary considerably. The extent to which an individual equine clinic implements biosecurity practices is contingent on a number of factors that include size and type of caseload, facility size and design, personnel and economic issues, level of risk aversion, etc. Numerous excellent resources are available in the literature[3,8,10,27,33,51,53,67,73,77] and online[1,2,23,56,57,69] that review in detail all aspects of biosecurity and help guide veterinary personnel in the design of an effective program. It is appropriate to briefly enumerate items likely to be key aspects of any biosecurity program here, but where more detail is required it is recommended that additional references be consulted.

Preventive measures

Segregation by risk

When establishing a biosecurity program, patients should be divided into risk categories; high, medium, or low are convenient and easily understood designations. Low risk comprises elective cases while medium risk would include non-GI emergencies (although some neurological cases should be considered high risk) and inpatients that receive antimicrobials for >72 h. In some cases, the high-risk categorization is mainly predicated on vulnerability to infection and susceptibility to all HAI, as is the case, for example, in neonates, particularly those that are critically ill. For other patients, high risk indicates that either because of known or suspected infection or because of past experience with similar patients, the animal represents a risk to other patients, potentially the hospital environment, and to personnel in the case of zoonotic agents.[56] In the case of equine colics there is ample evidence to indicate that they are a dual threat because they are at both high risk of developing various types of infection[36,40,49,50] and at high risk of shedding organisms such as *Salmonella*[5,19,30,32,34,36,45,46,61,64,71,72,76] and *Clostridia*.[10,11] Wherever possible, patients in different risk categories should be housed separately and cross-traffic of both animals and people should be limited or even prohibited, for example, cross-traffic with isolated patients.[3,27,53,67,77] Should the risk status of a patient change during hospitalization, it is critical that the client is informed immediately and that any such communications are properly documented in the medical record. Every large animal clinic should have an area designated for isolation of a patient. Ideally this would be in an area physically separated from lower risk animals. At a minimum, a stall(s) away from high traffic areas should be designated for isolation use. When occupied, access can be limited by placing barriers around the stall or between it and other areas of the hospital; although less than ideal, something as simple as cones and tape can work.

Cleaning and disinfection

Effective cleaning and disinfection are critical in preventing transmission of infectious agents between patients or from contaminated environments. To aid in this process, it is highly desirable that surfaces in animal housing and clinical spaces are cleanable and nonporous; this can be very simple such as ensuring that wood surfaces are properly sealed and painted or more complex like the installation of monolithic flooring systems. Critical evaluation of the hospital environment is essential. At a minimum, cleaning and disinfection protocols should include the following steps: (1) detergent to remove organic debris (critical to the efficacy of most disinfectants), (2) rinsing, (3) drying (optimum; or at a minimum water removal, as application of disinfectant to a water-logged area may result in dilution to the point of inefficacy), and (4) disinfectant application. Some, but not all, disinfectants require rinsing. Drying after cleaning and disinfection is always beneficial to pathogen control. Depending on the area to be covered, detergent and disinfectant solution can be delivered using a pump sprayer, power sprayer, hose-end sprayer or hose-end foamer such as a Hydrofoamer®. Hose-end sprayers or foamers should be set to deliver the appropriate dilution. It is important to check the accuracy of delivery prior to use, this is particularly true when using such devices for disinfectants as inappropriate concentrations can seriously impact the effectiveness of disinfection. If a power sprayer is used, a low pressure setting is generally preferred. Although higher pressures can assist in removing stubborn organic debris, they may also force debris and organisms into crevices or porous materials such as wood from which they can later emerge. Additionally, higher pressures cause more aerosolization and overspray that can potentially spread organisms widely, even into previously uncontaminated areas. In areas of high concern, multiple disinfectant steps may be useful. Care must be taken to ensure that the properties of the detergent and disinfectant are compatible. Disinfection protocols should be frequently reviewed and altered based on evidence gathered through patient and environment surveillance as bacterial resistance is a constant threat. Consideration should also be given to the effect of disinfectants (some of which are powerful oxidizers) on equipment, personnel, and the environment. A particular disinfectant may be more costly at the outset, but overall might be a prudent choice because of minimal destruction of equipment. If prolonged use of a disinfectant is found to damage surfaces an alternative should be sought, as loss of surface integrity defeats the object of maintaining sealed, cleanable surfaces in potentially critical areas. The use of prepackaged wipes containing glutaraldehyde or accelerated hydrogen peroxide disinfectants are a very convenient and effective means of disinfecting hand surfaces and certain types of equipment. It should go without saying that clippers, clipper blades, bandage or suture scissors, and all other equipment used on patients should be subject to appropriate cleaning and disinfection. There are several valuable resources covering cleaning protocols, and the properties and use of disinfectants.[5,8,26,27,31,35,53,56,63]

Hand hygiene

The importance of excellent hygiene[18] and overall cleanliness cannot be overemphasized. Strict hand hygiene should be stressed. As many veterinary facilities (particularly animal housing areas) were not constructed with infection control in mind, ready access to hand washing facilities is not always available. To correct this fundamental system error,[38] alcohol-based hand sanitizer should be prominently located throughout the facility. Sanitizing with alcohol-based products reduces the incidence of HAI in human medicine[18] and is also effective in veterinary hospitals.[74] The need for personal responsibility[38] and use of proper technique in hand hygiene (even when gloves are worn for patient handling) should be repeatedly emphasized to all personnel and clients as well.[18,38,48]

Barrier precautions and protective clothing

Barrier precautions in low- or medium-risk patient populations may be minimal, and should be based on incidence of infectious disease in this population. In general, protective apparel is not required for these patients but the need for excellent hand hygiene along with cleanliness of shoes (which should be safe, protective, and cleanable), clothes, and personal equipment such as stethoscopes is paramount. For higher risk patients personal protective equipment (PPE) may be required as well as the placement of disinfectant footbaths or footmats. Although footbaths may be effective in preventing the transmission of infectious agents,[6,28,54,68] opinions about the degree of such efficacy vary and there is little doubt that they can be difficult to manage and may be detrimental to the immediate environment in which they are placed. Nevertheless, at least in the case of isolated stalls, footbaths should be considered mandatory. In veterinary hospitals PPE usually includes the use of disposable gowns or coveralls, gloves, masks, caps, and boots. While opinions vary, our experience suggests that gowns usually do not sufficiently cover the lower leg and single-use disposable coveralls represent the best protection for working with isolated patients. Coveralls are available in several types. For cost-containment purposes we recommend a cheaper, nonwaterproof woven coverall for general use. However, where there is any risk of getting wet such as close contact with a diarrheic foal, working with an adult that has pipe-stream diarrhea, or any procedure that might require individuals to kneel on the stall floor, a more costly waterproof coverall, for example, Tyvek®, should be worn. In addition to coveralls, we routinely employ disposable plastic boots followed by rubber over-boots, gloves, and in specific cases (e.g., liquid diarrhea that may splash, cryptosporidium, methicillin-resistant *Staphylococcus aureus* [MRSA]) surgeon-type face masks and bouffant caps. No matter what type of PPE is used, it is important that all personnel understand the rationale behind such use and, most critically, the distinction between "clean" vs. "dirty" so that they either apply or remove PPE when necessary and move about the facility in an appropriate manner.[28,51,67,77]

Waste disposal

Infectious waste can be source of environmental contamination and of infection to patients, and personnel so management of infectious waste is an important part of biosecurity. All sharps should be placed in designated containers and disposed of according to local regulations. Other infectious materials can be autoclaved or incinerated where appropriate prior to final disposal. Acceptable ways of disposing of large volumes of waste bedding materials include composting, disposal at a designated landfill, or steaming.[27,53,67]

Antimicrobial use

Development of antimicrobial resistance among bacterial pathogens is an ever increasing problem and many of the pathogens associated with equine hospitals are MDR.[19,20,29,41,47,59,76,78] It should be part of an ICP to ensure that antimicrobials are used as conservatively as possible and in accordance with published guidelines. Development of an antibiotic use policy tailored to an individual clinic (using data gathered by monitoring trends in microbial resistance) is an excellent idea and if necessary enforced restriction of specific antimicrobials can be considered. It is inevitable, however, that organisms in hospital environments will be exposed to antimicrobials and disinfectants so implementation of infection control precautions must be used to help prevent the spread of agents in the environment, among patients, and personnel.

Other considerations

Other areas that should be considered for biosecurity purposes include the control of insects, rodents, birds, and other animals that might contact and transfer organisms of concern and how pastures and paddocks available for patient use are utilized. It is also necessary to consider controls for visitors and other foot traffic. It is highly recommended that an explicit visitor policy be developed that tightly restricts visits for high-risk cases in particular, or even forbids visits to isolated cases except in the most extreme circumstances such as when a patient is about to be euthanized.

Oversight and reporting

The ideal approach is to have an individual (or individuals) dedicated to biosecurity but this may only be feasible, or even warranted, in settings with a large multispecies caseload such as a university teaching hospital. Appointing a designated Biosecurity Officer with specialized training in epidemiology or infectious disease to oversee the program is best. However, in smaller hospitals with a component of emergency/critically ill patients, an individual capable of gathering, reviewing, and manipulating surveillance data and monitoring infection control activities on a daily basis, who then reports to a veterinarian responsible for making biosecurity policy, is a reasonable alternative. It is also helpful if the Biosecurity Officer has minimal to no clinical obligations; this eliminates conflict of interest regarding patient status and promotes the mind-set of "the hospital as a patient" for that individual.

Education

People working with animals in a hospital are likely to be exposed to a variety of infectious agents, including those with zoonotic potential,[56] even when this is not apparent. Training and education should be integral to any ICP so that everyone has awareness of these dangers and understands their specific responsibilities in reducing risk wherever possible. Educational efforts should focus on zoonotic and contagious diseases of importance and the routes of transmission by which the causative organisms spread,[69] steps necessary to maintain high standards of hygiene with particular emphasis on strict hand hygiene[18] and rigorous routine cleaning and disinfection, and proper use of PPE.[3,8,27,51,53,67,77]

Monitoring and surveillance

Patient

Patient monitoring and surveillance is a cornerstone of infection control.[52] Patient monitoring can include collection and collation of data with respect to HAI, such as catheter associated thrombophlebitis, anesthetic- or ventilator-associated pneumonia, or surgical site infections. It also should include reporting of any MRSA or vancomycin-resistant *Enterococcus* infections. In a referral hospital setting, monitoring and evaluation of MDR infections and trends in microbial resistance in isolates obtained from clinical submissions should also be part of the biosecurity effort.[3,27,52,53] The data generated can be used to make evidence-based decisions on the effectiveness of biosecurity protocols and to more accurately define the level of risk that different types of case represent. It may also be necessary to conduct routine patient surveillance of particularly problematic infectious organisms. In large animal referral hospitals principle among these would be *Salmonella*, though some also conduct active surveillance for MRSA. Surveillance data and identification of patients at risk both for disease transmission and nosocomial infection essentially directs many other biosecurity efforts in a hospital. Clearly, ensuring a good working relationship between those individuals involved in biosecurity and the diagnostic laboratory is essential to success.

Environment

Monitoring of the hospital environment is also critical to a successful biosecurity program. This does not always imply microbiological evaluation but should certainly encompass monitoring to ensure proper hygiene and control of clutter that might impede cleaning. Environmental sampling can, however, be useful in determining which patient populations, traffic patterns and protocols present a risk for hospital contamination, and in assessing how well containment efforts are performing.[3,52] Most commonly, large animal hospitals have used *Salmonella* as a general biosensor to evaluate ICPs,[12] but this does not preclude the investigation of other organisms under special circumstances or as needs change. If undertaken, high traffic areas, treatment areas, and facilities that house high-risk patients should be the focus of environmental surveillance.

Use of electrostatic wipes is an effective means of sample collection for large areas.[13] Establishment of a useful environmental sampling strategy requires collection of baseline data, without which it is not possible to assess the likelihood that particular infections are HAI, determine whether there has been an increase in such infections, or evaluate the efficacy of any interventions.

"Global"

Though not necessarily truly "global" in scope, it is essential that the individual(s) tasked with overseeing the program appreciates that just as disease-causing organisms evolve and change, evidence-based evolution of biosecurity protocols is inevitable and indeed crucial to ongoing program success. It is the responsibility of that individual to not only be aware of what is occurring in the hospital but also keep pace with infection threats outside the confines of the facility that may impinge on its activities. If necessary, the responsible individual should be prepared to adjust biosecurity protocols, the focus of surveillance, and any associated testing based on developments in the literature, knowledge of active outbreaks in the hospital referral area, regional, national, or even international infectious disease threats.

Biosecurity for the hospitalized equine colic patient

Specific concerns

A number of studies have identified hospitalized horses with the presenting complaint of colic to be at high risk of shedding *Salmonella*.[43,45,60,61,66,70] In addition, other factors associated with *Salmonella* shedding are common to many hospitalized equine colics such as transportation,[46,61,66,70] change in diet[71] or days of feed restriction,[45] feeding of alfalfa,[46] number of days feeding bran mash,[45] antimicrobial therapy,[43,45,61,66,70] abdominal surgery,[32,61,66,70] diarrhea at admission[71] or within 6 h of hospitalization,[46] fever during hospitalization,[71] leukopenia within 6 h of hospitalization,[46] neutropenia,[22] nasogastric intubation[43,61,66,70] or abnormal results of nasogastric intubation,[46] mean daily temperature,[45] and season.[15] In addition in separate studies diagnoses of both large[45] and small[65] colon impaction have been associated with *Salmonella* shedding. Abdominal surgery is most commonly performed on an emergency basis for diagnosis and treatment of horses with acute gastrointestinal disease. In those colics that undergo surgery, common complications include infections such as incisional infection, colitis, septic thrombophlebitis, pneumonia and peritonitis.[40,49,50] Because of their infection risk, well-documented propensity to shed *Salmonella*, and the fact that *Salmonella* is the most important cause of nosocomial outbreaks of disease at large animal hospitals,[12,19] the equine colic deserves special attention in ICPs.

Patient management

Preventive measures

Horses that present with colic but are subsequently determined to have enteritis should be isolated with full barrier precautions and PPE. Similarly, horses that develop diarrhea[24] (defined as liquid feces retaining no shape in the bedding passed more than twice in 12 h) particularly if accompanied by fever, leukopenia (or leukocytosis), inappetence, and nasogastric reflux (see below) should also be isolated. In general, however, provided colics are housed in manner that limits exposure to the fecal material of other colic patients, stringent barrier precautions are probably unnecessary. Dedicated footwear, disposable plastic boots, gloves, and scrupulous attention to the hygiene of both caregivers and the environment are what we currently employ in our hospital. However, colics at New Bolton Center's Widener Hospital are housed in a new facility where each stall is completely self-contained with its own ventilation system and there is no contact with feces from other patients housed in the same unit. Where there is direct airborne contact between stalls, and particularly where mucking of stalls takes place into a central aisle that is also used by animals and personnel, it may be necessary to apply more stringent barriers and PPE. All colics should be provided with their own equipment such as thermometers, grooming equipment, lead shank, hoof pick, ice boots, and equipment needed to check for nasogastric reflux. The designated equipment should stay with the patient for the duration of their hospitalization and be not used for other animals. It should be obvious that nasogastric intubation is a high-risk procedure and all equipment must be subject to rigorous cleaning and disinfection. As far as the tubes are concerned there are several options. Each client can be required to purchase a new tube if needed, tubes can be gas sterilized, or they can be subject to multistage cleaning and disinfection. For both the latter options it is important that the tubes are thoroughly dry. Once a patient is discharged, the stall and equipment used for that animal should be thoroughly cleaned and disinfected before being used for the next patient. Some institutions, including our own, also submit environmental samples from the stall for *Salmonella* testing before the stall is reused.

In the case of incisional infections, management factors at the time of surgery are likely to be important. For example, use of staples may be a risk factor for infection and covering of the incision with a protective dressing during recovery from anesthesia may be protective. Ensuring that perioperative antimicrobials are used appropriately may also be critical. A recent study conducted at New Bolton Center[36] indicated that only 40% of 113 surgical colics received antimicrobials within 1 h of the first incision. To maintain adequate tissue levels of antimicrobial during the recovery period most of the horses should also have been redosed intraoperatively, but only 2/113 received intraoperative antimicrobials. Although there were apparently no associations between antimicrobial timing and infection in this group of horses, in reality we do not know how much difference antimicrobials might be making because in the majority of cases they were not administered according to current guidelines.[14]

In some cases of incisional infection or thrombophlebitis (which has itself been associated with being positive for *Salmonella*[21]), MRSA is identified as the causative organism. Although all infections caused by MDR bacteria should be handled with great care, the zoonotic potential (primarily manifest as skin infections) and the possibility of developing nasal carrier status by MRSA warrant special precautions.[78] Full barriers should be applied to animals that are culture positive for MRSA and if possible they should be isolated, particularly where there is drainage from the infected site. In addition to the PPE described above, face masks and bouffant caps should always be worn. Use of a face mask limits the risk of transfer via hand-to-nose contact, thereby reducing the risk of nasal colonization in caregivers and subsequent transfer to other animals or people.[8,77,78]

Monitoring and surveillance

Many hospitals choose to conduct active surveillance for *Salmonella* in colic patients. If standard culture methods are used for detection,[19] individuals responsible for biosecurity must be cognizant of the lag time of 3–5 days between sample submission and return of results that could lead to widespread environmental contamination before an animal is identified as positive. Moreover, although definitive data on the sensitivity and specificity of the various culture methods in routine use are lacking, it is increasingly recognized that while specific (95–99%), they likely have sensitivities only in the 30–60% range at best. There are more sensitive standardized methods available such as those described by the International Organization for Standardization,[4,19] but these techniques are costly and can take at least 5 days or long as 7 days or more to complete. If PCR is available it should be considered as a screening test. It is almost certainly significantly more sensitive than regular culture and, even though overnight enrichment of samples is still required for reliable detection, PCR is capable of providing results 18–24 h after sample submission (Aceto *et al.* unpublished observations). We have successfully used PCR screening with culture follow-up using a modified ISO method[19] on PCR positive samples to identify *Salmonella* in both patient and environmental samples. Follow-up culture is necessary to confirm the presence of viable organisms. Isolates can then be used to identify the *Salmonella* serovar involved, test for antimicrobial susceptibility (crucial in clinical cases requiring therapeutic intervention), and may be required for more advanced characterization in epidemiological investigations, especially in possible outbreak situations. However, many hospitals may not have ready access to either culture or PCR detection techniques and must rely on clinical presentation to increase the index of suspicion that an animal is shedding *Salmonella*. Although fever, diarrhea,[24] and leukopenia have classically been associated with salmonellosis, in our experience clinical signs may be more subtle and varied so that these endpoints are not always adequate to identify animals that may be shedding. Fever in particular occurs commonly in colics without an infection being identified.[36] Nonetheless, patients should be monitored for development of fever and diarrhea. Additional clinical findings that should be considered include abnormal white blood cell count (i.e., leukopenia or leukocytosis), inappetence (particularly where the patient was eating and becomes inappetent), depression, persistent nasogastric reflux, and whether or not the patient had abdominal surgery. In our experience and that of others,[32,34] being *Salmonella* positive is associated with abdominal surgery in colics but this has not been demonstrated in all studies.[71,72]

To aid in the control of *Salmonella* and other infections, the clinical progress of colic patients should be monitored on a daily basis by infection control personnel as well as by the attending clinician so that where necessary, steps to contain infectious agents can be promptly initiated.

Biosecurity for the equine colic patient at home

General recommendations for isolating a horse at home

Not every colic patient discharged from the hospital with an infection that can be managed at home requires isolation, but every infected animal should be handled with care and the importance of general hygiene and hand hygiene in particular should be emphasized with the client. There are two conditions where isolation/barrier precautions should be recommended. Namely, horses found to be shedding *Salmonella* in their feces and horses identified with MRSA infections where there is drainage from the infected area(s). The recommendations below are designed to limit cross-contamination but as facilities tend to vary considerably, it may be necessary to devise a specific customized plan in consultation with the client and/or their referring veterinarian. Ideally, the affected animal should be housed in a separate building but as this is frequently not possible, placing it in an end stall or similar area where traffic is minimal, or at least can be easily controlled, is a reasonable option. The following general recommendations can be readily adapted or personalized and supplied to clients or other caregivers that will be managing isolated patients at home.

- *Always deal with the isolated horse last*
  After working with an isolated horse clothing should be changed or laundered and footwear should be changed or cleaned before doing anything with other animals.
- *Always wash hands*
  Disposable single-use plastic gloves should be worn and hands thoroughly washed or sanitized (even when gloves have been worn) after handling the affected horse or anything that it has been in contact with. Alcohol-based hand

sanitizers can be readily placed stallside and are effective provided an individual's hands are not grossly dirty, in which case they must be washed with soap and water.

- *Use a disinfectant footdip*
  A dip-tub or footmat containing disinfectant should be placed in front of the isolated stall. However, footdip management can be difficult. Dip-tubs must be changed daily or sooner if they become dirty and footmats should be recharged similarly. Typically, disinfectants will not work if there are high levels of organic material such as shavings, straw, dirt, or feces present. Diluted household bleach (8 fl oz [1 cup] per 1 gal of water) is cheap and effective but it is readily inactivated in the presence of organic debris so it *must* be changed regularly. Other types of disinfectant that have better activity in the face of organic debris can be purchased from a veterinary supply store. Whatever the disinfectant choice, clients must be instructed to carefully follow the directions for proper mixing and disposal, and observe any special precautions indicated on the label. If it seems likely that footdips will not receive proper attention or if you are familiar with the home environment and know that they will become dirty very quickly, it may be better to recommend that a pair of dedicated over-boots be placed stallside for use with that patient until it no longer represents a significant biosecurity risk.
- *Clean other stalls before that of the isolated animal*
  The isolated stall should be cleaned last preferably using a set of tools (pitchfork, shovel, broom, etc.) dedicated to that stall, or else ensure that the equipment is thoroughly cleaned and disinfected before using it on the stalls of other animals. Equipment should be cleaned using a detergent and a brush to remove gross debris followed by immersion of the equipment's head in bleach (8 fl oz [1 cup] per gallon of water) or some other disinfectant solution and wiping down of the handles. Drying in the sun is helpful.
- *Do not share buckets and feed tubs*
  While the horse is isolated, make sure that the same bucket and feed tub and any other equipment stays with that animal and does not get used for others.

- *Carefully dispose of materials that come into contact with the isolated animal*
  Provide a plastic bag to allow for separate disposal of gloves and any materials used in treatment of the isolated animal. Feces, used bedding, and uneaten feed should be collected separately and should not be placed on pastures unless they will be unused for at least a month. Manure and bedding should not be placed in an area that would allow direct drainage into any water system. Ideal disposal methods for feces, bedding, and feed would include proper composting or burying the material. Field spreading with prolonged exposure to sunlight is acceptable as long as the areas will not be used for feed or animals for at least 30 days.
- *Removing the animal from isolation*
  Once any clinical signs (e.g., fever, diarrhea, drainage from sites of infection) that may have been present have been resolved and in the absence of testing, an additional 7–10 days of confinement should be recommended before removing the horse from the isolated area; although it may be reasonable to consider hand-walking at this time, provided the isolated horse will not come into direct contact with other animals, and any feces deposited during the walk is immediately cleaned up. If cultures were submitted (see below), once the horse is negative it can be moved out of isolation. The area should then be thoroughly cleaned. If possible, it is a good idea to leave the area vacant for a while. It may not be practical to leave an area vacant for prolonged period but at a minimum it should be left until *completely* dry.

Recommendations for cleaning and disinfection

It is important to bear in mind that whether it be *Salmonella*, MRSA, or some other agent of concern, anything a shedding horse touches could potentially be contaminated; including all stall surfaces, waterers, and feeders. It is unlikely that everything in the isolated animal's environment is completely cleanable. A fully cleanable surface is one that is nonporous. Porous surfaces with intact finishes such as painted or varnished wood can also be cleaned. However, damaged finishes make such surfaces harder to clean effectively. Dirt floors in stalls are also impossible to clean completely. However, in the case of *Salmonella* which, with the exception of spore forming organisms, is about the most difficult organism to eliminate from equine environments, experience shows that such floors can be decontaminated to the point where organisms can no longer be isolated by standard culture methods. Moreover, our own experience and that of others[42] indicates that stablemates of horses infected with *Salmonella enterica* do not appear to have increased risks of gastrointestinal disease subsequent discharge.

- *Walls and other surfaces*
  After the stall is stripped and as much organic material as possible has been removed the walls and surfaces within an isolated animal's environment can be scrubbed with a plain anionic detergent such as laundry detergent (2–4 fl oz per 1 gal of water). All surfaces must be disrupted during this stage of cleaning. Surfaces should then be rinsed, and disinfected with, for example, dilute bleach (8 fl oz [1 cup] per 1 gal of water). The bleach can be poured or mopped onto surfaces and rinsed off 1 h later. This cleaning procedure can also be used on trailers. There are many other choices for disinfectants and another safe and excellent choice for both stalls and trailers are disinfectants that combine glutaraldehyde with the detergency and penetrating activity of quaternary ammonium disinfectants, for example, Synergize®. Whatever the disinfectant choice, the effect will only be optimum if surfaces are already cleaned and free of organic debris.
- *Buckets and feed tubs*
  Provided they are in good condition, these items can be effectively cleaned and disinfected by scrubbing with a detergent solution as above followed by rinsing and application of a disinfectant solution. Be sure that the equipment has adequate contact time with the disinfectant (at a minimum 10 min or longer according to label instructions). Finally, items used for the delivery of feed and water should always be rinsed with clean water. If, however, the surfaces of buckets or other equipment are damaged and cracked it may not be possible to clean and disinfect them effectively and some consideration should be given to discarding damaged items.

Salmonella

Preventive measures

All of the general guidelines outlined above are applicable to the home management of horses found to be shedding *Salmonella* in their feces. The key to containing such fecal organisms is limiting environmental accumulation. So in addition, removal of any fecal material visible to the naked eye is important. Feces should be removed from the stall of the isolated patient as often as possible to minimize contamination of noncleanable surfaces (2–3 times daily is adequate). Proper composting of fecal material is a good disposal method as a compost pile generating adequate heat will ensure destruction of organisms in a relatively short time (12–24 h).

Monitoring shedding status

In animals and people, *Salmonella* status is generally assessed by means of bacterial culture. *Salmonella* is shed in the feces of infected animals, many of which have no signs of illness and are apparently perfectly healthy, as is often the case with recovered colic patients.

Both three and five consecutive negatives have been suggested to demonstrate that an animal is not actively shedding *Salmonella*. There is ample evidence to indicate that animals shed intermittently[60,61] but the lack of sensitivity of many standard culture methods may also contribute to apparent "intermittent" shedding when only small numbers of organisms are present. In any case, neither five nor three cultures has been examined systematically in this context, although there is one study showing that submission of three samples identified more animals as positive than did a single culture.[25] As more sensitive detection methods become routinely available, three samples may ultimately be demonstrated as sufficient. Suffice to say at this point that *at least* three negative fecal cultures in a row are needed to say that the horse is not actively shedding *Salmonella*. This is not a guarantee that the horse will not shed in the future; however, it is an accepted protocol. At our hospital, for discharged colics that are *Salmonella* positive we have found it helpful to supply clients with a "kit" to make the process of collecting and submitting samples easier. The kit contains instructions (summarized below) fecal cups and lids, disposable gloves, and, if they will be sending samples to our microbiology laboratory, preprinted labels the same as those used when their horse was hospitalized. Recommendations for sampling are as follows.

A fresh fecal ball should be collected and placed into a plastic container. The sample should be refrigerated until shipment to the microbiological laboratory. Samples should be stored in a refrigerator that is not used for food. If a nonfood refrigerator is unavailable, samples can be stored in an insulated styrofoam or similar container with ice packs; but freezing should be avoided. At any point, if the fecal culture is still positive, it is recommended to wait 3–5 days before collecting and submitting another sample. As soon as a negative result is obtained, two more fresh fecal samples can be collected on consecutive days; there must be an interval of 24 h between samples. The samples can be submitted in pairs but they should be shipped to arrive at the lab within 48 h of collection as longer storage times may affect the accuracy of the results. Samples should be shipped for same or next day delivery along with one or more ice packs. To contain any spills during shipping, samples should be placed in closed double bags; if fecal cups are used they should also be placed into a closed plastic bag. Be sure to advise clients to date and label each sample and include sample information (date and time of collection, horse's name) and their contact details on accompanying paperwork. As soon as there have been at least three consecutive negative fecal culture results, it is unlikely that the horse is actively shedding *Salmonella*, and isolation protocols can be discontinued.

MRSA

Even if a colic with, for example, an incisional infection has been identified as positive for MRSA, provided there is no longer active drainage from the site of infection no special biosecurity precautions need be taken after the patient is discharged. It is, however, always prudent to remind clients that whenever they handle their horse, or any other animal for that matter, they should always wash or sanitize their hands. If there is still drainage from the infected area, caregivers at home should wear gloves when handling the affected horse and wash or sanitize hands after they are done. In addition, clients should be counseled that anyone handling the horse should avoid touching their face or nose until after they have washed their hands. Staphylococcal bacteria including MRSA are susceptible to most disinfectants and the practice of good basic hygiene is important in controlling this and many other microorganisms in the animal's environment. In particular, any item of equipment that may be shared between animals should be properly cleaned and disinfected. Until active drainage has ceased, the affected horse is best handled as described above for home isolation. Once the infection has cleared and there is no longer obvious drainage (this determination can be made with the assistance of the referring veterinarian), the stall and other equipment should be thoroughly cleaned. Additional resources about MRSA infections in horses designed for horse-owners are available online.[7] Quizzes for each chapter, additional clinical scenarios, and video demonstrations of surgical procedures are available online at www.wiley.com/go/southwood.

References

1. AAEP Biosecurity guidelines. Available at http://www.aaep.org/pdfs/control_guidelines/Biosecurity_instructions%201.pdf: accessed 20 November 2011.
2. AAEP Biosecurity guidelines for suspected cases of diarrheal disease. Available at http://www.aaep.org/pdfs/control_guidelines/Diarrheal%20Guidelines.pdf: accessed 20 November 2011.
3. Aceto, H.W. & Dallap Schaer, B.L. (2008) Biosecurity for equine hospitals: Protecting the patient and the hospital. In: *The Equine Hospital Manual* (eds K. Corley & J. Stephen), pp. 180–200. Wiley-Blackwell, Chichester, U.K.
4. Aceto, H., Miller, S.A. & Smith, G. (2011) Onset of diarrhea and pyrexia, and time to detection of *Salmonella* in feces in experimental studies of *Salmonella* infection *per os* in large animals. *Journal of the American Veterinary Medical Association*, **238**, 1333–1339.
5. Alinovi, C.A., Ward, M.P., Couëtil, L.L. & Wu, C.C. (2003) Detection of *Salmonella* organisms and assessment of a protocol for removal of contamination in horse stalls at a veterinary teaching hospital. *Journal of the American Veterinary Medical Association*, **223**, 1640–1644.
6. Amass, S.F., Arighi, M., Kinyon, J.M., Hoffman, L.J., Schneider, J.L. & Draper, D.K. (2006) Effectiveness of

using a mat filled with peroxygen disinfectant to minimize shoe sole contamination in a veterinary hospital. *Journal of the American Veterinary Medical Association*, **228**, 1391–1396.

7. Anderson, M.E. & Weese, J.S. (2008) MRSA for horse owners. Available at http://www.equidblog.com/uploads/file/JSW-MA2%20MRSA%20-%20Equine.pdf: accessed 20 November 2011.

8. Bain, F.T. & Weese, J.S. (eds) (2004) *The Veterinary Clinics of North America: Equine Practice—Infection Control*. WB Saunders, Philadelphia, Pennsylvania. *Veterinary Clinics of North America: Equine Practice*, **20**(3): 507–674.

9. Baker, J.R. (1969) An outbreak of salmonellosis involving veterinary hospital patients. *Veterinary Record*, **85**, 8–10.

10. Båverud, V. (2004) *Clostridium difficile* diarrhea: Infection control in horses. *Veterinary Clinics of North America: Equine Practice*, **20**, 615–630.

11. Båverud, V., Gustafsson, A., Franklin, A., Lindholm, A. & Gunnarsson, A. (1997) *Clostridium difficile*-associated with acute colitis in mature horses treated with antibiotics. *Equine Veterinary Journal*, **29**, 279–284.

12. Benedict, K.M., Morley, P.S. & Van Metre, D.C. (2008) Characteristics of biosecurity and infection control programs at veterinary teaching hospitals. *Journal of the American Veterinary Medical Association*, **233**, 767–773.

13. Burgess, B.A., Morley, P.S. & Hyatt, D.R. (2004) Environmental surveillance for *Salmonella enterica* in a veterinary teaching hospital. *Journal of the American Veterinary Medical Association*, **225**, 1344–1348.

14. Bratzler, D.W. & Houck, P.M. (2004) Antimicrobial prophylaxis for surgery: An advisory statement from the national surgical infection prevention project. *Clinical Infectious Disease*, **38**, 1706–1715.

15. Carter, J.D., Hird, D.W., Farver, T.B. & Hjerpe, C.A. (1986) Salmonellosis in hospitalized horses: Seasonality and case fatality rates. *Journal of the American Veterinary Medical Association*, **188**, 163–167.

16. Castor, M.L., Wooley, R.E., Shotts, E.B., Brown, J. & Payeur, J.B. (1989) Characteristics of *Salmonella* isolated from an outbreak of equine salmonellosis in a veterinary teaching hospital. *Equine Veterinary Science*, **9**, 236–241.

17. Centers for Disease Control and Prevention. (2009) Salmonella outbreak investigations: Timeline for reporting cases. Centers for Disease Control and Prevention, Atlanta, Georgia. Available at www.cdc.gov/salmonella/reportingtimeline.html: accessed 20 November 2011.

18. Centers for Disease Control and Prevention. (2002) Guideline for hand hygiene in health-care setting. Centers for Disease Control and Prevention, Atlanta, Georgia. MMWR 51: No. RR-16. Available at http://www.cdc.gov/mmwr/PDF/rr/rr5116.pdf: accessed 20 November 2011.

19. Dallap Schaer, B.L., Aceto, H. & Rankin, S.C. (2010) Outbreak of salmonellosis caused by *Salmonella enterica* serovar Newport MDR-AmpC in a large animal veterinary teaching hospital. *Journal of Veterinary Internal Medicine*, **24**, 1138–1146.

20. Dargatz, D.A. & Traub-Dargatz, J.L. (2004) Multidrug resistant *Salmonella* and nosocomial infections. *Veterinary Clinics of North America: Equine Practice*, **20**, 587–680.

21. Dolente, B.A., Beech, J., Lindborg, S. & Smith, G. (2005) Evaluation of risk factors for development of catheter-associated jugular thrombophlebitis in horses: 50 cases (1993–1998). *Journal of the American Veterinary Medical Association*, **227**, 1134–1141.

22. Dorn, C.R., Coffman, J.R. & Schmidt, D.A. (1975) Neutropenia and salmonellosis in hospitalised horses. *Journal of the American Veterinary Medical Association*, **166**, 65–67.

23. Ducel, G., Fabry, J. & Nicolle, L. (eds) (2002) *Prevention of Hospital-Acquired Infections: A Practical Guide*, 2nd edn. World Health Organization, Geneva, Switzerland. Available at http://www.who.int/csr/resources/publications/drugresist/whocdscsreph200212.pdf: accessed 20 November 2011.

24. van Duijkeren, E., Sloet van Oldruitenborgh-Oosterbann, M.M., Houwers, D.J., van Leeuwen, W.J. & Kalsbeek, H.C. (1994) Equine salmonellosis in a Dutch veterinary teaching hospital. *Veterinary Record*, **135**, 248–250.

25. van Duijkeren, E., Flemming, C., Sloet van Oldruitenborgh-Oosterbann, M.M., Kalsbeek, H.C. & van der Giessen, J.W. (1995) Diagnosing salmonellosis in horses: Culturing of multiple versus single faecal samples. *Veterinary Quarterly*, **17**, 63–66.

26. Dunowska, M., Morley, P.S. & Hyatt, D.R. (2005) The effect of Virkon-S® fogging on survival of *Salmonella enterica* and *Staphylococcus aureus* on surfaces in a veterinary teaching hospital. *Veterinary Microbiology*, **105**, 281–289.

27. Dunowska, M., Morley, P.S., Traub-Dargatz, J.L. & Van Metre, D.C. (2006) Biosecurity. In: *Equine Infectious Diseases* (eds D.C. Sellon & M.T. Long), pp. 528–539. Saunders Elsevier, St. Louis, Missouri.

28. Dunowska, M., Morley, P.S., Patterson, G., Hyatt, D.R. & Van Metre, D.C. (2006) Evaluation of the efficacy of a peroxygen disinfectant-filled footmat for reduction of bacterial load on footwear in a large animal hospital setting. *Journal of the American Veterinary Medical Association*, **228**, 1935–1939.

29. Dunowska, M., Morley, P.S., Traub-Dargatz, J.L., Hyatt, D.R. & Dargatz, D.A. (2006) Impact of hospi-

talization and antimicrobial drug administration on antimicrobial susceptibility patterns of commensal *Escherichia coli* isolated from the feces of horses. *Journal of the American Veterinary Medical Association*, **228**, 1909–1917.

30. Dunowska, M., Morley, P.S., Traub-Dargatz, J.L., *et al.* (2007) Comparison of *Salmonella enterica* serotype Infantis isolates from a veterinary teaching hospital. *Journal of Applied Microbiology*, **102**, 1527–1536.

31. Dvorak, G. (2005) Disinfection 101. Available at http://www.cfsph.iastate.edu/BRM/resources/Disinfectants/Disinfection101Feb2005.pdf: accessed 20 November 2011.

32. Ekiri, A.B., Mackay, R.J., Gaskin, J.M., *et al.* (2009) Epidemiologic analysis of nosocomial *Salmonella* infections in hospitalized horses. *Journal of the American Veterinary Medical Association*, **234**, 108–119.

33. Ekiri, A.B., Morton, A.J., Long, M.T., MacKay, R.J. & Hernandez, J.A. (2010) Review of the epidemiology and infection control aspects of nosocomial *Salmonella* infections in hospitalized horses. *Equine Veterinary Education*, **22**, 631–641.

34. Ernst, N.S., Hernandez, J.A., MacKay, R.J., *et al.* (2004) Risk factors associated with fecal *Salmonella* shedding among hospitalized horses with signs of gastrointestinal tract disease. *Journal of the American Veterinary Medical Association*, **225**, 275–281.

35. Ewart, S.L., Schott, H.C., II, Robison, R.L., Dwyer, R.M., Eberhart, S.W. & Walker, R.D. (2001) Identification of sources of *Salmonella* organisms in a veterinary teaching hospital and evaluation of the effects of disinfectants on detection of *Salmonella* organisms on surface materials. *Journal of the American Veterinary Medical Association*, **218**, 1145–1151.

36. Freeman, K.D., Southwood, L.L., Lane, J., Lindborg, S. & Aceto, H.W. (2011) Post operative infection, pyrexia and perioperative antimicrobial drug use in surgical colic patients. *Equine Veterinary Journal*. doi: 10.1111/j.2042-3306.2011.00515.x. [Epub ahead of print].

37. Garner, J.S., Jarvis, W.R., Emori, T.G., Horan, T.C. & Hughes, J.M. (1988) CDC definitions for nosocomial infections. *American Journal of Infection Control*, **16**, 128–140.

38. Goldmann, D. (2006) System failure versus personal accountability: The case for clean hands. *New England Journal of Medicine*, **355**, 121–123.

39. Glabman, M. (2004) The top ten malpractice claims (and how to minimize them). *Hospitals and Health Networks*, **78**, 60–66.

40. Hackett, E.S. & Hassel, D.M. (2008) Colic: Nonsurgical complications. *Veterinary Clinics of North America: Equine Practice*, **24**, 535–555.

41. Hartmann, F.A., Callan, R.F., McGuirk, S.M. & West, S.E. (1996) Control of an outbreak of salmonellosis caused by drug-resistant *Salmonella* anatum in horses at a veterinary hospital and measures to prevent future infections. *Journal of the American Veterinary Medical Association*, **209**, 629–631.

42. Hartnack, A.K., Van Metre, D.C. & Morley, P.S. (2012) The risk of gastrointestinal disease and death among horses infected with *Salmonella enterica* during hospitalization and among their stable mates. *Journal of the American Veterinary Medical Association*, **240**, 726–733.

43. Hird, D.W., Pappaioanou, M. & Smith, B.P. (1984) Case-control study of risk factors associated with isolation of *Salmonella saint paul* in hospitalized horses. *American Journal of Epidemiology*, **120**, 852–864.

44. Horan, T.C. & Gaynes, R.P. (2004) Surveillance of nosocomial infections. In: *Hospital Epidemiology and Infection Control* (ed C.G. Mayhall), 3rd edn., pp. 1659–1702. Lippincott Williams & Wilkins, Philadelphia, Pennsylvania.

45. House, J.K., Mainar-Jaime, R.C., Smith, B.P., House, A.M. & Kamiya, D.Y. (1999) Risk factors for nosocomial *Salmonella* infection among hospitalized horses. *Journal of the American Veterinary Medical Association*, **214**, 1511–1516.

46. Kim, L.M., Morley, P.S., Traub-Dargatz, J.L., Salman, M.D. & Gentry-Weeks, C. (2001) Factors associated with *Salmonella* shedding among equine colic patients at a veterinary teaching hospital. *Journal of the American Veterinary Medical Association*, **218**, 740–748.

47. Koterba, A., Torchia, J., Silverthorne, C., Ramphal, R., Merritt, A.M. & Manucy, J. (1986) Nosocomial infections and bacterial antibiotic resistance in a university equine hospital. *Journal of the American Veterinary Medical Association*, **189**, 185–191.

48. Larson, E. (2001) Hygiene of the skin: When is clean too clean? *Emerging Infectious Diseases*, **7**, 225–230.

49. Mair, T.S. & Smith, L.J. (2005a) Survival and complication rates in 300 horses undergoing surgical treatment of colic. Part 2: Short-term complications. *Equine Veterinary Journal*, **37**, 303–309.

50. Mair, T.S. & Smith, L.J. (2005b) Survival and complication rates in 300 horses undergoing surgical treatment of colic. Part 3: Long-term complications and survival. *Equine Veterinary Journal*, **37**, 310–314.

51. Morley, P.S. (2002) Biosecurity of veterinary practices. *Veterinary Clinics of North America: Food Animal Practice*, **18**, 133–155.

52. Morley, P.S. (2004) Surveillance for nosocomial infections in veterinary hospitals. *Veterinary Clinics of North America: Equine Practice*, **20**, 561–576.

53. Morley, P.S. & Weese, J.S. (2008) Biosecurity and infection control for large animal practices. In: *Large*

Animal Internal Medicine (ed B.P. Smith), 3rd edn., pp. 1524–1550. Mosby Elsevier, St. Louis, Missouri.

54. Morley, P.S., Morris, S.N., Hyatt, D.R. & Van Metre, D.C. (2005) Evaluation of the efficacy of disinfectant footbaths as used in veterinary hospitals. *Journal of the American Veterinary Medical Association*, **226**, 2053–2058.

55. Meyerson, L.A. & Reaser, J.K. (2002) Biosecurity: Moving toward a comprehensive approach. *Bioscience*, **52**, 593–600.

56. National Association of State Public Health Veterinarians, Veterinary Infection Control Committee. (2010) Compendium of veterinary standard precautions for zoonotic disease prevention in veterinary personnel. *Journal of the American Veterinary Medical Association*, **237**, 1403–1422. Available at http://www.nasphv.org/Documents/VeterinaryPrecautions.pdf: accessed 20 November 2011.

57. National Association of State Public Health Veterinarians, Veterinary Infection Control Committee. (2010) Model infection control plan for veterinary practices. Available at http://www.nasphv.org/Documents/ModelInfectionControlPlan.doc: accessed 20 November 2011.

58. Ogeer-Gyles, J., Mathews, K.A., Sears, W., Prescott, J.F., Weese, J.S. & Boerlin, P. (2006) Development of antimicrobial resistance in rectal *Escherichia coli* isolates from dogs hospitalised in an intensive care unit. *Journal of the American Veterinary Medical Association*, **229**, 694–699.

59. Ogeer-Gyles, J.S., Mathews, K.A. & Boerlin, P. (2006) Nosocomial infections and antimicrobial resistance in critical care medicine. *Journal of Veterinary Emergency and Critical Care*, **16**, 1–18.

60. Palmer, J.E. & Benson, C.E. (1984) *Salmonella* shedding in the equine. In: *Proceedings of the International Symposium on Salmonella*, New Orleans, Louisiana, pp. 161–163.

61. Palmer, J.E., Benson, C.E. & Whitlock, R.H. (1985) *Salmonella* shed by horses with colic. *Journal of the American Veterinary Medical Association*, **187**, 256–257.

62. Paré, J., Carpenter, T.E. & Thurmond, M.C. (1996) Analysis of temporal and spatial clustering of horses with *Salmonella* krefeld in an intensive care unit of a veterinary hospital. *Journal of the American Veterinary Medical Association*, **209**, 626–628.

63. Patterson, G., Morley, P.S., Blehm, K.D., Lee, D.E. & Dunowska, M. (2005) Efficacy of directed misting application of a peroxygen disinfectant for environmental decontamination of a veterinary hospital. *Journal of the American Veterinary Medical Association*, **227**, 597–602.

64. Ravary, B., Fecteau, G., Higgins, R., Paré, J. & Lavoie, J.P. (1998) Prevalence of infections caused by *Salmonella* spp. in cattle and horses at the Veterinary Teaching Hospital of the Faculty of Veterinary

Medicine of the University of Montreal. *Canadian Veterinary Journal*, **39**, 566–572.

65. Rhoads, W.S., Barton, M.H. & Parks, A.H. (1999) Comparison of medical and surgical treatment for impaction of the small colon in horses: 84 cases (1986–1996). *Journal of the American Veterinary Medical Association*, **214**, 1042–1047.

66. Schott, H.C., Ewart, S.L., Walker, R.D., *et al.* (2001) An outbreak of salmonellosis among horses at a veterinary teaching hospital. *Journal of the American Veterinary Medical Association*, **218**, 1152–1159.

67. Smith, B.P., House, J.K., Magdesian, K.G., *et al.* (2004) Principles of an infectious disease control program for preventing nosocomial gastrointestinal and respiratory tract diseases in large animal veterinary teaching hospitals. *Journal of the American Veterinary Medical Association*, **225**, 1186–1195.

68. Stockton, K.A., Morley, P.S., Hyatt, D.R. *et al.* (2006) Evaluation of the effects of footwear hygiene protocols on nonspecific bacterial contamination of floor surfaces in an equine hospital. *Journal of the American Veterinary Medical Association*, **228**, 1068–1073.

69. The Center for Food Security and Public Health. (2011) Infection control for veterinarians. The Center for Food Security and Public Health, Iowa State University, Ames, Iowa. Available at http://www.cfsph.iastate.edu/Infection_Control/overview-of-infection-control-for-veterinarians.php: accessed 20 November 2011.

70. Tillotson, K., Savage, C.J., Salman, M.D., *et al.* (1997) Outbreak of *Salmonella* infantis infection in a large animal veterinary teaching hospital. *Journal of the American Veterinary Medical Association*, **211**, 1554–1557.

71. Traub-Dargatz, J.L., Salman, M.D. & Jones, R.L. (1990) Epidemiologic study of salmonellae shedding in feces of horses and potential risk factors for development of the infection in hospitalized horses. *Journal of the American Veterinary Medical Association*, **196**, 1617–1622.

72. Traub-Dargatz, J.L., George, J.L., Dargatz, D.A., Morley, P.S., Southwood, L.L. & Tillotson, K. (2002) Survey of complications and antimicrobial use in equine patients at veterinary teaching hospitals that underwent surgery because of colic. *Journal of the American Veterinary Medical Association*, **220**, 1359–1365.

73. Traub-Dargatz, J.L., Dargatz, D.A., Morley, P.S. & Dunowska, M. (2004) An overview of infection control strategies for equine facilities, with an emphasis on veterinary hospitals. *Veterinary Clinics of North America: Equine Practice*, **20**, 507–520.

74. Traub-Dargatz, J.L., Weese, J.S., Rousseau, J.D., Dunowska, M., Morley, P.S. & Dargatz, D.A. (2006) Pilot study to evaluate 3 hygiene protocols on the reduction of bacterial load on the hands of veterinary

staff performing routine equine physical examinations. *Canadian Veterinary Journal*, **47**, 671–676.

75. Walker, R.L., Madigan, J.E., Hird, D.W., Case, J.T., Villanueva, M.R. & Bogenrief, D.S. (1991) An outbreak of equine neonatal salmonellosis. *Journal of Veterinary Diagnostic Investigation*, **3**, 223–227.

76. Ward, M.P., Brady, T.H., Couëtil, L.L., Liljebjelke, K., Maurer, J.J. & Wu, C.C. (2005) Investigation and control of an outbreak of salmonellosis caused by multidrug-resistant *Salmonella typhimurium* in a population of hospitalized horses. *Veterinary Microbiology*, **107**, 233–240.

77. Weese, J.S. (2004) Barrier precautions, isolation protocols and personal hygiene in veterinary hospitals. *Veterinary Clinics of North America: Equine Practice*, **20**, 543–559.

78. Weese, J.S. (2010) Methicillin resistant *Staphylococcus aureus* in animals. *Institute of Laboratory Animal Research Journal*, **51**, 233–244.

21 Special Considerations

Louise L. Southwood

Department of Clinical Studies, New Bolton Center, School of Veterinary Medicine, University of Pennsylvania, Kennett Square, PA, USA

Chapter Outline

Foals	**278**	Causes of colic	285
Causes of colic	279	Management considerations and complications	286
Neonates	279	**Geriatric horses**	**286**
Young foals and weanlings	280	Causes of colic	286
Management considerations and complications	281	Management considerations and complications	287
Pregnant mares	**282**	**Miniature horses, ponies,**	
Causes of colic	282	**and donkeys**	**287**
Management considerations and complications	283	Causes of colic	287
		Management considerations and complications	288
Postpartum mares	**284**	Hyperlipemia	288
Causes of colic	284	Postoperative intraperitoneal	
Management considerations	285	adhesions	289
Colts and stallions	**285**		

It is important to recognize that the vast majority of horses with colic will have the typical presentation, causes, response to treatment, and disease course. There are some groups of equine patients, however, that require special consideration when being evaluated and treated for colic.

Foals

There are several aspects of clinical disease and treatment that should be taken into consideration when managing foals with colic. It is difficult to compare reports in the literature because the

Practical Guide to Equine Colic, First Edition. Edited by Louise L. Southwood.
© 2013 John Wiley & Sons, Inc. Published 2013 by John Wiley & Sons, Inc.

definition of foal is variable. Neonates are generally considered <30 days old although types of disease tend to be different within the first 14 days of birth than foals older than 14 days.[28] Young foals (or sucklings) are generally considered to be 1–6 months and weanlings 6–12 months. Colic is relatively uncommon in young foals and weanlings.

Causes of colic

The typical causes of colic in foals vary considerably with age and are different to that observed commonly in adult horses. It is important to recognize that tympanic colic and impaction is a common cause of colic in any age horse, including foals.

Neonates

In neonates, colic is often associated with concurrent disease[28] including the following:

- Sepsis
- Hypoxic-ischemic encephalopathy
- Neonatal nephropathy
- Failure of passive transfer of maternal antibodies
- Umbilical remnant infection or patent urachus

Concurrent disease does not overall significantly impact survival[28] but does contribute to the expense associated with treatment and the prognosis varies depending on the specifics of the concurrent disease. Neonates with colic should also be examined carefully and thoroughly to assess the role, if any, that a concurrent disease plays in the overall clinical presentation.

Signs of colic in neonatal foals can be different to that in adult horses. Foals will often become quite, recumbent, and rotate their head only or roll up onto their back. Concurrent disease may also have an impact on colic signs and these foals need to be monitored carefully.

Common causes of colic in equine neonates are meconium-associated colic, enterocolitis, necrotizing enterocolitis, and transient medical colic with etiology unknown.[28] Surgical lesions are uncommon (~10% of foals admitted to a referral hospital) with small intestinal strangulating obstruction (SISO, p. 209) (e.g., volvulus, intussusceptions, herniation) being the most common

lesion observed at surgery.[5,28,56] Urogenital problems including ruptured bladder or urachus should be considered in neonates presenting for colic and require surgical repair. Foals also appear to have a relatively high incidence of perforated gastric ulcers compared to adults.[5,28,56]

Meconium-associated colic includes meconium impaction and meconium retention (Jon Palmer DVM, Personal Communication). Meconium impaction is associated with signs of persistent colic, abdominal distension, tail flagging, straining to defecate, decreased to absent fecal output, meconium palpable on digital rectal examination, abdominal palpation, and/or visible on sonographic examination.[28] Meconium retention is marked by decreased to absent fecal output and after 48 h of age meconium palpable on digital rectal examination, abdominal palpation or visualized on sonographic examination (p. 125). Meconium retention may be accompanied by episodic colic responsive to enemas or the neonate may show no signs of discomfort.[28] Meconium-associated colic can be managed medically with supportive care (enteral and intravenous [IV] fluids and nutritional support, enemas, and analgesia). The prognosis for survival is excellent (~100%) with the vast majority of foals responding to medical treatment.[28,56]

Enterocolitis is primarily manifest as diarrhea with mild signs of colic that are responsive to analgesic drugs. Foals with enterocolitis may also have reflux and intolerance to feeding. Sonographically there is evidence of fluid accumulation in the colon. In the majority of neonates, the etiological agent is not identified but can include *Clostridium* sp., *Salmonella* sp., rotavirus, and coronavirus. Enterocolitis is typically managed with supportive care (IV fluids, plasma, parenteral nutrition, systemic antimicrobial drugs, antidiarrheal medication, gastric decompression, and restricted access to nursing if the foal is intolerant to feeding). The prognosis for foals with enterocolitis is good to excellent. Neonates with necrotizing enterocolitis have sonographic, surgical or necropsy evidence of *pneumatosis intestinalis*[28] and possible gastroduodenal reflux (may contain blood), intolerance to enteral feeding, and diarrhea (may be hemorrhagic). Foals with necrotizing enterocolitis typically have abdominal distention. Necrotizing enterocolitis is also managed with supportive care. The prognosis for foals with necrotizing enterocolitis is less favorable than other causes of colic in neonates (~35%).[28] Occasionally, a neonate that is being managed for enterocolitis can develop a surgical lesion such as a small intestinal intussusceptions or volvulus.

Surgical lesions typically affecting equine neonates are jejunal intussusceptions and volvulus (p. 213), hernias (inguinal or scrotal (p. 285), diaphragmatic (p. 136)), meconium-associated colic, enterocolitis, and uroperitoneum.[5,28,56] Medically managed diseases (e.g., meconium-associated colic and enterocolitis) can be challenging to differentiate from lesions requiring surgery particularly without the ability to perform palpation per rectum. Transabdominal palpation can be useful. Abdominal sonographic evaluation can be used to diagnose many causes of colic in the neonate.[36] Neonates with a SISO are more likely to have severe or persistent pain that is unresponsive to analgesic drugs compared to other causes of colic in neonates.[28] Foals with strangulating obstruction typically have abnormal oral mucous membranes. Abdominal distention is also a feature for foals with a small intestinal volvulus; however, is also seen with meconium impaction and necrotizing enterocolitis. Early referral and surgical treatment when necessary is important for a favorable outcome.[5] Owners and veterinarians, however, are often reluctant to pursue surgery because of the reported low long-term prognosis and risk for adhesion formation. Overall short-term survival for neonates following colic surgery has previously reported to be between 25% and 75% and overall long-term survival 10–56% and between 33% and 75% for those surviving to discharge.[5,46,56] Recently, Mackinnon et al.[28] reported a short-term survival rate of 100% for neonates that were recovered from general anesthesia following colic surgery and none of the foals had been euthanized for colic at long-term follow-up which may be a reflection of earlier referral and treatment.

Overo lethal white syndrome is observed in neonates from parents with white overo patterning. Foals are homozygous for the mutated overo lethal white gene (Ile118Lys endothelin receptor B). Phenotypically the foals have an all white hair coat and will present with colic signs because the genetic mutation affects melanocytes and intestinal ganglia. The disease is fatal. Intestinal atresia has also been reported in equine neonates. The most consistent finding on physical examination with

atresia colic is the absence of meconium staining following repeated enemas. The large, transverse and/or small colon were involved in all foals.[60] Atresia coli may occur concurrently with atresia ani and renal aplasia or hypoplasia. An attempt can be made to resect or bypass the segment of atresia. However, the affected segment may be long and concurrent aganglionosis or hypoganglionosis, which can be diagnosed using histological evaluation of a biopsy sample, will result in ileus and recurrent abdominal pain.[41]

Young foals and weanlings

Young and weanling foals can have causes of colic that are also somewhat distinct from that caused by adult horses. Ascarid impaction (p. 208, 321) should be considered in a weanling foal with signs of acute colic and recent history of anthelmintic administration.[5,56] Ascariasis can also be associated with volvulus, intussusception, abscessation, peritonitis, adhesion formation, and intestinal rupture. Foals often have concurrent signs of lethargy, inappetence, coughing, nasal discharge, and failure to thrive. A tentative diagnosis can be made based on identification of ascarids in the feces or reflux but a definitive diagnosis is made at surgery or necropsy. Ascarid impactions can be managed medically with IV fluids, lubricants administered via a nasogastric tube, and analgesia. Surgery is often required. Prognosis is fair with surgery.[10,51]

Young foals and weanlings with an umbilical hernia can have a small segment of intestine become entrapped in the hernia and cause strangulation. Foals and weanlings with umbilical hernias should be monitored closely for signs of colic and the hernia palpated at least daily to ensure that it remains soft and reducible. Surgical repair of large umbilical hernias or hernias that have not resolved spontaneously by the time the foal is about 4 months old is recommended. The use of a hernia clamp should be avoided because of the potential for complications. A parietal hernia (also called Richter's or Littre's hernia) occurs when only the antimesenteric wall of the intestine becomes incarcerated. Necrosis of the intestinal wall associated with a parietal hernia can result in abscessation and enterocutaneous fistula formation. Foals and weanlings with strangulating umbilical hernias usually present with an acute onset of mild to moderate signs of colic. Clinical examination of the umbilical hernia reveals in increase in hernia size, firmness, edema, and/or pain on palpation. Parietal hernias do not cause a complete intestinal obstruction and while signs of colic may be observed initially, following intestinal necrosis these signs may subside. An enterocutaneous fistula can be diagnosed on examination with ingesta seen at the umbilicus and marked periumbilical edema and inflammation. An uncomplicated umbilical hernia is treated surgically by enlarging the hernia and freeing the entrapped intestine followed by herniorrhaphy. Resection and anastomosis of the affected bowel is often not necessary if the lesion is acute. The prognosis for survival is excellent. Surgical treatment of an enterocutaneous fistula requires en bloc resection of the affected body wall and intestine with anastomosis of the adjacent unaffected bowel. The prognosis for survival is good to excellent.

Pyloric and duodenal ulcers (p. 205) can cause stricture with subsequent gastric outflow obstruction and are seen most often in foals 3–6 months old. Bruxism and ptyalism are the most common clinical signs.[8,61] Spontaneous reflux, diarrhea, postprandial colic, and lack of fecal production are also observed. Diagnosis is made based on clinical signs and confirmed with abdominal sonographic and contrast radiographic examination (p. 158). Some foals can be managed medically by withholding feed or providing small-volume frequent feeding, IV fluids, parenteral nutrition, or antiulcer medication (i.e., sucralfate, omeprazole, ranitidine, and prostaglandin analogues). Gastroduodenostomy or gastrojejunostomy with or without jejunojejunostomy may be required in some foals.[61]

Proliferative enteropathy associated with *Lawsonia intracellularis* infection is a cause of colic in young foals and weanlings typically 3–9 months old. Clinical signs include diarrhea, weight loss or failure to thrive, and colic.[23,29,44] Hypoproteinemia and markedly thickened small intestine identified on sonographic examination support the tentative diagnosis. Diagnosis can be confirmed antemortum with fecal PCR and serum antibody titers and postmortem based on the gross and histological appearance of the affected intestine. Proliferative enteropathy is treated with supportive care and erythromycin, azithromycin, oxytetracycline then doxycycline, or chloramphenicol.[44]

Management considerations and complications

Particularly, care should be taken with regard to use of certain potentially toxic drugs in the neonate. Nonsteroidal anti-inflammatory drugs (NSAIDs) are not typically used to manage colic signs in equine neonates because of their gastrointestinal and renal toxicity (p. 53). Butorphanol (p. 55) is the most commonly used analgesic drug and is adequate to control pain except in patients requiring surgical treatment.[28] Similarly, care should be taken with the use of aminoglycosides because of the potential for nephrotoxicity with these drugs. When aminoglycosides are used, plasma peak and trough levels should be monitored and dose rate and treatment interval altered accordingly. Ceftiofur at a higher dose rate than that used in adult horses can be used as an alternative to aminoglycosides. The cardiovascular effects of alpha-2 agonists (p. 55) can be more clinically relevant in neonates particularly if there is another underlying disease.

While nutrition is important in any hospitalized patient, neonates cannot have nutrition withheld for a period beyond several hours. Parenteral nutrition should be provided in foals not capable of enteral nutrition. When feeding the postoperative colic patient, milk can be offered soon after surgery and gradually increased to meet the foal's nutritional requirements. See Chapter 23 on Nutrition (p. 301). Fluid and electrolyte requirements for foals are different to that in adult horses[37] and are covered in Chapter 11 on Intravenous Catheterization and Fluid Therapy (p. 99).

The main postoperative complication that is considered particularly important in the equine neonate is intraperitoneal adhesion formation. Neonatal abdominal surgery can be challenging because the mesentery and blood vessels are more easily damaged compared to adult horses and, subjectively, the intestine becomes inflamed quickly and with less manipulation than that of the adult horse. Fibrin accumulation with formation of fibrinous adhesions can occur even during surgery particularly with long-standing lesions and prolonged surgery time making early surgical intervention and efficient and meticulous surgical technique critical. Whether or not equine neonates are more prone to adhesion formation compared to their mature adult counterparts is debated. Foals <30 days old were more likely to develop adhesions from even minimal intestinal manipulation compared with foals >30 days.[25] Cable *et al.*[5] reported that 33% of foals (<1 year) examined after abdominal surgery had intra-abdominal adhesions and adhesions caused a clinical problem in 19% of foals. Sucklings (16 days to 5.9 months) were reported to form adhesions more frequently (21%) than weanlings (6–11.9 months, 3.5%) and yearlings (12–23.9 months, 3.6%).[46] There was no difference in adhesion formation between neonates and other age groups.[46] On the other hand, although 10% of horses aged <2 years died of complications associated with postoperative intraperitoneal adhesions, there was no association between age and adhesion formation.[49] Postoperative colic and peritoneal adhesions were not an important reason for euthanasia in the most recent study evaluating colic in equine neonates,[28] which is likely a reflection of early surgical intervention and adhesion prevention methods used. See Chapter 19 on Postoperative Complications (p. 244).

Pregnant mares

Causes of colic

Colic in later term pregnant mares can be challenging to diagnose and manage. Obtaining a tentative diagnosis preoperatively for mares in their last trimester can be difficult. Palpation per rectum is often unrewarding because of the vast size and position of the fetus and abdominocentesis should not be performed without sonographic guidance because of the risk of abortion associated with inadvertent amniocentesis.[47] Abdominal sonographic examination can be particularly useful in these patients to assess the need for surgery and evaluate the fetus. Uterine and body wall pain as well as mild intestinal or colonic displacement or compression can cause signs of colic particularly in maiden mares. Common causes of colic in pregnant mares include large colon volvulus (p. 220); right dorsal

displacement (p. 220); proximal enteritis (PE) and ileus (p. 207); tympany; cecal (p. 214), large colon (p. 217), and small colon impaction (p. 221); small intestinal strangulation (p. 209); uterine torsion;[2,17] body wall tear; and hemorrhage into the broad ligament. Uterine torsion, body wall tear, and hemorrhage are specific for the periparturient mare.

Uterine torsion should be considered as a differential diagnosis for any mare in the last trimester of pregnancy (particularly between 9 and 10 months gestation) showing mild to moderate signs of colic. Diagnosis can be made based on palpation per rectum with the broad ligament of the uterus identified coursing across the caudal abdomen (p. 34). Uterine torsion can be corrected by (1) rolling the mare while she is under general anesthesia by maintaining the uterus/fetus in position with a plank ("plank in the flank") and rolling the mare in the direction of the torsion;[58] (2) via a flank laparotomy;[38] or (3) via a ventral midline celiotomy.[21] The overall mare survival following uterine torsion correction was recently reported to be 84% (gestation <320 days survival was 97% and ≥320 days survival was 72%). The overall foal survival was 54% (gestation <320 days foal survival was 65% and ≥320 days foal survival was 32%) with 83% of mares discharged from the hospital with a viable fetus delivering a live and healthy foal.[6] Abortion rates following uterine torsion were previously reported to be 40%.[2]

Colic and ventral edema are the most common presenting complaints for mares with body wall tears.[43] Body wall tears occur late in gestation and are classically associated with draft breeds and twins; however, in a recent report that was not observed.[43] There may be a decrease in foal survival with decrease in gestational age. Sonographic evaluation of the body wall is diagnostic and can be used to identify specific defects.[43] Sonography is also important to identify hydrops allantois or amnion (associated with poor fetal survival) and placentitis.[43] Placentitis should be treated with antimicrobial drugs (e.g., trimethoprim sulfa). Conservative management strategies that avoid induction of parturition or elective cesarean section are recommended and include stall confinement, an abdominal support wrap, and analgesic drugs (NSAIDs). The fetus should be monitored using electrocardiography and sonography. The mare should be checked frequently for signs of impending parturition and assisted vaginal delivery performed if necessary. A body wall hernia usually results from the tearing and mesh herniorrhaphy may be necessary. Rebreeding is not recommended.

Hemorrhage into the broad ligament can be a cause of colic during pregnancy. Diagnosis and management is the same as that for postpartum hemorrhage (see below), namely, per rectum palpation and sonographic evaluation and supportive care.

Management considerations and complications

The abortion rate in pregnant mares associated with colic and colic surgery is reported to be 11–22% for medically managed mares and 20–46% with surgery.[2,7,13,45] Abortion was higher during early gestation (<40 days) compared to later in gestation (340 days) in one study[13] but not in another.[45] Abortion is higher in medically managed mares with more severe disease[45] and in horses with clinical signs of endotoxemia.[2] During the first 2 months of gestation, endotoxin-induced prostaglandin F2 (PGF-2) secretion results in pregnancy failure due to regression of the corpus luteum, which is the main source of progesterone during early pregnancy.[11] Later in gestation, the corpus luteum is no longer responsible for progesterone production for maintenance of pregnancy.[11] However, it is possible that prolonged exposure of the gravid uterus to high levels of PGF-2 during endotoxemia leads to myometrial contractions and abortion. Potential detrimental effect of PGF-2 on the gravid uterus can be blocked by increasing progesterone levels. Exogenous progesterone (300 mg/day) or altrenogest (44 mg (20 mL)/day, ReguMate®) is recommended in pregnant mares with more than just mild colic, particularly if associated with signs of endotoxemia.[11] Treatment should be continued at least until the clinical signs of endotoxemia have resolved for late-term pregnant mares. If treating a mare during early gestation, progesterone supplementation should be maintained until the latter part of gestation when the placenta becomes the source of progesterone for pregnancy maintenance.[11] Endotoxemia should be managed by treating or removing the source of endotoxin and with NSAIDs, anti-endotoxin drugs (e.g., polymixin B), and supportive care (p. 246).

Nutritional requirements of the late-term pregnant mare are an important consideration during the management of colic. The fetus gains 45% of its final birth weight after 270 days gestation and has a high glucose uptake at this time.[48] When feed was withdrawn from mares experimentally for >30 h, 5/8 mares delivered prematurely within 1 week of the last period of feed withdrawal, highlighting the potential consequences of inadequate or intermittent feeding on premature delivery.[48] There was no association, however, between feed withdrawal and abortion in a clinical study of pregnant mares with colic.[2] Early referral and treatment is clearly important to avoid prolonged feed restriction. Management with parenteral nutrition, which may be as simple as the addition of glucose (1.25–5%) to the IV fluids, is recommended (see Chapter 23 on Nutrition [p. 301]).

Surgery can be challenging in the late-term pregnant mare. Every effort should be made to make surgery time as short as possible. Having the mare clipped and prepared prior to induction of general anesthesia can decrease the time the mare is in dorsal recumbency. Urinary catheterization and placement of a temporary Caslick's suture to appose the vulva lips may prevent vaginal contamination during surgery and ascending placentitis. Even in mares at term and mares that are anticipated to have postoperative complications, it is not recommended to perform a cesarean section because foal viability is better if the fetus has an opportunity to mature in readiness for birth. Prolonged duration of surgery (≥3 h), intraoperative hypotension,[7] and intraoperative hypoxia particularly during the last 60 days of pregnancy[45] was associated with abortion or delivery of a nonviable foal. Intranasal oxygen may be beneficial in the immediate postoperative period.

Postoperatively the fetus should be checked for viability and the placenta evaluated for evidence of placentitis or separation from the endometrium. Placentitis can be treated with antimicrobial drugs (e.g., trimethoprim sulfa). It is rare for mares to have incisional problems associated with late-term pregnancy and parturition even if it occurs soon after surgery; however, use of an abdominal support bandage is recommended. Mares should be monitored for hypertriglyceridemia (p. 288). Supportive care during the postoperative period is critical particularly in the late-term pregnant mare (see Chapter 11 on Intravenous Catheterization and Fluid Therapy [p. 99], Chapter 18 on Postoperative Patient Care [p. 230], Chapter 19 on Postoperative Complications [p. 244], and Chapter 23 on Nutrition [p. 301]).

Postpartum mares

Causes of colic

Colic is relatively common in postpartum mares and can be caused by as simple a problem as uterine involution or pneumouterus[24] through to large colon volvulus or fatal hemorrhage. Typical signs of colic may not be readily observed because maternal behavior may override typical pain behavior. Postpartum mares need to be monitored frequently and carefully to avoid treatment delay.[12] Gastrointestinal, urogenital, and body cavity problems should be considered as causes of colic in postpartum mares.[12]

While colic in postpartum mares can be caused by a wide array of lesions, large colon volvulus and hemorrhage were the most common reasons for emergency admission at a referral hospital.[12] Hemorrhage can occur into the broad ligament (middle uterine, utero-ovarian artery), peritoneal cavity (middle uterine, utero-ovarian artery, uterus), uterus (intraluminal or intramural), or vagina. The incidence of hemorrhage increases with increase in age of the mare.[12] Horses generally present early during the postpartum period (24–48 h) and often have anemia, hypoproteinemia, and hypofibrinogenemia.[12] The diagnosis is often made on palpation per rectum (p. 34) with or without sonography. Mares are managed conservatively with analgesia and sedation (p. 51) and supportive care (p. 99). A low-dose of acepromazine may be beneficial. Administration of oxytocin will not reduce hemorrhage from a uterine artery. It should not be given if there is a hematoma in the broad ligament as the induced uterine contraction and associated pain may disrupt the clot. Naloxone is an opiod antagonist which may be beneficial in hemorrhagic shock by attenuating the effect of opiods. Epsilonaminocaproic acid, prevents the activation of plasminogen to plasmin and, therefore, prevents fibrinolysis of the clot. Antimicrobials are often recommended. Blood transfusion may be necessary in some mares. Prognosis for survival is excellent (88%) for mares that survived to admission at a referral hospital.[12] Differentiation of a broad ligament hematoma from a large colon volvulus is important because immediate surgical intervention is necessary for successful management of a horse with a large colon volvulus. Mares with a large colon volvulus typically have moderately to severe signs of pain and abdominal distention. Careful palpation per rectum and sonography can be used to differentiate between the two problems.

Gastrointestinal causes of colic in postmartum mares include:[12]

(1) Large colon volvulus (most common) (p. 220)
(2) Colonic displacements
    (a) Nephrosplenic ligament entrapment (p. 219)
    (b) Right dorsal displacement (p. 220)
(3) Small intestinal lesions
    (a) Jejunal volvulus (p. 212)
    (b) Incarceration in a mesenteric rent (see below)
    (c) Segmental jejunal necrosis associated with mesenteric tear (see below)
(4) Cecal impaction (p. 214) or perforation (p. 215)
(5) Small colon and mesocolon trauma (p. 222)

Mesenteric rents can occur as a result of trauma associated with pregnancy and parturition and can lead to either tearing of the arcuate vessel(s) and avascular necrosis of the adjacent intestine or strangulation of a segment of intestine through the mesenteric defect. While broodmares are affected more frequently, horses of any age, breed or gender can be affected by jejunal strangulation through a mesenteric rent. Mares with vascular damage and jejunal necrosis can present with a hemoabdomen and/or signs consistent with intestinal necrosis (mild colic, tachycardia, injected membranes, fever, nasogastric reflux, septic peritonitis). Mares with jejunal strangulation through a mesenteric rent have clinical signs consistent with a small intestinal strangulating obstruction (p. 209) (moderate and persistent colic, tachycardia, dilated small intestine palpable per rectum or identified sonographically, nasogastric reflux, and serosanguinous peritoneal fluid). Early recognition and surgical treatment involving resection of the affected intestinal segment (p. 193, 199) is important for a favorable outcome. Mesenteric defect closure is recommended.

Vaginal tearing can also result in herniation of intestine through the rent. Diaphragmatic hernia (p. 136) should also be on the differential diagnosis list of postpartum mares presenting for colic.

Rectal prolapsed can occur in association with parturition. A type IV prolapse is where the peritoneal rectum and a variable amount of small colon intussuscepted through the anus and almost invariably results in tearing of the mesocolon and detachment of the small colon vascular supply with subsequent small colon necrosis. Small colon necrosis causes small colon obstruction, signs of abdominal pain, peritonitis, and shock. A tentative diagnosis is made based on a history of rectal prolapsed and clinical signs and can be confirmed during exploratory celiotomy, laparoscopy, or at necropsy.

Other considerations in postpartum mares presenting for signs of colic and shock include: uterine tear, metritis, and ruptured bladder. A uterine tear can be diagnosed based on uterine palpation. Mares with a uterine tear are often leukopenic[12] and septic peritonitis can be diagnosed sonographically (p. 133) and based on peritoneal fluid analysis (p. 87). Clinical signs of uterine tear may not be initially apparent in mares with retained fetal membranes if the membranes are intact at the site of the tear. While conservative management may be successful in an occasional mare, surgical repair of the tear is recommended. Metritis occurred most frequently following dystocia and mares and is treated with antimicrobial drugs, uterine lavage, and supportive care. Ruptured bladder is uncommon.

Management considerations

The main management considerations revolve around the foal. The decision to wean the foal is based on the critical illness of the mare and the availability of a nurse mare. The foal should be monitored closely to determine if its nutrient requirements are being met (i.e., monitoring weight gain, frequency of nursing, and resting). Nutritional supplementation of the foal may be necessary (p. 304). Neonatal foals should also be evaluated and monitored closely for problems. An abdominal support bandage should be placed on the mare to avoid trauma to the surgical site during nursing.

Colts and stallions

Causes of colic

Colts and stallions have causes of colic similar to mares and geldings; however, can also have inguinal or scrotal hernia and rarely testicular torsion as a cause of colic. Inguinal herniation of bowel can rarely occur in geldings. Inguinal or scrotal hernia can be direct or indirect. An indirect hernia involves the herniation of small intestine (or omentum) through vaginal ring into vaginal tunic (most common). A direct hernia involves the passage of small intestine (or omentum) through a rent in the peritoneum and transverse fascia adjacent to the vaginal ring to lie in subcutaneous tissue of the scrotum and prepuce (more common in foals than adults) i.e. "directly" through the body wall. Strenuous exercise, breeding, and trauma are predisposing factors for acquired hernias. Standardbreds and Tennessee walking horses are reported to be most commonly affected. Evisceration is more common in Standardbreds after an open castration compared to other breeds. In adults, indirect inguinal hernias are usually nonreducible, and involve a very short loop of intestine, which becomes strangulated resulting in signs of abdominal pain, and causes venous (and arterial) occlusion with secondary edema and swelling of the affected testis. A loop of distended small intestine can usually be palpated per rectum entering the inguinal ring. Palpation per rectum (p. 28) is usually diagnostic in combination with clinical signs of colic and an enlarged scrotum/testis. Sonographic examination can also be useful; however, is often not necessary. Hernia reduction by massaging the small intestine back through the inguinal ring with the horse under general anesthesia may be successful in some horses. Surgery usually involves an inguinal and/or ventral midline approach, with hernia reduction, resection and anastomosis of the nonviable intestine, unilateral castration, and closure of the vaginal ring (p. 199). Bilateral castration is recommended if the horse is not going to be used for breeding to prevent herniation on the contralateral side. Laparoscopic closure of the contralateral inguinal ring is recommended if the other testis is to be left in place. The prognosis for survival is excellent. Congenital indirect inguinal or scrotal hernias in foals are usually reducible (strangulation is uncommon), and involve a variable length of intestine. These hernias usually resolve by 3–6 months of age, but if the hernia is increasing in size or becomes non-reducible, surgical correction is indicated. Direct or ruptured inguinal hernias usually occur at 4–48 hours of age, and foals are colicky, dull, and have severe scrotal and preputial swelling. Although the intestine is usually not strangulated, these are surgical emergencies. In addition to hernia reduction, surgery involves repair of the rent in the fascia or muscle. The vaginal ring can be closed laparoscopically in some cases.

Torsion of the spermatic cord (testicular torsion) is rare. Torsions <180° are considered an incidental finding and are not associated with clinical signs. Torsion is reported to occur more frequently in trotting Standardbreds and may affect retained testes more frequently. Horses with torsion of 360° have signs of acute inguinal pain which may be manifest as colic. Venous occlusion results in edema and enlargement of the affected testes and cord. Arterial occlusion can cause testicular infarction. Torsion is thought to occur as a consequence of a long ligament of the tail of the epididymis or proper ligament of the testis. Diagnosis of the torsion is based on clinical signs and by identification of a firm, enlarged testis. Sonographic evaluation may be helpful. Inguinal hernia is considerably more common and should be ruled-out. Removal of the affected testis is usually necessary. Breeding soundness should be maintained following unilateral castration. If the ligamentous structures of the contralateral testis are long, orchiopexy can be performed to prevent torsion.

Management considerations and complications

Fertility is unaffected by unilateral castration. Complications are similar to those occurring with other horses (p. 244). In addition, re-herniation of intestine through the inguinal canal or herniation through the contralateral inguinal canal can occur.

Geriatric horses

Causes of colic

Colic was one of the most common reasons for admission of geriatric horses to referral hospitals[4]

and the second most common reason for euthanasia of geriatric horses with 24% of geriatric horses being euthanized for lameness and 21% for colic.[20] Because of the aging equine population,[3] it is not uncommon for horses to live and be functional well into their 20s which is a testament to ongoing advances in nutrition, management, and veterinary care. The definition of geriatric is somewhat ill defined and likely to vary between horse breeds and even between individual horses. Generally, geriatric is considered either ≥16 or ≥20 years of age.

While geriatric horses can colic for various reasons, it is important to recognize that strangulating (small) intestinal lesions occur more commonly in geriatric compared to mature nongeriatric horses.[22,52,53] Strangulating pedunculated lipoma (p. 209) is a common cause of colic in geriatric horses. There is a tendency for geriatric horses to show less dramatic signs of pain compared to younger horses. A geriatric horse with a strangulating lesion may just flank stare and paw occasionally. Nostril flare and tachypnea are common manifestations of pain. Therefore, a strangulating lesion should be high on the differential diagnosis list and ruled-out with abdominal palpation per rectum (p. 27) and sonographic examination (p. 128), and peritoneal fluid analysis (p. 87) in horses in their late teens or older examined in the field or admitted for colic. Early referral and surgical intervention are critical for a favorable outcome in patients with strangulating intestinal lesions. Large colon impaction is also a frequently observed cause of colic in the geriatric horses,[4] particularly over the winter months. Gastric lesions (ulceration and neoplasia) were also relatively common.[4]

An important observation is that although geriatric horses presenting with colic were more likely than mature horses to be euthanized without surgery (i.e., lower survival with medical treatment) or during surgery, the survival of geriatric horses with a strangulating lesion or requiring jejunojejunostomy was not different to that for mature horses. Geriatric horses undergoing surgery for a large intestinal simple obstruction did have a lower survival than that of mature horses; however, the survival for mature horses was almost 100% and that of geriatric horses ~80%. The reason for the lower survival rate with large intestinal simple obstruction was not apparent upon reviewing the cases.[53]

Management considerations and complications

Aging in horses is associated with alterations in markers of inflammation with a shift toward a proinflammatory state.[31] Geriatric horses (≥16 years old) had increased expression of interleukin (IL)-6, IL-8, and interferon-γ as well as an increase in TNF-α release from peripheral blood mononuclear cells after lipopolysaccharide (endotoxin) stimulation.[31] Circulating TNF-α is cytotoxic[26,27] and high levels have been associated with morbidity and mortality in equine colic patients.[1] Geriatric horses of 20–35 years were found to have a reduction in digestion of crude protein, phosphorus, and fiber compared to younger horses, which was thought to be associated with ongoing intestinal damage from parasites.[42] The immune impairment associated with aging (immunosenescence) can lead to an increase in morbidity (and mortality) as a result of infectious disease.[39] There is also evidence of altered wound healing associated with changes in fibroblast function with aging[18,54] and older horses had a higher celiotomy complication rate compared to yearlings in one study.[59] Despite these age-related changes, complications in geriatric horses undergoing colic surgery are not typically higher than younger mature horses.

There was no difference in the proportion of geriatric and mature horses with postoperative fever, leukopenia, diarrhea, incisional infection, incisional dehiscence, colic, repeat laparotomy, or laminitis.[50] There were actually fewer geriatric than mature horses with a high fever and jugular vein thrombophlebitis. Overall there was a higher proportion of geriatric than mature horses with postoperative reflux and inappetence. However, there was no difference in the proportion of geriatric and mature horses with small intestinal strangulating lesions having postoperative reflux or inappetence.[50] There was no difference in the mortality between geriatric and mature horses developing postoperative complications.[50] Based on these results as well as clinical experience, euthanasia of a geriatric horse with signs of colic requiring surgery because "the horse is old and will not do well" has no basis. Long-term survival of these patients needs to be evaluated as does the impact of concurrent disease (e.g., pituitary pars intermedia dysfunction, PPID).

Postoperative nutrition (p. 301) is an important consideration in all horses following colic surgery, particularly geriatric horses that may have poor dentition[4] and a preexisting low body condition score. Geriatric horses were also more likely to be inappetent postoperatively compared to mature horses. Parenteral nutrition (p. 306) should be considered early during the postoperative period in geriatric horses should inappetence or reflux develop as a complication. Older horses can do well on a complete pelleted senior feed if they are willing to eat such a diet. Most horses indicate a desire for hay. The addition of corn oil to the diet may help with regaining and maintaining body condition.

Miniature horses, ponies, and donkeys

Causes of colic

An important consideration for small ponies and miniature horses is that because of their small body size, the expense associated with treating colic and colic surgery should be considerably reduced making economics somewhat less of a reason for euthanasia. Causes of colic in miniature horses also tend to be impaction-types which generally have a better prognosis and less expense association with postoperative management.[19,30] In a recent report, the most common surgical lesion in American miniature horses was a fecalith (~70%) located primarily within the small colon and most frequently diagnosed in horses age <6 months.[16] A fecalith causes a complete obstruction leading to persistent signs of mild to moderate colic and abdominal distension that can become severe. Focal pressure necrosis of the small (or large) colon at the site of obstruction can occur fairly rapidly. Surgical correction involves either breaking down the fecalith using gentle massage of the well lubricated bowel or removal through an enterotomy (p. 190). Resection of nonviable bowel is indicated with anastomosis of adjacent healthy bowel (p. 192). While more common in miniature horses, fecalith formation can occur in horses of any breed. Strangulating lesions are uncommon. Short-term survival to hospital discharge for miniature horses recovered from anesthesia was 98–100% with the most common postoperative complications being diarrhea and inappetence. Most (87%) were alive at least 12 months after surgery.[16,40] Therefore, the prognosis for these patients is excellent.

Ponies present for colic for similar reasons to horses. Ponies tend to have a longer life expectancy and, therefore, have colic signs caused by strangulating lipoma or impaction.

Presentation of donkeys for colic is relatively uncommon. Diagnosis of colic in donkeys can be more difficult than in horses because donkeys show few overt signs of abdominal pain and colic may not be identified until the donkey is in the terminal stages of the disease.[9] The incidence of colic in donkeys at a Donkey Sanctuary in the UK was not different to that of horses.[9] Impaction, particularly at the pelvic flexure, was the most common cause of colic in donkeys (~55% of colic episodes). Older donkeys, lighter body weight, those fed extra rations, donkeys with musculoskeletal problem and dental disease, and those that previously suffered colic were at increased risk of impaction. There was also a different incidence between farms. The mortality for donkeys with colic (51%) was higher than that for horses.[9] The high mortality rate was attributed to the age of the donkeys (predominantly geriatric with a mean age of 25 years), the progressed disease state when donkeys were identified with colic, underlying disease, and surgery rarely being performed when deemed necessary.[9]

Management considerations and complications

Hyperlipemia

Hyperlipemia is a life-threatening complication that can develop insidiously in ponies, miniature horses, and donkeys with colic. Hyperlipemia describes the gross observation of lipid in the plasma (lipemia) and is typically associated with a plasma triglyceride concentration >500 mg/dL and fatty infiltration of the liver and other organs.[34,35] Hyperlipidemia is used to describe a triglyceride concentration 50–500 mg/gL, is not associated with lipemia or fatty infiltration of organs, and is a less severe form of the disease.[34,35] Hypertriglyceridemia is any increase in plasma triglyceride concentration above the reference limit (11–52 mg/dL).[34,35] Recently, severe hypertriglyceridemia was defined in horses as serum triglyceride concentrations >500 mg/dL and no signs of gross lipemia.[14] Horses had triglyceride concentrations between 541 and 1604 mg/dL.

Hypertriglyceridemia can occur in any inappetent or critically ill equine patient.[14,57] Mild to moderate hypertriglyceridemia (100–300 mg/dL) occurs in almost all horses following colic surgery[55] which is similar to that observed in fasting horses.[14,35] Hypertriglyceridemia rapidly resolves following reintroduction of feed.[55] Ponies, miniature horses, and donkeys as well as obese animals, however, are at high risk.[32,33] Problems are also observed in pregnant and lactating mares.[14,57] Endotoxemia and the associated increase in TNF-α and systemic inflammatory response cause an increase in lipolysis with triglyceride overproduction and possibly insulin resistance predisposing to hypertriglyceridemia.[14,57] Azotemia causes a decrease in renal clearance of triglycerides and has also been associated with hypertriglyceridemia.[14,57] Patients affected by hypertriglyceridemia commonly have a primary disease associated with the gastrointestinal tract (enteritis/colitis or colic) or postpartum complications (retained fetal membrane, metritis, uterine tear).[14,32,33,57]

Clinical signs associated with hypertriglyceridemia are nonspecific and include dull mentation, lethargy, and inappetence or anorexia.[32] If not treated, hypertriglyceridemia can progress to hepatic lipidosis, liver failure, multiple organ dysfunction, and death.[14,57]

Serum or plasma triglyceride concentrations should be monitored every 1 to 3 days in patients at high risk for developing hypertriglyceridemia. Routinely including IV dextrose (2.5–5%) as part of the treatment plan in these patients is recommended to prevent hypertriglyceridemia.

Resolution of hypertriglyceridemia involves treatment of the underlying disease process, enteral nutrition and/or dextrose administration with or without insulin. Enteral nutrition is the preferred form of calorie provision, particularly in patients with mild to moderate hypertriglyceridemia, and can be in the form of commercially prepared low-residue diets.[33] If provision of enteral nutrition is not possible because of the underlying gastrointestinal disease, calories can be provided with IV dextrose. IV dextrose is typically administered as a 2.5–5% solution at a maintenance (plus losses) fluid rate.[57] Dunkel and McKenzie[14] reported using 50% dextrose in water at an average rate of 10 kcal/kg/day, which was 125 mg dextrose/kg/h and 0.25 mL/kg/h of 50% dextrose. Partial parenteral nutrition can be provided if it is perceived that the patient would benefit from the addition of amino acids;

however, lipids should be avoided. Blood and urine glucose concentration should be monitored in patients receiving IV dextrose with or without insulin. Insulin inhibits fat mobilization by inhibiting hormone-sensitive lipase activity and promotes the uptake of triglycerides into peripheral tissues by stimulating lipoprotein lipase activity.[57] Regular insulin can be administered as an IV constant rate infusion at 0.05 U/kg/h[14] or bolus 0.2 U/kg IV every 1–6h for up to 24 hours.[57] Ultralente insulin can be given 0.4 U/kg subcutaneously every 24h.[57] Insulin should be discontinued once the triglycerides are observed to decrease toward reference values. Exogenous insulin hastens the clearance of triglycerides from the blood but does not necessarily impact survival.[57] Heparin has been used as an adjunctive treatment because of its ability to act as a cofactor for endothelium-bound lipoprotein lipase; however, is not commonly used.[14]

The majority of patients respond favorably to treatment, particularly if the problem is identified early. Hypertriglyceridemia was not associated with failure to survive to discharge from the hospital,[57] which may have been confounded by the impact of the underlying disease process on fatality. Miniature horses with a peak serum triglyceride concentrations >1200mg/dL died or were euthanatized, whereas almost all horses with a peak serum triglyceride concentrations <1200mg/dL survived.[32]

Postoperative intraperitoneal adhesions

Intraperitoneal adhesions (p. 255) were identified in 25–40% of miniature horses requiring a second celiotomy,[16,40] which has led to the suggestion that these patients are predisposed to postoperative intraperitoneal adhesion formation. However, they have a preponderance for small colon lesions, which have a somewhat under recognized risk for adhesion formation. Nonetheless, adhesion prevention measures (p. 255) should be undertaken in miniature horses and ponies requiring surgery. Quizzes for each chapter, additional clinical scenarios, and video demonstrations of surgical procedures are available online at www.wiley.com/go/southwood.

References

1. Barton, M.H. & Collatos, C. (1999) Tumor necrosis factor and interleukin-6 activity and endotoxin concentration in peritoneal fluid and blood of horses with acute abdominal disease. *Journal of Veterinary Internal Medicine*, **13**, 457–464.
2. Boening, K.J. & Leendertse, I.P. (1993) Review of 115 cases of colic in the pregnant mare. *Equine Veterinary Journal*, **25**, 518–521.
3. Brosnahan, M.M. & Paradis, M.R. (2003) Assessment of clinical characteristics, management practices, and activities of geriatric horses. *Journal of the American Veterinary Medical Association*, **223**, 99–103.
4. Brosnahan, M.M. & Paradis, M.R. (2003) Demographic and clinical characteristics of geriatric horses: 467 cases (1989–1999). *Journal of the American Veterinary Medical Association*, **223**, 93–98.
5. Cable, C.S., Fubini, S.L., Erb, H.N. & Hakes, J.E. (1997) Abdominal surgery in foals: A review of 119 cases (1977–1994). *Equine Veterinary Journal*, **29**, 257–261.
6. Chaney, K.P., Holcombe, S.J., LeBlanc, M.M., et al. (2007) The effect of uterine torsion on mare and foal survival: A retrospective study, 1985–2005. *Equine Veterinary Journal*, **39**, 33–36.
7. Chenier, T.S. & Whitehead, A.E. (2009) Foaling rates and risk factors for abortion in pregnant mares presented for medical or surgical treatment of colic: 153 cases (1993–2005). *Canadian Veterinary Journal*, **50**, 481–485.
8. Coleman, M.C., Slovis, N.M. & Hunt, R.J. (2009) Long-term prognosis of gastrojejunostomy in foals with gastric outflow obstruction: 16 cases (2001–2006). *Equine Veterinary Journal*, **41**, 653–657.
9. Cox, R., Proudman, C.J., Trawford, A.F., Burden, F. & Pinchbeck, G.L. (2007) Epidemiology of impaction colic in donkeys in the UK. *BMC Veterinary Research*, **3**, 1–11.
10. Cribb, N.C., Cote, N.M., Bouré, L.P. & Peregrine, A.S. (2006) Acute small intestinal obstruction associated with *Parascaris equorum* infection in young horses: 25 cases (1985–2004). *New Zealand Veterinary Journal*, **54**, 338–343.
11. Daels, P.F. (2004) Hormonal therapy in pregnant mare. In: *Proceedings of the Annual Meeting for Italian Association Equine Veterinary*, Perugia, Italy.
12. Dolente, B.A., Sullivan, E.K., Boston, R. & Johnston, J.K. (2005) Mares admitted to a referral hospital for postpartum emergencies: 163 cases (1992–2002). *Journal of Veterinary Emergency and Critical Care*, **15**, 193–200.
13. Drumm, N.K., Embertson, R.M., Hopper, S.A., et al. (2011) Foaling rates and factors associated with fetal outcome after colic surgery in pregnant Thoroughbred mares in central Kentucky. In: *Proceedings of American College of Veterinary Surgeons Symposium*, Chicago, Illinois.
14. Dunkel, B. & McKenzie, H.C. (2003) Severe hypertriglyceridemia in clinically ill horses: Diagnosis, treatment and outcome. *Equine Veterinary Journal*, **35**, 590–595.

15. Frazer, G., Burba, D., Paccamonti, D., *et al.* (1997) The effects of parturition and peripartum complications on the peritoneal fluid composition of mares. *Theriogenology*, **48**, 919–931.

16. Haupt, J.L., McAndrews, A.G., Chaney, K.P., Labbe, K.A. & Holcombe, S.J. (2008) Surgical treatment of colic in the miniature horse: A retrospective study of 57 cases (1993–2006). *Equine Veterinary Journal*, **40**, 364–367.

17. Hillyer, M.H., Smith, M.R. & Milligan, P.J. (2008) Gastric and small intestinal ileus as a cause of acute colic in the post parturient mare. *Equine Veterinary Journal*, **40**, 368–372.

18. Holm-Pedersen, P., Fenstad, A.M. & Folke, L.E. (1974) DNA, RNA and protein synthesis in healing wounds in young and old mice. *Mechanisms of Ageing and Development*, **3**, 173–185.

19. Hughes, K.J., Dowling, B.A., Matthews, S.A. & Dart, A.J. (2003) Results of surgical treatment of colic in miniature breed horses: 11 cases. *Australian Veterinary Journal*, **81**, 260–264.

20. Ireland, J.L., Clegg, P.D., McGowan, C.M., Platt, L. & Pinchbeck, G.L. (2011) Factors associated with mortality of geriatric horses in the United Kingdom. *Preventive Veterinary Medicine*, **101**, 204–218.

21. Jung, C., Hospes, R., Bostedt, H. & Litzke, L.F. (2008) Surgical treatment of uterine torsion using a ventral midline laparotomy in 19 mares. *Australian Veterinary Journal*, **86**, 272–276.

22. Krista, K.M. & Kuebelbeck, K.L. (2009) Comparison of survival rates for geriatric horses versus nongeriatric horses following exploratory celiotomy for colic. *Journal of the American Veterinary Medical Association*, **235**, 1069–1072.

23. Lavoie, J.P., Drolet, R., Parsons, D., *et al.* (2000) Equine proliferative enteropathy: A cause of weight loss, colic, diarrhoea and hypoproteinaemia in foals on three breeding farms in Canada. *Equine Veterinary Journal*, **32**, 418–425.

24. Livesey, L.C., Carson, R.L. & Stanton, M.B. (2008) Postpartum colic in a mare caused by pneumouterus. *Veterinary Record*, **162**, 626–627.

25. Lundin, C., Sullins, K.E., White, N.A., Clem, M.F., Debowes, R.M. & Pfeiffer, C.A. (1989) Induction of peritoneal adhesions with small intestinal ischaemia and distention in the foal. *Equine Veterinary Journal*, **21**, 451–458.

26. MacKay, R.J. (1992) Association between serum cytotoxicity and selected clinical variables in 240 horses admitted to a veterinary hospital. *American Journal of Veterinary Research*, **53**, 748–752.

27. MacKay, R.J., Merritt, A.M., Zertuche, J.M., Whittington, M. & Skelley, L.A. (1991) Tumor necrosis factor activity in the circulation of horses given endotoxin. *American Journal of Veterinary Research*, **52**, 533–538.

28. MacKinnon, M.C., Southwood, L.L., Burke, M.J. & Palmer, J.E. (2012) Causes, management, and outcome of equine neonates presenting with colic: 137 foals (2000–2010). *Journal of the American Veterinary Medical Association*, (submitted).

29. McClintock, S.A. & Collins, A.M. (2004) Lawsonia intracellularis proliferative enteropathy in a weanling foal in Australia. *Australian Veterinary Journal*, **82**, 750–752.

30. McClure, J.T., Kobluk, C., Voller, K., Geor, R.J., Ames, T.R. & Sivula, N. (1992) Fecalith impaction in four miniature foals. *Journal of the American Veterinary Medical Association*, **200**, 205–207.

31. McFarlane, D. & Holbrook, T.C. (2008) Cytokine dysregulation in aged horses and horses with pituitary pars intermedia dysfunction. *Journal of Veterinary Internal Medicine*, **22**, 436–442.

32. Mogg, T.D. & Palmer, J.E. (1995) Hyperlipidemia, hyperlipemia, and hepatic lipidosis in American miniature horses: 23 cases (1990–1994). *Journal of the American Veterinary Medical Association*, **207**, 604–607.

33. Moore, B.R., Abood, S.K. & Hinchcliff, K.W. (1994) Hyperlipaemia in 9 miniature horses and miniature donkeys. *Journal of Veterinary Internal Medicine*, **8**, 376–381.

34. Naylor, J.M. (1982) Hyperlipemia and hyperlipidemia in horses, ponies and donkeys. *Compendium on Continuing Education for the Practicing Veterinarian*, **4**, 321–326.

35. Naylor, J.M., Kronfeld, D.S. & Acland, H. (1980) Hyperlipemia in horses: Effects of undernutrition and disease. *American Journal of Veterinary Research*, **6**, 899–905.

36. Neal, H.N. (2003) Foal colic: Practical imaging of the abdomen. *Equine Veterinary Education*, **15**, 263–270.

37. Palmer, J.E. (2004) Fluid therapy in the neonate: Not your mother's fluid space. *Veterinary Clinics of North America: Equine Practice*, **20**, 63–75.

38. Pascoe, J.R., Meagher, D.M. & Wheat, J.D. (1981) Surgical management of uterine torsion in the mare: A review of 26 cases. *Journal of the American Veterinary Medical Association*, **179**, 351–354.

39. Pawelec, G. (2006) Immunity and aging in man. *Experimental Gerontology*, **41**, 1239–1242.

40. Ragle, C.A., Snyder, J.R., Meagher, D.M. & Honnas, C.M. (1992) Surgical treatment of colic in American miniature horses: 15 cases (1980–1987). *Journal of the American Veterinary Medical Association*, **201**, 329–331.

41. Rakestraw, P.C. & Hardy, J. 2006. Large intestine. In: *Equine Surgery*, 3rd edn. (eds Auer, J.A. & Stick, J.A.), pp. 436–478. Saunders, Elsevier, St. Louis, Missouri.

42. Ralston, S.L., Squires, E.L. & Nockels, C.F. (1989) Digestion in the aged horse. *Journal of Equine Veterinary Science*, **9**, 203–205.

43. Ross, J., Palmer, J.E. & Wilkins, P.A. (2008) Body wall tears during late pregnancy in mares: 13 cases (1995–2006). *Journal of the American Veterinary Medical Association*, **232**, 257–261.

44. Sampieri, F., Hinchcliff, K.W. & Toribio, R.E. (2006) Tetracycline therapy of Lawsonia intracellularis enteropathy in foals. *Equine Veterinary Journal*, **38**, 89–92.

45. Santschi, E.M., Slone, D.E., Gronwall, R., Juzwiak, J.S. & Moll, H.D. (1991) Types of colic and frequency of postcolic abortion in pregnant mares: 105 cases (1984–1988). *Journal of the American Veterinary Medical Association*, **199**, 374–377.

46. Santschi, E.M., Slone, D.E., Embertson, R.M., Clayton, M.K. & Markel, M.D. (2000) Racing performance of Thoroughbred horses after colic surgery as juveniles: 206 cases. *Equine Veterinary Journal Supplements*, **32**, 332–332.

47. Schmidt, A.R., Williams, M.A., Carleton, C.L., Darien, B.J. & Derksen, F.J. (1991) Evaluation of transabdominal ultrasound-guided amniocentesis in the late gestational mare. *Equine Veterinary Journal*, **23**, 261–265.

48. Silver, M. & Fowden, A.L. (1982) Uterine prostaglandin F metabolite production in relation to glucose availability in late pregnancy and a possible influence of diet on time of delivery in the mare. *Journal of Reproduction and Fertility Supplement*, **32**, 511–519.

49. Singer, E.R. & Livesey, M.A. (1997) Evaluation of exploratory laparotomy in young horses: 102 cases (1987–1992). *Journal of the American Veterinary Medical Association*, **211**, 1158–1162.

50. Southwood, L.L. (2010) Colic in the geriatric horse. In: *Proceedings of American College of Veterinary Surgeons Symposium*, Seattle, Washington.

51. Southwood, L.L., Ragle, C.A., Snyder, J.R. & Hendrickson, D.A. (1996) Surgical treatment of ascarid impactions in horses and foals. In: *Proceedings of the 42nd Annual Convention of the American Association of Equine Practitioners*, Denver, Colorado, pp. 258–263.

52. Southwood, L.L., Gassert, T. & Lindborg, S. (2010) Colic in geriatric compared to mature nongeriatric horses. Part 1: Retrospective review of clinical and laboratory data. *Equine Veterinary Journal*, **42**, 621–627.

53. Southwood, L.L., Gassert, T. & Lindborg, S. (2010) Colic in geriatric compared to mature nongeriatric horses. Part 2: Treatment, diagnosis and short-term survival. *Equine Veterinary Journal*, **42**, 628–635.

54. Sussman, M.D. (1973) Aging of connective tissue: Physical properties of healing wounds in young and old rats. *American Journal of Physiology*, **224**, 1167–1171.

55. Underwood, C., Southwood, L.L., Walton, R.M. & Johnson, A.L. (2010) Hepatic and metabolic changes in surgical colic patients: A pilot study. *Journal of Veterinary Emergency and Critical Care*, **20**, 578–586.

56. Vatistas, N.J., Snyder, J.R., Wilson, W.D., Drake, C. & Hildebrand, S. (1996) Surgical treatment for colic in the foal (67 cases): 1980–1992. *Equine Veterinary Journal*, **28**, 139–145.

57. Waitt, L.H. & Cebra, C.K. (2009) Characterization of hypertriglyceridemia and response to treatment with insulin in horses, ponies, and donkeys: 44 cases (1995–2005). *Journal of the American Veterinary Medical Association*, **234**, 915–919.

58. Wichtel, J.J., Reinertson, E.L. & Clark, T.L. (1988) Nonsurgical treatment of uterine torsion in seven mares. *Journal of the American Veterinary Medical Association*, **193**, 337–338.

59. Wilson, D.A., Baker, G.I. & Boero, M.J. (1995) Complications of celiotomy incisions in horses. *Veterinary Surgery*, **24**, 506–514.

60. Young, R.L., Linford, R.L. & Olander, H.J. (1992) Atresia coli in the foal: A review of six cases. *Equine Veterinary Journal*, **24**, 60–62.

61. Zedler, S., Embertson, R., Barr, B., Bernard, W.V. & Boston, R.C. (2009) Surgical treatment of gastric outflow obstruction in 40 foals: 1986–2004. *Veterinary Surgery*, **38**, 623–630.

22 Long-term Recovery and Prevention

Louise L. Southwood

Department of Clinical Studies, New Bolton Center, School of Veterinary Medicine, University of Pennsylvania, Kennett Square, PA, USA

Chapter Outline

Long-term recovery	292	Long-term complications following colic surgery	294
Postoperative management following hospital		Long-term survival following colic surgery	294
discharge	292	Return to use	295
Monitoring	292	**Prevention**	**295**
Incisional care	293		
Feeding	294		

Long-term recovery

Postoperative management following hospital discharge

An outline of discharge instructions are shown in Table 22.1. The main concerns with regard to management following hospital discharge are to return the gastrointestinal tract to normal function and ensure body wall healing. Horses need to be monitored closely for long-term complications particularly during the first month and then the first year following colic surgery.

Monitoring

Postoperative colic patients need to be monitored following hospital discharge for:

- incisional problems;
- appetite;
- water consumption;
- fecal and urine output;
- body weight;
- demeanor;
- signs of colic;
- signs of laminitis (uncommon);

Table 22.1 Typical discharge instructions following colic surgery.

Monitoring	Monitor your horse's demeanor/attitude, appetite, water consumption, and manure and urine production. Your horse should be monitored closely for signs of colic and incisional complications (see below)
Exercise	Stall rest for 4 weeks. Hand walking and grazing is encouraged. The horse can then be moved to a stall and small run for an additional 4 weeks. After the initial 8 weeks of rest, the horse can be turned out into a pasture area and be used for light exercise if there have been no complications with incisional healing. Gradually return the horse to his/her intended use after 12 weeks of convalescence if the incision is healing
Incisional care	The incision should be monitored for signs of infection including excessive swelling, pain on palpation, or drainage. If there are any concerns contact your veterinarian or surgeon
Feeding	Return the horse to his/her regular diet over a 2 week period. Monitor body weight and condition and adjust diet accordingly. Provide good quality hay and water at all times for your horse. Access to pasture may decrease the risk for colic
Medication	None

If any signs of illness occur, the horse's rectal temperature should be taken. Differential diagnoses for a horse with a fever following hospital discharge are similar to the immediate postoperative period during hospitalization and include incisional infection, salmonellosis, pneumonia, viral infection, and rarely peritonitis. See Chapter 19 on Postoperative Complications (p. 244).

Horses are not typically discharged with any medication. Antimicrobial drug use should be confined to the perioperative period. Treatment with nonsteroidal anti-inflammatory drugs (NSAIDs) is usually discontinued at least 24–48 h prior to hospital discharge. Some surgeons may treat horses with an incisional infection with antimicrobial drugs; however, any benefit of antimicrobial drugs for resolution of celiotomy incisional infection remains to be demonstrated.

Incisional care

Following hospital discharge, patients should be confined to a stall for 4 weeks followed by a stall with a small run for an additional 4 weeks to allow the body wall to heal. Hand walking and grazing should be encouraged during this period of recovery. Horses should then be turned out for an additional 4 weeks prior to commencing training. Light riding can also be performed during this time period if there have been no incisional complications.

The incision should be monitored for signs of infection including excessive edema formation, pain on palpation, and drainage (see Chapter 19 on Postoperative Complications [p. 244]). If incisional drainage is observed following hospital discharge, the area should be prepared and a sample collected for bacterial culture and sensitivity testing. While systemic antimicrobial drugs are not used by many surgeons to treat incisional infection, it is potentially useful to monitor trends for infecting bacteria and antimicrobial sensitivity patterns. Typical organisms causing postceliotomy surgical site infection and antimicrobial drug resistance patterns vary between hospitals.

Management of incisional infections involves opening the skin wound adequately to allow sufficient drainage and keeping the surgical site clean by scrubbing with a chlorhexidine- or povidone-iodine-based scrub and saline. Alcohol can be used on the skin around the wound but should not be allowed to contact the subcutaneous tissue. Infected surgical wounds tend to drain for several weeks and probably until the suture material used to close the body wall and subcutaneous tissue is resorbed. There have been no studies investigating any benefit of antimicrobial drugs on resolution of postceliotomy surgical site infection.

The main complications following incisional infection are hernia formation[23,29,30] and possibly adhesion formation between the bowel and body wall incision.[30,32] Hernia formation was about 60 times more likely in horses with an incisional infection compared to horses without an incisional infection[23] and was reported to occur in 8% of postoperative colic patients.[30] Current recommendations for preventing hernias in postoperative colic patients with an infection and then managing body wall hernias is the CM™ Heal Hernia Belt (CM Equine Products).[25] Measurements necessary to fit the hernia belt are (1) girth, (2) largest part of the abdomen, and (3) from the base of the whither, along the top line, to just in front of the flank (www.cmequineproducts.com).

Body wall hernias that are large and do not respond to treatment with a hernia belt can be surgically repaired either primarily or using mesh herniorrhaphy. The primary apposition of incisional hernias in horses without the use of mesh support has a shorter surgical time, duration of hospitalization, and appears to result in a good cosmetic outcome while avoiding the complications associated with mesh implantation.[51] Horses can return to athletic activity and even breeding with even moderately sized abdominal hernias (David Freeman DVM, Rolf Embertson DVM, Donnie Slone DVM, personal communication).

Feeding

Horses should be reintroduced to their normal diet gradually over a period of days to weeks depending on the change necessary. Horses should be monitored closely for weight loss or weight gain and the diet modified accordingly. It is common for horses to lose some body weight and condition following colic surgery particularly if they developed postoperative complications (e.g., salmonellosis, postoperative reflux).[47] However, horses should regain weight within 6 months following surgery. Some horses may require dietary modification following colic surgery depending on the primary lesion and surgical procedure performed including feeding a complete pelleted feed or corn oil to increase body weight. See Chapter 23 on Nutrition (p. 301).

Long-term complications following colic surgery

The most common long-term complications are related to recurring gastrointestinal disease and incisional problems including colic, postoperative intraperitoneal adhesions, and incisional hernia formation.[30]

Colic occurs in approximately 25–35% of horses following hospital discharge after colic surgery,[30,47] with most horses having sporadic or recurrent colic (three or fewer episodes) and only a small percentage having >4 colic episodes or with signs severe enough

to require hospital readmission (8%) or a second surgery (3%).[4,30] Most colic episodes occur within the first 2–3 months after surgery.[4] Serosanguinous peritoneal fluid, small intestinal obstruction, intestinal resection, and postoperative ileus were associated with signs of colic long-term. Large colon displacements and volvulus have about a 15% recurrence rate.[12,45,46] If these lesions recur, colopexy (p. 202),[16] large colon resection (p. 195), or nephrosplenic space ablation[13,14,41] can be performed to prevent recurrence. Importantly, horses with large colon displacement or volvulus that have experienced an episode of colic prior to the episode necessitating surgery are significantly more likely to have an episode of colic after surgery compared with horses that have not experienced a previous colic episode indicating an underlying predisposition.[46] Horses with small intestinal lesions tend to develop complications associated with stenosis at the anastomosis site or adhesion formation. Stenosis can occur typically with side-to-side anastomosis techniques and requires a second surgical procedure with revision of the anastomosis.

Postoperative intraperitoneal adhesions (p. 255) occur in approximately 8% of horses after colic surgery[30] and in up to 20% of horses with small intestinal lesions. Severity of pain at admission, serosanguinous peritoneal fluid, small intestinal lesions, intestinal resection, postoperative ileus, incisional complications, and repeat celiotomy are associated with adhesion formation.[30] Adhesions can occasionally be managed medically using analgesic drugs as needed (e.g., flunixin meglumine or firocoxib) and nutritional modification (e.g., pasture and pelleted feed). Horses with persistent signs of colic associated with adhesion formation require either a repeat laparotomy or laparoscopic adhesiolysis.

Incisional infection can also occur as a long-term complication following hospital discharge (typically at ~10–14 days postoperatively), with abdominal hernia formation and adhesions between the bowel and body wall being the most important long-term complications following incisional infection (see Incisional care [p. 293]).

Long-term survival following colic surgery

Long-term survival (>1 year) is typically about 80–90% of horses that are discharged from the hospital following colic surgery.[30,47] The survival rates at 6, 12, 24, 36, 48, and 60 months were recently reported to be 95%, 87%, 81%, 77%, 62%, and 58%, respectively, in one study,[5] which is about 10–20% lower than that reported previously[35–37,39] when considering that only horses discharged from the hospital were included in the analysis. Comparison to a similarly aged population that had not undergone colic surgery would provide useful information with regard to the impact of colic and colic surgery on long-term survival. Clinical features associated with decreased long-term survival for horses with large intestinal lesion were increasing age, admission heart rate, admission packed cell volume (PCV), relaparotomy, and resection and for horses with small intestinal lesions, admission PCV, admission total plasma protein (TPP), duration of surgery, and relaparotomy.[38,39] Horses that have long-term problems with colic not surprisingly have a higher long-term mortality compared to horses that do not (26% vs. 12%, respectively).[30] Colic is the reason for euthanasia in the majority of horses following colic surgery (60–70%).[30,47]

Return to use

Short-term survival has improved substantially over the past 20 years and is generally good to excellent for horses with most types of lesions. Recent studies have focused not only on long-term survival but also the ability of the postoperative colic patient to return to their intended use including athletic performance. A large majority of horses (85–90%) resume or start sporting activities after colic surgery,[5, 26] with 84% of owners reporting that horses achieve the same or better performance after surgery.[5] Most horses (68%) perform at their intended use by 6 months following colic surgery and 56% at or above their preoperative performance level.[11] At 12 months following surgery, 76% of horses return to their intended use and 69% at or above their previous performance level.[11] Similarly, 70% of Thoroughbred racehorses return to racing following colic surgery. Racehorses undergoing colic surgery performed as well as their cohorts from the race preceding surgery from annual quarter Q3 to Q12 postoperatively.[17] Age, admission heart rate, admission TPP, and blood lactate were associated with failure to return to racing following

colic surgery.[17] Juvenile Thoroughbreds (<2 years old) that had a celiotomy were significantly less able to race (63%) than their unaffected siblings (82%), with age at the initial surgery being associated with the percentage of horses racing. However, affected foals that were able to race won as much money, raced as often, and made as many starts as their siblings.[42]

Horses that require surgery for colic during hospitalization for treatment of another performance-limiting problem (e.g., musculoskeletal or upper respiratory tract disease) may not return to their previous level of performance.[11] Laminitis, a relatively uncommon postoperative complication (<1% horses),[29] may also impact the ability of a horse to return to performance.[11] Horses with incisional hernia formation and postoperative diarrhea are less likely to return to their intended use by 6 months.[11] A similar percentage of horses with salmonellosis (75%) return to their intended use postoperatively compared to horses that did not have salmonellosis (81%).[47] Based on this data, owners should not be discouraged from performing colic surgery on athletic horses and every effort should be made to prevent complications that may limit a horse's ability to return to their previous performance level.

Prevention

Prevention of colic is a challenge facing equine veterinarians and horse owners. Some horses appear to be either predisposed or at high risk for recurrent problems with colic. Recurrent colic was reported to occur in 37% of horses within 1 year of a colic episode,[43] with approximately 12% of horses with recurrent colic requiring surgery and 12% requiring euthanasia.[43] Recurrent colic was associated with known dental problems and aerophagia (crib-biting or wind sucking).[43] In another study, 44% of horses showing signs of colic were reported to have had colic previously, 11% within the previous year.[49] Despite the predisposition for individual horses to colic, the importance of a genetic predisposition to colic has received little attention. In general the reason for recurrent colic continues to be elusive. A reduced number of interstitial cells of Cajal (interstitial cells that serve as a pacemaker creating the basal electrical rhythm leading to smooth muscle contraction)[15] and a reduction in myenteric plexus number and neuron density and an increase in enteroglial cells (cellular support of enteric nerves)[44] were observed in horses undergoing surgery for large intestinal disease. Idiopathic fibrosis of the muscularis of the large intestine has been identified in horses with chronic colic associated with the large intestine[31] and highlights the importance of obtaining an intestinal biopsy in horses with recurrent signs of colic.

A seasonal pattern to colic has been reported with spring (and autumn) overall being the season with the highest observed incidence.[21,34,49] Impaction colic is more commonly observed over the winter months as is epiploic foramen impaction.[2] The seasonal distribution of colic is likely related to management factors such as diet and diet change, exercise regimen, and housing.[1]

Several management factors have been indentified that appear to increase the risk of horses for colic. Minimizing exposure of horses to these risk factors may help prevent colic. Some risk factors associated with colic are listed in Table 22.2. In general, allowing horses access to a well-managed pasture, feeding good quality hay, access to fresh water at all times, dental care, strategic deworming, avoiding sand ingestion, minimizing stereotypic behavior such as aerophagia, and making any changes to the diet or exercise regimen gradually over time are likely important preventive measures.

Diet has not surprisingly been associated with signs of colic. While there are reports that did not identify any association between colic and type of dried forage or frequency of feeding forage,[49] other studies have demonstrated associations with the type and quality of feed. Regional differences exist with regard to the type of feed and causes of colic. Coastal Bermuda grass hay is fed in the south eastern part of the United States and has been associated with colic, in particular ileal and cecal impaction.[6,27,33] Providing a pelleted feed in addition to forage was recommended to prevent ileal impaction.[27] Feeding hay from round bales has been associated with colic.[22] The association between colic and forage is attributed to poor hay quality or the presence of mold. The types of hay associated with increased risk of colic are high fiber and low protein content and, therefore, less digestible.[8,22] In Texas and California, feeding alfalfa hay has been associated with enterolithiasis.[9,18,19] Feeding less alfalfa and more grass hay and

Table 22.2 Risk factors for colic and colonic obstruction and distention that were identified in epidemiological studies in Texas and the United Kingdom.

Location	Risk factor
Texas[3–5]	Change in diet, type or batch of hay, type of grain, or concentrate fed
	Less exposure to pasture
	Feeding >2.7 kg of oats per day, hay from round bales, coastal Bermuda grass hay
	Change in housing or weather
	Thoroughbred and Arabian breeds
	Aged >8 or 10 years
	Having had a previous episode of colic or having undergone an exploratory celiotomy for colic
	Recent (<7 days previously) administration of an anthelmintic (Note: Regular anthelmintic administration reduced the risk of colic)
United Kingdom[8]	Hours spent in a stable
	Residing at the present stable for <6 months
	Change in exercise regimen
	Travel within the preceding 24 h
	Having had a previous episode of colic
	Absence of administration of an ivermectin or moxidectin anthelmintic within the previous 12 months
	Infrequent teeth checks
	Aerophagia (crib-biting, wind sucking)

increasing daily access to pasture grazing were recommended to decrease enterolithiasis in horses residing in high-risk areas.[18,19] Dietary modifications promoting acidification of colonic contents and dilution of minerals (e.g., increasing the grain:hay ratio or supplementation with apple cider vinegar) might also be beneficial to prevent enterolithiasis.[18,19] In general, a higher concentrate intake has been associated with an increased risk of colic, including gastric ulceration.[22,48] Recent change in hay or concentrate has also been associated with colic.[8,21,22,48] Although equine grass sickness is associated with a longer duration of access to pasture in the United Kingdom and Europe,[1] in general, an increase of time on pasture and less time in a stall has been associated with a decreased risk of colic.[21,22] Care must be taken, however, in horses residing in sandy regions and it is recommended to not feed horses on sandy ground, limit access to sandy pastures, feed a high bulk diet, and supplement with psyllium mucilloid in these regions. These studies overall support the notion that attention needs to be paid to risk factors in specific geographical regions and that horses should be provided ample access to good quality pasture and hay with any dietary changes being made slowly.

Recently, the importance of colonic microbiota has been investigated with an observed increase in lactic-acid producing bacteria (*Bacillus-Lactobacillus-Streptococcus*) in grain-fed horses and horses with colic caused by simple colonic obstruction/distention compared to horses fed grass only.[10] Importantly, there was no associated increase in lactate utilizing bacteria (*Veillonellaceae* spp.) associated with the documented increase in colonic lactate concentration, which may be important in colic associated with simple colonic obstruction/distention.[10] Further investigation into the impact of diet and change in diet on colonic microbiota, its importance in gastrointestinal disease, and methods to restore and maintain normal colonic function while maintaining the dietary energy requirements of athletes are warranted.

Gastrointestinal parasites have long been associated with colic. While the importance of *Strongylus vulgaris* has declined with the use of ivermectin-based anthelmintics, tapeworms, cyathostomes, and ascarids are considered to play a role in some causes of colic. Despite conflicting results in the literature, using a targeted deworming program is likely important in colic prevention in some horses. An increased risk of colic was associated with horses not on a regular deworming program[8] and an absence of administration of moxidectin/ivermectin anthelmintic in the previous 12 months was associated with simple colonic obstruction and distention.[21] Other studies have identified no association between colic and anthelmintic used and parasite control programs.[7,20,49] It is most likely that a combination of parasite burden, the host response to the parasite, and other management factors play a role in parasite-related colic. Anthelmintic administration can be associated with colic and is likely associated with sudden and rapid death of parasites in horses with a heavy burden. For example, an increased risk of colic was observed in the 7 day period following anthelmintic treatment,[8] particularly in horses with serological evidence of a heavy tapeworm burden.[3] This further emphasizes the importance of a targeted deworming program at selected times to prevent the formation of a heavy parasite burden while preserving parasite anthelmintic sensitivity. Anthelmintic resistance is a continually emerging problem making pasture management strategies an important component of parasite control including rotation or co-grazing with ruminants, removal of feces from pastures, and composting of stall manure and bedding before spreading it on pastures.[28] See Chapter 24 on Gastrointestinal Parasitology and Anthelmintics (p. 316).

Exercise regimen has been associated with colic. Some of the key findings include (1) an increased risk of colic in horses being exercised at least once a week compared to those turned out with no ridden exercise,[8] (2) simple colonic obstruction/distention associated with a recent change in a regular exercise program,[21] and (3) the association between intensive exercise and gastric ulceration.[1] Horses that have been subject to recent stall confinement do appear to be particularly predisposed to colic. Horses that spend all of their time in a stall are at increased risk of colic when compared to horses at pasture.[22] More hours spent in a stall were also associated with increased risk of simple colonic obstruction/distention, particularly in the 14 days following a change in housing. A large increase in risk of colic was observed in horses stalled >19 h/day.[21]

Water deprivation has been associated with colic, particularly large colon impaction.[40,50] Horses with access to ponds or a water source other than buckets, troughs, or tanks are at decreased risk of colic.[7,24] Water mineral content analysis is recommended in high-risk areas for enterolithiasis.[18,19] Provision of fresh, clean, palatable water at all times is important for colic prevention.

Transportation has been associated with colic.[21,50] The exact reasons for colic following transportation are not necessarily clear but are likely related to feed and water intake, confinement, management changes, as well as stress.[1] Recognition of horses that are predisposed to colic associated with transportation and taking particular care with provision of feed and water and even providing water and mineral oil via a nasogastric tube may prevent colic in these horses.

Epidemiological studies have indicated that horses should be kept at pasture, allowed free access to water, provided good quality hay, and not fed concentrates, which is generally in conflict with the athletic demands placed on this species. Future studies should be directed toward optimizing diet and management for performance while maintaining gastrointestinal function. Dental care is recommended as a component of a colic prevention program,[21,43,50] along with a targeted deworming program. As part of any colic prevention program, particular attention should be paid to risk factors for colic in specific geographical areas and preventative measures undertaken that are relevant to these regions.

References

1. Archer, D.C. & Proudman, C.J. (2006) Epidemiological clues to preventing colic. *Veterinary Journal*, **172**, 29–39.
2. Archer, D.C., Pinchbeck, G.L., Proudman, C.J. & Clough, H.E. (2006) Is equine colic seasonal? Novel application of a model based approach. *BMC Veterinary Research*, **2**, 27.
3. Barrett, E.J., Blair, C.W., Farlam, J. & Proudman, C.J. (2005) Postdosing colic and diarrhoea in horses with serological evidence of tapeworm infection. *Veterinary Record*, **156**, 252–253.
4. Burford, J.H., Tudur-Smith, C., Smith, J., *et al.* (2011) The incidence of post-operative colic in 1412 horses discharged following exploratory laparotomy for investigation of acute gastrointestinal disease. In: *Proceedings of the 10th Equine Colic Research Symposium*, Indianapolis, Indiana, pp. 126–127.
5. Christophersen, M.T., Tnibar, A., Pihl, T.H., Andersen, P.H. & Ekstrøm, C.T. (2011) Sporting activity following colic surgery in horses: A retrospective study. *Equine Veterinary Journal*, **43**(Suppl 40), 3–6.
6. Cohen, N.D. & Peloso, J.G. (1996) Risk factors for history of previous colic and for chronic, intermittent colic in a population of horses. *Journal of the American Veterinary Medical Association*, **208**, 697–703.
7. Cohen, N.D., Matejka, P.L., Honnas, C.M. & Hooper, R.N. (1995) Case-control study of the association between various management factors and development of colic in horses. Texas Equine Colic Study Group. *Journal of the American Veterinary Medical Association*, **206**, 667–673.
8. Cohen, N.D., Gibbs, P.G. & Woods, A.M. (1999) Dietary and other management factors associated with colic in horses. *Journal of the American Veterinary Medical Association*, **215**, 53–60.
9. Cohen, N.D., Vontur, C.A. & Rakestraw, P.C. (2000) Risk factors for enterolithiasis among horses in Texas. *Journal of the American Veterinary Medical Association*, **216**, 1787–1794.
10. Daly, K., Proudman, C.J., Duncan, S.H., Flint, H.J., Dyer, J. & Shirazi-Beechey, S.P. (2011) Alterations in microbiota and fermentation products in equine large intestine in response to dietary variation and intestinal disease. *British Journal of Nutrition*, **5**, 1–7.
11. Davis, W., Fogle, C.A., Blikslager, A.T. & Gerard, M.P. (2011) A retrospective analysis of return to function following colic surgery in 195 cases (2003–2010). In: *Proceedings of the 10th Equine Colic Research Symposium*, Indianapolis, Indiana, p. 205.
12. Embertson, R.M., Cook, G., Hance, S.R., Bramlage, L.R., Levine, J. & Smith, S. (1996) Large colon volvulus: Surgical treatment of 204 horses (1986–1995). In: *Proceedings of the 42nd Convention of the American Association of Equine Practitioners*, Denver, Colorado, pp. 254–255.
13. Epstein, K.L. & Parente, E.J. (2006) Laparoscopic obliteration of the nephrosplenic space using polypropylene mesh in five horses. *Veterinary Surgery*, **35**, 431–437.
14. Farstvedt, E. & Hendrickson, D. (2005) Laparoscopic closure of the nephrosplenic space for prevention of recurrent nephrosplenic entrapment of the ascending colon. *Veterinary Surgery*, **34**, 642–645.
15. Fintle, C., Hudson, N.P.H., Mayhew, I.G., Edwards, G.B., Proudman, C.J. & Pearson, G.T. (2004) Interstitial cells of Cajal (ICC) in equine colic: An immunohistochemical study of horses with obstructive disorders of the small and large intestines. *Equine Veterinary Journal*, **36**, 474–479.
16. Hance, S.R. & Embertson, R.M. (1992) Colopexy in broodmares: 44 cases (1986–1990). *Journal of the American Veterinary Medical Association*, **201**, 782–787.
17. Hart, S., Southwood, L.L., Lindborg, S. & Aceto, H.W. (2011) Retrospective analysis of the impact of abdominal surgery on return to function in racing Thoroughbreds. *Journal of the American Veterinary Medical Association*, (submitted).
18. Hassel, D.M., Rakestraw, P.C., Gardner, I.A., Spier, S.J. & Snyder, J.R. (2004) Dietary risk factors and colonic pH and mineral concentrations in horses with enterolithiasis. *Journal of Veterinary Internal Medicine*, **18**, 346–349.
19. Hassel, D.M., Aldridge, B.M., Drake, C.M. & Snyder, J.R. (2008) Evaluation of dietary and management risk factors for enterolithiasis among horses in California. *Research in Veterinary Science*, **85**, 476–480.

20. Hillyer, M.H., Taylor, F.G. & French, N.P. (2001) A cross-sectional study of colic in horses on thoroughbred training premises in the British Isles in 1997. *Equine Veterinary Journal*, **33**, 380–385.

21. Hillyer, M.H., Taylor, F.G.R., Proudman, C.J., Edwards, G.B., Smith, J.E. & French, N.P. (2002) Case control study to identify risk factors for simple colonic obstruction and distension colic in horses. *Equine Veterinary Journal*, **34**, 455–463.

22. Hudson, J.M., Cohen, N.D., Gibbs, P.G. & Thompson, J.A. (2001) Feeding practices associated with colic in horses. *Journal of the American Veterinary Medical Association*, **219**, 1419–1425.

23. Ingle-Fehr, J.E., Baxter, G.M., Howard, R.D., Trotter, G.W. & Stashak, T.S. (1997) Bacterial culturing of ventral median celiotomies for prediction of postoperative incisional complications in horses. *Veterinary Surgery*, **26**, 7–13.

24. Kaneene, J.B., Miller, R., Ross, W.A., Gallagher, K., Marteniuk, J. & Rook, J. (1997) Risk factors for colic in the Michigan (USA) equine population. *Preventive Veterinary Medicine*, **30**, 23–36.

25. Klohnen, A. (2011) Evaluation of post-operative abdominal incisional complications treated with a new hernia belt: 85 horses (2011–2005). In: *Proceedings of the 10th Equine Colic Research Symposium*, Indianapolis, Indiana, pp. 154–155.

26. Launois, T., Heiles, P.H., Desbrosse, F., Perrin, R., Rossignol, F. & Scicluna, C. (2006) Sports activity after colic surgery: Postoperative outcome of 100 procedures. In: *Proceedings of the 9th International Congress of the World Equine Veterinary Association*, Marrakech, Morocco, pp. 279–281.

27. Little, D. & Blikslager, A.T. (2002) Factors associated with development of ileal impaction in horses with surgical colic: 78 cases (1986–2000). *Equine Veterinary Journal*, **34**, 464–468.

28. Lyons, E.T., Drudge, J.H. & Tolliver, S.C. (2000) Larval cyathostomiasis. *Veterinary Clinics of North America: Equine Practice*, **16**, 501–513.

29. Mair, T.S. & Smith, L.J. (2005) Survival and complication rates in 300 horses undergoing surgical treatment of colic. Part 2: Short-term complications. *Equine Veterinary Journal*, **37**, 303–309.

30. Mair, T.S. & Smith, L.J. (2005) Survival and complication rates in 300 horses undergoing surgical treatment of colic. Part 3: Long-term complications and survival. *Equine Veterinary Journal*, **37**, 310–314.

31. Mair, T.S., Pearson, G.R., Fews, D., *et al.* (2011) Idiopathic fibrosis of the muscularis of the large intestine in five horses with colic. In: *Proceedings of the 10th Equine Colic Research Symposium*, Indianapolis, Indiana, pp. 97–98.

32. Morello, S., Southwood, L., Engiles, J., *et al.* (2012) Effect of intraperitoneal PERIDAN™ Concentrate Adhesion Reduction Device on clinical findings,

infection, and tissue healing in an adult horse jejuno-jejunostomy model. *Veterinary Surgery*, (in press).

33. Plummer, A.E., Rakestraw, P.C., Hardy, J. & Lee, R.M. (2007) Outcome of medical and surgical treatment of cecal impaction in horses: 114 cases (1994–2004). *Journal of the American Veterinary Medical Association*, **231**, 1378–1385.

34. Proudman, C.J. (1991) A two year, prospective survey of equine colic in general practice. *Equine Veterinary Journal*, **24**, 90–93.

35. Proudman, C.J., Smith, J.E., Edwards, G.B. & French, N.P. (2002) Long-term survival of equine surgical colic cases. Part 1: Patterns of mortality and morbidity. *Equine Veterinary Journal*, **34**, 432–437.

36. Proudman, C.J., Smith, J.E., Edwards, G.B. & French, N.P. (2002) Long-term survival of equine surgical colic cases. Part 2: Modeling postoperative survival. *Equine Veterinary Journal*, **34**, 438–443.

37. Proudman, C.J., Smith, J.E., Edwards, G.B. & French, N.P. (2002) Long-term survival of equine surgical colic cases. Part 1: Patterns of mortality and morbidity. *Equine Veterinary Journal*, **34**, 432–437.

38. Proudman, C.J., Edwards, G.B., Barnes, J. & French, N.R. (2005) Factors affecting long-term survival of horses recovering from surgery of the small intestine. *Equine Veterinary Journal*, **37**, 360–365.

39. Proudman, C.J., Edwards, G.B., Barnes, J. & French, N.P. (2005) Modeling long-term survival of horses following surgery for large intestinal disease. *Equine Veterinary Journal*, **37**, 366–370.

40. Reeves, M.J., Salman, M.D. & Smith, G. (1996) Risk factors for equine acute abdominal disease (colic): Results from a multi-centre case control study. *Preventive Veterinary Medicine*, **26**, 285–301.

41. Röcken, M., Schubert, C., Mosel, G. & Litzke, L.F. (2005) Indications, surgical technique, and long-term experience with laparoscopic closure of the nephrosplenic space in standing horses. *Veterinary Surgery*, **34**, 637–641.

42. Santschi, E.M., Slone, D.E., Embertson, R.M., Clayton, M.K. & Markel, M.D. (2000) Colic surgery in 206 juvenile Thoroughbreds: Survival and racing results. *Equine Veterinary Journal Supplements*, **32**, 32–36.

43. Scantlebury, C.E., Archer, D.C., Proudman, C.J. & Pinchbeck, G.L. (2011) Recurrent colic in the horse: Incidence and risk factors for recurrence in the general practice population. *Equine Veterinary Journal*, **43**(Suppl 39), 81–88.

44. Schusser, G.E. & White, N.A. (1997) Morphologic and quantitative evaluation of the myenteric plexuses and neurons in the large colon of horses. *Journal of the American Veterinary Medical Association*, **210**, 928–934.

45. Smith, L.J. & Mair, T.S. (2010) Are horses that undergo an exploratory laparotomy for correction of a right

dorsal displacement of the large colon predisposed to post operative colic, compared to other forms of large colon displacement. *Equine Veterinary Journal*, **42**, 44–46.

46. Southwood, L.L., Bergslien, K., Jacobi, A., *et al.* (2002) Large colon displacement and volvulus in horses. In: *Proceedings of the 7th International Equine Colic Research Symposium*, Manchester, pp. 32–33.

47. Southwood, L.L., Lindborg, S. & Aceto, H.W. (2011) Long-term complications and survival of horses with salmonellosis compared to horses without salmonellosis following colic surgery. Preliminary data. In: *Proceedings of the 10th Equine Colic Research Symposium*, Indianapolis, Indiana, pp. 226–227.

48. Tinker, M.K., White, N.A., Lessard, P., *et al.* (1997) A prospective study of equine colic risk factors. *Equine Veterinary Journal*, **29**, 454–458.

49. Traub-Dargatz, J.L., Kopral, C.A., Seitzinger, A.H., Garber, L.P., Forde, K. & White, N.A. (2001) Estimate of the national incidence of and operation-level risk factors for colic among horses in the United States, spring 1998 to spring 1999. *Journal of the American Veterinary Medical Association*, **219**, 67–71.

50. White, N.A. (1997) Risk factors associated with colic. In: *Current Therapy in Equine Medicine* (ed. N.E. Robinson), 4th edn., pp. 174–179. W.B. Saunders Co, Philadelphia, Pennsylvania.

51. Whitfield-Cargile, C.M., Rakestraw, P.C., Hardy, J., Cohen, N.D. & Davis, B.E. (2011) Comparison of primary closure of incisional hernias in horses with and without the use of prosthetic mesh support. *Equine Veterinary Journal*, **43**(Suppl 39), 69–75.

23

Nutrition

Brett S. Tennent-Brown,[1] Kira L. Epstein,[2] and Sarah L. Ralston[3]

[1]Equine Centre, University of Melbourne Veterinary Hospital, Werribee, Victoria, Australia
[2]Department of Large Animal Medicine, College of Veterinary Medicine, University of Georgia, Athens, GA, USA
[3]Department of Animal Science, School of Environmental and Biological Sciences, Rutgers, The State University of New Jersey, New Brunswick, NJ, USA

Chapter Outline

Feeding the postoperative colic	
patient	**302**
General considerations	302
How much to feed	302
Energy requirements	302
Protein requirements	303
Enteral or parenteral nutrition	303
Enteral nutrition	303
Guidelines for administration of enteral	
nutrition to adult horses	303
Blender diets	303
Compositional diets	303
Special considerations for foals	304
An approach to enteral feeding in the adult	
horse after colic	305
Parenteral nutrition	306
Dextrose solutions	307
Partial parenteral nutrition	307
Total parenteral nutrition	307
Carbohydrates (dextrose)	307
Lipids	307

Protein (amino acids)	307
Vitamins and trace minerals	308
Composing parenteral nutrition	
formulations	308
Guidelines for the preparation and	
administration of parenteral nutrition	308
Complications associated with parenteral	
nutrition	309
Hyperglycemia	309
Hypertriglyceridemia	310
Electrolyte abnormalities	310
Monitoring	310
Plasma triglyceride concentrations	310
Blood or plasma glucose concentration	310
Plasma electrolyte concentrations	310
Blood urea nitrogen	311
Long-term nutritional management	
of the postcolic patient	**311**
General considerations	311
Postsurgical colic long-term concerns	313
Postoperative weight gain	314

Practical Guide to Equine Colic, First Edition. Edited by Louise L. Southwood.
© 2013 John Wiley & Sons, Inc. Published 2013 by John Wiley & Sons, Inc.

Feeding the postoperative colic patient

General considerations

If insufficient calories are provided in the form of dietary carbohydrate or fat, endogenous proteins are catabolized to meet energy requirements. Malnutrition impairs immune function, delays wound healing, and increases patient morbidity and mortality. Therefore, the primary goal of a nutritional support protocol is to provide sufficient calories, in the form of carbohydrate or fat (lipid), to prevent or reduce endogenous protein catabolism. The inclusion of an exogenous protein source (usually provided as amino acids) will further help preserve endogenous proteins.

Most healthy adult horses will tolerate 3–5 days of fasting without adverse effect; however, pregnant or lactating mares, critically ill horses, horses in poor body condition, and foals are unable to tolerate even brief periods of feed deprivation. Nutritional support should be instituted immediately in animals with increased energy requirements or limited reserves (including foals). Nutritional support should be considered for any animal whose intake has been (or is expected to be) decreased for 48 h and must be instituted sooner rather than later to optimize patient outcome.

How much to feed

Energy requirements

The energy requirements of healthy horses are determined by age, lean body mass, activity level, gender, reproductive status, and ambient temperature. Maintenance Energy Requirements (MER) are defined as the energy required for zero body weight (BW) change during normal activity in non-working horses. Resting Energy Requirements (RER) are defined as the energy required to meet basal requirements plus the energy required for thermogenesis and are typically about 70% of maintenance requirements. Equations to calculate MER and RER for adult horses have been developed from metabolic studies (Table 23.1). Energy requirements of foals are considerably higher than those of adults; for example, the RER for foals are approximately twice that of mature horses

Table 23.1 Formulae and guidelines used to estimate energy and protein requirements for adult horses and foals.

Energy requirements	
Adult (Mcal/day)	
Resting*	0.975 + 0.021 (BW)
Maintenance	
Horses weighing 200–600 kg	1.4 + 0.03 (BW)
Horses weighing >600 kg	1.82 + 0.0383 (BW) $- 1.5 \times 10^{-5}$ (BW)[1]
Foal (kcal/kg/day)	
Resting[†]	45–50
Maintenance and growth[‡]	120–145
Protein requirements	
Adult (g/day)	
Maintenance	40 × MER
	1.26 × BW
Foals (g/kg/day)[§]	
Maintenance	2–3
Maintenance and growth	5–6

Nutritional programs should aim to provide resting energy requirements and maintenance protein requirements. Bodyweight is measured in kilograms (1 kg = 2.204 lb). Energy requirements may be expressed in Joules using the conversion factor of 4.184 (i.e., 1 cal is equivalent to 4.184 J). Note differences in units for adult and foal recommendations.
*Calculated from horses weighing between 125 and 856 kg.
[†]The RER were measured by indirect calorimetry in sedated foals.
[‡]Estimated from average milk intakes of foals.
[§]The exact protein requirements for healthy foals are unknown (see text for details). BW, body weight; MER, maintenance energy requirements; RER, resting energy requirements.

(Table 23.1). This increased energy requirement is largely related to rapid growth as foals increase their bodyweight by 1–4% daily during the first weeks of life and will consume between 120 and 150 kcal/kg of energy per day (Table 23.1).

Although some disease conditions (e.g., burns, neoplasia, and severe sepsis) increase energy requirements, severely ill patients frequently have decreased energy requirements, due in part to their decreased level of activity. Therefore, for most patients meeting RER is sufficient to prevent weight loss and protein catabolism. Furthermore, the provision of energy in excess of requirements can be as detrimental as providing insufficient energy. For these reasons, it is recommended to use RER for a starting point in nutritional support. It is critical to recognize that static calculations of energy requirements are an estimate and should only be used as a starting point. Adjustments in the amount of energy provided should be based on frequent and careful clinical monitoring of the patient.

Protein requirements

In contrast to energy, current recommendations call for the provision of maintenance levels of crude protein to patients receiving nutritional support to preserve endogenous proteins and optimize recovery. Estimates for maintenance of crude protein requirements for adults and foals are given in Table 23.1. The exact protein requirement for healthy foals is not known. Based on milk intake, growing, healthy foals will consume between 5 and 6 g/kg per day. For sick foals receiving parenteral nutrition, 2–3 g/kg per day has been suggested as a target and appears appropriate.

Enteral or parenteral nutrition

The provision of nutrition enterally rather than parenterally is physiologically more appropriate and less expensive.[4,11] Because the enterocytes obtain their nutrients from the gastrointestinal lumen rather than from the circulation, some level of enteral nutrition is important to maintain gastrointestinal integrity and function. As a result, enteral nutrition is preferred if the gastrointestinal tract is accessible and functional.

Enteral nutrition

Horses with a poor appetite should be offered a variety of feed stuffs to tempt them to eat. It is often more important to get these animals to eat something rather than becoming overly concerned with specific dietary requirements. Many horses with a poor appetite for hay or commercially prepared concentrates will readily consume fresh grass if it is offered or they are allowed to graze.

Animals that are completely inappetent but have a functional gastrointestinal tract can be fed liquid diets via a nasogastric tube.[4,10] Dysphagic horses (animals with pharyngeal dysfunction, foals with a poorly developed suck reflex) should also be fed via a nasogastric tube. If nasogastric intubation is not possible or practical, animals can be maintained with an esophageal feeding tube.

Guidelines for administration of enteral nutrition to adult horses

A nutritional program should initially aim to meet RER or ~70% of the patient's MER, and meals should be small and frequent (i.e., fed every 4–6 h).[4,10] Feeding should begin at ~25% of the final target nutritional allowance and gradually increased over 2–3 days. One to two cups of vegetable oil per day (~1.6 Mcal per cup or 240 mL) can be added to the diet if additional calories are required without increasing bulk. Note that supplemental fat should not be given to hyperlipemic animals. Supplemental feeding is gradually decreased once the patient begins to voluntarily consume food.

Blender diets

Liquid diets, which can be easily prepared from commercially produced pelleted rations, have the advantage of being readily available and inexpensive. Pellets designed as a complete feed should provide a nutritionally balanced meal and contain the fiber that is an important energy source for horses. While fiber is important for colonic health, it does make these diets slightly more difficult to administer and large diameter nasogastric tubes (5/8 in. external diameter or larger) are usually required. The quantity of feed provided is based on the caloric content of the specific feed used and should aim to meet RER or ~70% of MER. Individual meals should be softened in 2–3 L of water, pulverized in a blender and then made up to a final volume of 6–8 L for a full-sized adult horse. An example of a blender diet and its associated feeding regimen are given in Table 23.2.[4]

Compositional diets

Commercially available human liquid diets (e.g., Osmolite, Vital, or Jevity available from Abbott Nutrition, Columbus, OH) have been used for horses. These diets are expensive, provide insufficient protein, and do not contain fiber which often results in a self-limiting diarrhea. However, these diets are easily prepared and administered

Table 23.2   Example of a blender diet using a complete pelleted feed (Equine Senior available from Purina Mills, St. Louis, MO) and recommended tube feeding schedule for a 450 kg horse to provide approximately resting energy requirements (10.5 Mcal/day).

	Day			
	1	2	3	4
Percentage full allowance (%)	25	50	75	100
Pelleted feed (g)*	700	1400	2100	2900
Vegetable oil (mL)†	100	200	300	400
Digestible energy (Mcal)	2.6	5.1	7.7	10.5

The day's ration should be administered as four to six meals. The use of vegetable oil increases the caloric content without increasing bulk.
*Equine Senior (Purina Mills, St. Louis, MO) provides ~2.7 Mcal/kg.
†Vegetable oil contains ~0.67 Mcal/100 mL.
Source: Modified from Fascetti and Stratton-Phelps (2003).

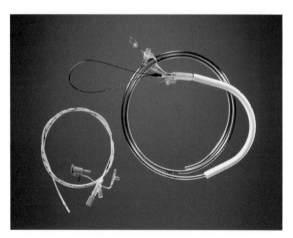

Figure 23.1   16 French (90 cm in length) and 14 French (125 cm in length) nasogastric tubes suitable for use as indwelling feeding tubes (MILA International, Inc., Florence, KY). Fluids and liquid diets are easily administered through these tubes and patients are able to eat and drink around them. The tubes are easily secured to the muzzle using tape or suture.
Source: Courtesy of MILA International, Inc., Florence, KY.

through small nasogastric tubes (12–18 French [4–6 mm internal diameter] 108–250 cm length available from MILA International, Inc., Florence, KY; Figure 23.1) that can be left in place as long as required. Although a slurry of alfalfa meal can be added to provide fiber, this will necessitate using a larger bore nasogastric tube. A liquid diet has been specifically developed for horses (Critical Care Meals available from MD's Choice Nutritional Products, Louisville, TN) and a "homemade"

compositional diet has also been designed for horses (Table 23.3).[10] Both of these diets can be tailored to meet individual patient's requirements and can be composed to provide a source of fiber.

Recently, Purina® Horse Feed has developed a a low-bulk, nutrient-dense powdered, complete nutritional supplement. WellSolve® Well-Gel®, is a palatable, concentrated source of nutrients with easily digestible protein, vitamins and minerals. WellSolve® Well-Gel® is fortified with glutamine, and provides 100% of NRC protein, vitamin and mineral requirements when fed as directed. It provides digestible fiber and is suitable for horses requiring a soluble carbohydrate-restricted diet. It can be given via a nasogastric tube, or fed as a slurry or as a dry top-dress supplement.

Special considerations for foals

Healthy young foals consume ~20–25% of their BW (10–13 L for a 50 kg foal) in milk daily. Although the volume relative to their BW decreases as they age, the absolute volume of milk ingested increases steadily and peaks at ~18 L per day around 3 months of age. Normal foals begin to consume small amounts of hard feed at about 10 days of age and this gradually increases to contribute a greater proportion to the foal's nutrition. Between 2 and 6 months of age, healthy foals consume 2.4–2.8% of their bodyweight in dry matter daily. In spite of these high dietary intakes, foals have limited reserves of energy and tolerate fasting poorly.

Table 23.3 Example of a liquid compositional diet developed for enteral feeding.

	Day						
	1	2	3	4	5	6	7
Water (L)	21	21	21	21	21	21	21
Electrolyte mix (g)*	230	230	230	230	230	230	230
Dextrose (g)	300	400	500	600	700	800	900
Caesin (g)†	300	450	600	750	900	900	900
Dehydrated alfalfa meal (g)	2000	2000	2000	2000	2000	2000	2000
Digestible energy (Mcal)	7.4	8.4	9.4	10.4	11.8	11.8	12.2

Each day's allowance should be divided and administered as four to six meals. Note that this diet will meet resting energy requirements for a 450 kg horse by day 4 and this is sufficient in most cases. Provision of energy in excess of resting energy requirements should be based on continued loss of weight or body condition.
*Composition of electrolyte mix: sodium chloride (NaCl) 10 g; sodium bicarbonate (NaHCO$_3$) 15 g; potassium chloride (KCl) 75 g; potassium phosphate (K$_2$HPO$_4$) 60 g; calcium chloride (CaCl$_2$) 45 g; magnesium oxide (MgO) 25 g.
†Casein (Sigma-Aldrich, St. Louis, MO) or edible acid casein-90 (American Casein Company, Burlington, NJ).
Source: Modified from Naylor et al. (1984).

Following colic surgery, foals that are still nursing can be allowed to nurse for 1–2 min every 2 h and muzzled between meals or separated from the mare. The length of time allowed for nursing is gradually increased as the foal improves clinically. Although this is easy and the most physiologically appropriate way to feed foals, it is obviously impossible to precisely regulate how much milk is ingested as hungry foals may gorge themselves. Milking the mare before nursing can limit this although it is not completely effective. If a more controlled approach is required, the foal should be fed small meals from a bottle or pan or via a nasogastric feeding tube.

When providing enteral nutrition to the foal following colic surgery, we recommend providing mare's milk or reconstituted mare's milk replacer at 3–5% of bodyweight (i.e., 1.5–2.5 L/day for a 50 kg foal) divided into small meals fed every 2 h (i.e., ~120–200 mL per meal). If two or three of these small meals are tolerated, the volume fed is then increased to 10% of bodyweight daily. For foals with mild gastrointestinal disease or that have been off feed for a limited time, feeding can usually be started at a higher rate (e.g., 10% of bodyweight). The rate at which the volume of milk fed is increased will depend on the clinical progression of the foal; the target daily allowance for young foals (<4–6 weeks of age) should be 20–25% of bodyweight. For older foals that have begun to consume hard feed and are tolerating milk meals, we recommend

feeding small, frequent meals of complete pelleted feeds designed for foals. The manufacturer's directions are used to guide the amount offered.

If mare's milk is not available, commercial milk replacers (e.g., Mare's Match, Land O'Lakes Animal Milk Products, Shoreview, MN; Mare's Milk Plus, Buckeye Nutrition, Dalton, OH; Foal Lac, PetAg, Inc., Hampshire, IL) can be used and fed at the same rates. Although very good, some of these products contain high concentrations of sodium and other electrolytes and occasionally may cause problems with water balance. Pasteurized cow's milk (2% fat with ~20 g of dextrose added per liter) has been used without any ill effects in foals up to a few weeks of age. Although goat's milk can be more difficult to locate, it is also well tolerated and does not require alteration.

An approach to enteral feeding in the adult horse after colic

There are no hard and fast rules on "refeeding" horses with gastrointestinal disease and individual veterinarians have preferences based on their clinical experiences. The need to meet the horse's energy requirements while avoiding further disruption of the gastrointestinal flora (i.e., overgrowth of bacteria such as Clostridium spp. and Salmonella spp.) must be balanced against providing sufficient time for the gastrointestinal tract to return to normal function.

For horses with nonstrangulating intestinal obstructions that have responded to medical management (e.g., impactions and spasmodic colic), clinical signs are used to determine when to begin refeeding. There should have been no signs of colic for at least 12 h and the horse should be passing feces before refeeding is initiated. If mineral oil has been administered, oil-coated feces should be observed within 24 h of administration. If an impaction has been diagnosed, resolution of the impaction should be monitored and confirmed by repeated examination per rectum. The type of feed to offer initially varies among clinicians and with the type of lesion. For impactions, particularly those of the small intestine (ileum) or small colon, many clinicians begin feeding small volumes of a low residue feed, such as fresh green grass or a complete pelleted meal. The quantity fed and interval between meals is then gradually increased to more closely resemble the horse's normal diet. This approach should be continued as long as the patient remains comfortable and continues to pass feces. If tolerated, horses can usually be returned to their normal diet over 2–3 days. It is important to remember that fecal production will decrease as a result of reduced feed intake but should not stop completely for prolonged periods.

Refeeding protocols for horses after abdominal surgery will depend on the portion of gastrointestinal tract involved and the surgical procedure performed. For horses with nonstrangulating gastrointestinal obstructions (i.e., large colon displacements or impactions), the approach to refeeding is similar to that used for horses with medically managed nonstrangulating obstructions. Generally, these horses can be offered feed within 12 h of recovery as long as they are comfortable and passing feces (fecal production will depend on the amount of ingesta remaining in the gastrointestinal tract after surgery). Although the type and quantity of feed offered are dependent on clinician preference and lesion location, beginning with frequent, small volume meals and increasing the volume offered relatively quickly (i.e., over 1–2 days) depending on the progression of the horse's clinical signs is well tolerated. Horses recovering from a large colon volvulus are often fed in a similar manner to those that had a nonstrangulating obstruction. In contrast, horses recovering from small intestinal strangulating obstructions are at an increased risk for postoperative ileus or

obstruction, and many clinicians prefer to withhold feed from these patients for 12 to 24 h and monitor for signs of colic and production of gastric reflux. If signs of ileus or obstruction do not develop (or have resolved), starting to refeed the horse with small volumes of a low residue diet (e.g., 250–500 g of a complete pelleted diet or limited grazing of fresh green grass) is effective. If this approach is tolerated, hay can be added, the amount of feed increased, and the frequency of meals decreased to return the horse to its routine diet over 2–3 days. Some horses do not tolerate hay postoperatively and develop signs of colic, reflux, and/or inappetence. This appears to be particularly true for horses that required a jejunocecostomy or have developed adhesions. These horses can often be maintained on a complete pelleted diet with access to fresh green pasture but not hay.

In horses with inflammatory disease of the gastrointestinal tract, refeeding is dependent upon the portion of the gastrointestinal tract involved. Horses with typhlitis, typhlocolitis, or colitis should be encouraged to eat throughout the course of the disease to promote enterocyte health and maintain bulk and fiber for fecal consistency. As noted above, a variety of feedstuffs should be offered to patients with decreased appetites. In horses with proximal enteritis, feed must be withheld until the small intestine regains normal function and gastric reflux ceases. Withholding feed for at least 12 h after gastric reflux has stopped and beginning refeeding with small amounts of a low residue diet (e.g., 250–500 g of a complete pelleted diet or limited grazing of fresh green grass) offered frequently (every 2–3 h) is recommended. If the horse tolerates refeeding (no signs of colic or gastric reflux), then changes can be made to return the horse to its normal diet over 2–3 days.

Parenteral nutrition

Intravenous (IV) or parenteral nutrition should be considered in: horses with gastrointestinal dysfunction in which a prolonged recovery is anticipated; horses with limited reserves or increased nutritional demands but limited ability to increase feed intake; horses in which the gastrointestinal tract is not easily accessible (e.g., pharyngeal or esophageal injury); and recumbent horses.[3,6]

Parenteral nutrition formulations aim to meet patients' nutrient requirements with combinations of carbohydrates (dextrose), lipids, and amino acids. Because enterocytes obtain their nutrients from the bowel lumen, animals receiving parenteral nutrition should also receive small enteral ("trophic") meals to help maintain normal gastrointestinal function if at all possible.[3,6]

Dextrose solutions

Dextrose administered at a rate of 2 mg/kg/min to an average sized horse (i.e., 5% dextrose solution at ~1 L/h) provides ~4 Mcal/day or 45% of RER. Many clinicians administer dextrose solutions to horses that have a decrease in nutritional intake but are not completely inappetent or those in which the decrease in nutritional intake is expected to be of short duration. However, administration of dextrose solutions alone might not be particularly protein-sparing, causing some authorities to question their value. Despite widespread use, there is no evidence that the administration of dextrose solutions alone alters outcome in equine patients. Many critically ill horses become hyperglycemic at even low rates of dextrose infusion and poorly regulated hyperglycemia is thought to be detrimental in human critical care patients. Therefore, blood glucose concentrations should be monitored closely and the rate of infusion altered or insulin administered as required to avoid hyperglycemia.[3,6]

Partial parenteral nutrition

The administration of dextrose and amino acid combinations is thought to better preserve endogenous protein than administration of dextrose alone. The use of dextrose/amino acid solutions avoids the complications associated with lipid administration and is less expensive than total parenteral nutrition formulations. In addition, commercially available combinations (e.g., Aminosyn II, Hospira, Lake Forest, IL; Travasol, Baxter Healthcare, Deerfield, IL) are packaged such that they are easily prepared sterilely without specialized facilities. These solutions are hypertonic (~1500 mOsmol/L for 5% amino acids/25% dextrose solutions) and should be administered into a large vein or concurrently with fluids. Dextrose/amino acid solutions should be administered at a rate that provides the desired

carbohydrate (energy) load. As with dextrose solutions, some horses might not tolerate high infusion rates initially and administration should begin at 25–50% of the final target rate. The infusion rate can then be increased gradually (e.g., by 25% of the final target allowance every 6–24 h) if blood glucose concentrations remain within normal limits.

Total parenteral nutrition

Total parenteral nutrition (TPN) formulations contain combinations of carbohydrate (dextrose), fat (lipid), and protein (amino acids) to meet energy and protein requirements.[3,6] Total parenteral nutrition formulations used in equine medicine have largely been adapted from human medicine. When the differences between the diets of horses and humans are considered, it is clear that these formulations may not be optimal for critically ill equine patients. Although there is very limited information supporting (or refuting) their benefit in equine medicine, TPN formulations appear to be well tolerated clinically. The components of TPN formulations are:

Carbohydrates (dextrose)
Dextrose should provide the majority (50–70%) of the nonprotein calories. The low caloric density of dextrose requires that concentrated solutions (50% dextrose) with correspondingly high osmolarities (2520 mOsmol/L) are used.

Lipids
Lipid is provided as emulsions of long-chain fatty acids derived from safflower, canola, or soybean oil. The addition of lipid to parenteral solutions increases caloric density, reduces osmolarity, and confers a metabolic advantage over the administration of dextrose alone. In most formulations, lipids provide 30–50% of nonprotein calories. Lipids should be used with caution in horses with hypertriglyceridemia or not at all in hyperlipemic patients.

Protein (amino acids)
Amino acids are provided as 8.5% or 10% solutions. The quantity of nitrogen (in grams) provided can be calculated by multiplying the weight of protein (in grams) by 0.16. This value can then be used to calculate the ratio of nonprotein calories (i.e., calories from dextrose and lipids) to nitrogen. The

ideal ratio of nonprotein calories to nitrogen (kcal:g) in equine patients is unknown; ratios of 120:1 to 150:1 have been suggested for healthy humans and lower ratios of 80:1 to 90:1 are recommended for critically ill humans. Ratios of approximately 100:1 appear to be well tolerated clinically in horses.

Vitamins and trace minerals

The vitamin and trace element requirements of critically ill adult horses and foals are not known. Multivitamin (e.g., Multi-Vitamin Infusion, Mayne Pharma, Paramus, NJ) and trace mineral (e.g., Multitrace-5 Concentrate, American Regent, Inc., Shirley, NY) mixtures are empirically added to parenteral nutrition formulations.

Composing parenteral nutrition formulations

Parenteral nutrition formulations should aim to meet RER and maintenance crude protein requirements.[3,6] Protein requirements should be calculated first and the remaining calories provided by a combination of dextrose and lipid. Alternatively, the entire energy requirement can be met with dextrose and lipid and the caloric contribution of the administered protein ignored. An example worksheet for a TPN formulation providing 70% of nonprotein calories with dextrose and 30% with lipid is given in Table 23.4. This formulation has a nonprotein calorie to nitrogen ratio of ~90:1. Examples of TPN formulations suggested by other authors for adult horses and foals are given in Table 23.5.

Guidelines for the preparation and administration of parenteral nutrition

Sterility is essential when preparing parental nutrition, and solutions should be mixed in a laminar flow hood. Dextrose solutions are acidic (pH 3.2–6.5) and hypertonic, which can cause destabilization of lipid emulsions. Therefore, the dextrose and amino acids should be mixed first and lipids added last. Parenteral nutrition formulations containing lipids can be prepared ahead of time if they are refrigerated, but should not be stored for longer than 24 h. If the lipid component of the solution separates and cannot be remixed, the solution should be discarded. Even with the addition of lipid emulsions, parenteral nutrition solutions are hypertonic and should be adminis-

Table 23.4   Example of a worksheet for a total parenteral formulation to meet resting energy and maintenance protein requirements for adult horses.

Bodyweight (kg)
  Maintenance crude protein requirements (g/day)
  1.26 (BW) (1)
  Resting energy requirements (kcal/day)
  975 + 21 (BW) (2)

Parenteral nutrition formulation
  Energy (kcal) supplied by protein (amino acids)*
  Protein (g) × 4 (kcal/g) (3)
  Energy (kcal) to be supplied by dextrose and lipid[†]
  Subtract value for (3) from (2) (4)
  Volume of amino acid solution required[‡]
  8.5% solution: protein (g)/0.085 (g/mL)
  10% solution: protein (g)/0.1 (g/mL)
  Volume (mL) of 50% dextrose required to provide 70% of calories (either value 2 or 4)[§]
  0.7 × ((Energy [kcal]/3.4 [kcal/g])/0.5 [g/mL])
  Volume (mL) of lipid solution required to provide 30% of calories (either value 2 or 4)**
  10% solution: 0.3 × ((Energy [kcal]/11 [kcal/g])/0.1 [g/mL])
  20% solution: 0.3 × ((Energy [kcal]/11 [kcal/g])/0.2 [g/mL])

This formulation provides 70% of the nonprotein calories with dextrose and 30% with lipid and has a nonprotein calorie to nitrogen ratio of ~90:1. If 10% lipid solutions are used, the final osmolarity is ~1200 mOsmol/L. Minerals and trace elements are added empirically to the final solution.
*Protein (or amino acids) provides 4 kcal/g of energy.
[†]This step can be left out if all calories are to be provided by dextrose and lipid and the caloric contribution of the administered protein is ignored.
[‡]An 8.5% amino acid solution provides 0.085 g/mL of protein; a 10% solution provides 0.1 g/mL.
[§]Each gram of carbohydrate (dextrose) provides 3.4 kcal of energy.
**A 10% lipid solution provides 0.1 g/mL of protein; a 20% solution provides 0.2 g/mL. Each gram of lipid provides 11 kcal of energy.

tered into a central vein in foals. Administration into the jugular vein appears to be well tolerated by adult horses.

Parenteral nutrition solutions, especially those containing lipid, should be administered via a dedicated port. Parenteral nutrition IV lines should not be used to administer medications or to collect blood samples. Long-term, multilumen catheters are preferred and reduce the possibility of incompatibilities among different medications. Strict attention to sterility is required when placing IV catheters for use with parenteral nutrition.

Table 23.5 Examples of parenteral nutrition formulations for adult horses (450 kg) and foals (50 kg) providing 24 h of nutrition when administered at target rate.

	Adults (450 kg)		Foals (50 kg)		
50% dextrose (mL) (% nonprotein calories)	2500 (53)	4500 (61)	1000 (76)	1000 (61)	1500 (61)
10% lipids (mL) (% nonprotein calories)*	3500 (47)	4500 (39)	500 (24)	1000 (39)	1500 (39)
10% amino acids (mL)[†]	6000	9000	1000	1500	1500
Osmolarity (mOsm/L)	1040.5	1134.3	1412.4	1172.3	1223.0
Protein (g) (nitrogen [g])[‡]	600 (96)	900 (144)	100 (16)	150 (24)	150 (24)
Nonprotein calorie:nitrogen (kcal:g)	84:1	88:1	140:1	116:1	175:1
Target rate (mL/h)[§]	500	750	104	146	188
Mcal/day**	10.5	16.2	2.7	3.4	4.8
kcal/kg/day**	23.3	36.0	53.0	68.0	96.0

*Available as Liposyn II, Hospira, Lake Forest, IL; or Intralipid, Baxter Healthcare, Deerfield, IL.
[†]Available as Aminosyn II, Hospira, Lake Forest, IL; or Travasol, Baxter Healthcare, Deerfield, IL.
[‡]One gram of amino acids contains 0.16 g of nitrogen.
[§]If no additional fluids added.
**Includes calories from amino acid solutions (calories from amino acids can be excluded if desired).

IV lines carrying parenteral nutrition are ideally changed every 24 h if the formulation includes lipid and every 72 h if dextrose/amino acid solutions are used. Lines should not be disconnected between changes, and gloves and masks should be worn whenever IV lines are handled. Inline filters (0.22 μm) should be used to remove particulate matter and microorganisms from dextrose/amino acid solutions. Because these filters can become clogged when used with lipid-containing solutions, 1.2 μm filters are recommended; however, the latter filters will not remove microorganisms.

Parenteral nutrition formulations should be administered by an infusion pump to ensure accurate delivery. Infusions should begin at 25–50% of the final calculated target rate and the rate increased by 25% every 6–24 h if the animal remains euglycemic and does not become markedly hypertriglyceridemic. The calculated target allowance should be exceeded only if there is continued loss of weight or body condition.

Complications associated with parenteral nutrition

The most serious complication associated with administration of parenteral nutrition is infection. Dextrose and amino acid solutions are a poor growth media for bacteria but can support fungi. In contrast, lipid emulsions are an excellent growth medium for both bacteria and fungi. However, the most commonly encountered complication with administration of parenteral nutrition is hyperglycemia. Hypertriglyceridemia is not uncommon and abnormalities in electrolyte, trace element, or vitamin concentrations can also occur. Abrupt discontinuation of IV dextrose administration can lead to a profound hypoglycemia because of increased endogenous insulin activity. Therefore, animals receiving TPN should be gradually weaned once they are voluntarily consuming sufficient feedstuffs to provide their RER.

Hyperglycemia
Many critically ill horses become hyperglycemic even at very low dextrose infusion rates. Euglycemia might also be difficult to maintain in horses with pre-existing insulin resistance (e.g., horses with Pituitary Pars Intermedia Dysfunction [Cushing's disease] or Equine Metabolic Syndrome). The risk of hyperglycemia is reduced by gradual introduction to parenteral nutrition. Although there is evidence in human medicine that hyperglycemia may be detrimental to outcome, mild hyperglycemia is probably acceptable in most equine patients provided that glucose concentrations do not exceed the renal threshold (~180–220 mg/dL). Hyperglycemia can be controlled by decreasing the rate of administration or dextrose content of the solution, although this obviously

decreases the energy delivered to the patient. Exogenous insulin can be administered to control hyperglycemia either as single injections of ultralente insulin (0.2–0.3 IU/kg SC every 12–24 h) or as a continuous infusion of regular insulin (0.002–0.02 IU/kg/h). Changes in dextrose and insulin infusion rates should be made incrementally and gradually to avoid large swings in plasma glucose concentrations.

Hypertriglyceridemia
Hypertriglyceridemia (serum triglyceride concentration >100 mg/dL) occurs in some patients, particularly neonates and those with severe sepsis. If persistent hyperlipemia occurs, the rate of administration or the lipid content of the solution can be decreased although this too will reduce the energy delivered to the patient. Administration of heparin (40 IU/kg SC every 12 h) increases lipoprotein lipase activity and might be of some benefit in controlling hypertriglyceridemia. Parenteral solutions containing lipids should probably not be administered to patients with existing hyperlipemia and hepatic lipidosis.

Electrolyte abnormalities
The most common electrolyte abnormality experienced by horses receiving parenteral nutrition is hypokalemia, but hypomagnesemia, hypocalemia, and hypophosphatemia are not uncommon. Hypophosphatemia can be potentiated by exogenous insulin therapy.

Monitoring

Careful and frequent monitoring is required to ensure the efficacy of a nutritional program and avoid complications. Monitoring bodyweight is probably the most efficacious way to monitor the adequacy of a nutrition program especially in foals. In the first weeks of life, healthy foals gain ~1–1.5 kg in bodyweight daily (and occasionally more). Daily weight gain then slows, averaging ~0.8 kg/day between 3 and 6 months of age and 0.7 kg/day between 6 and 9 months of age. Sick foals should not be expected to gain weight at these rates, even when they are provided with apparently adequate nutrition; however, it is important that sick foals do not lose weight. Adult horses should also be monitored closely to ensure that they are not losing weight.

Catheter sites should be checked at least twice daily for signs of swelling, heat or pain and the vein palpated carefully for indications of thrombosis. If there is any suggestion of infection, the catheter must be removed and replaced. Ideally, the catheter tip should be collected sterilely and cultured.

The following clinical pathology variables should also be checked frequently in animals receiving enteral or parenteral nutrition:

Plasma triglyceride concentrations
Animals in a negative energy balance become hyperlipidemic as endogenous lipids are metabolized for use as an energy source. It is especially important to measure plasma triglyceride concentrations in patients predisposed to hyperlipidemia (i.e., ponies, donkeys, and miniature breeds p. 287). Pregnancy and pituitary pars intermedia dysfunction (Equine Cushing's Disease) exacerbate insulin resistance and also increase the likelihood of developing hyperlipidemia. Septic animals frequently become hyperlipidemic when administered exogenous lipids, necessitating changes in their nutritional plan. We typically measure plasma triglyceride concentrations every 2–3 days in animals at risk for developing hyperlipidemia.

Blood or plasma glucose concentration
Although common in malnourished foals, hypoglycemia occurs infrequently in malnourished adults and euglycemia does not ensure that a nutritional program is adequate. Excessive or prolonged hyperglycemia (i.e., plasma glucose concentrations exceeding ~180–220 mg/dL) and glucosuria should be avoided in both foals and adults. Glucose concentrations should initially be measured frequently (i.e., every 2–6 h) in horses receiving dextrose infusions or insulin. Once the patient and glucose concentration stabilize, the frequency of measurement can be decreased to every 12–24 h.

Plasma electrolyte concentrations
Plasma concentrations of potassium, calcium, magnesium, and phosphorous should be checked frequently (i.e., every 24–72 h) in critically ill horses, particularly those receiving parenteral nutrition. Hypokalemia, hypocalcemia, and hypomagnesemia are commonly identified in animals held off feed for even relatively short periods. All of these electrolytes are easily

supplemented; however, it is important to avoid over supplementation. Hypophosphatemia is not uncommon in animals receiving parenteral nutrition and is well recognized in human patients that require exogenous insulin to control blood glucose concentrations.

Blood urea nitrogen

Measurement of blood urea nitrogen (BUN) concentration can provide some information regarding protein metabolism. In animals catabolizing endogenous proteins, BUN concentration can become increased in the face of a normal creatinine concentration. Increases in BUN concentration in animals receiving parenteral formulations containing amino acids might also indicate protein intolerance.

Long-term nutritional management of the postcolic patient

Once a horse has survived a bout of colic, whether or not surgical correction was necessary, the primary concern is always how to prevent a reoccurrence. It has been documented repeatedly that risk of colic is increased after the horse has experienced at least one episode, especially if the first episode required surgical correction.[2,5] A secondary concern, especially if surgical correction and resection was involved, is how the digestive capabilities of the horse might have been altered. Horses that have had gastrointestinal surgery also frequently suffer significant loss of weight and condition in the immediate postoperative period due to prolonged periods where oral intake was restricted or prohibited in addition to bouts of peritonitis. The increased metabolic rates recorded in other species after surgical intervention and/or septic events can cause rapid and severe catabolism and loss of muscle and fat masses. Though the exact metabolic changes are not yet documented scientifically in horses, the weight and muscle loss observed in other animals is commonly seen after colic surgery, especially those with complicated recoveries.

In this part of the chapter the general considerations for prevention of reoccurrence, digestive alterations, feeding recommendations, and refeeding strategies for weight gain will be discussed.

General considerations

It is important to carefully evaluate the precolic management and feeding practices to determine if there were any of the established risk factors (Table 23.6) for spasmodic/gas and impaction colic[2] present that could be modified or eliminated. Recent changes in environment, feed or hay, lack of exercise (in a stall 12–24 h per day), inadequate water access/intake, inadequate forage intake (<1.0–1.5% BW per day), poor quality forages, excessive grain-based concentrate intakes are all associated with an increased risk of abdominal malaise, especially in sensitive horses or if in combinations (i.e., stalled horses fed poor quality hay, high grain rations). In one epidemiological study[7] of the 50 horses that had access to round bales of hay, 31 had developed colic. Horses maintained on good quality pastures and/or with free access to good quality hay, salt, and water with minimal amounts of grain-based concentrates and other supplements will have the lowest risk of colic.

Changes in environment and diet frequently cannot be avoided, and many horses cannot be given free access to pasture or turnout on a regular basis. Horses given an abrupt feed change from grass hay to grass silage or grass haylage from the same crop did not have any adverse changes in their colonic ecosystem during the first 28 h but adjustments in the colonic bacterial populations were observed over the next 3 weeks.[9] If abrupt changes in the feed type or quantity must be made, care must be taken to minimize stress as much as possible and to monitor the horse's intake and fecal output carefully for at least 2 weeks. If feed intakes must be restricted for whatever reason it is important to divide the total daily intake into as many small, frequent feedings as possible to avoid fasts longer than 3–4 h.

If it is not possible provide regular exercise and free access to forages, at least insure intake of a minimum of 20 g of forage per kg BW per day.[1] This would be a *minimum* of 10 kg hay for a 500 kg horse. Individual meals of high starch feeds (grains and sweet feeds) are recommended not to exceed 3 g of concentrate/kg BW (1.5 kg per meal for a 500 kg horse). Obviously many horses have been regularly fed amounts of grain-based concentrates that exceed this recommendation without adverse

Table 23.6   Dietary and management risk factors for colic and potential solutions.

Documented risk factor[2]	Potential solutions
Recent change in diet	Slowly introduce new feeds to sensitive horses over the course of 3 or 4 days, adding <25% of the total to eventually be fed at a time
Inadequate access to water	If possible provide free access to unfrozen water at all times, especially in stalls. Use of a single water bucket filled only twice a day is often inadequate and automatic waterers need to be checked regularly for malfunction
Inadequate voluntary intake of water	Soak feeds in water, add small amounts of salt (2–3 oz) to feeds (not the water bucket), add flavoring to water (apple juice, grape juice, peppermint oil, etc.)
Recent change in type of hay	Slowly introduce new hay to sensitive horses over the course of 3–4 days, adding <25% of the total to eventually be fed at a time
Recent change in housing/location	When moving to a new location try to bring along sufficient hay/feed/water from "home" for at least 2 or 3 days. Monitor feed and water intakes and manure production carefully for the first week
Lack of access to pasture or forage	If at all possible maximize the time the horse is turned out on pasture or drylot with hay feeders. If it is not possible to provide regular exercise and free access to forages at least insure intake of a minimum of 20 g of forage per kg BW per day (Coenen et al. 2011)
Nontraditional hays/round bales	Use of Sudan grass, sorghum, red-top cane, peanut, haygrazer hay, and access to round bales were associated with increased risk of colic. These should be avoided in colic-prone horses
>2.6 kg oats/day	Feed only as much grain-based concentrate as necessary to maintain good body condition and limit individual high starch meals to <3 g/kg BW
Toxic plant ingestion	Check hay and pastures (including perimeter trees and shrubs)

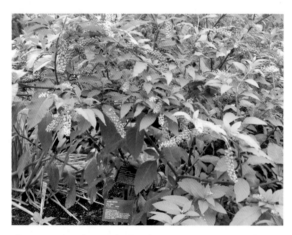

Figure 23.2   Pokeweed (*Phytolacca americana*). Cornell University School of Veterinary Medicine Toxic Plant Garden. Source: Photo by Sarah Ralston.

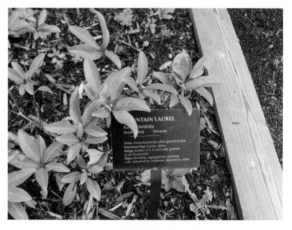

Figure 23.3   Mountain laurel (*Kalmia latifolia*). Cornell University School of Veterinary Medicine Toxic Plant Garden. Source: Photo by Sarah Ralston.

consequences but in colic-prone horses it is prudent to be more conservative.

Horses usually avoid ingesting toxic plants, however if weeds are incorporated into hay, or there is inadequate forage available, horses may eat them. It is always important to check hay and

pastures for the plants that will cause colic if ingested in sufficient quantities. Pokeweed (*Phytolacca americana*) (Figure 23.2), Moutain Laurel (*Kalmia latifolia*) (Figure 23.3), field bindweed (Morning glory) (*Convolvulus arvensis* spp.) (Figure 23.4), Castor oil plant (*Ricinus communis*)

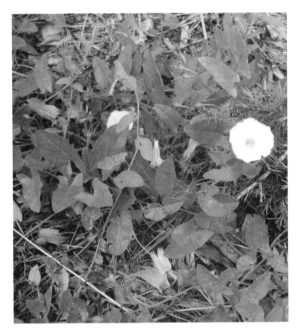

Figure 23.4 Bindweed (Morning glory) (*Convolvulus arvensis*)
Source: Photo by Sarah Ralston.

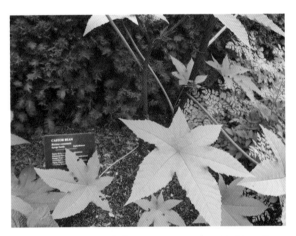

Figure 23.5 Castor oil plant (*Ricinus communis*). Cornell University School of Veterinary Medicine Toxic Plant Garden.
Source: Photo by Sarah Ralston.

are present it is important to look for evidence that they might have been "tasted."

In horses prone to impaction colic the key is to maintain optimal gastrointestinal hydration and avoid excessively coarse hay (i.e., overly mature Coastal Bermuda). However, feeding large quantities (>1% BW) of highly digestible pelleted or textured concentrates will decrease voluntary water intake and can also lead to impactions[12]. Again, offering good quality forages free choice with free access to unfrozen water and salt and as much turnout as possible is the best recommendation. If inadequate voluntary water intake is a concern, salt (NaCl 60–120 g/day) can be added to the ration. If excessive amounts are added, however, salt may decrease voluntary intake of feed so the amounts need to be adjusted to the individual horse's preference. Adding preferred flavors, such as apple or grape juice or peppermint oils to water buckets, especially during and after transport to a new location, can also entice finicky horses to drink more water. Though horses prefer, if given a choice, to drink cold water, they will actually consume more warm (>7°C) water if it is the only choice. Contrary to popular belief, wheat bran is not laxative. The traditional benefits associated with regular feedings of bran mashes were due to the water content of the mash and not the bran itself. Soaking any of the feeds offered to the horse in water, especially shredded beet pulp, will help increase intake without unbalancing mineral nutrition. Recommending daily bran mashes will only serve to put the horse at risk of nutritional secondary hyperparathyroidism due to the high phosphorus content of bran.

Postsurgical colic long-term concerns

If no intestine was resected or the horse had only a typhlectomy or resection of <50% of the small or large intestines, there are no significant nutritional changes needed once the horse has recovered fully from the surgery.[13] If chronic diarrhea is present after the first week or two, the use of probiotic/prebiotic formulations may be warranted. However few, if any, have been proven scientifically to result on "normal" fermentative activity in the colon and many contain bacterial species not native to the horse. Live yeast culture

(Figure 23.5), Jimson weed, potato or tomato plants (*Solanaceae* spp.), Oak trees (*Quercus* spp.), horse chestnut and buckeye trees (*Aesculus* spp.), and curly dock (*Rumex* spp.) are common culprits. Horses have been known to develop acquired preference for weeds such as pokeweed. If these

(*Saccharomyces* spp.) supplementation, however, has been reported to have small but significant benefit to horses switched from high fiber to high starch rations.[8] Some studies have reported that use of probiotics in horses with normal feces (indicative of normal colonic function) may actually disrupt the bacterial/protozoal populations. It is not recommended that postcolic horses with normal fecal output be given probiotics. Similarly, if the small intestine was the site of the initial insult probiotics/prebiotics will not provide any digestive benefits to this site. An old but also unverified technique to restore colonic microbial populations is to dose the affected horse via nasogastric tube with "fecal tea," a slurry of fresh feces obtained by rectal grab from a healthy horse known to be free of disease or intestinal parasites. Recent work from France has shown that significant numbers of bacterial delivered intragastrically will survive passage to the large intestine.

If >50% of the large colons were removed, the horse will require higher than maintenance protein and phosphorus, decreased fiber intake, and possibly increased B-vitamins.[13] The large colons do contribute significantly to protein balance under normal circumstances and are the primary site of phosphorus absorption/reabsorption. Alfalfa or alfalfa/grass mix hay is the forage of choice but should be offered in limited quantities initially (1–1.5% BW divided into three or more feedings). Pelleted or extruded feeds formulated to be fed without hay ("complete feeds") are the best choice if the horse does not tolerate being fed hay. Most of the "complete" formulations are not high calories, because they are designed to be fed in relatively large amounts (1.5–2.0% BW per day). The total amount offered in a single day should be divided into at least 3, preferably more feedings to maximize digestive efficiency. If weight loss is a problem adding a high protein (>16%)/higher fat (>7%) supplement may help. These horses need higher quality proteins, such as alfalfa or soybean meal sources. Edible oils can be used for added calories, since the ileum is still intact for fat absorption. A mixture of 0.25 kg wheat bran (for protein and phosphorus) with 0.5 kg dry beet pulp (for the calcium) soaked in water and fed three times a day might help in horses that do not tolerate long stem hays due to

adhesions or strictures. It could be fed before or after feeding the concentrates.

Major small intestinal resection (>60%) is best managed by avoidance of large amounts of grain. High quality legume hay and beet pulp-based complete feeds are recommended, placing the emphasis on digestion and absorption in the large intestines. If the ileum is intact, edible oils may be used to increase caloric intake but should be introduced slowly and no more than 100–200 mL per feeding.

Ileal bypass/resection will dictate the need for increased fat-soluble vitamins A and E, and perhaps K (only if bleeding problems develop) since it is the primary site of fat absorption. There also will be an increased need for calcium since the ileum is also the primary site of absorption for that mineral. High fat feeds and edible oils should not be included in the ration. Good quality alfalfa or alfalfa/grass mix hays should be the primary component of the ration with grain-based, low fat extruded or pelleted feeds added as needed for weight gain or maintenance. Synthetic water-soluble forms of Vitamin E and A may be necessary for long-term maintenance. If evidence of A and/or E deficits develop (recurrent infections and/or rhabdomyolysis, ocular defects, reproductive failure, etc.) periodic parenteral administration of these normally fat-soluble vitamins may be necessary. It is advisable to monitor blood concentrations of A and E on a monthly or every 2 month schedule.

Postoperative weight gain

Giving free access to alfalfa or alfalfa/grass mix hay or hay cubes (introduced slowly as above) will usually optimize gain in condition without need for extra supplements, if tolerated by the horse. However if consumption of alfalfa or legume hays results in diarrhea or recurrence of abdominal malaise, another source of good quality protein and calories will be needed in addition to good quality grass hay/pasture. Pelleted or extruded feeds designed for young, growing horses are optimally suited for encouraging weight gain in the postsurgical horse. If extra calories are needed to add weight/condition, the use of edible oils (e.g., soybean, corn, or safflower) is indicated if the horse has normal hepatic and digestive function. Fats or edible oils, however, should not exceed 10% of the total caloric intake per day (<350 mL per 500 kg horse per day divided into at least two feedings).

References

1. Coenen, M., Kienzle, E., Vervuert, I. & Zeyner, A. (2011) Recent German developments in the formulation of energy and nutrient requirements of horses and the resulting feeding recommendations. *Journal of Equine Veterinary Science*, **31**, 219–229.
2. Cohen, N., Gibbs, P. & Wods, A.M. (1999) Dietary and other management factors associated with colic in horses. *Journal of the American Veterinary Medical Association*, **215**, 53–60.
3. Dunkel, B.M. & Wilkins, P.A. (2004) Nutrition and the critically ill horse. *Veterinary Clinics of North America: Equine Practice*, **20**, 107–126.
4. Fascetti, A.J. & Stratton-Phelps, M. (2003) Clinical assessment of nutritional status and enteral feeding in the acutely ill horse. In: *Current Therapies in Equine Medicine 5* (ed. N.E. Edward Robinson), pp. 705–710. Saunders, Philadelphia, Pennsylvania.
5. Goncalves, S., Julliand, V. & Leblond, A. (2002) Risk factors associated with colic in horses. *Veterinary Research*, **33**, 641–652.
6. Hardy, J. (2003) Nutritional support and nursing care of the adult horse in intensive care. *Clinical Techniques in Equine Practice*, **2**, 193–198.
7. Hudson, J.M., Cohen, N.D., Gibbs, P. & Thompson, J.A. (2001) Feeding practices associated with colic in horses. *Journal of the American Veterinary Medical Association*, **219**, 1419–1425.
8. Jouany, J.-P., Medina, B., Bertin, G. & Julliand, V. (2009) Effect of live yeast culture supplementation on hindgut microbial communities and their polysaccharidase and glycoside hydrolase activities in horses fed a high-fiber or high-starch diet. *Journal of Animal Science*, **87**, 2844–2852.
9. Muhonen, S., Julliand, V., Lindberg, J.E., Bertilsson, J. & Jansson, A. (2009) Effects on the equine colon ecosystem of grass silage and haylage diets after an abrupt change from hay. *Journal of Animal Science*, **87**, 2291–2298.
10. Naylor, J.M., Freeman, D.E. & Kronfield, D.S. (1984) Alimentation of hypophagic horses. *Compendium on Continuing Education for the Practicing Veterinarian*, **6**, S93–S99.
11. Paradis, M.R. (2003) Nutritional support: Enteral and parenteral. *Clinical Techniques in Equine Practice*, **2**, 87–95.
12. Ralston, S. (1992) Regulation of feed intake in the horse in relation to gastrointestinal disease. *Pferdeheilkunde* (1st European Conference on Horse Nutrition), 15–18.
13. Ralston, S.L. (1997) Nutrition of horses before and after surgery. In: *The Veterinarian's Practical Reference to Equine Nutrition* (ed K.N. Thompson), pp. 131–134. Purina Mills and American Association of Equine Practitioners, St. Louis, Missouri.

24 Gastrointestinal Parasitology and Anthelmintics

Louise L. Southwood

Department of Clinical Studies, New Bolton Center, School of Veterinary Medicine, University of Pennsylvania, Kennett Square, PA, USA

Chapter Outline

Gastrointestinal parasitology	**316**	*Parascaris equorum*	**321**
Anoplocephala perfoliata	**318**	Definition	321
Definition	318	Life cycle	321
Life cycle	318	Pathology and clinical disease	322
Pathology and clinical disease	318	Diagnosis and management	322
Diagnosis and management	319	*Strongylus vulgaris*	**322**
Cyathostomes	**320**	Definition	322
Definition	320	Life cycle	322
Life cycle	320	Pathology and clinical disease	323
Pathology and clinical disease	320	Diagnosis and management	323
Diagnosis and management	320	**Anthelmintics**	**323**

Gastrointestinal parasitology

Equine species are hosts to numerous gastrointestinal parasites. The most importantly recognized when considering colic are *Anoplocephala perfoliata*, cyathostomes/cyathostomins, *Parascaris equorum*, and *Strongylus vulgaris*. The association between colic and gastrointestinal parasites is constantly up for debate. While it is generally accepted that small parasite burdens are unlikely to cause clinical disease, heavily parasitized horses can have intestinal damage leading to altered motility and signs of colic, weight loss, and colitis.[15] Causes of colic that have been associated with gastrointestinal parasitism include gas/spasmodic colic, colitis (p. 215), ileal and cecal impaction (p. 208, 214), ileocecal and cecocolic intussusceptions (p. 213, 214), and ascarid impaction (p. 208). While there are other parasites that infect the equine gastrointes-tinal tract (e.g., *Gasterophilus* spp. (bots can cause gastric irritation), *Oxyuris equi* (pinworms can cause perianal irritation and pruritus), and *Strongyloides westeri* (threadworm may cause diarrhea in neonates 10–14 days old)), these are generally not associated with gastrointestinal disease causing colic.

Recommendations for parasite control have changed recently with the continuing emergence of parasite resistance to many anthelmintic drugs.[5,6] Routine anthelmintic administration on a frequent and rotating schedule has been replaced with the recommendation to monitor fecal egg counts (FECs) and to perform regular fecal egg count reduction tests (FECRT) with a targeted selective deworming approach. A targeted selective deworming approach involves anthelmintic administration to horses with FEC above a certain threshold or those with evidence of parasitic disease.[17] Targeted selective treatment is *not* recommended for yearlings or foals as these animal should be dewormed routinely.[17] One concern is the lack of association between the numbers of strongyle eggs shed in the feces and the magnitude of the strongyle infection, which may mean that heavy undetected parasite burdens could lead to clinical disease in an individual horse. However, if the goal is to minimize pasture contamination, FECs may be a good indication of the need for individual anthelmintic treatment. Parasite control programs need to optimize the balance between preventing disease in the individual animal and providing a sustainable parasite management program for the herd and farm.

FECs are based on various modifications of the McMaster, Stoll, and Wisconsin techniques.[17] These techniques use a counting chamber which enables a known volume of fecal suspension (known weight of feces and a known volume of flotation fluid) to be examined microscopically allowing the number of eggs per gram of feces (EPG) to be calculated.[17] Flotation fluids are based on solutions of zinc or magnesium sulfate, sodium chloride, and/or sugars (e.g., sucrose). Passive flotation and flotation obtained by centrifugation are used.[17] The technique is varied slightly to increase the specificity for different parasites. Commercially available kits obtainable online may help reduce the expense of FEC monitoring to owners/managers of large farms. Using composite or group samples

from animals of the same age group as well as identifying horses that are high and low egg shedders and targeting deworming programs toward these horses may also be used to optimize parasite management programs without them being financially prohibitive.[17] Parasites detected with a plain FEC include strongyle eggs, *P. equorum*, *Strongyloides westeri*, *Eimeria leuckarti*, *O. equi* (occasional), and *A. perfoliata* (occasional). Serological methods have been developed for *A. perfoliata*.[17] Larval culture is used for species differentiation of strongyle eggs.[17] FECRT are considered the gold standard for detecting anthelmintic resistance with a fecal egg count reduction <90% being diagnostic for resistance.[17] A minimum of six horses should be evaluated, with FEC performed at the time of treatment and then 14 days posttreatment. FECRT can be labor intensive. Alternatively, FECs can be performed 2 weeks posttreatment with the persistence of parasite eggs prompting a more involved FECRT.

Pasture management is also advocated: pasture hygiene performed weekly or biweekly, mixed or alternate grazing with ruminants, mid-summer movement, and pasture rotation in warm climates.[17] Dose and move strategies are controversial because they can decrease the size of the parasite refugium (i.e., parasites not exposed to the anthelmintic) on the fresh pasture which may contribute to anthelmintic resistance.

There are several features of parasite control programs that can contribute to resistance. A high frequency of anthelmintic administration is efficacious in the short term but not sustainable because of the development of anthelmintic resistance, particularly if the dosing interval is shorter than the prepatent period for the parasite which leads to the subsequent parasite generation being resistant.[14] Frequent dosing may also impair the ability of young horses to mount an acquired immune response.[16] Frequent drug rotations can contribute to the development of anthelmintic resistance; however, annual drug class rotation may be effective for a sustainable parasite control program particularly if formulated for an individual farm.[17] Underestimation of body weight and subsequent use of an insufficient anthelmintic dose is an important cause of anthelmintic resistance. Use of a girth tape to estimate body weight is advocated and when treating a large herd dose should be based on the heaviest horse.[17] Anthelmintic drugs formulated for horses should be used according to the manufacturer's directions.[17] Pharmacokinetics of formulations for other species may not be appropriate for the horse and can contribute to anthelmintic resistance.[17] Despite the apparent importance of anthelmintic resistance, outbreaks of clinical disease associated with resistant parasites have not to date been reported.[8,17]

In order to prevent complications with possible parasite-associated colic, it is recommended to deworm several weeks ahead of an elective surgery and in cases of emergency surgery, deworming should be delayed until the horse has returned to their normal diet and gastrointestinal function (2–4 weeks).[17]

Anoplocephala perfoliata

Definition

Three species of cestodes (flatworms or tapeworms), namely, *A. perfoliata* (cecal tapeworm), *A. magna* (largest tapeworm, distal small intestine), and *Paranoplocephala mamillana* (smallest tapeworm, proximal small intestine), can be found in horses in the United States. *A. perfoliata* is the most common tapeworm in the horse and it has been associated with causes of colic localized to the ileocecal region.

Life cycle

A. perfoliata has an indirect life cycle that involves the oribatid mite as an intermediate host. The infected mite is ingested by grazing horses. The cysticercoid from the infected mite develops into an adult tapeworm in the equine intestine (prepatent period 2–4 months). Adult tapeworms have a scolex (head) for attachment to the intestinal mucosa and strobila (body) composed of proglottids (segments) which are either mature with reproductive organs or gravid and containing eggs. Gravid proglottids and embryonated eggs are passed into the feces and on to the pasture. Eggs are ingested by the oribatid mite with laval tapeworm (cysticercoid) development in the body cavity of the mite which is found on the pasture especially in warm humid weather.[24]

Pathology and clinical disease

A. perfoliata attaches to the cecal mucosa near the ileocecal valve.[24] The presence of large numbers of the parasite causes mucosal ulceration, pseudomembranous formation, local inflammation that may be transmural, and development of fibrous connective tissue.[24] A significant relationship between parasite burden and mucosal/submucosal injury has been shown in conjunction with hypertrophy of the circular muscle layer and injury to the enteric nervous system with moderate to high parasite burdens.[19] Injury to the enteric nervous system included degenerative-regressive changes in the neuronal cells and a decrease in the number of myenteric ganglia and neuronal cells.[19] The local effect of the tapeworms is thought to alter motility in the ileocecal area and impair movement of ingesta from the distal small intestine into the cecum. Colic associated with *A. perfoliata* has included tympanic colic, ileal impaction (p. 208), ileocecal (p. 213) and cecocolic intussusception (p. 214), cecal impaction (p. 214), and cecal perforation (p. 215).[2,8,18,20,21,23,26,32]

A serological assay (see below) was used as part of a colic-outbreak investigation where a strong association between tapeworm infection and colic with evidence of a dose–response relationship was observed. Treatment with anticestode anthelmintics led to a decrease in the incidence of colic and a fall in antibody levels.[21] The study showed that the risk of ileal impaction colic and spasmodic colic increases with tapeworm infection intensity.[21] In another study,[23] cases of spasmodic colic were much more likely to be associated with *A. perfoliata* infection detected coprologically than controls (odds ratio [OR] 8) and based on serological diagnosis an increase in intensity of infection correlated with an increased risk of colic; 22% of spasmodic colic cases were estimated to be tapeworm-associated. No significant association was found between colic and strongyle egg counts.[23] Similarly, a strong association between ileal impaction and *A. perfoliata* was diagnosed using coprological (OR 34) and serological (OR 26) methods; 81% of the horses with ileal impaction were estimated to be tapeworm-associated.[23] These studies are supported by clinical observational studies.[2,8,18,26,32]

Table 24.1   Anthelmintics used in the management of equine gastrointestinal parasites.

Anthelmintic drug	Commercial products	Mechanism of action	Regimen
Ivermectin (avermectin)	Zimecterin®, Meriel Zimecterin® Gold, Meriel* Equimax®, Bimeda† Eqvalan®, Meriel	Macrolytic lactones (avermectins and milbemycins) interfere with GABA-mediated neurotransmission, causing paralysis and death of the parasite	200 µg/kg once Ineffective against cestodes and encysted cyathostomes
Moxidectin (milbemycin)	Quest®, Fort Dodge Quest® Plus, Fort Dodge‡	See above	400 µg/kg once Ineffective against cestodes
Praziquantel	Zimecterin® Gold, Meriel* Equimax®, Bimeda† Quest® Plus, Fort Dodge‡	Mostly unknown but may increase permeability of tapeworm cell membranes to calcium causing paralysis in the contracted state with the parasites being destroyed by the host immune system. Likely impairs the function of mucosal attachment	Deworming for tapeworms should be based on egg counts and horses dosed at 1 mg/kg once
Fenbendazole	Panacur PowerPak®, Intervet Safeguard®, Merck	Benzimidazoles bind to the beta tubulin subunit and interfere with microtubule formation, essential for energy metabolism	10 mg/kg once
Oxibendazole	Anthelcide EQ, Pfizer	See above	10 mg/kg once
Pyrantel pamoate	Strongid®, Pfizer Various generics	Tetrahydropyrimidines, nicotinic agonists, mimic the activity of acetylcholine, initiating muscular contraction. The parasite is unable to feed and quickly starves. Tetrahydropyrimidines only affect adult populations of worms	6.6 mg/kg once
Pyrantel tartrate	Strongid C®, Pfizer Continuex 2X, Farnam	See above	2.64 mg/kg daily
Piperazine	Variable generics	Agonist effects upon the inhibitory GABA (γ-aminobutyric acid) receptor paralyzing parasites, which allows the host body to easily expel the parasite	88 mg/kg once

*Zimecterin® Gold—ivermectin 1.55% and praziquantel 7.75% w/v.
†Equimax®—ivermectin 1.87% and praziquantel 14.03% w/v.
‡Quest® Plus—moxidectin 2% and praziquantel 12.5% w/v.

Diagnosis and management

A targeted deworming program is recommended. Serological tests for detecting tapeworm infection have been developed based on the IgG(T) subtype antibody response to the 12/13 kDa component of the parasite excretory/secretory (E/S) antigen which is positively correlated with parasite intensity.[22] These tests are available in Europe and have not gained widespread use in the United States. The assay is useful at a group level, but with the high variability it is not reliable for diagnosis in a specific horse.[22] The practical application of the anti-12/13 kDa IgG(T) ELISA was demonstrated in a colic-outbreak investigation.[21] High false positive results, however, have been reported.[7] Horses can be antibody positive for up to 5 months posttreatment and a lack of specificity for A. perfoliata has been identified.[17] A fecal egg count using a semiquantitative centrifugation/flotation technique whereby feces mixed with tap water are filtered through gauze and centrifuged then the pellet re-suspended in flotation fluid (saturated saline and 50% glucose) was more reliable for evaluation of an individual horse for targeted deworming.[7]

Praziquantel is 100% effective against *A. perfoliata* at a dose rate ≥1 mg/kg[28,29] and pyrantel pamoate at 13.2 mg/kg is >95% effective (Table 24.1).[25] Tapeworms are usually passed in the feces within 48 h treatment.[28,29] Ivermectin and moxidectin are *not* effective against cestodes. The most common management program involves two treatments per year; however, the optimal seasonal timing has not yet been determined and should be based on FEC and tailored to the needs of each farm.[24]

Cyathostomes

Definition

Cyathostomes, or small strongyles, are nematode gastrointestinal parasites. There are reportedly over 50 species of small strongyles; however, about 10 species are considered important in horses.[9] The role of cyathostomes in equine gastrointestinal disease has become more apparent with the decline in disease associated with the large strongyles particularly *S. vulgaris* (p. 322). Their importance lies in their high prevalence in the equine population, pathogenicity, and anthelmintic resistance.

Life cycle

Cyathostomins have a five-stage, direct life cycle (i.e., there is no intermediate host). Horses become infected via ingestion of infective third-stage larvae (L3) which enter the mucosa and submucosa of the large intestine. The L3 develop through several encysted stages (early L3, late L3, and developing fourth-stage larvae [L4]). The L4 emerge into the intestinal lumen and develop into fifth-stage larvae (L5) or adult male and female worms. The adult worms reside in the large intestine and produce eggs which are passed in the horse's feces onto the pasture. An embryo develops in the egg to the first larval stage (L1) prior to hatching. Development is optimal under warm moist conditions and can be inhibited by extreme heat or cold, dry conditions, and sunlight. Embryonated eggs and L3 are more resistant to environmental conditions than are L1 and L2.[9] Once hatched, the larvae develops to L2 and then the ensheathed infective L3.[9,15] The prepatent period is 6–12 months; however, it can be longer when development of encysted larvae in the intestinal wall is inhibited.[15] The most favorable environmental conditions for development are spring and fall in northern temperate areas and the winter in warmer, subtropical regions.[9]

Pathology and clinical disease

Clinical disease associated with cyathostomins is thought to be caused by sudden eruption of large numbers of encysted larvae from the intestinal mucosa into the lumen. The sudden eruption can cause extensive damage to the intestinal mucosa causing signs of colic, weight loss, colitis (diarrhea and pyrexia), and even sudden death.[9] Ventral edema, hypoalbuminemia, and leukocytosis may also be observed. The clinical syndrome is referred to as larval cyathostominosis and typically occurs in winter or early spring and is more common in younger animals.[9,12] Aged ponies have also been observed to have episodes of recurrent diarrhea and weight loss.[13] The cause for emergence of encysted larvae is essentially unknown and may include alterations in the host immune response, anthelmintic administration possibly associated with removal of luminal stages triggering release of encysted cyathostomes, as well as seasonal and dietary changes.[9] Diarrhea has also been associated with mucosal penetration by infective L3 strongyles and the presence of encysted larvae may also cause alterations in intestinal motility.[9]

Diagnosis and management

The goal of management is to minimize the parasite burden and prevent disease. Complete elimination of the parasite may be detrimental because (1) failure of the host to develop an acquired immune response could result in more serious clinical disease, and (2) the parasite refugium (including encysted larvae) is thought to be important for preventing anthelmintic resistance.

Pasture management and anthelmintic treatment are strategies used to control cyathostomes. When designing a management plan, consideration of the individual animal needs to be weighed against the sustainability of the plan with respect to the development of anthelmintic resistance.

The goal of pasture management is to destroy embryonated eggs and larvae. Pasture management includes harrowing and mowing to expose eggs and larva to sunlight and desiccation, rotation, alternating pastures with ruminants, removal of fecal material, and composting straw and feces prior to applying to the pasture.[9]

Anthelmintic drugs used for cyathostomes include benzimidazoles (fenbendazole, oxbendazole), macrocyclic lactones (ivermectin, moxidectin), piperazine, and pyrantel (Table 24.1).[24] Anthelmintic resistance is a problem. There is a high prevalence of resistance to benzimidazoles and resistance to pyrantel and ivermectin has been documented.[10,31] Cyathostomes are sensitive to moxidectin and resistance has not been reported. Multidrug resistance of cyathostomes to fenbendazole, pyrantel, and ivermectin has been observed on one farm.[31] Treatment with fenbendazole at 10 mg/kg for 5 days or moxidectin at 400 μg/kg is currently efficacious against encysted larvae.[9] Ivermectin even at a high dose rate is ineffective against encysted larvae. Moxidectin had >90% efficacy against ascarids, cyathostomes, strongyles, bots, and larval pinworms.[3] Rotation of anthelmintics is controversial with respect to whether rotation between drug classes should occur with each treatment or the same drug class used for several consecutive treatments.[9] Strategic use of drugs on a seasonal basis (spring and autumn) is recommended over treating all horses every 6–8 weeks.[9] A reduction in the egg reappearance interval, particularly in foals, is considered the first indication of cyathostome resistance.[17]

Strongyle FECs have a high degree of variation due to an uneven distribution in the feces and there is a poor correlation between parasite burden and FEC. Therefore, some animals could have a high parasite burden and be at risk for clinical disease with little evidence based on the FEC.[17] There is currently no method to detect encysted cyathostome larvae.[15] Serological tests are being developed and investigated to identify the encysted cyathostome larvae but are not yet available.[15,17] However,

consistency in level of shedding in individual horses over time indicates that some adult horses require fewer prophylactic treatments than other horses to prevent pasture contamination. FEC are more reliable during the grazing season because encysted larvae accumulate over the autumn and winter and adult female worms shed fewer eggs in the nongrazing season.[17]

The parasite refugium is considered important for prevention of anthelmintic resistance. Free-living stages on the pasture are a major part of the refugium as are encysted cyathostomins when treated with nonlarvicidal anthelmintics. However, treatment against encysted larvae with moxidectin and a 5 day course of fenbendazole may decrease the parasite refugium and contribute to the development of anthelmintic resistance and should be taken into consideration when managing cyathostome infection on a farm.[17]

Parascaris equorum

Definition

P. equorum is the large round worm in the horse. Adult worms are ~4 mm in diameter and 10–50 cm long.[26] A heavy burden may involve several hundred ascarids.

Life cycle

P. equorum has a direct life cycle with a free-living and parasitic phase. Ascarid infections are acquired through ingestion of larvated eggs from the environment. The eggs hatch in the small intestine and the larvae enter the portal circulation and are carried to the liver. Following intrahepatic migration (1 week), the larvae reenter the circulation and travel to the lungs. The larvae leave the circulation, penetrate the alveoli, travel up the bronchial tree, and are swallowed. Once in the small intestine, the larvae molt into adults in the duodenum and proximal jejunum. Eggs are observed in the feces 75–80 days postinfection (prepatent period).[24] Acquired immunity to *P. equorum* is excellent in horses with infections being limited to young foals, weanlings, and yearlings and rarely a horse >2 years old.[24]

Pathology and clinical disease

Large ascarid burdens can cause impaction (p. 208). Jejunal volvulus (p. 212), intussusceptions (p. 213), abscessation, and rupture can also be associated with intestinal ascarids.[4,30] Ascarid impaction is typically observed in foals, median age at presentation 5 (range 3–24) months.[4,30] Foals are more likely to present in autumn with colic associated with *P. equorum* infection than in any other season which is likely a reflection of the age of the foal at this time of the year. Recent deworming is often associated with signs of colic caused by an ascarid impaction.[4,30] Foals typically present with mild to severe signs of colic, nasogastric reflux often with ascarids is obtained, and distended loops of jejunum may be palpated per rectum or observed sonographically. It is important to note that ascarids are not typically seen on abdominal sonographic examination. Peritoneal fluid may be serosanguinous. A tentative diagnosis is made based on the age and clinical features and identification of ascarids in the reflux or feces. A definitive diagnosis is made at surgery or necropsy. Ascarid impactions can be managed medically or surgically. The short-term prognosis for survival is reported to be 50–64% and long-term prognosis 10–25%.[4,30]

Note that *P. equorum* infection is also associated with lethargy, inappetence, decreased weight gain, hypoproteinaemia, coughing, and nasal discharge in young horses associated with the migratory phase of the life cycle.

Diagnosis and management

Ascarid impaction is a serious cause of colic making prevention of ascariasis important. Resistance to ivermectin and moxidectin has been reported. Anthelmintics that have been used against *P. equorum* include fenbendazole, oxibendazole, ivermectin, moxidectin, pyrantel pamoate, pyrantel tartrate, and piperazine (Table 24.1). Resistance to macrocyclic lactones as well as pyrantel pamoate have been observed.[24] Efficacies (average) for foals ranged for fenbendazole (10 mg/kg) from 50% to 100% (80%), for oxibendazole (10 mg/kg) from 75% to 100% (97%), and for pyrantel pamoate at 1× (6.6 mg/kg) from 0% to 71% (2%) and at 2× (13.2 mg/kg) 0% to 0% (0%). A significant reduction

of ascarid infections for fenbendazole and oxibendazole was observed but not for pyrantel pamoate.[11] Moxidectin had >90% efficacy against ascarids, cyathostomes, strongyles, bots, and larval pinworms.[3]

FECs in mares and foals should be monitored. Routine anthelmintic treatment of foals should begin no earlier than 60–70 days of age and treatment repeated at the greatest interval that minimized environmental contamination with ascarid eggs.[24] Treatment every 60 days is the maximum dosing interval for ascarid control and may not prevent environmental contamination; however, more frequent treatment increases selection pressure for anthelmintic resistance.[24] Monitoring drug efficacy on individual farms at least annually is strongly recommended. Stabling for a few days after treatment for *P. equorum* may help prevent recontamination of a clean pasture.[17] Pasture management (see above) in addition to steam cleaning of the stalls is advocated.

Benzimidazoles are thought to be the least likely group of anthelmintics to cause ascarid-impaction colic if a foal has a heavy parasite burden.[1] Benzimidazoles starve ascarids by interfering with synthesis of β-tubulin, and have a slower mode of action than anthelmintics such as ivermectin and pyrantel pamoate that work on neuromuscular transmission (Table 24.1). Therefore, foals suspected of having a heavy ascarid burden (i.e., no previous deworming history, high *P. equorum* egg counts, and abdominal enlargement) should be dewormed with fenbendazole.[3,24,30] Careful monitoring for signs of colic and concurrent administration of mineral oil via a nasogastric tube is also recommended for heavily parasitized foals.

Strongylus vulgaris

Definition

S. vulgaris is the best-known large strongyle or large red worm.[24]

Life cycle

S. vulgaris has a direct life cycle. Infection with *S. vulgaris* occurs when horses ingest infective L3 from the environment. The larvae pass through the stomach, exsheath, and invade the small intestinal mucosa where they molt to L4. The L4 penetrate local arterioles, burrow into the tunica intima, and migrate to the cranial mesenteric artery, which is the site of greatest larval accumulation and pathology. The larvae reside in the cranial mesenteric artery for 4 months where they mature into the L5 stage. The L5 migrate through the vasculature back to the cecum where they form submucosal nodules which eventually rupture after which the parasites return to the intestinal tract as young adults. The young adults mature into sexually mature adults over ~6 weeks and begin to shed eggs. The prepatent period is 6–7 months.[24]

Pathology and clinical disease

The presence of L4/L5 in the cranial mesenteric artery causes a verminous arteritis with the formation of extensive thrombi within the lumen, hypertrophy of the tunica media, and cranial mesenteric artery enlargement. Activation of coagulation and platelet aggregation occur as a result of the presence of the L4/L5. Chemical mediators of vasoconstriction and alterations of intestinal motility have also been proposed as causes of colic associated with S. vulgaris.[27,33,34]

Cranial mesenteric artery enlargement may be detected on palpation per rectum in small horses and arteritis diagnosed sonographically in some cases. Serological tests for S. vulgaris thus far have had considerable cross-reactivity with other nematodes and a lack of specificity. A poymerase chain reaction (PCR) technique for the identification of S. vulgaris DNA in blood is being investigated.[17,24]

Cranial mesenteric arteritis may be associated with chronic intermittent colic. Thromboembolic colic can occur when thrombi from the cranial mesenteric artery occlude the arterial supply to the intestine. Intestinal ischemia causes severe signs of colic pain and horses rapidly develop signs of shock. While segmental ischemic necrosis may be manageable with intestinal resection, often there is extensive ischemia necessitating euthanasia.

Diagnosis and management

Large strongyles have been eradicated from most well-managed farms. Treatment with fenbendazole,

ivermectin, or moxidectin is effective against strongyle larvae and adults (Table 24.1). Nemocidal activity may take up to 5 weeks. Anthelmintic resistance has not been observed. Because the prepatent period is 6 months, patent S. vulgaris infections resulting in pasture contamination would not be observed for 6 months after treatment. Therefore, treatment every 6 months should completely prevent pasture contamination. The maximum duration of survival of infective larval stages in the environment is ~12 months. Therefore, no source of reinfection would exist with the implementation of this regimen for 18+ months.[17,24] Naïve hosts, however, may be extremely sensitive to the presence of S. vulgaris.[17,24]

Anthelmintics

Frequently used anthelmintics against common equine gastrointestinal parasites, their mechanisms of action, and recommended dose rate are included in Table 24.1. Quizzes for each chapter, additional clinical scenarios, and video demonstrations of surgical procedures are available online at www.wiley.com/go/southwood.

References

1. Austin, S.M., DiPietro, J.A. & Foreman, J.H. (1990) *Parascaris equorum* infections in horses. *Compendium on Continuing Education for the Practicing Veterinarian*, **12**, 1110–1119.
2. Barclay, W.P., Phillips, T.N. & Foerner, J.J. (1982) Intussusception associated with *Anoplocephala perfoliata* infection in five horses. *Journal of American Veterinary Medical Research*, **180**, 752–753.
3. Cleale, R.M., Edmonds, J.D., Paul, A.J., et al. (2006) A multicenter evaluation of the effectiveness of Quest® Gel (2% moxidectin) against parasites infecting equids. *Veterinary Parasites*, **137**, 119–129.
4. Cribb, N.C., Cote, N.M., Bouré, L.P. & Peregrine, A.S. (2006) Acute small intestinal obstruction associated with *Parascaris equorum* infection in young horses: 25 cases (1985–2004). *New Zealand Veterinary Journal*, **54**, 338–343.
5. Kaplan, R.M. (2002) Anthelmintic resistance in nematodes of horses. *Veterinary Research*, **33**, 491–507.
6. Kaplan, R.M., Klei, T.R., Lyons, E.T., et al. (2004) Prevalence of anthelmintic resistant cyathostomes on horse farms. *Journal of the American Veterinary Medical Association*, **225**, 903–910.
7. Kjaer, L.N., Lungholt, M.M., Nielsen, M.K., Olsen, S.N. & Maddox-Hyttel, C. (2007) Interpretation of serum

antibody response to *Anoplocephala perfoliata* in relation to parasite burden and faecal egg count. *Equine Veterinary Journal*, **39**, 529–533.

8. Little, D. & Blikslager, A.T. (2002) Factors associated with development of ileal impaction in horses with surgical colic: 78 cases (1986–2000). *Equine Veterinary Journal*, **34**, 464–468.

9. Lyons, E.T., Drudge, J.H. & Tolliver, S.C. (2000) Larval cyathostomiasis. *Veterinary Clinics of North America: Equine Practice*, **16**, 501–513.

10. Lyons, E.T., Tolliver, S.C. & Collins, S.S. (2009) Probable reason why small strongyle EPG counts are returning "early" after ivermectin treatment of horses on a farm in Central Kentucky. *Parasitology Research*, **104**, 569–574.

11. Lyons, E.T., Tolliver, S.C., Kuzmina, T.A. & Collins, S.S. (2011) Further evaluation in field tests of the activity of three anthelmintics (fenbendazole, oxibendazole, and pyrantel pamoate) against the ascarid *Parascaris equorum* in horse foals on eight farms in Central Kentucky (2009–2010). *Parasitology Research*, **109**, 1193–1197.

12. Mair, T.S. (1993) Recurrent diarrhea in aged ponies associated with larval cyathostomiasis. *Equine Veterinary Journal*, **25**, 161–163.

13. Mair, T.S. (1994) Outbreak of larval cyathostomiasis among a group of yearling and two-year-old horses. *Veterinary Record*, **135**, 598–600.

14. Matthee, S. & McGeoch, M.A. (2004) Helminths in horses: use of selective treatment for the control of strongyles. *Journal of the South African Veterinary Association*, **75**, 129–136.

15. Matthews, J.B. (2011) Review article: HBLB's advances in equine veterinary science and practice. *Equine Veterinary Journal*, **43**, 126–132.

16. Monahan, C.M., Chapman, M.R., Taylor, H.W., French, D.D. & Klei, T.R. (1997) Foals raised on pasture with or without daily pyrantel tartrate feed additive: Comparison of parasite burdens and host responses following experimental challenge with large and small strongyle larvae. *Veterinary Parasitology*, **73**, 277–289.

17. Nielsen, M.K., Fritzen, B., Duncan, J.L., *et al.* (2010) Practical aspects of equine parasite control: A review based upon a workshop discussion consensus. *Equine Veterinary Journal*, **42**, 460–468.

18. Owen, R., Jagger, D.W. & Quan-Taylor, R. (1989) Caecal intussusceptions in horses and the significance of *Anoplocephala perfoliata*. *Veterinary Record*, **124**, 34–37.

19. Pavone, S., Veronesi, F., Genchi, C., Fioretti, D.P., Brianti, E. & Mandara, M.T. (2011) Pathological changes caused by *Anoplocephala perfoliata* in the mucosa/submucosa and in the enteric nervous system of equine ileocecal junction. *Veterinary Parasitology*, **176**, 43–52.

20. Proudman, C. & Edwards, G. (1993) Are tapeworms associated with equine colic? A case control study. *Equine Veterinary Journal*, **25**, 224–226.

21. Proudman, C.J. & Holdstock, N.B. (2000) Investigation of an outbreak of tapeworm-associated colic in a training yard. *Equine Veterinary Journal Supplements*, **32**, 37–41.

22. Proudman, C.J. & Trees, A.J. (1996) Correlation of antigen specific IgG and IgG(T) responses with *Anoplocephala perfoliata* infection intensity in the horse. *Parasite Immunology*, **18**, 499–506.

23. Proudman, C., French, N.P. & Trees, A.J. (1998) Tapeworm infection is a significant risk factor for spasmodic colic and ileal impaction colic in the horse. *Equine Veterinary Journal*, **30**, 194–199.

24. Reinemeyer, C.R. & Nielsen, M.K. (2009) Parasitism and colic. *Veterinary Clinics of North America: Equine Practice*, **25**, 233–245.

25. Reinemeyer, C.R., Hutchens, D.E., Eckblad, W.P., Marchiondo, A.A. & Shugart, J.I. (2006) Dose-confirmation studies of the cestocidal activity of pyrantel pamoate paste in horses. *Veterinary Parasitology*, **138**, 234–239.

26. Roberts, C.T. & Slone, D.E. (2000) Caecal impactions managed surgically by typhlotomy in 10 cases (1988–1998). *Equine Veterinary Journal Supplements*, **32**, 74–76.

27. Sellers, A.F., Lowe, J.E., Drost, C.J., Rendano, V.T., Georgi, J.R. & Roberts, M.C. (1982) Retropulsion-propulsion in equine large colon. *American Journal of Veterinary Research*, **43**, 390–396.

28. Slocombe, J.O.D. (2006) A modified critical test and its use in two dose titration trials to assess efficacy of praziquantel for *Anoplocephala perfoliata* in equids. *Veterinary Parasitology*, **136**, 127–135.

29. Slocombe, J.O., Heine, J., Barutzki, D. & Slacek, B. (2007) Clinical trials of efficacy of praziquantel horse paste 9% against tapeworms and its safety in horses. *Veterinary Parasitology*, **144**, 366–370.

30. Southwood, L.L., Ragle, C.A., Snyder, J.R. & Hendrickson, D.A. (1996) Surgical treatment of ascarid impactions in horses and foals. *Proceedings of the American Association of Equine Practitioners*, **54**, 338–343.

31. Traversa, D., von Samson-Himmelstjerna, G., Demeler, J., *et al.* (2009) Anthelmintic resistance in cyathostomin populations from horses yards in Italy, UK and Germany. *Parasites and Vectors*, **2**, S2.

32. Trotz-Williams, L., Physick-Sheard, P., McFarlane, H., Pearl, D.L., Martin, S.W. & Peregrine, A.S. (2008) Occurrence of *Anoplocephala perfoliata* infection in horses in Ontario, Canada and association with colic and management practices. *Veterinary Parasitology*, **153**, 73–84.

33. White, N.A. (1981) Intestinal infarction associated with mesenteric vascular thrombotic disease in the horse. *Journal of the American Veterinary Medical Association*, **178**, 259–262.

34. Wright, A.I. (1972) Verminous arteritis as a cause of colic in the horse. *Equine Veterinary Journal*, **4**, 169.

Appendix A

Clinical Scenarios

Quizzes for each chapter, additional clinical scenarios, and video demonstrations of surgical procedures are available online at www.wiley.com/go/southwood.

Clinical scenario 1

Signalment: 10 year old Thoroughbred gelding
Presenting complaint: Colic

History: The horse had been observed to lie down more than normal during the previous 24–36 h and had been slow to come into the stall to be fed. On careful questioning of the owner, the horse had never been observed to paw, roll, flank stare, or kick at his abdomen during this period of illness.

Pertinent admission physical examination and laboratory findings: The horse was recumbent, unable to stand, and had an abnormal mentation. Unfortunately the horse was sedated prior to examination making assessment of colic versus neurological signs difficult to discern. had a marked tachycardia (80 beats/min), dark pink oral mucous membranes; packed cell volume (PCV) 64%, total plasma protein (TPP) 5.6 g/dL, peripheral leukocyte count 2900 cells/μL, and marked hyperammonemia (370 μmol/L).

Differential diagnoses: Acute colitis (p. 215), gastrointestinal perforation (p. 171), large colon volvulus (p. 220), neurological disease

Management: Abdominal sonographic examination revealed a markedly thickened large colon. A tentative diagnosis of severe acute colitis with secondary intestinal hyperammonemic encephalopathy was made. The horse was euthanized for financial reasons. Necropsy confirmed the diagnosis of severe acute colitis of unknown etiology.

Comment: The lack of clinical signs specific for colic in this case made typical causes of colic such as a strangulating obstruction less likely and were more consistent with acute colitis. Laboratory data supported the diagnosis of colitis (relative hypoproteinemia and leucopenia). Sonographic evidence of a thick large colon (≥9 mm) is not necessarily specific for large colon volvulus. Recumbent horses should be carefully examined prior to sedation to obtain an accurate representation of the clinical signs being shown.

Clinical scenario 2

Signalment: Yearling Standardbred colt
Presenting complaint: Colic

History: The yearling had a 3 h history of colic that was unresponsive to treatment with flunixin meglumine. He had a 1 month history of mild intermittent colic (three episodes) which was responsive to treatment with flunixin meglumine. The farm has a history of high fecal egg counts for *Anoplocephala perfoliata* and does not treat horses

Practical Guide to Equine Colic, First Edition. Edited by Louise L. Southwood.
© 2013 John Wiley & Sons, Inc. Published 2013 by John Wiley & Sons, Inc.

with praziquantel tartrate or pyrantel pamoate prior to 1 year of age.

Pertinent admission physical examination findings: Persistent mild signs of colic, mild tachycardia (56 beats/min), decreased intestinal borborygmi, and distended and thickened small intestine on palpation per rectum.

Tentative diagnosis: Ileocecal intussusception (p. 213)

Management: Exploratory celiotomy confirmed the diagnosis of ileocecal intussusception. The 4 cm intussusception was nonreducible and an ileocecostomy was performed to completely bypass the obstruction. The yearling recovered well from surgery and recommendations were made regarding management of tapeworm burdens in young horses.

Comment: The tentative diagnosis of ileocecal intussusception was made based on the signalment and history of intermittent colic episodes. The tentative diagnosis was supported by the parasite management history and palpation per rectum findings. Horses with chronic ileocecal intussusception often have thickened small intestine due to muscular hypertrophy associated with the long-standing partial obstruction.

Clinical scenario 3

Signalment: 4 year old Warmblood gelding

Presenting complaint: Colic

History: The horse had been showing mild to moderate signs of colic for 6 h that had become unresponsive to treatment with flunixin meglumine and xylazine/butorphanol. He had sustained a puncture wound to the sole of his hoof and had been confined to a stall and treated with trimethoprim sulfa and phenylbutazone for 7 days prior to presentation. He also had a history of being surgically treated for a NSLE 2 years prior to presentation.

Pertinent admission physical examination findings: Palpation per rectum findings were consistent with a NSLE. Other physical examination and laboratory findings were unremarkable.

Tentative diagnosis: NSLE (p. 219)

Management: Treatment with phenylephrine hydrochloride was unsuccessful. Exploratory celiotomy confirmed the diagnosis of NSLE. There

was also an omental adhesion to the previous pelvic flexure enterotomy site. The horse recovered well and ablation of the nephrosplenic space via a standing laparoscopic approach recommended to prevent reentrapment.

Comment: The history of previous NSLE and recent stall confinement were useful in forming a tentative diagnosis which was supported by the findings on palpation per rectum. Sonographic evaluation of the nephrosplenic area could have been used to confirm the diagnosis but was deemed unnecessary because of the convincing findings on palpation per rectum, primarily the identification of the caudal pole of the left kidney with the caudodorsal border of the spleen palpated ventrally and slightly displaced from the left body wall and large colon entrapped between the kidney and the caudodorsal border of the spleen.

Clinical scenario 4

Signalment: 12 year old Thoroughbred broodmare

Presenting complaint: Colic

History: Colic of unknown duration.

Pertinent admission physical examination and laboratory findings: Severe signs of colic; bright and alert; heart rate 60 beats/min; extremity temperature within normal limits; jugular refill and pulse quality very good; PCV 61%, TPP 7.8 g/dL; plasma lactate concentration 8.2 mmol/L; plasma creatinine concentration 2.2 mg/dL; plasma glucose concentration 139 mg/dL.

Tentative diagnosis: Large colon volvulus (p. 220)

Management: The diagnosis of a large colon volvulus was confirmed at surgery and the colon derotated and a pelvic flexure enterotomy performed. The mare had no postoperative complications and was discharged 72 h post admission.

Comment: Despite the laboratory values indicating a less than favorable prognosis, physical examination findings (extremity temperature, jugular refill, pulse quality) in this case were more indicative of cardiovascular status and predictive of outcome. The case also exemplifies the importance of monitoring multiple indices as well as trends over time and the benefit of exploratory celiotomy to determine prognosis.

Clinical scenario 5

Signalment: 14 year old Missouri Fox Trotter mare

Presenting complaint: Colic/pelvic flexure impaction

History: 24 h history of colic, with a possible pelvic flexure impaction identified on palpation per rectum.

Pertinent admission physical examination and laboratory findings: Quiet and alert, heart rate 56 beats/min, respiratory rate 40 breaths/min, rectal temperature 101.5°F; palpation per rectum pelvic flexure impaction; no nasogastric reflux (NGR); hyperlactatemia (5.9 mmol/L); plasma creatinine concentration 3.7 mg/dL; hyperglycemia (391 mg/dL); hypochloremia (88 mmol/L).

Tentative diagnosis: Pelvic flexure impaction (p. 217)

Management: Because the horse's demeanor, tachycardia, tachypnea, and laboratory findings (plasma creatinine, glucose, and chloride concentration) were not consistent with a pelvic flexure impaction, abdominal sonographic examination and abdominocentesis was performed revealing distended loops of small intestine and serosanguinous peritoneal fluid with a high nucleated cell count (11 000/μL) and total protein (TP) (4.8 g/dL) and lactate concentration (14 mmol/L). Exploratory celiotomy revealed an epiploic foramen entrapment (p. 211) and a resection and jejunoileostomy was performed. The horses developed postoperative ileus that responded to medical treatment with erythromycin and was discharged 11 days postoperatively and doing well at long-term follow-up.

Comment: Physical examination findings and laboratory data which are inconsistent with the tentative diagnosis should prompt further diagnostic tests. The impacted pelvic flexure was secondary to sequestration of fluid in the proximal gastrointestinal tract associated with the strangulation and is more consistent with dried out ingesta than a true impaction.

Clinical scenario 6

Signalment: 2 year old Thoroughbred filly

Presenting complaint: Colic

History: Colic of several hours duration that was unresponsive to treatment with analgesia drugs.

Pertinent admission physical examination and laboratory findings: Mild signs of colic at admission, no abdominal distention, heart rate 40 beats/min, and intestinal borborygmi within normal limits; palpation per rectum revealed a pelvic flexure impaction with a small amount of feces in the rectum. Limited laboratory data was performed (PCV, TPP, plasma lactate concentration) and was within normal limits.

Diagnosis: Pelvic flexure impaction (p. 217)

Management: Oral water and electrolytes (4–5 L every 2 h) were given. Pain was managed using intravenous (IV) firocoxib and sedation with IV xylazine as needed. The filly became increasingly painful. An IV catheter was placed for drug administration and IV fluids were given at a maintenance rate. Despite the severity and persistence of pain, she had no abdominal distention, continued to pass feces, had good intestinal borborygmi, and did not develop reflux. She responded to treatment over about 36–48 h and was discharged from the hospital.

Comment: Horses with a large colon impaction can become moderately painful but if they are not developing abdominal distention based on abdominal contour and palpation per rectum, have good intestinal borborygmi, and are passing even a small amount of feces, medical management can be pursued. The filly may not have needed IV fluids; however, placement of an IV catheter did facilitate administration of analgesic drugs. Surgery for correction of large colon impaction following administration of large volumes of fluid for several days is challenging and can result in colonic rupture. Surgery, however, is indicated for horses that do not appear to be responding to medical treatment (i.e., absent intestinal borborygmi, no fecal output, abdominal/colonic distention) or when a displacement or volvulus occurs as a complication.

Clinical scenario 7

Signalment: 14 year old Thoroughbred cross gelding

Presenting complaint: Colic

History: Mild persistent colic signs of 24 h duration.

Pertinent admission physical examination and laboratory findings: Sweating, muscle fasciculation, reluctant to ambulate, weak, injected sclera, pale purple oral mucous membranes, cool extremities, poor jugular refill, pulse not palpable, tachypnea, and tachycardia. Several loops of distended small intestine were identified on palpation per rectum and a floating sensation typical of positive pressure within the peritoneal cavity was appreciated. PCV 65%, TPP 6 g/dL; severe hyperlactatemia (14 mmol/L); and peripheral leukocyte count 500/µL. Peritoneal fluid brown with large numbers of bacteria.

Tentative diagnosis: Gastrointestinal perforation (p. 171)

Management: Euthanasia. No necropsy was performed.

Comment: The horse presented with classic signs of gastrointestinal perforation. Minimal laboratory data was performed for economical reasons but the profound leucopenia is typical of horses with septic peritonitis secondary to gastrointestinal perforation. The hyperlactatemia and high PCV with a relative hypoproteinemia are also typical for a horse with gastrointestinal rupture and indicate a poor prognosis. Sonographic evaluation could also have been performed to confirm the diagnosis.

Clinical scenario 8

Signalment: 7 year old Quarter Horse gelding

Presenting complaint: Colic

History: Acute colic then dull mentation, inappetence, 8 L NGR.

Pertinent admission physical examination and laboratory findings: Not painful, heart rate 40 beats/min, capillary refill time (CRT) >3 s; duodenal distention on palpation per rectum; 8 L NGR; PCV 49%, TPP 6.8 g/dL; mild hyperlactatemia (2.2 mmol/L), plasma creatinine concentration 2.2 mg/dL; moderate hyperglycemia (224 mg/dL); hyponatremia/hypochloremia; nonsegmented neutrophils identified. Peritoneal fluid was red tinged with 101 000 cells/µL, TP 4.6 g/dL, and lactate concentration 6.1 mmol/L.

Differential diagnoses: Proximal enteritis (p. 207), strangulating small intestinal obstruction (p. 209), septic peritonitis (p. 169), neoplasia (p. 223)

Management: Abdominal sonographic examination was unremarkable. The horse was treated with IV polyionic isotonic fluids and IV potassium

penicillin and gentamicin. NGR ceased shortly after hospital admission. The horse responded well to medical treatment, and was discharged from the hospital 4 days following admission. One year later the horse was doing well.

Comment: Care needs to be taken with interpretation of laboratory values particularly peritoneal fluid analysis. More information is needed on peritoneal fluid lactate concentration in horses with peritonitis/enteritis. Abdominal sonographic evaluation was useful for deciding to pursue medical treatment. Careful monitoring of the patient's response to medical management provides substantial information with regard to the need for surgical treatment.

Clinical scenario 9

Signalment: 10 year old Thoroughbred broodmare

Presenting Complaint: Colic

History: Colic 3 days postpartum.

Pertinent admission physical examination and laboratory findings: Dull mentation, heart rate 48 beats/min, rectal temperature 100.1°F, intestinal borborygmi reduced; 1 L NGR; PCV 49%, TPP 7.4 g/dL, peripheral leukocyte count 13 000/µL, fibrinogen concentration 617 mg/dL. Peritoneal fluid orange and cloudy with 130 600 nucleated cells/µL and TP 6 g/dL.

Tentative diagnosis: Septic peritonitis (p. 169) secondary to uterine or intestinal injury

Management: An exploratory celiotomy was pursued and was within normal limits. The mare drained large volumes of fluid from the celiotomy incision immediately postoperatively necessitating drain placement. She recovered well without further complications and was doing well at long-term follow-up.

Comment: Clinical features consistent with horses with septic peritonitis that will respond to medical management include an absence of colic signs, normal or improving intestinal borborygmi, normal feces, NGR <2 L, and yellow-orange peritoneal fluid. In retrospect, the mare should have been monitored for several hours to determine the response to therapy and surgery may have been avoided. Horses with peritonitis with moderate-severe pain, fever, absent intestinal borborygmi, lack of fecal output, and distended small intestine are likely to have a concurrent lesion and surgery is recommended. Abdominal sonographic evaluation may have facilitated patient evaluation and decision-making in this case.

Clinical scenario 10

Signalment: 2 year old Thoroughbred colt

Presenting complaint: Colic

History: Colic with 10 L NGR.

Pertinent admission physical examination and laboratory findings: No signs of colic, heart rate 52 beats/min, rectal temperature 101.9°F; 10 L NGR; distended small intestine on palpation per rectum. PCV 53%, TPP 8.2 g/dL; peripheral leukocyte count 12 740/μL; plasma creatinine concentration 3.2 mg/dL, hyperglycemia (215 mg/dL), and hypochloremia (90 mmol/L).

Differential diagnoses: Proximal enteritis (p. 207), strangulating or nonstrangulating small intestinal obstruction (p. 208–213)

Management: Treatment for proximal enteritis was pursued because of the lack of colic signs, mild fever, and large volumes of NGR and included IV polyionic isotonic fluids, flunixin meglumine, polymyxin B, metronidazole, plasma, IV lidocaine, sucralfate, prophylactic cooling of hooves for laminitis prevention, and frequent gastric decompression. Abdominal sonography was performed and revealed minimal anechoic fluid, multiple loops of small intestine with abnormal motility. Abdominocentesis was attempted but the spleen was punctured. The horse did not show signs of colic. The NGR was positive for clostridium toxins. The horse continued to reflux ~100 L/day for 2–3 days.

Because of the large volumes of reflux, an exploratory celiotomy was recommended. A jejunal stricture associated with an omental adhesion was identified and resection of the affected intestinal and jejunojejunostomy was performed. Unfortunately the horse succumbed to salmonellosis during the postoperative period.

Comment: The horse had typical signs of proximal enteritis and the case highlights the usefulness of surgery as a diagnostic as well as a therapeutic tool. The minimal peritoneal fluid identified sonographically placed a strangulating intestinal obstruction lower on the differential diagnosis list.

Appendix B

Drug Dosages used in the Equine Colic Patient

Practical Guide to Equine Colic, First Edition. Edited by Louise L. Southwood.
© 2013 John Wiley & Sons, Inc. Published 2013 by John Wiley & Sons, Inc.

Table B.1 Drug dosages used in the equine colic patient.

Drug	Use	Complications	Dose rate	Amount 500 kg horse[a] typically used
Acepromazine	Alpha-1 adrenergic antagonist Sedation Motility stimulant	Vasodilation causing hypotension; avoid in shock or with hemorrhage	0.02–0.06 mg/kg IV or 0.03–0.1 mg/kg IM 0.01 mg/kg IM q4–6 h (motility)	10–30 mg (1–3 mL) IV 15–50 mg (1.5–5 mL) IM 5 mg (0.5 mL) IM q4–6 h
Acetylcysteine	Retention enema for meconium impaction in neonates		200 mL of 4% solution; 40 mL of 20% solution with 160 mL warm water*	NA
Adrenalin (see epinephrine)				
ε Aminocaproic acid	Inhibitor of fibrinolysis and indicated to control hemorrhage	Contraindicated in disseminated intravascular coagulopathy (DIC)	Bolus: 20–40 mg/kg IV q6h CRI: 3.5 mg/kg/min for 15 min, then 0.25 mg/kg/min[†]	20 g in 1 L saline IV over 30–60 min followed by 10 g IV every 6 h until bleeding has stopped
Altrenogest	Maintenance of pregnancy during endotoxemia		0.044–0.088 mg/kg PO q24h	22–44 mg (10–20 mL) PO q24h
Amikacin	Antimicrobial (gram negative bacteria)	Nephrotoxic	Adults 10 mg/kg IV q24h Foals 25 mg/kg IV q24h	5 g (20 mL) IV q 24h (not commonly used systemically in adult horses because of expense)
Ampicillin sodium	Antimicrobial	Diarrhea	20 mg/kg IV q6–8h	10 g IV q8h
Aspirin	Prevent platelet aggregation	Gastrointestinal and renal side-effects	10–100 mg/kg PO q48h[‡]	
Azithromycin	Antimicrobial against *L. intracellularis*		10 mg/kg PO q24h for 5 days then 10 mg/kg PO q48h	
Bethanechol	Motility stimulant (not currently used)	Abdominal pain, diarrhea, salivation, and gastric secretion	0.025 mg/kg	
Equine Bio-sponge® (see DTO smectite)				
Bismuth subsalicylate	Antidiarrheal		0.5–1 mL/kg PO q4–6 h[‡]	250–500 mL PO q4–6 h
Buprenorphine	Opiate sedative analgesic (not commonly used)		0.004–0.01 mg/kg IV[‡]	
Butorphanol	Opiate sedative analgesic	Decrease in gastrointestinal motility; excitation if used alone	0.01–0.1 mg/kg IV or IM CRI: 13 µg/kg/h Neonate: 0.02–0.04 mg/kg IV or IM	5–10 mg (0.5–1 mL) IV with xylazine

[a]NOTE: Check concentration of drug preparation being used. Concentrations may vary.

(continued)

Table B.1 (cont'd)

Drug	Use	Complications	Dose rate	Amount 500 kg horse typically used
N–butylscopolammonium bromide (Buscopan®)	Spasmolytic analgesic	Ileus and colic with repeated doses; tachycardia	0.3 mg/kg IV once	150 mg (7.5 mL)
Calcium borogluconate 23%	Calcium supplementation for hypocalcemia		0.2–1 mL/kg IV over 2–3 h	100–500 mL IV over 2–3 h. Usually administered in IV fluids.
Ceftiofur	Antimicrobial	Diarrhea	Adult: 2.2 mg/kg IV q12h Neonate: 10 mg/kg IV q6h	1 g (20 mL) IV q12h
Charcoal (activated)	Prevent absorption of toxins for gastrointestinal tract		1–3 g/kg PO via nasogastric tube	0.5–1.5 kg
Chloramphenicol (palmitate or base)	Antimicrobial against *L. intracellularis;*** incisional infection	Diarrhea; aplastic anemia (humans)	50 mg/kg PO q6–8h for 14d	
Cimetidine	Antiulcer medication (H₂ receptor antagonist)		6.6 mg/kg IV q6h 16–20 mg/kg PO q8h	
Detomidine	Alpha-2 agonist sedative analgesic	Cardiovascular effects; decreased GI motility; hyperglycemia; increased urine production; profuse sweating; ataxia; tachypnea in febrile horses	0.01–0.02 mg/kg IV 0.02–0.04 mg/kg IM CRI: 6–15 μg/kg bolus then 0.6 μg/kg/min (halve rate every 15 min)	5–10 mg (0.5–1 mL) IV 10–20 mg (1–2 mL) IM
Dexamethasone	Corticosteroid anti-inflammatory	Infection and impaired tissue healing; laminitis	0.05–0.2 mg/kg IV q24h 0.02–0.2 mg/kg PO q24h	25–100 mg IV q24h 10–100 mg PO q24h
Diazepam	Sedation for neonates; induction of general anesthesia with ketamine; control of seizure activity	Excitation in foals/horses if used alone	0.02–0.1 mg/kg IV 0.1–0.2 mg/kg IM	10–50 mg (2–10 mL) IV NOTE: never use without prior sedation with an alpha-2 agonist because will cause excitation
Dimethyl sulfoxide (DMSO)	Anti-inflammatory; endotoxemia; ischemia-reperfusion injury; adhesion prevention; acute neurological disease	Hemolysis if given IV as concentrated solution (>10%)	0.02–0.1 g/kg (gastrointestinal) 1 g/kg (neurological) given IV diluted to a 10% solution in isotonic fluids	~50 g (~50 mL of 90% solution) 500 g (~500 mL of 90% solution). Always diluted and given as a 10% solution.
Dioctyl sodium sulfosuccinate (DSS)	Fecal softener/laxative	Diarrhea and colic	10–50 mg/kg in 2 L water delivered via nasogastric tube§	5–10 g in 2 L water delivered via nasogastric tube one time only. NOTE: strongly recommend staying at low end of dose range.

Drug	Indication/Action	Adverse effects/Cautions	Dose	Dose (per horse)
Diphenhydramine Antihistamine			0.5–1 mg/kg IV or IM	
Dipyrone	Anti-inflammatory analgesic; antipyretic		5–22 mg/kg IV or IM	
Dobutamine	ß1 agonist used to improve cardiac output	Tachycardia, arrhythmias	CRI: 2–20 µg/kg/min	
Dopamine	Support of blood pressure and cardiac output		CRI: 3–25 µg/kg/min	
Domperidone	Poor milk production in postparturient mares		1.1 mg/kg PO q24h	
Doxycycline (see tetracycline)				
DTO smectite	Endotoxin absorption from intestinal lumen; antidiarrheal	Only use in horses with good intestinal motility		0.5–1.5 kg per horse initially then 0.5 kg q8–24h for 1–4 days
Enrofloxacin	Antimicrobial drug	Diarrhea; arthropathy in young horses	5.5 mg/kg IV q24h 7.5 mg/kg PO q24h	
Epinephrine	Anaphylactic reaction; resuscitation; blood pressure support	Tachyarrhythmias	0.01–0.02 mg/kg IV q 3–5 minutes (for CPR)‡ CRI: 0.1–2 µg/kg/min	5–10 mg IV
Erythromycin stearate (also phosphate, ethylsuccinate, estolate)	Antimicrobial against L. intracellularis		15–25 mg/kg PO q6–8h for 21 days	
Erythromycin lactobionate	Motility stimulant; motilin agonist	Diarrhea, colic; tachyphylaxis	1–2 mg/kg diluted in 1L saline given IV over 60min every 6h	0.5–1 g diluted in 1 L IV over 1 h
Fenbendazole	Anthelmintic		10mg/kg PO once	
Firocoxib	COX-1 sparing NSAID		0.27 mg/kg IV loading dose then 0.09 mg/kg IV q24h	45 mg (6.75 mL) IV loading dose then 45 mg (2.25 mL) IV q24h
Flumazenil	Benzodiazepam antagonist		0.5–2 mg slow IV‡	
Flunixin meglumine	Nonsteroidal anti-inflammatory drug; analgesia	Nephrotoxic; gastrointestinal ulceration; right dorsal colitis; clostridium myositis if given IM	0.25 mg/kg IV q6–8h (antiendotoxic) 0.5 mg/kg IV q6–8h or 1 mg/kg IV q12h (anti-inflammatory, analgesic)	125 mg (2.5 mL) q6–8h 250 mg (5 mL) q6–8h 500 mg (10 mL) q12h
Furosemide	Diuretic; pulmonary edema	Electrolyte disturbances	0.5–2 mg/kg IV once	250–500 mg (5–10 mL) IV once

(continued)

333

Table B.1 (cont'd)

Drug	Use	Complications	Dose rate	Amount 500 kg horse typically used
Gentamicin	Antimicrobial (gram negative spectrum)	Nephrotoxic (peak and trough plasma concentrations should be monitored); neuromuscular blockade	Adult: 6.6–8.8 mg/kg IV q24h Neonate: 12 mg/kg IV q24h	3.3–4.4 g (33–44 mL) IV q24h
Guaifenesin	Centrally acting muscle relaxant for induction of general anesthesia		25–100 mg/kg	Given to effect
Heparin	Anticoagulant used for adhesion prevention; DIC; prevention of thromboembolic disease	Decrease in PCV caused by erythrocyte agglutination	40–60 U/kg IV or SQ q8–12h	Concentration varies but 20 000 U (2 mL of 10 000 U/mL) SQ q8–12h for adhesion prevention
Hetastarch	Colloid support	Coagulopathy with >10 mL/kg/day	2–10 mL/kg IV	1–5 L IV
Hypertonic saline 7–7.5%	Resuscitation fluid	Cellular dehydration if not followed up by 5–10× volume of isotonic crystalloids	2–4 mL/kg once	1–2 L once
Insulin	Hyperglycemia; hypertriglyceridemia	Hypoglycemia	Regular: 0.1–0.5 U/kg SQ q12h CRI: 0.01–0.2 U/kg/h Protamine zinc: 0.1–0.3 U/kg SQ q12h	
Ivermectin	Anthelmintic		0.2 mg/kg PO once	
Ketamine	Induction of general anesthesia (GA); analgesic	Excitation	1.7–2.2 mg/kg (GA) 0.2–0.8 mg/kg IV or 1–2 mg/kg IM (analgesic) CRI: 0.5–1 mg/kg bolus then 0.4–0.8 mg/kg/h (analgesic)	850–1100 mg (~8–10 mL) (GA)
Ketoprofen	Nonsteroidal anti-inflammatory drug		2.2 mg/kg IV q24h	
Lidocaine epidural	Analgesia	Collapse; ataxia	0.22 mg/kg	5 mL of a 2% solution
Lidocaine IV	Analgesia; anti-inflammatory; motility modification through anti-inflammatory effects	Collapse and seizure; possibly incisional infection; avoid in hepatic toxicity	1.3 mg/kg loading dose over 15 min 0.05 mg/kg/min CRI IV	

Drug	Indication	Side effects	Dose	
Lidocaine enema	Facilitate palpation per rectum			60 mL 2% lidocaine placed topically in rectum using extension tubing or 12 mL 2% lidocaine in 50 mL of water
Magnesium sulfate	Laxative	Diarrhea	0.5–1 g/kg in water via a nasogastric tube	250–500 g in water via a nasogastric tube
Medetomidine	Sedative analgesic		0.004–0.01 mg/kg IV; 0.01–0.02 mg/kg IM	
Meloxicam			0.6 mg/kg IV or IM q24h	300 mg IV or IM q24h
Metoclopramide	Motility stimulant (dopamine D2 agonist)	Extrapyramidal side effects (excitation)	Bolus: 0.25 mg/kg IV q6h in 0.5–1 L saline given over 1 h; CRI: 0.04 mg/kg/h IV	125 mg in 1 L saline IV q6h
Metronidazole	Antimicrobial (anaerobic bacteria including *Clostridium* spp.)		25 mg/kg PO q12h	12.5 g PO q12h
Misoprostol	Synthetic prostaglandin	Colic (not reported in horses)	1–4 µg/kg PO q24h	0.5–2 mg PO q24h
Mineral oil	Lubricant, laxative		5–10 mL/kg PO	Up to 4 L
Naloxone	Opiate antagonist; abdominal hemorrhage; motility stimulant		0.01–0.05 mg/kg IV	
Neostigmine methylsulfate	Motility stimulant; cholinesterase inhibitor	Colic	0.0044 mg/kg SQ every 0.5–1 h. Dose rate can be increased incrementally to a maximum dose rate of 0.02 mg/kg	~2 mg SQ q0.5–1h
Norepinephrine	β1 and α adrenergic agonist used for blood pressure support through		0.1–5 µg/kg/min	
Omeprazole	Proton pump inhibitor; prevention and treatment of gastric ulcers		4 mg/kg PO q24h (treatment); 1 mg/kg PO q24h (prevention); 0.5–1.5 mg/kg IV q24h	2 g PO q24h; 0.5 g PO q24h
Oxibendazole	Anthelmintic		10–15 mg/kg PO once	
Oxytetracycline (see tetracycline)				
Penicillin procaine	Antimicrobial (gram positive and anaerobic bacteria)	Procaine reaction causing excitation	20000 U/kg IM q12h	10×10^6 U (33 mL) IM q12h

(continued)

335

Table B.1 (cont'd)

Drug	Use	Dose rate	Complications	Amount 500kg horse typically used
Potassium penicillin	Antimicrobial (gram positive and anaerobic bacteria)	20000 U/kg IV q6h	Give slowly IV because high potassium concentration	10×10^6 U (20mL) IV q6h of 500 000 U/mL preparation
Pentastarch	Colloid support	2–15mL/kg IV q24h		1–7.5 L IV q24h
Pentoxyphylline	Possibly for treatment of endotoxemia	10mg/kg PO q12h		5 g PO q12h
Phenylbutazone	Nonsteroidal anti-inflammatory analgesic drug	2.2–4.4 mg/kg IV q12–24h	Nephrotoxicity; gastrointestinal ulceration; right dorsal colitis	1–2 g (5–10mL) q12–24h
Phenylephrin	Alpha-1 adrenergic agonist causing vasoconstriction for treatment of NSLE; used during general anesthesia for controlling hypotension	3 µg/kg/min for 15 min IV (NSLE)[‡]; 0.25–2 µg/kg/min (general anesthesia)	Bradycardia; uticarcia; fatal hemorrhage	~20mg diluted in 30–60mL saline given over 15 min (NSLE)
Piperazine	Anthelmintic	88–110mg/kg once		
Plasma	Provision of coagulation factors during hemorrhage; antiendotoxic; colloidal support	6–20mL/kg IV until hemorrhage stops (hemorrhage); 4–6mL/kg (antiendotoxic, J5 plasma); ~20–40mL/kg to increase TPP 1g/dL (10g/L)	Hypersensitivity reaction	3–10L (hemorrhage); 2–3 L (antiendotoxic); 10–20L (colloidal support)
Polymixin B	Antiendotoxin	1 000–5 000 U/kg administered in 1 L 5% dextrose over 15–30min q8–12h	Nephrotoxicity; collapse and death if administered IV undiluted	Typically 1.5–3 $\times 10^6$ U IV q8–12h
Praziquantel	Anthelmintic (tapeworms)	0.5–1 mg/kg PO once		250–500mg PO once
Prednisolone	Corticosteroid anti-inflammatory	0.2–4.4mg/kg PO or IM q12–24h	Infection; delayed tissue healing; laminitis	100–2200 mg PO or IM q 12–24h
Progesterone	Maintain pregnancy			300mg IM q24h
Psyllium mucilloid	Fiber used for clearance of sand from the GI tract	1g/kg PO q6–24h		500g PO q6–24h
Pyrantel pamoate	Anthelmintic	6.6mg/kg PO once		3.3 g PO once
Ranitidine	H_2 receptor agonist for treatment of gastric ulcers primarily in foals	6.6mg/kg PO q8h; 1.5 mg/kg IV q8h		

Drug	Indication	Side effects	Dose	Dose (alternate)
Romifidine	Sedation		0.05–0.12 mg/kg IV 0.1–0.2 mg/kg IM	
Sucralfate	Antiulcer medication		20–40 mg/kg PO q6–8h	5–10 g (5–10 tablets) PO q6–8h
Tetracycline	Antimicrobial against *L. intracellularis* also, Potomac Horse Fever (Neorickettsia risticii)		Oxytetracycline 6.6 mg/kg IV q12h for 7 days; then doxycycline 10 mg/kg PO q12h for 8–17 days (L. intracellularis) Oxytetracycline 6.6 mg/kg IV q12h for 5 days (N. risticii)	
Trimethoprim sulfonamide	Braodspectrum antimicrobial drug	Diarrhea	30 mg/kg PO q12h	
Vasopressin	Blood pressure support	Decrease perfusion to gastrointestinal tract	0.25 U/kg/min and increased to effect	
Vinegar	Enterolith prevention			250 mL PO q24h
Xylazine	Alpha-2 adrenergic agonist; sedative analgesic drug	Cardiovascular effects; decreased GI motility; hyperglycemia; increased urine production; profuse sweating; ataxia; tachypnea in febrile horses	0.2–1.1 mg/kg IV 0.4–2.2 mg/kg IM CRI: 1 mg/kg bolus then 12 µg/kg/min	Typically 100–200 mg (1–2 mL) IV with butorphanol
Xylazine epidural	See above	Collapse	0.17 mg/kg in 6–10 mL sterile saline or 2% lidocaine	0.75 mL
Yohimbine	Motility stimulant		0.075 mg/kg IV	
Yunan Baiyou	Controlling hemorrhage			4 g per adult horse orally q6h

*Pusterla et al. (2004).
†Ross et al. (2007).
‡Corley and Stephen (2008).
§Freeman et al. (1992).
**Sampieri et al. (2006).
††Hardy et al. (1994).

References

Pusterla, N., Magdesian, K.G., Maleski, K., Spier, S.J. & Madigan, J. (2004) Retrospective evaluation of the use of acetylcysteine enemas in the treatment of meconium retention in foals: 44 cases (1987–2002). *Equine Veterinary Education*, **16**, 133–136.

Ross, J., Dallap, B.L., Dolente, B.A. & Sweeney, R.W. (2007) Pharmacokinetics and pharmacodynamics of epsilon-aminocaproic acid in horses. *American Journal of Veterinary Research*, **68**, 1016–1021.

Corley, K. & Stephen, J. (2008) *The Equine Hospital Manual*, pp. 655–669. Blackwell Publishing, Chichester.

Freeman, D.E., Ferrante, P.L. & Palmer, J.E. (1992) Comparison of the effects of intragastric infusion of equal volumes of water, dioctyl sodium sulfosuccinate, and magnesium sulfate on fecal composition and output in clinically normal horses. *American Journal of Veterinary Research*, **53**, 1347–1353.

Sampieri, F., Hinchcliff, K.W. & Toribio, R.E. (2006) Tetracycline therapy of Lawsonia intracellularis enteropathy in foals. *Equine Veterinary Journal*, **38**, 89–92.

Hardy, J., Bednarski, R.M. & Biller, D.S. (1994) Effect of phenylephrine on hemodynamics and splenic dimensions in horses. *American Journal of Veterinary Research*, **55**, 1570–1578.

Appendix C

Normal Ranges for Hematology and Palsma Chemistry and Conversion Table for Units

Table C.1   Normal ranges for hematology in adult horses and neonatal foals.

Hematology	Adult*	Neonate 24 h[‡]	Neonate 1 month[†]
White blood cell count (×10³ cells/μL)	4.9–10.3	4.9–11.7	5.3–12.2
Segmented neutrophils (×10³ cells/μL)	2.2–8.1	3.4–9.6	2.8–9.3
(%)	28.0–82.8		
Nonsegmented (band) neutrophils (×10³ cells/μL)			
(%)	0-0.2 (0–2)		
Lymphocytes (×10³ cells/μL)	1.7–5.8	0.7–2.1	1.4–2.3
(%)	19.8–58.9		
Monocytes (×10³ cells/μL)	0–1.0	0.07–0.4	0.03–0.5
(%)	1.4–10.5		
Eosinophils (×10³ cells/μL)	0–0.8	0–0.02	0–0.1
(%)	0–8.7		
Basophils (×10³ cells/μL)	0–0.3	0–0.03	0–0.08
(%)	0–2		
Platelets (×10³ cells/μL)	72–183	129–409	136–468
Red blood cells (×10⁶ cells/μL)	6.2–10.2	8.2–11.0	7.9–11.1
Hematocrit (%)	31–50	32–46	29–41
Hemoglobin (g/dL)	11.4–17.3	12.0–16.6	10.9–15.3
(g/L)	114–173	120–166	109–153

*Normal values from New Bolton Center clinical pathology laboratory.
[†]Axon & Palmer (2008) and Harvey (1990).

Practical Guide to Equine Colic, First Edition. Edited by Louise L. Southwood.
© 2013 John Wiley & Sons, Inc. Published 2013 by John Wiley & Sons, Inc.

Table C.2   Normal ranges for plasma biochemistry for adult horses and neonatal foals.

Biochemistry	Adult*	Neonate 24 h[†]	Neonate 1 month[†]
Albumin (g/dL)	2.5–4.2	2.0–5.0	0.9–3.5
(g/L)	25–42	20–50**	9–35**
Alkaline phosphatase (ALP) (U/L)	109–315	861–2671[§]	210–866[§]
Ammonia (µg/dL)	19–94	low	low
(µmol/L)	11–55		
Antithrombin III (%)	150–220		
Aspartate aminotransferase (AST) (U/L)	205–555	146–340**	252–440**
Bile acids (enzymatic) (µg/mL)	0.4–3.5	10.6–30.2[‡,***]	3.7–6.9[‡]
(µmol/L)	1.0–8.6	26–74	9–17
Bilirubin (total) (mg/dL)	0.1–1.9	1.6–5[‡,***]	1.0–1.6[‡]
(µmol/L)	1.7–32.5	27.4–85.5	17.1–27.4
Blood urea nitrogen (mg/dL)	8–27	9–40**	6–21**
(mmol/L)	2.9–9.6	3.2–14.3	2.1–7.5
Calcium (mg/dL)	10.7–13.4	9.5–13.4	10.7–13.1
(mmol/L)	2.7–3.4	2.4–3.4**	2.7–3.3**
Carbon dioxide (TCO$_2$) (mEq/L or mmol/L)	24–31	21–34	22–32
Chloride (mEq/L or mmol/L)	94–102	90–114**	97–109**
Cholesterol (mg/dL)	51–109	11.7–58.8	7.4–23.5
(mmol/L)	1.3–2.8	0.3–1.5[†]	0.2–0.6[§]
Creatine kinase (U/L)	90–270	40–909**	81–585**
Creatinine (mg/dL)	0.6–1.8	0.11–0.38**	0.10–0.16**
(µmol/L)	53.1–159.2	9.7–33.6	8.8–14.1
Fibrinogen (mg/dL)	150–375	50–430	140–660
(g/L)	1.5–3.7	0.5–4.3[§§]	1.4–6.6[§§]
Gamma glutamyltransferase (GGT) (U/L)	12–45	11–50[§,***]	14–44[‡]
Glucose (mg/dL)	72–114	121–223	130–216
(mmol/L)	4.0–6.3	6.7–12.4	7.2–12.0
Lactate (mmol/L)	<1.0	0.6–1.1[††]	
Magnesium (mg/dL)	1.6–2.5	0.6–3.9	0.9–2.7
(mmol/L)	0.7–1.0	0.3–1.7**	0.4–1.2**
Phosphorous (mg/dL)	1.9–5.4	3.7–7.4	5.0–9.3
(mmol/L)	0.6–1.7	1.2–2.4**	1.6–3.0**
Potassium (mEq/L or mmol/L)	2.7–4.9	3.6–5.6**	3.8–5.4**
Sodium (mEq/L or mmol/L)	132–141	123–159**	136–154**
Sorbitol dehydrogenase (SDH) (U/L)	0.3–7.0	1.0–18.0[†,†††]	0–6.1[‡]
Total plasma protein (g/dL)	4.6–6.9	5.2–8.0	5.1–7.1
(g/L)	46–69	52–80[‡‡]	51–71[‡‡]
Triglycerides (mg/dL)	11–52	4–154[‡,***]	14–134[‡]
(mmol/L)	0.12–0.59	0.05–1.74	0.16–1.51

*Normal values from New Bolton Center clinical pathology laboratory.
[†]Axon and Palmer (2008).
[‡]Barton and LeRoy (2007).
[§]Bauer et al. (1989).
**Bauer (1990).
[††]Butters (2008).
[‡‡]Harvey (1990).
[§§]Harvey et al. (1990).
***2 days old.
[†††]7 days old.

Table C.3   Plasma antimicrobial drug concentrations.*

Antimicrobial drug	Timing	Concentration (µg/mL)
Gentamicin	30 min peak	32–40
	12 h trough	<1–2
Amikacin	30 min peak	50–60
	12 h trough (adults)	<2–5
	24 h trough (neonates)	<2–5

*Values New Bolton Center clinical pathology laboratory.

Table C.4   Conversion from conventional units to SI units for clinical laboratory data

	Conventional Unit	Conversion Factor	SI Unit
Albumin	g/dL	10	g/L
Alkaline phosphatase (ALP)	units/L	1.0	U/L
Ammonia	µg/dL	0.587	µmol/L
Antithrombin III	mg/dL	10	mg/L
Aspartate Aminotransferase (AST)	units/L	1.0	U/L
Bile acids	µg/dL	2.45	µmol/L
Bilirubin	mg/dL	17.1	µmol/L
Blood urea nitrogen	mg/dL	0.357	mmol/L
Calcium	mg/dL	0.25	mmol/L
	mEq/L	0.5	mmol/L
Carbon dioxide (total)	mEq/L	1.0	mmol/L
Chloride	mEq/L	1.0	mmol/L
Cholesterol	mg/dL	0.0259	mmol/L
Creatine kinase	units/L	1.0	U/L
Creatinine	mg/dL	88.4	µmol/L
Fibrinogen	g/dL	10	g/L
Gamma glutamyltransferase (GGT)	units/L	1.0	U/L
Glucose	mg/dL	0.0555	mmol/L
Lactate	mg/dL	0.111	mmol/L
Magnesium	mg/dL	0.411	mmol/L
	mEq/L	0.50	mmol/L
Phosphorous	mg/dL	0.323	mmol/L
Potassium	mEq/L	1.0	mmol/L
Sodium	mEq/L	1.0	mmol/L
Sorbitol dehydrogenase (SDH)	units/L	1.0	U/L
Total plasma protein	g/dL	10	g/L
Triglycerides	mg/dL	0.0113	mmol/L
White blood cell count	x 10^3/µL	1.0	x 10^9/L

• to convert from the conventional unit to the SI unit, **multiply** by the conversion factor;
• to convert from the SI unit to the conventional unit, **divide** by the conversion factor.
Adapted from: http://www.unc.edu/~rowlett/units/scales/clinical_data.html

References

1. Axon, J.E. & Palmer, J.E. (2008) Clinical pathology of the foal. *Veterinary Clinics of North America: Equine Practice*, **24**, 357–385

2. Barton, M.H. & LeRoy, B.E. (2007) Serum bile acid concentrations in healthy and clinically ill neonatal foals. *Journal of Veterinary Internal Medicine*, **21**, 508–513.
3. Bauer, J.E. (1990) Normal blood chemistry. In: *Equine Clinical Neonatology* (eds A.M. Koterba,

W.H. Drummond & P.C. Kosch), pp. 602–614. Lea & Febiger, Philadelphia, Pennsylvania.

4. Bauer, J.E., Asquith, R.L. & Kivipelto, J. (1989) Serum biochemical indicators of liver function in neonatal foals. *American Journal of Veterinary Research*, **50**, 2037–2041.

5. Butters, A. (2008) Medical and surgical management of uroperitoneum in a 4 day old foal. *Canadian Veterinary Journal*, **49**, 401–403.

6. Harvey, J.W. (1990) Normal hematologic values. In: *Equine Clinical Neonatology* (eds A.M. Koterba, W.H. Drummond & P.C. Kosch), pp. 561–570. Lea & Febiger, Philadelphia, Pennsylvania.

7. Harvey, R.W., Asquith, R.L., McNulty, P.K., Kivipelto, J. & Bauer, J.E. (1984) Haematology of foals up to one year old. *Equine Veterinary Journal*, **16**, 347–353.

Index

abdominal palpation per rectum
  abnormal findings, 26–7
    cecum, 28, 30–31
    kidney and spleen, 35
    large colon distention, 28–9, 32–3
    peritoneal cavity, 35–6
    rectal tear, 33–4
    small (descending) colon, 33
    small intestine, 27–9
    urogenital tract, 34–5
  complications, 36–7
  diagnoses, 28
  differential diagnoses, 27
  indications, 22–3
  indications for referral, 74
  mild colic, 46
  normal anatomy
    abdominal cavity, 25
    bladder, 24
    cecum, 25
    inguinal rings, 25
    kidney and spleen, 25
    large colon, 26
    pelvic region, 24
    rectum, 24
    small (descending) colon, 25–6
    uterus and ovaries, 25
  preparation
    lubrication, 23
    materials required, 23
    rectal relaxation, 23–4
    rectal sleeve, 23
    restraint, 23
    sedation, 24
  procedure, 24–36
abdominal radiography
  diaphragmatic hernia, 157
  enterolithiasis, 155–6
  equipment
    cassettes/detector and holder, 150–152
    radiolucent markers, 151
    safety equipment, 151
    X-ray generator, 150
  foals, 157–9
  gut fill, 152
  indications, 149–50
  intestinal sand accumulation, 156–7
  metallic foreign material, 157
  sedation/restraint, 152
abdominal sonographic evaluation
  gastric distension and impaction, 131–4
  indications, 117
  intussusceptions, 127
  large colon displacements

Practical Guide to Equine Colic, First Edition. Edited by Louise L. Southwood.
© 2013 John Wiley & Sons, Inc. Published 2013 by John Wiley & Sons, Inc.

abdominal sonographic evaluation (*cont'd*)
   large colon volvulus, 122–3
   left dorsal displacement, 121–2
   right dorsal displacement, 120–121
   large intestinal impactions
   large colon or cecal impaction, 123–4
   meconium retention, 125
   sand impactions, 124
   small colon impactions, 124
   patient preparation, 117
   procedure
   abdominal examination (complete), 118–20
   FLASH, 118
   transrectal examination, 120
   right dorsal colitis, 125–6
   small intestinal lesions
   adhesions, 130–131, 134
   idiopathic small intestinal muscular
      hypertrophy, 130, 133
   strangulating *vs.* nonstrangulating
      obstruction, 128–30
   transducer selection, 117
abdominocentesis
   complications, 89–90
   indications, 87–8
   preparation, 88
   procedure, 88–9
acid-base imbalances, 80–81
adhesions
   long-term recovery, 294
   miniature horses, 289
   postoperative complication, 255–6
   previous colic surgery, 9
   sonographic evaluation, 130–131
adult horses
   abdominal radiography
   caudodorsal radiograph, 153–4
   caudoventral radiograph, 153, 156
   cranioventral radiograph, 153, 155
   metallic foreign objects, 157
   mid-abdominal radiograph, 153, 155
   antimicrobial drug concentrations, 339
   arterial blood pressure, 102
   biochemistry in, 338
   colloid oncotic pressure, 100
   drug dosages, 329–35
   energy and protein requirements for, 302, 308
   enteral nutrition, 303
   fecal output, 7
   glucose homeostatic dysfunction, 83

heart rate, 16
hematology in, 337
IV catheterization, 104, 107
IV fluid therapy
   electrolyte replacement, 110
   maintenance fluid rate, 110
   replacement/resuscitation fluid, 109
   colloids, 112–14
Landis-Pappenheimer equation for, 100
mild colic, 46–8
parenteral nutrition formulations for, 309
physical examination, 14–21
postoperative patient care
   central venous pressure, 234
   fluid therapy plan, 237
   mean arterial pressure, 235
   patient assessment, 231
   physical examination, 232
   urine-specific gravity, 234
sonographic examination, 118–20
urine output, 102
water consumption, 7
alkaline phosphatase (ALP), 82
alpha-2 adrenergic agonists, 17, 239
   adverse effects and contraindications, 55
   alpha-2 antagonists, 55
   clinical use, 54–5
   dose rates, 330, 335
   mechanism of action, 54
aminoglycosides
   dose rates, 329, 332
   toxicity, 9
   for young foals and weanlings, 281
analgesia
   alpha-2 adrenergic agonists
   adverse effects and contraindications, 55
   alpha-2 antagonists, 55
   clinical use, 54–5
   dose rates, 330, 335
   mechanism of action, 54
   hyoscine-N-butylbromide
   adverse effects and contraindications, 59
   clinical use, 58–9
   dose rate, 330
   mechanism of action, 58
   indications, 51–2
   intravenous lidocaine
   adverse effects and contraindications, 58
   clinical use, 57–8
   complications, 58

dose rate, 332
mechanism of action, 57
mild colic, 46–7
nonsteroidal anti-inflammatory drugs
adverse effects and contraindications, 53
clinical use, 52–3
dose rate, 331–4
mechanism of action, 52
mild colic, 46–7
opioids
adverse effects and contraindications, 56–7
antagonists, 56
clinical use, 56
dose rate, 329
mechanism of action, 55
postoperative use, 238–40, 249–50
Anoplocephala perfoliata (tapeworms)
definition, 318
diagnosis and management, 319–20
life cycle, 318
prevention of colic, 297
pathology and clinical disease, 318
cecal perforation, 215
cecocolic intussusception, 215
ileal impaction, 208
ileocecal intussusception, 213
anthelmintics, 319
gastrointestinal parasite control, 8–9
Anoplocephala perfoliata, 318
ascarid impaction, 322
cyathostomes, 320–321
fecal egg count reduction test, 317
pasture management, 317
Strongylus vulgaris, 323
resistance, 297, 317
arrhythmia, 17
arterial oxygen content (CaO$_2$), 101
ascariasis, 321–2
impaction, 208–9
prevention, 209, 322
prevention of colic, 297
treatment, 209
young foals and weanlings, 280
ascarid impaction, 208–209
aspartate transaminase (AST), 82

benzimidazole anthelmintics, 209, 321, 322
biosecurity program
vs. biocontainment, 263
definition and terminology, 263

for equine colic patient at home
cleaning and disinfection, 271–2
general recommendations, 270–271
MRSA, 273
shedding *Salmonella*, 272–3
for hospitalized equine colic patient
monitoring and surveillance, 269–70
preventive measures, 269
shedding *Salmonella*, 268
hospital acquired infections, 263–4
infection control programs, 264
monitoring and surveillance
hospital environment, 268
patient, 267–8
preventive measures
antimicrobial use, 267
barrier precautions and protective clothing, 266
Biosecurity Officer, 267
cleaning and disinfection, 265–6
hand hygiene, 266
high and low risk patients, 265
training and education, 267
waste disposal, 266–7
broad ligament hematoma
abdominal palpation, 27, 34–5
cause of colic and treatment, 282–4
sonographic examination, 120, 136
broodmares
postpartum mares, 284–5
pregnant mares, 284
Buscopan®
abdominal palpation per rectum, 23, 24
adverse effects and contraindications, 59
clinical use, 58–9
dose rate, 330
mechanism of action, 58
mild colic, 47
butorphanol *see also* opioids
dose rate, 329
for young foals and weanlings, 281
mild colic, 46–7
postoperative pain, 250
postoperative patient care, 239
trocharization, 161

cardiac output (Q), 101
cecal impaction, 9, 10
abdominal palpation per rectum, 28, 30–31
clinical signs, 214
medical treatment, 214

cecal impaction (*cont'd*)
  necropsy, 215
  sonography, 123–4
  surgical treatment, 168, 214
  typhlotomy, 190
cecal perforation, 168, 215
cecal tympany, 28, 30–31
cecocecal intussusception, 214–15 *see also* cecocolic
    intussusception
cecocolic intussusception, 198, 214
  abdominal palpation per rectum, 28, 30–31
  clinical signs, 215
  sonographic evaluation, 127, 130
  surgical treatment, 215
cecum
  abdominal palpation per rectum, 28, 30–31
  celiotomy, 178–9
ceftiofur, 330
  colic surgery, 175
  for young foals and weanlings, 281
  postoperative patient care, 240
celiotomy *see also* colic surgery
  abdominal organs, 181–2
  approaches
    ventral, 177
    lateral, 185
  cecum, 178–9
  indications (general), 164–6
  large colon, 182–3
  small colon, 182
  small intestine, 179–81
  transverse colon, 182
central venous pressure (CVP), 102
clinical laboratory data
  clinical chemistry
    acid-base evaluation, 80–81
    electrolyte imbalance, 81–2
    hepatobiliary assessment, 82–3
    metabolic indicators, 83
    renal parameters, 83
  coagulation
    inhibitors, 84–5
    platelets, 83–4
    secondary hemostasis, 84
  hematology
    erythrogram, 79
    leukogram, 79–80
  indications, 78–9
coagulation
  inhibitors, 84–5
  platelets, 83–4

  secondary hemostasis, 84
colic
  donkeys
    causes, 285–6
    hyperlipemia, 288–9
  drug dosages, 329–35
  geriatric horses
    causes, 286
    management and complications, 287
  mild (*see* mild colic)
  miniature horses
    causes, 287
    management and complications, 287–8
  ponies
    causes, 287
    management and complications, 287–8
  postpartum mares, 284–5
  pregnant mares, 282–4
  risk factors and prevention
    colonic microbiota, 297
    dental care, 298
    diet, 296–7
    exercise regimen, 297
    gastrointestinal parasites, 297
    genetic predisposition, 295
    recurrent colic, 295
    risk factors, 296–7
    seasonal pattern, 296
    transportation, 297
    water deprivation, 297
colic surgery
  anastomosis, 192
    end-to-end technique, 195–7
    ileocecostomy, 194–5
    jejunocecostomy, 193–4
    jejunoileostomy, 193
    jejunojejunostomy, 193
    side-to-side anastomosis, 197
    small colon resection, 197–202
  colopexy, 202
  complications
    diarrhea, 248–9
    endotoxemia and the associated SIRS, 246–8
    fever, 244–6
    incisional complications, 256–8
    ischemia-reperfusion injury, 246
    postoperative ileus, 251–3
    postoperative intraperitoneal adhesions,
      255–6
    recurrent colic, 249–51
    septic peritonitis, 253–4

diagnosis and correction, 198–201
enterotomy, 190–191
indications, 164–6, 174
laparoscopy, 177, 187–8
lateral approaches, 196–7
    body wall closure, 186–7
    celiotomy, 186
    incision, 185–6
long-term recovery
    complications, 294
    feeding, 294
    incisional care, 293–5
    postoperative management, 292–4
    return to use, 295
    survival, 294–5
needle decompression, 189
partial typhlectomy, 191–2
surgical preparation
    analgesic drugs, 174–5
    anesthesia, 175
    antimicrobial drugs, 175
    cardiovascular stabilization, 174
    surgical site preparation, 176
ventral approaches, 176
    body wall closure, 183–5
    celiotomy (see celiotomy)
    incision, 177–8
colitis, 9, 10, 169, 215–6 see also diarrhea
colopexy, 202
COX see cyclooxygenase (COX)
CVP see central venous pressure (CVP)
cyathostomes
    clinical disease, 320
    definition, 320
    diagnosis and management, 320–321
    life cycle, 320
    pathology, 320
    prevention of colic, 297
cyclooxygenase (COX), 46
    ischemia-reperfusion injury, 246
    non-steroidal anti-inflammatory drugs, 46,
        52–4
    right dorsal colitis, 216

detomidine, 52, 54–5, 74, 165, 239 see also alpha-2
        agonists
    abdominal palpation per rectum, 74
    causing bradycardia, 17
    causing tachypnea, 20
    dosage rate, 330
    mild colic, 46

postoperative pain, 250–251
postoperative patient care, 239
diaphragmatic hernia
    laparoscopy, 177, 188
    postpartum mares, 285
    radiography, 157
    sonographic evaluation, 136, 138
diarrhea see also enterocolitis; colitis
    cyathostomins, 320
    enteral fluid therapy, 68
    enterocolitis, 279
    in postoperative colics, 231
    IV fluid therapy
        acidosis, 111
        electrolyte abnormalities, 110
        maintenance fluid rate, 110
    postoperative
        prevalence, 248
        prevention, 248
        treatment, 248–9
    small colon impaction, 221–2
    ventral midline celiotomy, 248–9
dimethyl sulfoxide, 53, 330
dioctyl sodium sulfosuccinate (DSS), 330
    laxative, 66
    mild colic, 47

early referral see referral
electrolytes
    abnormality
        hypernatremia, 68, 110
        hypocalcemia, 68, 82, 111
        hypochloremia, 68, 82
        hypokalemia, 82
        hypomagnesemia, 68, 82
        hyponatremia, 65, 109, 110
        parenteral nutrition, 310
    enteral fluid therapy, 68
    imbalance, 81–2
    IV fluid therapy, 110–111
endotoxemia
    electrolyte imbalances, 82, 111
    fluid distribution, 100
    fluid therapy, 111–14
    hetastarch, 113
    hypertonic saline solution, 112
    hypertriglyceridemia, 288
    injected oral mucous membranes, 17–18
    lactate concentration, 81
    leukopenia, 80
    lidocaine (IV), 57

endotoxemia (*cont'd*)
 NSAID, 52
 platelets, 83–4
 pregnant mares, 283
 prevention, 246–7
 pyrexia, 19
 secondary hemostatic system, 84
 shock, 73, 101
 treatment, 247–8
enrofloxacin, 331
 colic surgery, 175
 dose rate, 331
 postoperative patient care, 240
enteral fluid therapy
 complications
  diarrhea, 68
  electrolyte disturbances, 68
  mild colic, 67–8
  nasogastric tube-associated problems, 68–9
 contraindications, 64
 enteral fluids composition
  balanced electrolyte solution, 65
  dioctyl sodium sulfosuccinate (DSS), 66
  laxatives or cathartics, 66
  magnesium sulfate, 66
  mineral oil, 66
  oral rehydration solutions, 65
  tap water, 64–5
 fluids and electrolytes absorption, 62–3
 indications, 63–4
 technique
  continuous infusions, 66–7
  intermittent boluses, 66
enterocentesis
 abdominocentesis, 89
 peritoneal fluid analysis, 90
enterocolitis *see also* diarrhea; colitis
 decreased AT activity, 85
 electrolyte abnormalities, 82
 leukopenia, 80
 necrotizing enterocolitis
  sonographic evaluation, 120
  neonatal foals, 4, 279–80
 postoperative patient care, 231
 triglyceride abnormalities, 83
enterolithiasis, 218–9
 diet, 7, 296
 palpation per rectum, 27, 28
 radiography, 155–6
 recurrent colic, 9, 73

 risk factors, 218
 signs, 219
 sonography, 141
 treatment of, 219
 water source, 8, 297
epiploic foramen entrapment, 211
equine grass sickness, 209
erythrogram, 79
esophageal trauma, NGT, 44
exploratory celiotomy *see* colic surgery

fast localized abdominal sonography of horses
  (FLASH), 118
fecal egg count reduction tests (FECRT), 317
fecal egg counts (FECs), 317
FECRT *see* fecal egg count reduction tests (FECRT)
FECs *see* fecal egg counts (FECs)
fenbendazole, 209, 319, 321–3, 333
fever
 biosecurity, 270
 geriatric and mature horses, 287
 postoperative complication, 244–6
 postoperative patient care, 232
 rectal temperature, 19
firocoxib, 331 *see also* non-steroidal anti-
  inflammatory drugs (NSAID)
 clinical use, 53
 ischemia-reperfusion injury, 246
 mechanism of action, 52
 mild colic, 46
 postoperative pain, 250
 postoperative patient care, 239
FLASH *see* fast localized abdominal sonography
  of horses (FLASH)
fluid distribution, 99–101
 colloid oncotic pressure, 100–101
 dehydration, 101
 endotoxemia and hypoproteinemia, 100
 hypovolemia, 101
 Landis-Pappenheimer equation, 100
 Starling-Landis equation, 100
fluid therapy
 enteral (*see* enteral fluid therapy)
 IV (*see* intravenous (IV) fluid therapy)
 mild colic, 47
flunixin meglumine, 6, 36, 57, 72, 83, 331, 333 *see
  also* non-steroidal anti-inflammatory drugs
 adhesion prevention, 255, 256
 adverse effects and contraindications, 53
 clinical use, 52

endotoxemia (treatment), 247, 249
indications
    for referral, 72
    for surgery, 165–6
mechanism of action, 52
mild colic, 46–7
postoperative pain, 250
postoperative patient care, 238–9
preparation for surgery (analgesia), 174
foals, 279–81
    adhesions, 255–6
    aminoglycoside plasma concentration, 339
    abdominocentesis
        omental herniation, 89
    biochemistry, 338
    causes of colic, 279–81
        ascarid impaction, 208–9
        cecal impaction, 214
        gastric ulceration, 205
        jejunal volvulus, 212
        meconium retention, 222–3
    colloid oncotic pressure (COP), 100
    colic, 278–9
        management, 283–4
        neonates, 279–80
        postoperative complication, 283
        young foals and weanlings, 280–281
    colic surgery
        incision, 177
        needle decompression, 189
        preparation, 175
    drug dosages, 329–35
    energy and protein requirements for, 302
    fluid therapy, 109–111
    gamma glutamyl transferase (GGT), 82
    hematology, 337
    IV catheterization, 103–9
    mean arterial blood pressure, 102
    nasogastric tube, 39, 40
    nutrition
        energy requirements, 302
        enteral nutrition, 304–5
        general, 302
        parenteral nutrition, 308–10
        protein requirements, 303
    Parascaris equorum, 321–2
    peritoneal fluid
        nucleated cell count, 93
    physical examination
        heart rate, 16

rectal temperature, 19
prognosis for racing, 295
radiography, 155, 157–9
sonography, 46, 117, 119–20
    abscess, 138–40
    jejunojejunal intussusception, 127
    meconium retention or impaction, 125
    stomach, 132

gamma glutamyltransferase (GGT), 82–3
gas colic, 4, 9, 45, 49 see also mild colic; spasmodic
        colic
gastric disease
    gastric impaction, 205–6
    gastric rupture, 206–7
    gastric ulceration, 205
gastrointestinal parasitology
    Anoplocephala perfoliata, 318–19
    anthelmintics, 319, 323
    cyathostomes, 320–321
    FECs and FECRT, 317
    Parascaris equorum, 321–22
    parasite control programs, 317–18
    parasites, 316–17
    Strongylus vulgaris, 322–3
gastrosplenic ligament entrapment, 211–12
gentamicin, 162, 240, 240, 332
geriatric horses, 286–7

heart rate
    assessment, 16–17
    hyoscine-N-butylbromide, 59
    packed cell volume, 79
    postoperatively, 232
    shock, 73
hemorrhage
    effusions, 96, 97
    epiploic foramen entrapment, 211
    hemangiosarcoma, 142
    intra-abdominal, 134
    intraluminal uterine, 136
    IV fluid therapy, 109
    mesenteric trauma, 222
    nasogastric intubation, 43–4
    pale mucous membranes, 18
    peritoneal fluid, 90, 97
    periparturient, 135
    postoperatively, 233
    postpartum mares, 34, 170, 284
    pregnant mares, 284

hemorrhage (*cont'd*)
   shock, 101
   trocharization, 163
hepatobiliary assessment, 82–3
hetastarch, 108, 113–14, 332
   postoperative patient care, 236–7
   preparation for colic surgery, 174
Holliday-Segar formula, 110
HSS *see* hypertonic saline solution (HSS)
hyoscine-N-butylbromide *see also* Buscopan®
   adverse effects and contraindications, 59
   clinical use, 58–9
   mechanism of action, 58
hyperglycemia, 83
   parenteral nutrition, 309–10
   postoperative patient care, 234
hyperlipemia
   parenteral nutrition, 310
   ponies, miniature horses, and donkeys, 288–9
hypermagnesemia, enteral fluid therapy, 68
hypernatremia
   electrolyte disturbances, 68
   IV fluid therapy, 110
hypertonic saline solution (HSS), 111–12, 235, 248, 332
hypertriglyceridemia
   parenteral nutrition, 309–10
   ponies, miniature horses, and donkeys, 288–9
   postoperative patient care, 334
   triglycerides, 83
hypocalcemia, 82
   enteral fluid therapy, 68
   IV fluid therapy, 111
hypochloremia, 68, 82
hypoglycemia, 83
hypokalemia, 82
hypomagnesemia, 68, 82
hyponatremia
   colitis, 216
   enteral fluids, 65, 68
   IV fluid therapy, 109, 110

ileal impaction, 208
   Anaplocephala perfoliata, 9, 318
   geographical regions, 8
   indications for surgery, 167
   palpation per rectum, 27, 28
   prevention, 296
   sonography, 130
   surgery, 199
   tapeworms, 9, 318

ileal muscular hypertrophy *see* idiopathic small intestinal muscular hypertrophy
idiopathic small intestinal muscular hypertrophy, 129, 130, 133, 151, 208
ileocecal intussusceptions, 213–14
   Anoplocephala perfoliata, 9, 10, 318
   palpation per rectum, 27
   signalment, 4
   sonography, 127, 129
   surgery, 199
   tapeworms, 9, 10, 318
ileocecostomy, 194–5
impaction colic *see* ileal impaction; cecal impaction; large colon impaction; small colon impaction
incisional complications, 256–8
inguinal hernia, 28, 29, 199
intestinal borborygmi, 19
intestinal obstruction
   complete/partial intestinal, 165–6
   early referral, 73–4
   hypochloremia, 82
   small intestine, 131
intestinal resection and anastomosis, 192
   ileocecostomy, 194–5
   jejunocecostomy, 193–4
   jejunoileostomy, 193
   jejunojejunostomy, 193
   large colon resection
      end-to-end technique, 195–7
      side-to-side anastomosis, 197
   small colon resection, 197–202
intra-abdominal or intra-peritoneal adhesions *see* adhesions
intravenous (IV) catheterization
   complications, 107, 109
   indications, 103
   preparation
      catheters, 103–4
      materials required for, 103
      skin preparation, 104
   procedure
      IV catheter care, 106–7
      over-the-needle technique, 105–6
      over-the-wire (Seldinger) technique, 106–7
intravenous (IV) fluid therapy
   colloid replacement
      hydroxyethyl starch, 113–14
      plasma, 112
   hypertonic saline solution (HSS), 111–12

oxygen delivery
  central venous pressure, 102
  hypovolemia, 101
  hypoxia, 102
  mean arterial blood pressure, 102–3
  plasma creatinine concentration, 102
  shock, 101–2
  SvO₂ and venous oxygen tension, 102
  urine output, 102
  polyionic isotonic fluids
    electrolyte replacement, 110–111
    maintenance fluid rate, 110
    replacement/resuscitation, 109–10
intravenous (IV) fluids, 108
intravenous (IV) lidocaine, 57–8 *see also*
        analgesia
  clinical use, 57–8
  complications, 58
  dose rate, 332
  ischemia-reperfusion injury, 246
  mechanism of action, 57
  postoperative ileus, 251–3
  postoperative pain, 250
  postoperative patient care, 239
ischemia-reperfusion injury, 246
  adhesions, 255
  dimethylsulfoxide (DMSO), 330
  early referral, 71, 72
  flunixin meglumine and, 53
  hypocalcemia, 82, 111
  hypomagnesemia, 82, 111
  ileus, 251
  intravenous (IV) lidocaine and, 57–8, 239
  lactate, 79, 81, 92
  leukopenia, 80, 245
  magnesium sulfate, 111
  postoperative complication, 246
intussusception *see* ileocecal intussusception;
        jejunojejunal intussusception; cecocolic
        intussusception
ivermectin-based anthelmintics, 9, 209, 296, 297,
        319, 320–322, 332

jejunal intussusception, 213
jejunal volvulus, 4, 14, 27, 180, 194, 198, 212, 246,
        279–80, 322
jejunocecostomy, 193–4
jejunoileostomy, 193
jejunojejunal intussusception, 4, 27, 127, 128, 181,
        209, 210, 213, 279–80, 322

jejunojejunostomy, 193
jugular refill time, 18

ketamine, 239, 250, 332, 334
kidney
  palpation per rectum, 25, 26
  nephrosplenic ligament entrapment, 29, 31,
        35, 219
  non-steroidal anti-inflammatory drugs,
        53, 239
  sonographic evaluation, 118–20
    nephrosplenic ligament entrapment, 121–2
    neoplasia, 141
    urolithiasis, 143–5
  surgical anatomy, 183, 186, 188

laminitis, 5, 20–21, 169, 208, 216, 232, 233, 248, 255,
        292, 295
laparoscopy, 37, 177, 187–8, 199–201, 212, 255, 256,
        258, 285, 294
large colon disease
  abdominal palpation per rectum, 28–9, 32–3
  inflammatory disease, 215–6
  simple obstruction
    ascending colon impaction, 216
    enterolithiasis, 218–19
    nephrosplenic ligament entrapment, 219–20
    right dorsal displacement, 220
    sand colopathy, 217–18
  sonographic evaluation
    large colon volvulus, 122–3
    left dorsal displacement, 121–2
    right dorsal displacement, 120–121
  strangulating obstruction, 220–221
large colon volvulus (LCV), 220–221, 324
  clinical signs, 6
  CVP measurement, 102
  history, 9
  palpation per rectum, 32
  plasma lactate concentration, 170–171
  postpartum mare, 4, 170, 284, 285
  prognostic indices, 170
  referral, 72
  sonographic evaluation, 120–123
  surgery, 195, 221
Lawsonia intracellularis infection, 281
laxatives, 47, 66
LCV *see* large colon volvulus (LCV)
left dorsal displacement see nephrosplenic
        ligament entrapment leukogram, 79–80, 337

lidocaine *see also* intravenous lidocaine
　enema
　　forpalpation per rectum, 23–4
　　for rectal tear, 36
　intravenous catheterization, 103, 106
　nasogastric intubation, 42
　trocharization, 161
lipopolysaccharide *see* endotoxin

Magnesium, 338
　hypermagnesemia, 68
　hypomagnesemia, 68, 82
　IV fluid therapy, 111
magnesium sulfate, 333
　enteral fluid therapy, 66
　ischemia-reperfusion injury, 111
　mild colic, 47
mean arterial blood pressure (MAP), 102–103
Meckel's diverticulum, 212–13
meconium-associated colic, 222–3, 279–80
　radiographic evaluation, 158
　signalment, 4
　sonographic evaluation, 120, 125
meloxicam, 53 *see also* non-steroidal anti-
　　inflammatory drugs
　ischemia-reperfusion injury, 246
　mild colic, 46
　postoperative patient care, 239
mesenteric rent, 199, 222
mesodiverticular band, 213
metabolic indicators, 83
mild colic
　clinical indications, 45–6
　enteral fluid therapy, 67–8
　management
　　analgesia, 46–7
　　fluid therapy, 47
　　frequent monitoring, 48
　　laxatives, 47
　　nutrition, 48
　　spasmolytic drugs, 47
　practical perspective, 45
miniature horses, 288–9

N -butylscopolammonium bromide *see* Buscopan®
nasogastric intubation *see also* nasogastric tube (NGT)
　complications
　　hemorrhage, 43–4
　　pharyngeal and esophageal trauma, 44
　　tracheal intubation, 44
　early referral, 75
　gastric impaction, 43
　indications, 38
　preparation
　　buckets and water, 39
　　head-neck ventroflexion, 39
　　materials required, 38, 39
　　medications, 39
　　nasogastric tube, 39, 40
　　short-acting sedative, 39
　　stomach pump, 39
　procedure
　　nasogastric tube passage, 40–42
　　reflux assessment, 42–3
　　sedation, 39–40
　proximal enteritis, 43
nasogastric tube (NGT) *see also* nasogastric
　　intubation
　passage of
　　esophagus, 41
　　nasal passage, 41
　　pharynx, 41
　　stomach, 41–2
　　trachea, 41–2
　permanent marks, 39–40
　problems with, 44
　types of, 39–40
necrotizing enterocolitis, neonatal foals,
　　279–80
needle technique, abdominocentesis, 88–9
neonatal foals *see also* foals
　causes of colic, 279
　colloid oncotic pressure (COP), 100
　fluid therapy, 110–111
　gamma glutamyltransferase (GGT), 82
　hematology in, 337
　management, 281
　meconium retention, 222
　mixed venous oxygen, 102
　plasma antimicrobial drug concentrations,
　　339
　plasma biochemistry for, 338
　sonographic evaluation, 117, 119–20, 132
nephrosplenic ligament entrapment (NSLE), 183,
　　219–20
　abdominal palpation per rectum, 29, 32
　diagnosis, 219
　sonographic diagnosis, 121–2
　surgical correction, 200
　prevention, 294

nonsteroidal anti-inflammatory drugs
        (NSAIDs)
    adverse effects and contraindications, 53–4
    clinical use, 52–3
    mechanism of action, 52
    mild colic, 46
    postoperative patient care, 238–9
    for young foals and weanlings, 281
nostril flare, 19–20
NSAIDs *see* nonsteroidal anti-inflammatory drugs
        (NSAIDs)
NSLE *see* nephrosplenic ligament entrapment
        (NSLE)

omental herniation, 89–90
opioids
    adverse effects and contraindications, 56–7
    analgesic therapy, 46
    antagonists, 56
    clinical use, 56
    mechanism of action, 55
oral mucous membranes
    dry, 18
    hemorrhagic shock, 18
    injected membranes, 17–18
    normal, 17
    tacky, 18
over-the-needle technique, 105–6
over-the-wire (Seldinger) technique, 106–7

Parascaris equorum, 9, 321–2 *see also* ascariasis
partial typhlectomy, 191–2
patient's history
    clinical presentation, 323–7
    clinical significance, 1–3
    detailed history
        appetite, 6–7
        defecation and urination, 7
        exercise regimen, 8
        feeding regimen, 7
        gastrointestinal parasite control, 8–9
        housing location, 8
        pasture access and housing, 8
        recent transportation, 8
        vaccination history, 9
        water consumption, 7
        water source, 7–8
    initial history
        clinical signs, 6
        colic signs and duration, 6

    dull mentation and inappetence, 5–6
    mare's reproductive status, 6
    recumbency, 5
medical history
    crib biting/ windsucking, 10
    current/recent medication, 9–10
    previous colic and colic surgery, 9
    recent medical problems, 10
signalment, 4
pelvic flexure (PF) impactions, 217
    enteral fluid therapy, 63–8
    indications for surgery, 167
    medical history, 6, 7, 9–10
    palpation per rectum, 32–3
    pelvic flexure enterotomy, 190
    physical examination, 14
    signalment, 4
    sonographic evaluation, 123
pelvic flexure enterotomy, 190
pentastarch, 113, 114
peritoneal cavity
    abdominal palpation per rectum, 35–6
    hematoma, 134, 135
peritoneal fluid analysis
    application of, 97
    biochemical evaluation
        D-dimer concentrations, 92
        lactate and glucose concentration, 92
        protein concentration, 91–2
    cells and cell counts
        erythrocytes, 93
        nucleated cells, 93–5
    effusion
        exudates, 97
        hemorrhagic, 97
        transudate, 95–7
    gross characteristics
        color and clarity, 90–91
        volume, 90
    indications, 87–8
    nonrepresentative sampling, 90
personal protective equipment (PPE), 266
pharyngeal trauma, nasogastric intubation, 44
physical examination
    admission physical examination sheet, 13
    cardiovascular status assessment
        dehydration, hypovolemia, and shock,
            15–16
        extremity temperature, 18
        heart rate, 16–17

physical examination (*cont'd*)
   jugular refill time, 18
   oral mucous membranes, 17–18
   pulse quality, 19
  checklist, 14
  clinical significance, 12–14
  digital pulses, 20–21
  gastrointestinal tract evaluation, 19
  initial patient observation
   abdominal distention, 14
   abrasions, 14
   body condition score, 14–15
   mentation/attitude, 14
   pain assessment, 14–15
   sweating, 14
  rectal temperature, 19
  respiratory system, 19–20
piperazine, 209, 319, 336
plasma, 112
pneumoperitoneum, 36
polyurethane catheters, 106, 107
ponies, 287–8
postoperative complications
  diarrhea, 248–9
  endotoxemia and SIRS, 246–8
  fever, 244–6
  incisional complications, 256–8
  intraperitoneal adhesion formation, neonates, 281
  intraperitoneal adhesions, 255–6
  ischemia-reperfusion injury, 246
  laminitis, 20–21, 295
  postoperative ileus, 251–3
  recurrent colic, 249–51
  septic peritonitis, 253–4
  small intestinal volvulus, 212
postoperative ileus, 251–3
postoperative intraperitoneal adhesions, 255–6
postoperative patient care
  monitoring
   arterial blood pressure, 234–5
   central venous pressure, 234
   laboratory data, 233–4
   patient assessment, 231–2
   physical examination, 232–3
  treatment
   anti-inflammatory and analgesic drugs, 238–40
   antimicrobial drugs, 239–41
   colloids, 236
   crystalloids, 235–6
   fluid therapy, 235, 237–8

hydroxyethyl starch, 236–7
plasma, 236
postoperative feeding and nutrition, 241
postpartum mares, 284–5
potassium supplementation, 110
PPE *see* personal protective equipment (PPE)
praziquantel, 9, 208, 214, 319, 320, 336
pregnant mares, 282–4
prevention of colic, 295–8
proliferative enteropathy *see Lawsonia intracellularis* infection
prostanoids, 52
proximal enteritis, 207–208
  gamma glutamyltransferase, 82–3
  indications for surgery, 167
  mild colic, 49
  nasogastric reflux, 43, 73
  sonographic evaluation, 129–30
psyllium mucilloid, 47, 297, 334
pulse quality, 19
PvO_2 *see* venous oxygen tension (PvO_2)

Radiography *see* abdominal radiography
RDD *see* right dorsal displacement (RDD)
rectal examination *see* abdominal palpation per rectum
rectal tear, 34
  emergency first aid, 36
  management, 37
recurrent colic, 9, 14, 46, 72–4, 143, 165, 170, 223, 249–51, 294–8
referral
  client
   financial considerations, 76
   referral hospital, 75–6
  clinical significance, 71–2
  indications
   abdominal pain, 72–3
   abdominal palpation per rectum, 74
   intestinal obstruction, 73–4
   nasogastric reflux, 73
   shock, 73
   tachycardia/ increasing heart rate, 73
  patient preparation
   analgesia, 74–5
   fluid therapy, 75
   nasogastric intubation, 75
   transportation, 75
   trocharization, 75
Rhodococcus equi intra-abdominal abscess, 140
right dorsal colitis, 216–17

medical history, 9
medical *vs.* surgical treatment, 169
non-steroidal anti-inflammatory drugs
        (NSAIDs), 53
    sonographic evaluation, 125–6
    surgery, 188
right dorsal colon (RDC) impactions, 33 *see also*
        large colon impaction
right dorsal displacement (RDD), 220
    colonic impaction and, 168
    gamma glutamyltransferase, 82
    medical history, 9
    palpation per rectum, 28–9, 32, 72
    postpartum mares, 284
    sonographic evaluation, 120–121
    surgical correction, 200

SDH *see* sorbitol dehydrogenase (SDH)
scrotal hernia, 137
septic peritonitis
    cecal perforation, 215
    postoperative patient care, 232
    postoperative complication, 253–4
SIRS *see* endotoxin
SISO *see* small intestinal strangulating obstruction
        (SISO)
small (descending) colon
    abdominal palpation per rectum, 33
    small (descending) colon impaction, 221–2
    meconium retention, 222–3
    mesenteric rent, 222
    neoplasia, 223
small colon enterotomy, 191
small intestinal enterotomy, 191
small intestinal strangulating obstruction (SISO),
        209–14
    clinical pathology, 80, 82–3
    neonates, 279
    postoperative feeding, 306
    referral, 71
sonography *see* abdominal sonographic
        evaluation
sorbitol dehydrogenase (SDH), 82, 338
spasmodic colic, 205, 306, 311, 316, 318 *see also* gas
        colic; mild colic
spasmolytic drugs, 47 *see also* Buscopan®
spleen
    abdominal palpation per rectum, 25, 26, 35
    nephrosplenic ligament entrapment, 29, 31
    gastrosplenic ligament entrapment,
        211–12

neoplasia, 223
nephrosplenic ligament entrapment, 219
sonographic evaluation, 119, 120
    abscess, 138, 139
    adhesions, 130
    gastric distention, 131, 132
    hematoma, 140
    hemorrhage, 134
    nephrosplenic ligament entrapment, 121–2
    neoplasia, 141
    surgical anatomy, 183, 186, 188
strangulating *vs.* nonstrangulating obstruction,
        128–30, 166–7
Strongylus vulgaris, 9, 322–3
surgical treatment *see also* colic surgery
    euthanasia without surgery, 170–171
        gastrointestinal tract perforation, 171
        prognostic indices, 170–171
    indications for
        cecal impaction, 168
        colitis, 169
        intestinal obstruction, 165–6
        large colon impaction, 167–8
        medical management response, 165
        peritoneal fluid analysis, 166
        peritonitis, 169–70
        persistent or severe abdominal pain, 165
        postpartum hemorrhage, 170
        small colon impaction, 168–9
        small intestinal lesions, 166–7
        sonographic examination, 166
SvO$_2$ *see* venous oxygen saturation (SvO$_2$)
systemic inflammatory response syndrome *see*
        endotoxemia

tachycardia, 16–8, 73, 167, 232, 323–5
    heart rate assessment, 16, 17, 232
tachypnea, 20, 55, 232
    respiratory rate assessment, 20
tapeworms *see Anoplocephala perfoliata*
teat cannula technique for abdominocentesis, 89
transudates, 95–7
trocharization
    complications, 162–3
    indications, 160–161
    preparation, 161
    prior to referral, 75
    procedure
        paralumbar approach, 161–2
        transrectal approach, 162
typhlotomy, 190–191

ultrasonography, 46, 121–2 *see also* abdominal
     sonographic evaluation
umbilical hernia, 138
urogenital tract
   abdominal palpation per rectum,
        34–5
   transrectal examination, 120
uterine hemorrhage, 136–7, 284–5
uterine torsion, 34–5, 282

venous oxygen saturation (SvO$_2$), 101, 102
venous oxygen tension (PvO$_2$), 101, 102
ventral midline celiotomy
   approach, 176–8
   closure, 183–5

xylazine, 54–5, 335
   bradycardia, 17
   colic surgery preparation, 175
   epidural, 36
   indications
      for referral, 72
      for surgery, 165
   mild colic, 46–7
   motility, 63, 117,
   nasogastric intubation, 39
   palpation per rectum, 24
   postoperative pain, 250
   postoperative patient, 239
   rectal tear, 36
   tachypnea with fever, 20

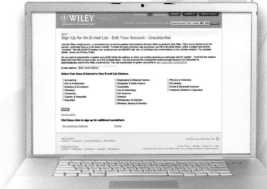
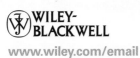